NEUROANATOMY

FOR SPEECH-LANGUAGE PATHOLOGY AND AUDIOLOGY

SECOND EDITION

MATTHEW H. ROUSE, SLP.D.

Associate Professor and Chair
Communication Disorders
Biola University, La Mirada, California

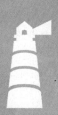

JONES & BARTLETT
LEARNING

World Headquarters
Jones & Bartlett Learning
5 Wall Street
Burlington, MA 01803
978-443-5000
info@jblearning.com
www.jblearning.com

Jones & Bartlett Learning books and products are available through most bookstores and online booksellers. To contact Jones & Bartlett Learning directly, call 800-832-0034, fax 978-443-8000, or visit our website, www.jblearning.com.

Substantial discounts on bulk quantities of Jones & Bartlett Learning publications are available to corporations, professional associations, and other qualified organizations. For details and specific discount information, contact the special sales department at Jones & Bartlett Learning via the above contact information or send an email to specialsales@jblearning.com.

15186-2

Production Credits

VP, Product Management: Amanda Martin
Director of Product Management: Laura Pagliuca
Product Assistant: Melissa Duffy
Director, Project Management: Jenny L. Corriveau
Project Specialist: Alex Schab
Project Manager, Navigate: Jessica deMartin
Digital Project Specialist: Rachel Reyes
Marketing Manager: Michael Sullivan
Product Fulfillment Manager: Wendy Kilborn
Composition: codeMantra U.S. LLC
Cover Design: Kristin E. Parker

Text Design: Kristin E. Parker
Director, Content Services and Licensing: Joanna Gallant
Rights & Media Manager: Shannon Sheehan
Rights & Media Specialist: John Rusk
Background of Cerebellum: © Image Source/Getty Images;
   Human brain being supported by fingers of a hand:
   © Dimitri Otis/Getty Images;
   Background with human brain and mechanical parts:
   © VeraPetruk/Getty Images
Printing and Binding: LSC Communications
Cover Printing: LSC Communications

Library of Congress Cataloging-in-Publication Data

Names: Rouse, Matthew H., author.
Title: Neuroanatomy for speech-language pathology and audiology / Matthew H. Rouse.
Description: Second edition. | Burlington, Massachusetts: Jones & Bartlett Learning, [2020] | Includes bibliographical references and index.
Identifiers: LCCN 2018052232 | ISBN 9781284151060
Subjects: | MESH: Communication Disorders | Neurologic Manifestations | Central Nervous System—anatomy & histology | Central Nervous System Diseases—pathology | Nervous System Physiological Phenomena
Classification: LCC RC423 | NLM WL 340.2 | DDC 616.85/5—dc23
LC record available at https://lccn.loc.gov/2018052232

6048

Printed in the United States of America
23 22 21 20 19   10 9 8 7 6 5 4 3 2

This book is dedicated to three sets of people:

To my wife, Chrissie, and my daughters, Torie and Lexie… thank you for your gracious gift of time to complete this work.

To my parents… thank you for your years of love, commitment, and encouragement.

To my neuroanatomy students… thank you for your feedback. You have all made this text better.

© VeraPetruk/Getty Images

Brief Contents

Contents

PART I Introductory Issues   1

Chapter 1   Introduction to Neurology 3

Chapter 2   Navigation and Organization of the Nervous System 27

Chapter 3   Development of the Nervous System 45

PART II General Neuroanatomy   59

Chapter 4   The Cells of the
Nervous System 61

Chapter 5   The Spinal Cord, Brainstem,
Cranial Nerves, and Cerebellum 93

Chapter 6   Diencephalon, Basal Ganglia,
and Brain Ventricles 131

**PART III   Neuroanatomy Applied
to Communication and
Communication Disorders 201**

**Chapter 9   Consciousness and Disorders
of Consciousness 203**

Preface

This text is primarily intended for graduate students studying communication sciences and disorders, but it is also written in an accessible way for junior or senior undergraduates preparing for graduate school. It is more important than ever for communication science and disorders students to understand the neurological underpinnings of communication disorders. As I think back on my own education, I did not have a standalone neuroanatomy class in either my undergraduate or graduate communication sciences and disorders training. At that time, this kind of information was imbedded over the span of a couple of weeks in an undergraduate anatomy of speech and hearing course. After graduate school, I entered the profession as a medical speech-language pathologist at a regional trauma center. It was here that I was challenged to learn about a variety of neurological disorders that I had previously learned little about. It has been over a quarter century since I completed my master's studies, and a lot has changed since that time. Now, nearly all graduate training programs have a full class in neuroscience to help students better understand, assess, and treat people with neurogenic communication disorders.

This text was born after a 15-year search for a neuroscience book focused on communication and communication disorders for my class. I adopted general neuroscience texts written by neurologists and neuroscientists, but I was unhappy with the lack of discussion about communication and communication disorders. I also tried texts written by communication scientists and others in communication disorders, but I found these to resemble the general neuroscience texts with some discussion of communication disorders sprinkled in here and there. Often, robust discussions of language or swallowing were entirely missing. I mentioned this frustrating search to a salesperson from Jones & Bartlett Learning, who asked "Have you ever thought about writing one?" The seed was planted and I realized that it was time to stop complaining and produce something that would at *least* help me in my class. My hope is that this text will be helpful to those of you who also teach this subject matter as well as helpful to your students.

▶ Organization of the Text

Neuroanatomy for Speech-Language Pathology and Audiology is organized into four main sections. The first three chapters, comprising Part I, Introductory Issues, introduce readers to the nervous system. Chapter 1 starts this process by taking the reader into the world of the nervous system. Important terms like *neurology* and *neuropathology* are explored, as well as the classification of neurological disorders and a brief introduction to the history of neuroscience. An introduction to imaging technology is included in this chapter because professionals in communication sciences and disorders are consumers of the reports generated by these studies. Chapter 2 introduces some basic orientation terms that will help in navigating around neurological structures as well as three methods for organizing the nervous system. Chapter 3 surveys the development of the neurological system through the life span, from conception to the last years of life.

Part II, General Neuroanatomy, includes Chapters 4 through 8. These chapters introduce the reader to the main neurological structures. This journey begins with the cells of the nervous system and ends with a review of the cerebral hemispheres. In Chapter 4, we take a microscopic approach and discuss the cells of the nervous system, both their structure and function. Chapter 5 zooms out to begin a macroscopic journey around the neurological structures (i.e., structures we can see and examine with the naked eye). More specifically, it looks at the spinal cord, brainstem, cranial nerves, and cerebellum. A close inspection of the 12 cranial nerves will occur in this chapter. The journey continues in Chapter 6 by examining structures above the brainstem and inside the brain—namely, the diencephalon and the surrounding thalamic structures and structures in close proximity, such as the brain's ventricles. The focus again moves in the next two chapters to the cerebral hemispheres. Chapter 7 discusses the overall structure of the cerebral hemispheres, such as their sulci, gyri, and blood supply. Chapter 8 then surveys important areas of the cerebral cortex using the Brodmann numbering system. Here we discuss the structure and function of various areas, such as Broca's and Wernicke's, two of several areas crucial in speech production and comprehension.

Part III, Neuroanatomy Applied to Communication and Communication Disorders, includes Chapters 9 through 15. I believe these chapters are unique when compared to other neuroscience texts for speech-language pathologists and audiologists because they specifically focus on the neurology of speech, language, hearing, cognition, emotion, and swallowing. These are the communication processes important to these professionals. Chapter 9 begins this third section by exploring consciousness. We say that speech is a voluntary, conscious activity, but what do we mean by consciousness? What are the disorders of consciousness (e.g., coma) that might affect communication? Chapter 10 is of special interest to audiologists because it explores the neurology of the hearing and balance systems and includes discussion of select disorders of these systems. Chapter 11 turns to the topic of speech. Here we look at neurological structures crucial for speech production and attempt to connect problems with these structures to various speech disorders observed in clinical practice. Language is the focus of Chapter 12. The neurological structures involved in speaking, listening, reading, and writing are explored as well as communication disorders associated with each of these modalities. Chapter 13 moves away from communication to swallowing. The cortical and subcortical controls of swallowing are surveyed as well as neurogenic swallowing problems. In recent years, speech-language pathologists have taken a more active role in what are called cognitive-communicative disorders. Chapter 14 focuses on cognition by looking at three main areas of cognition: attention, memory, and executive functions. Several cognitive-communicative disorders, like right hemisphere disorder, are examined through the lens of attention, memory, and executive functions. The final chapter of this section, Chapter 15, looks at the neurology of emotion. Children with autism have become more prevalent on caseloads, so there has been increased interest in how these children process and produce emotional responses. Chapter 15 discusses what we know about the neurology of emotion and the neurological differences between typical children and those with conditions like autism.

Finally, Part IV, Practicing Neuroanatomy, helps prepare students to apply what they have learned throughout the text. Chapter 16 discusses how a neurologist examines a person with a suspected neurological condition and looks at points of overlap with what a speech-language pathologist or audiologist would do in his or her assessment. A cranial nerve examination form is included in this chapter for students to practice this important exam. Also, major signs and symptoms of neurological conditions are surveyed.

▶ Features and Benefits

Each chapter includes a number of pedagogical features designed to enhance student learning. At the beginning of each chapter, you will find a Chapter Preview that offers a general introduction to the chapter's contents, an In This Chapter feature that lists main points discussed in the chapter, Learning Objectives that present the chapter's desired outcomes, and a Chapter Outline that lists the main headings for quick reference.

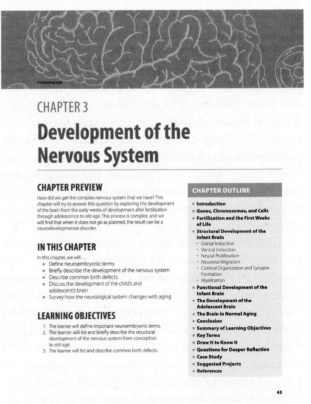

CHAPTER 3

Development of the Nervous System

CHAPTER PREVIEW

How did we get the complex nervous system that we have? This chapter will try to answer this question by exploring the development of the brain from the early weeks of development after fertilization through adolescence to old age. This process is complex, and we will find that when it does not go as planned, the result can be a neurodevelopmental disorder.

IN THIS CHAPTER

In this chapter, we will . . .
- Define neuroembryonic terms
- Briefly describe the development of the nervous system
- Describe common birth defects
- Discuss the development of the child's and adolescent's brain
- Survey how the neurological system changes with aging

LEARNING OBJECTIVES

1. The learner will define important neuroembryonic terms.
2. The learner will list and briefly describe the structural development of the nervous system from conception to old age.
3. The learner will list and describe common birth defects.

CHAPTER OUTLINE

- **Introduction**
- **Genes, Chromosomes, and Cells**
- **Fertilization and the First Weeks of Life**
- **Structural Development of the Infant Brain**
  - Dorsal Induction
  - Ventral Induction
  - Neural Proliferation
  - Neuronal Migration
  - Cortical Organization and Synapse Formation
  - Myelination
- **Functional Development of the Infant Brain**
- **The Development of the Adolescent Brain**
- **The Brain in Normal Aging**
- **Conclusion**
- **Summary of Learning Objectives**
- **Key Terms**
- **Draw It to Know It**
- **Questions for Deeper Reflection**
- **Case Study**
- **Suggested Projects**
- **References**

45

At the end of each chapter, the information related to the chapter's learning objectives is described in the Summary of Learning Objectives feature. Key Terms are also listed, the definitions of which can be found in the Glossary at the end of this text. Suggestions for drawing activities—critical for visual learners—are presented in the Draw It to Know It feature, and Questions for Deeper Reflection and Suggested Projects encourage students to delve deeper into the material.

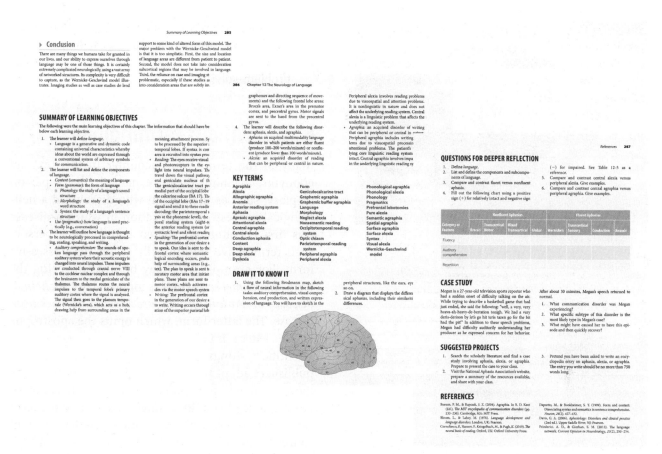

In addition to these activities, at least one Case Study is included in each chapter that allows students to apply what they are learning. Finally, References are included to credit sources cited in the chapter and to facilitate further study.

▶ Instructor Resources

In addition to the listed features within the text, supplemental learning materials are available for teachers through Jones & Bartlett Learning. They include the following:

- Test Bank, containing more than 250 questions
- Instructor's Manual, including sample answers for the Questions for Deeper Reflection and the Case Studies
- Slides in PowerPoint format, featuring more than 200 slides with select artwork from the text
- Image Bank, supplying key figures from the text
- Sample Syllabus, showing how a course can be structured around this text

Qualified instructors can gain access to these teaching materials by contacting their Health Professions Account Specialist at go.jblearning.com/findarep.

▶ What's New in This Edition?

The second edition of this text has been thoroughly updated. Some of these changes have come about through my own experience teaching with the text. Other changes have been made because of student feedback. Still other changes have been made due to feedback from colleagues. I highly value feedback from students and colleagues and am grateful for it.

The following is a list of the significant changes made in this edition of the text:

- The content from the previous edition's Chapter 3 has been divided into two chapters. Chapter 2 now covers the navigation and organization of the nervous system, while Chapter 3 more deeply explores nervous system development.
- Chapter 3 now takes a life span perspective, including information about the adolescent and adult brain.
- The content from the previous edition's Chapter 2 relating to the neurological exam has been moved to the end of the text (Chapter 16). This change came about because reviewers of the *First Edition* thought students would be better served to have

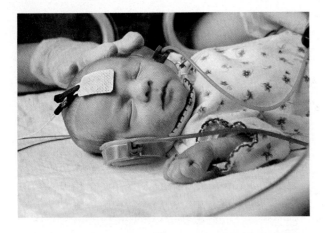

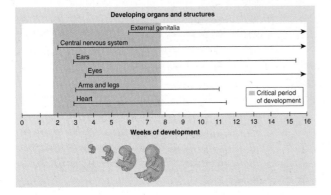

all the background information in place before thinking about how to apply it to a patient.

■ Information about neuroimaging has been moved to the first chapter to better continue the discussion of neuroscience's history.

■ All of the chapters have many additional figures, tables, and boxes to better enhance student learning.

■ Some of the figures from the *First Edition* have been updated and changed to better illustrate the text's discussion.

■ More information has been added about key neurogenic communication disorders and their connection to the nervous system. For example, Chapter 14, which covers the neurology of cognition, now has a substantial section on right hemisphere disorder as well as dementia.

■ Case Studies have been added to encourage problem-solving

▶ Eponymous Terminology

Many of the terms you encounter in this text are eponyms, meaning they are named after a person or place, such as the person who discovered a neurological process or the location in which a disease was first encountered. When named for a person, such terms have traditionally taken the possessive form. For example, you may be used to seeing the term *Alzheimer's disease* as opposed to *Alzheimer disease*, or *Parkinson's disease* instead of *Parkinson disease*. The latter form, which omits the apostrophe and the letter *s*, is increasingly preferred in medical and scientific writings, and as more organizations and publishers adopt this form, it will likely become the more familiar approach even in general contexts. For example, if you do an internet search of the term *Down syndrome*, you will notice that few current sources write this term as *Down's syndrome*, although the possessive spelling was quite common in the not-too-distant past.

In this edition of *Neuroanatomy for Speech-Language Pathology and Audiology*, eponymous terms are generally written in the nonpossessive form (e.g., Parkinson disease). Some terms may look odd to you (e.g., Bell palsy), but in the near future, such spellings may become the norm. That said, a few exceptions to this rule have been made throughout this text to allow for common usage within the field of neuroanatomy. There remains a clear preference to use the possessive form of the terms *Broca's area*, *Wernicke's area*, and *Exner's area*. To maintain a sense of consistency among these terms, the possessive form is used for all eponymous terms relating to Broca and Wernicke (e.g., Broca's aphasia).

About the Author

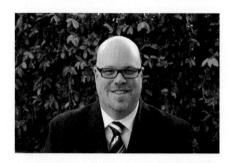

Matthew H. Rouse earned a BS in Biology from the University of Redlands in 1990 before he transitioned into the field of Communication Sciences and Disorders, earning an MS in Communication Disorders from the University of Redlands in 1992. After graduation, he worked in the hospital system as a medical speech-language pathologist from 1992 to 2000. In 1999, Dr. Rouse accepted a full-time teaching position at Biola University in the Communication Sciences and Disorders program and is currently the chair of the Department of Communication Sciences and Disorders. He earned his doctoral degree in Speech-Language Pathology in 2009 and wrote his dissertation on training students in empathetic counseling skills. His research interests include neuroscience, neurogenic communication disorders, and counseling. Matt lives in La Habra, California, with his wife Chrissie and their two children.

Reviewers

Vishwa Bhat, PhD
Associate Professor
William Paterson University

Marie E. Byrne, PhD
Professor
Mississippi University for Women

Carrie Childers, PhD, CCC-SLP
Assistant Professor
Marshall University

Joanne Christodoulou, EdD, CCC-SLP
Lecturer
Kean University

O'Neil Guthrie, PhD
Assistant Professor
Northern Arizona University

Peter Ivory, PhD, CCC-A
Professor and Director of Faculty Affairs
California State University, Los Angeles

Melissa Johnson, PhD
Assistant Professor
Nazareth College

Sharon Jones, PhD
Assistant Professor
Northeastern State University

Rik Lemoncello, PhD, CCC-SLP
Associate Professor
Pacific University

Thomas Linares, PhD
Program Director
Maryville University

Pamela Monaco, MD
Professor
Molloy College

Lori Newport, AuD
Associate Professor
Biola University

Kerri Phillips, SLPD, CCC-SLP
Professor and Program Director
Louisiana Tech University

Jayanti Ray, PhD, CCC-SLP
Professor
Southeast Missouri State University

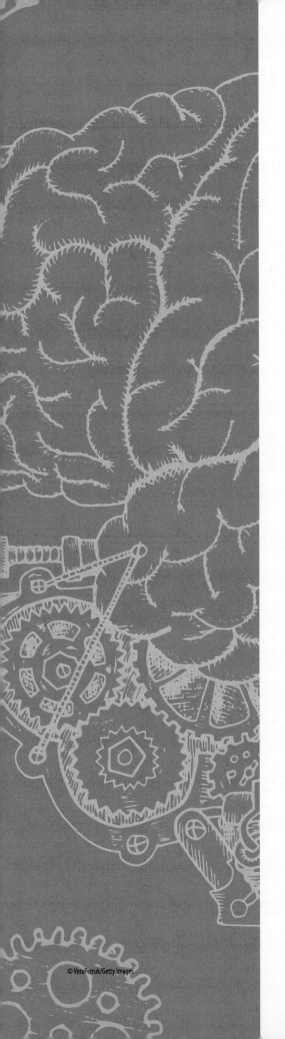

PART I

Introductory Issues

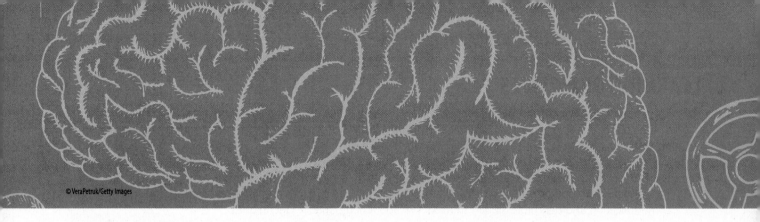

CHAPTER 1

Introduction to Neurology

CHAPTER PREVIEW

In this chapter we will begin our journey into the world of neuroscience. We will define important terms, like *neurology*, to help us begin to frame this world. We will then make a case on why it is important for a speech-language pathologist and audiologist to have a working knowledge of the nervous system. Lastly, we will examine theoretical perspectives and technologies that speak to the question: How does the brain work?

IN THIS CHAPTER

In this chapter, we will . . .

- Define the term *neurology*
- Discuss why speech-language pathologists and audiologists need to know and understand neurology
- Discuss why the neurological system is a precious resource
- Answer the question: What does neurology mean to me?
- Define the terms *function*, *activity*, and *participation barriers*
- Survey examples of famous people who have suffered neurological conditions
- Examine statistics concerning neurological disorders
- List various categories of neurological disorders
- Discuss basic theoretical perspectives as to how the brain works
- Survey important researchers in the history of neuroscience
- Compare and contrast neuroimaging techniques
- Discuss why these theoretical perspectives matter to fields associated with communication sciences and disorders

LEARNING OBJECTIVES

1. The learner will define the following terms: *neurology, anatomy, physiology,* and *pathology.*
2. The learner will be able to create an argument as to why speech-language pathologists and audiologists need neurological training.
3. The learner will be able to list various categories of neurological disorders and provide one example in each category.
4. The learner will be able to draw and explain the spectrum of belief as to how the brain works.
5. The learner will list and define structural and functional imaging techniques and list at least one reason why communication disorders professionals should know about neuroimaging techniques.

▶ Introduction: Defining Neurology

We begin our journey into the human nervous system with this question from the anthropologist Stephen Juan: "Have you ever wondered about how fantastic the human brain really is? Every thought, every action, every deed relies upon this incredible organ. Although we take the brain for granted, we couldn't wonder without it" (Juan, 1998, p. 1). The brain is the vehicle we use to wonder. It includes not only the brain but also those other parts of the neurological system that pertain to communication. **Neurology** is simply the study of the anatomy, physiology, and pathology of the nervous system. **Anatomy** is the study of structure, **physiology** is the study of function or structures in motion, and **pathology** is the study of disease processes that affect both anatomy and physiology. Put the prefix *neuro-* in front of each of these words and you get distinct yet highly related fields of study. **Neuroanatomy** is the study of the nervous system's structure. A neuroanatomical topic is a neuron (i.e., a nervous system cell) and its structure. When we want to talk about how a neuron functions, we have just entered into the area of **neurophysiology**. The study of nervous system diseases is called **neuropathology**. An example of neuropathology would be amyotrophic lateral sclerosis, or Lou Gehrig disease, which affects both the anatomy and physiology of neurons and leads to serious neurological problems. There are other fields in addition to these, including neurosurgery (removal of structures that impair normal nervous system functioning), neuroradiology (use of radiation therapy for nervous system tumors), and neuroembryology (normal and pathological development of the nervous system).

The **nervous system** is a series of organs that make communication between the brain and body possible in order for us to interact with the world around us. It is through the nervous system's connections to the body (and vice versa) that we think, feel, and act. The most well-known organ of the nervous system is the brain, followed by the spinal cord and then the various nerves (**FIGURE 1-1**). The purpose of this chapter is to give a broad overview of the nervous system as well as a brief survey of neuroscience's history and the important figures in that history. This chapter also explores modern neuroimaging techniques that have led to a better understanding of the brain and how it works.

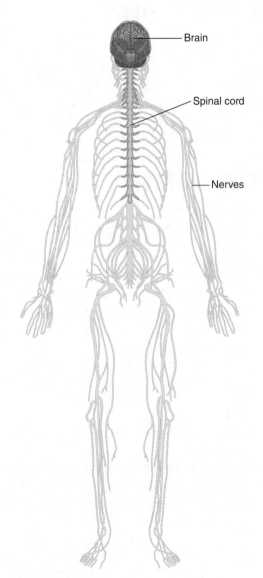

FIGURE 1-1 The brain, spinal cord, and nerves are the major components of the human nervous system.

▶ The Need for Neurological Training

Why should a speech-language pathologist (SLP) or audiologist be concerned about the anatomy, physiology pathology of the nervous system? What difference does this knowledge make to clinical practice?

Rubens (1977), a neurologist, outlined several reasons why SLPs and audiologists should know about neuroscience and neurology. First, he argued that these professionals should know how to speak the language of neurology so that they and neurologists could better communicate. Neurologists have their own language. When communication disorders professionals have knowledge of this language, they can communicate more easily with neurologists. In turn, neurologists may be more willing to learn the language of SLPs and audiologists. An example of this neurological language is the word *dyskinesia*, a general word for a disorder of movement. Neurologists also extensively use abbreviations (e.g., CVA for cerebral vascular accident, or stroke) and use them considerably in their charting. Knowing these terms and abbreviations can obviously help the SLP or audiologist understand the neurologist's assessment report and progress notes. Second, knowing about the nervous system and where a lesion is (e.g., frontal lobe versus occipital lobe) helps the SLP anticipate likely patient problems and choose appropriate initial testing instruments. For example, a patient with a focal left hemisphere stroke will be tested differently than someone with diffuse brain injury due to a traumatic brain injury. Third, knowing about neurological etiologies, such as stroke, traumatic brain injury, and brain tumor, helps an SLP or audiologist predict the kinds of problems patients are likely to face. For example, a patient with occlusion of the middle cerebral artery will have a different symptom complex (e.g., speech and language) than will a patient with posterior cerebral artery occlusion (e.g., visuospatial). Fourth, a working knowledge of neuroscience helps SLPs and audiologists document patient change and determine the efficacy of various treatment methods in rewiring the brain for improved communication. Fifth and connected to the previous point, knowledge of neural plasticity (i.e., the brain's ability to change and adapt after injury) helps the SLP plan therapy in a way that takes advantage of this phenomenon. One principle of neuroplasticity is that repetition matters, meaning repeated experience can help the brain learn new skills. This insight can obviously be used in therapy by giving numerous repetitions of certain sounds or words, thus improving a patient's likelihood of learning and generalizing these new skills.

SLPs and audiologists must do their part in fostering good relationships with neurologists and other doctors; one important way of gaining their colleagues' respect is by being excellent at what they do. Nothing elicits respect like a job well done. Though SLPs and audiologists are autonomous professionals (i.e., they are not supervised by neurologists or other doctors), they depend on neurologists for many things, such as referrals and important neurological information on the patient (LaPointe, 1977). Tending to their relationships with these physicians not only helps SLPs and audiologists in these areas, but also ultimately helps patients receive the important and specialized services that only SLPs and audiologists can provide. I often tell my students that no one—not even neurologists—will know more about speech, language, hearing, or swallowing than they will once they are through graduate school and their clinical fellowship. This is not said out of pride, but rather out of reality; no one has as much clinical training in these areas as a licensed, certified SLP or audiologist, just like no one has as much knowledge of neurology as a neurologist.

Some readers might be thinking, "Well, that's all fine, but I'm not going to work in a hospital or with neurologists. I'm going to work in a public school. What does all this matter to me?" Manasco (2017) offers a helpful maxim: "When you hear hoof beats, think horses, not zebras" (p. 5). What this adage is saying is that horses are the most likely explanation, while zebras are the outliers, the unexpected possibilities. Imagine you are working in a public school and a child walks into your office. Most likely, the child was sent to your office because he or she has a developmental language or speech sound disorder (i.e., a horse). However, it is possible the child was referred for testing because he or she has had a severe concussion or a stroke (i.e., a zebra). At some point, a child will walk into your office and your knowledge of neurology and neurogenic communication disorders will be needed to properly assess, diagnose, and treat that child. As Manasco explains, "You must be able to recognize and treat those problems in your field that are very out of the ordinary or even extraordinary" (2017, p. 5).

▶ A Broad Overview of the Nervous System

The Nervous System Is a Precious Resource

I remember watching the 2008 Summer Olympic Games on television with my 4-year-old daughters and seeing their joy and amazement as gymnasts Nastia

Liukin and Shawn Johnson moved with grace and precision on the vault, floor exercises, uneven bars, and balance beam (**FIGURE 1-2**). Nastia took the gold in the individual all-around and Shawn the silver. It was a proud moment for the U.S. Olympic squad and all Americans watching these amazingly skilled athletes contort their bodies in incredible ways. The precision, timing, and coordination of these athletes had come from years of training not only their muscles but also their nervous systems. Plans for motor (or movement) activity were developed through years of repetitive action. As the adage goes, "Practice makes perfect."

The nervous system is on full display in the works of our favorite composers and performers. They have fine-tuned their nervous systems through hours of practice to execute precisely the actions needed to perform a piece of music or create a piece of art. Itzhak Perlman (**FIGURE 1-3**), the famous violinist, began playing the violin at 3 years old and, although he contracted polio at an early age, practiced for numerous hours and became one of the world's most famous violinists. Great feats of the body are in part products of the nervous system. The nervous system is definitely a precious resource, one that works quietly in the background, unknown by us unless a disease develops.

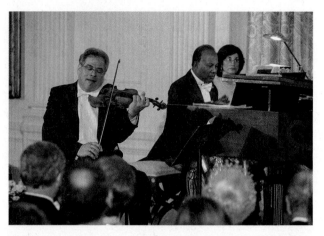

FIGURE 1-3 Itzhak Perlman playing at the White House for President George W. Bush and First Lady Laura Bush.
Courtesy of Shealah Craighead/George W. Bush Presidential Library and Museum.

What Does Neurology Mean to Me?

The nervous system is like an automatic transmission in a car; one does not need to think about shifting the gears. The nervous system comes into the forefront when something goes wrong with it. A **neurological disorder** involves a disease in the nervous system that impairs a person's health, resulting in some level of disability. The World Health Organization's (WHO's) *International Classification of Functioning, Disability and Health* (ICF) defines disability as "a universal human experience, sometimes permanent, sometimes transient" that affects the health and functioning of a person (WHO, 2014). We should not think of people in two categories (healthy versus disabled), but rather remember that we are all on a spectrum with health at one end and disability at the other end. There are times in our lives when we experience more health and less disability, and vice versa.

Earlier generations used the terms *impairment*, *disability*, and/or *handicap* when discussing people who had health issues, and these terms are still widely used in everyday language (e.g., think of how most people refer to parking spaces with a wheelchair sign). WHO has attempted to change this language by using the alternative terms *function*, *activity*, and *participation*. The older terms of *impairment*, *disability*, and *handicap* come from the medical model of disability that puts an emphasis on the person's health condition, his or her limitations due to this condition, and cures or treatment. The medical model does not include the role of society in disability and the barriers a society can erect for those with disabilities (i.e., the social model of disability). The focus of the medical model is on biological and medical answers. WHO's use of alternative terms is an attempt to blend the social model of disability, which

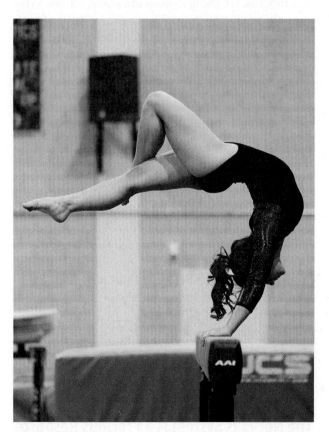

FIGURE 1-2 A gymnast on a balance beam illustrating how years of practice hone the nervous system.
Courtesy of Bill Evans/U.S. Air Force.

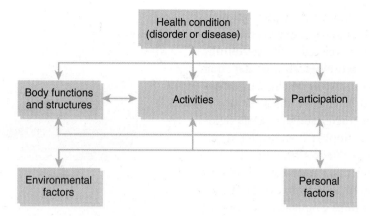

FIGURE 1-4 The interaction between functioning, disability, and health.

Modified from World Health Organization. (2011). *World report on disability*. Retrieved from http://whqlibdoc.who.int/publications/2011/9789240685215_eng.pdf

emphasizes the role of society and its barriers, with the medical model. WHO's model still has elements of the medical model by stressing a person's health condition (e.g., stroke) and how that condition has affected the structure and function of the body (e.g., paralysis). Issues with **function barriers** (formerly impairment) "are problems in body function or alterations in body structure" (WHO, 2011, p. 5). Examples of function issues include paralysis and blindness. In the area of communication disorders, examples include hearing loss and language impairment. **Activity barriers** (formerly disability) "are difficulties in executing activities" (WHO, 2011, p. 5), especially skills of daily living like walking or eating. For example, neurogenic communication disorders can lead to issues in the daily communication of needs and wants with other people or eating. Lastly, **participation barriers** (formerly handicap) "are problems with involvement in any area of life" (WHO, 2011, p. 5). These barriers include challenges participating in education and employment, often due to external barriers such as discrimination and transportation problems. It is important to note that not everyone who has a function barrier will have barriers in activity and/or participation. For example, a person who is deaf may technically have hearing dysfunction but have no issues with daily activities or involvement in other areas of life.

WHO's ICF also "looks beyond the idea of a purely medical or biological conceptualization of dysfunction, taking into account the other critical aspects of disability" (WHO, 2014), such as environmental and personal factors (**FIGURE 1-4**). Environmental factors describe the world in which people with neurological disorders live and interact. These factors can act as either facilitators or barriers and include products, technology, buildings, support, relationships, attitudes, services, systems, and policies. Personal factors relate directly to the person with a neurological disorder. For example, a person's motivation and self-esteem can play into his

or her interaction with the environment (WHO, 2011). **FIGURE 1-5** illustrates WHO's ICF applied to someone who has suffered a spinal cord injury.

It is likely that you have an acquaintance, friend, or family member who suffers from some sort of nervous system problem, such as Alzheimer or Parkinson disease, which may disable or handicap the person. If so, then neurology has personal significance to you. In other words, neurology is not a study that is distant from us; it affects our personal lives, especially when our loved ones or we ourselves experience a neurological disorder.

Famous People With Neurological Conditions

Neurological disorders do not discriminate. They strike the old and the young, the rich and the poor, and people of every color, culture, and nationality.

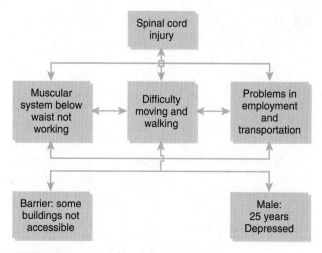

FIGURE 1-5 An example of the ICF applied to a case involving spinal cord injury.

Adapted from the Centers for Disease Control and Prevention. (n.d.). The ICF: An overview. Retrieved from https://www.cdc.gov/nchs/data/icd/icfoverview_finalforwho10sept.pdf

Many famous people have suffered from serious neurological conditions. Former president Ronald Reagan died from complications related to **Alzheimer disease**, a progressive neurological disorder that results in intellectual decline. Actor Michael J. Fox has **Parkinson disease**, a degenerative disorder of the central nervous system characterized by muscle rigidity and tremors. Actor Christopher Reeve suffered spinal cord injury in his upper neck after being thrown from a horse and was wheelchair bound and ventilator dependent until his death in 2004 from cardiac arrest. Stephen Hawking, the famous English physicist, was diagnosed at 21 years of age with an unusual form of amyotrophic lateral sclerosis (ALS; also known as Lou Gehrig disease); he struggled with this disease until his death in 2018 at 76 years old. Roy Horn, an entertainer from the famous Las Vegas tiger act known as Siegfried and Roy, suffered a stroke after his tiger Montecore bit him in the neck. Roy had fallen during a performance, and it is thought that Montecore was trying to pull him to safety. Most people suffer from neurological conditions privately, but these celebrities have had to endure their conditions in the public eye. Their willingness to share openly about their conditions has led to greater public awareness regarding conditions like ALS and Parkinson disease.

Prevalence, Incidence, and Cost of Neurological Disorders

Statistics regarding the **incidence** (i.e., the number of new cases per year in a given population) and **prevalence** (i.e., the total number of current cases in a given population at a point in time) of neurological

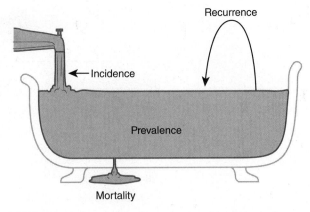

FIGURE 1-6 An illustration of important epidemiological terms.

disorders are challenging to obtain due to the relatively few available studies (**FIGURE 1-6** illustrates these important epidemiological terms). One study by Hirtz et al. (2007), summarized in **FIGURE 1-7**, estimated the incidence and prevalence of select neurological disorders in the United States. Because population statistics change rapidly, Hirtz et al.'s information is out of date for some conditions; for example, the Centers for Disease Control and Prevention (2018) and Baio et al. (2018) report that the prevalence rate for children with autism spectrum disorder is now 16.8/1,000, or 1 in 59 children.

Whatever the statistics, the number of people suffering from neurological disorders is great. In fact, WHO estimates that nearly one in six people worldwide, or about 1 billion people, suffer from a neurological disease (Bertolote, 2007).

In addition to the personal hardships of people affected, there is also a tremendous financial cost associated with the assessment and treatment of neurological

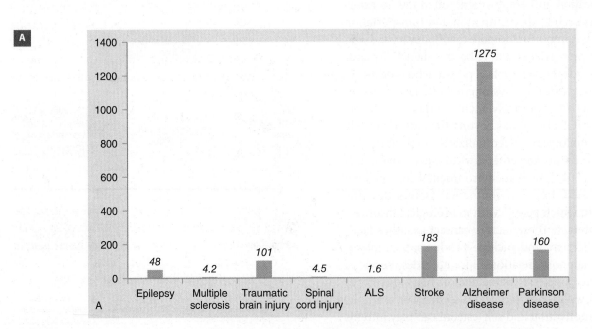

FIGURE 1-7A **A.** Incidence of select neurological disorders in the United States (new cases per 100,000).

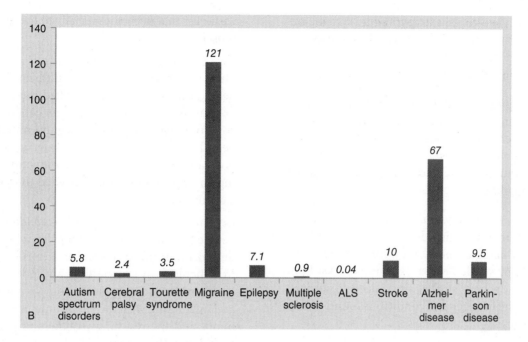

Data from: Hirtz, D., Thurman, D. J., Gwinn-Hardy, K., Mohamed, M., Chaudhuri, A. R., & Zalutsky, R. (2007). How common are the "common" neurologic disorders? *Neurology, 68,* 332.

FIGURE 1-7B B. Prevalence of select neurological disorders in the United States (total cases per 1,000). ALS = amyotrophic lateral sclerosis.

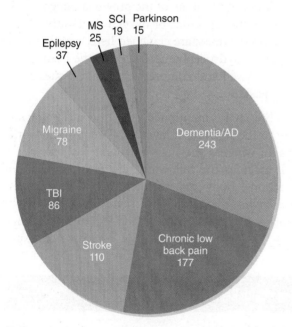

FIGURE 1-8 Annual cost of major neurological disorders in billions of dollars. AD = Alzheimer disease, MS = multiple sclerosis, SCI = spinal cord injury, TBI = traumatic brain injury.

Data from: Gooch, C. L., Pracht, E., & Borenstein, A. R. (2017). The burden of neurological disease in the United States: A summary report and call to action. *Annals of Neurology, 81*(4), 479–484.

disorders. Gooch, Pracht, and Borenstein (2017) report that the following disorders alone cost the United States approximately $800 billion per year: Alzheimer disease and other dementias, stroke, traumatic brain injury, chronic lower back pain, migraine, epilepsy, multiple sclerosis, spinal cord injury, and Parkinson disease (**FIGURE 1-8**). The treatment of Alzheimer disease led the list with an annual cost of approximately $243 billion.

Classification of Neurological Disorders

WHO has developed a classification system for diseases, including pathologies of the nervous system, called the International Statistical Classification of Diseases and Related Health Problems. This name is commonly shortened to the International Classification of Diseases and, because it is in its 10th edition, is abbreviated ICD-10. Under "Diseases of the Nervous System," there are 11 subcategories of neurological diseases (WHO, 2010). These categories are briefly described here:

Inflammatory diseases: These are neurological diseases caused by bacterial, viral, or parasitic pathogens. Two conditions under this category are encephalitis (brain infection) and meningitis (infection of membranes that surround the brain and spinal cord).

Systematic atrophies primarily affecting the central nervous system: Atrophy refers to a wasting away of something, in this case the nervous system. The progressive, hereditary disorder known as Huntington disease is an example of a condition in this category.

Extrapyramidal and movement disorders: The extrapyramidal system is that part of the nervous system that regulates our movements. The basal ganglia serve as a kind of control center for this system. Parkinson disease, a degenerative neurological disease involving rhythmic shaking, is an example.

Other degenerative diseases of the nervous system: Other conditions that are degenerative in nature, but do not involve the extrapyramidal system, are included in this category. An example is Alzheimer disease, which is a progressive neurological disorder involving gradual loss of cognitive abilities.

Demyelinating diseases of the central nervous system: Myelin is a white, fatty substance that insulates our nerve tracts; thus, demyelinating diseases like multiple sclerosis involve the stripping of myelin from the nerve tracts. This process leads to muscle weakness.

Episodic and paroxysmal disorders: This classification involves disorders that come and go instead of being chronic. They can also be characterized by sudden or paroxysmal attacks. Epilepsy, headaches, stroke, and sleep disorders make up the four general conditions found under this category.

Nerve, nerve root, and plexus disorders: These conditions involve nerves, nerve roots, and branching networks of nerves. One example is Bell palsy, which is a condition that affects the facial nerve and causes paralysis to one side of the face. Another example is phantom limb syndrome, in which amputees continue to have sensation from their absent limb.

Polyneuropathies and other disorders of the peripheral nervous system: The central nervous system involves the brain and spinal cord, and the peripheral nervous system involves all the nerves that connect the central nervous system with body structures, such as muscles, sense organs, and glands. Guillain-Barré syndrome is an acute polyneuropathy affecting the peripheral nervous system. It is life threatening due to the profound weakness that occurs, especially to the respiratory muscles.

Diseases of the myoneural junction and muscle: These disorders result from problems where a nerve and muscle connect, called the myoneural or neuromuscular junction. Myasthenia gravis is a condition whose name means grave muscle weakness. It is an autoimmune disorder in which the body attacks the neuromuscular junction, inhibiting an important chemical needed to make muscles contract.

Cerebral palsy and other paralytic conditions: Most people have heard of cerebral palsy, which occurs due to brain injury before or at birth and leads to difficulties in muscle tone and posture. These problems lead to struggles in completing activities and interacting with the environment. Spinal cord injury and the resulting weakness or paralysis is included in this category.

Other disorders of the nervous system: WHO has included this category to catch any pathology that does not fit in any of the previous categories. For example, episodes of oxygen deprivation, called anoxic events, are classified here. Another example is hydrocephalus, in which the brain ventricles swell and compress the brain tissues against the skull.

The ICF, mentioned earlier, is complementary to the ICD-10. It lays out a broad framework of health, whereas the ICD-10 focuses on disease. The ICF includes the following general categories: body functions, body structures, activities, participation, and environmental factors. There are several subcategories that are relevant to the SLP and audiologist; these are described in **BOX 1-1**. Readers can explore

---

BOX 1-1 International Classification of Functioning, Disability and Health Related to Communication

Body Functions

- *Chapter 2: Sensory Functions and Pain*
  - b210–b229 Seeing and related functions
  - b230–b249 Hearing and vestibular functions
- *Chapter 3: Voice and Speech Functions*
  - b310 Voice functions
  - b320 Articulation functions
  - b330 Fluency and rhythm of speech functions
  - b340 Alternative vocalization functions
  - b398 Voice and speech functions, other specified
  - b399 Voice and speech functions, unspecified

Body Structures

- *Chapter 1: Structures of the Nervous System*
  - s110 Structure of brain
  - s120 Spinal cord and related structures
  - s130 Structure of meninges
  - s140 Structure of sympathetic nervous system
  - s150 Structure of parasympathetic nervous system
  - s198 Structure of the nervous system, other specified
  - s199 Structure of the nervous system, unspecified

- *Chapter 2: The Eye, Ear, and Related Structures*
  - s210 Structure of eye socket
  - s220 Structure of eyeball
  - s230 Structures around eye
  - s240 Structure of external ear
  - s250 Structure of middle ear
  - s260 Structure of inner ear
  - s298 Eye, ear, and related structures, other specified
  - s299 Eye, ear, and related structures, unspecified
- *Chapter 3: Structures Involved in Voice and Speech*
  - s310 Structure of nose
  - s320 Structure of mouth
  - s330 Structure of pharynx
  - s340 Structure of larynx
  - s398 Structures involved in voice and speech, other specified
  - s399 Structures involved in voice and speech, unspecified

Activities and Participation
- *Chapter 3: Communication*
  - d310–d329 Communicating: receiving
  - d330–d349 Communicating: producing
  - d350–d369 Conversation and use of communication devices and techniques
  - d398 Communication, other specified
  - d399 Communication, unspecified

Reproduced from: *International classification of functioning, Disability and Health (ICF).* © World Heath Organization.

these subcategories in more detail by visiting the ICF website (www.who.int/classifications/icf/en/).

▶ A Brief History of Neuroscience

The history of neuroscience has been a quest to answer the question: How does the brain work? One attempt to answer this question has been that the brain works in bits and pieces, having discrete areas that handle specific functions. The other attempt to answer this question has been that it works more holistically (**FIGURE 1-9**). The holistic proponent would say that the brain works as an integrative whole and cannot be broken down into discrete areas. Having said this, there have been people throughout history who thought the brain did not have anything to do with mental functions. We now embark on a brief history of neuroscience.

Prehistory

Prehistory or prehistoric refers to a period before history was written down, a period prior to about 3500 BCE. What is known about this period comes from various artifacts that have been unearthed. Artifacts that shed light on prehistoric understandings of neuroscience include skulls with holes in them and the instruments used in making these

holes, called **trephines**. These were usually sharp stones used to create holes in skulls through cutting, scraping, and/or drilling. This procedure is known as **trephination** (**FIGURE 1-10**). Why would prehistoric people perform such procedures on each other? There is no written history to rely on, so we have to base our ideas on premodern and modern

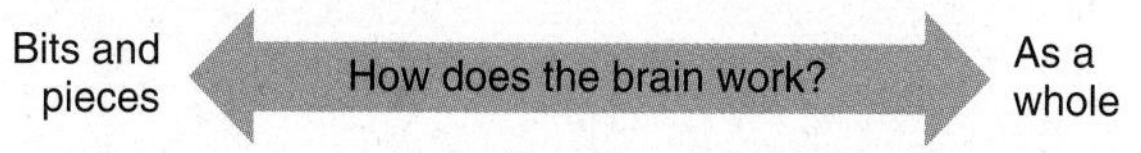

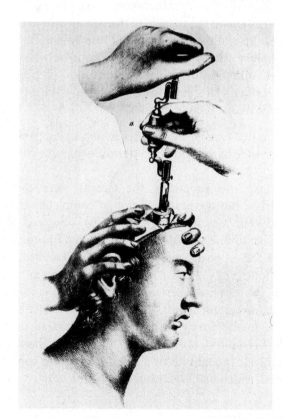

FIGURE 1-10 An example of trephination.
Courtesy of the National Library of Medicine.

Bits and pieces ◀——— How does the brain work? ———▶ As a whole

FIGURE 1-9 The spectrum of belief about brain function.

reasons for this procedure. We can guess that pre-historic people performed this procedure to treat headaches, seizures, posttraumatic brain injury, and perhaps even madness or beliefs in evil spirits. The bottom line is that these people knew there was something special about the head region and they continued to perform trephinations, probably because the procedure worked from time to time. For example, it is conceivable that the procedure successfully relieved pressure in the cranial cavity after a traumatic brain injury, bringing improved functioning to the patient.

Early History

The Egyptians were cardio-centrists, meaning they believed the seat of mental functions was in the organ we call the heart. However, they did make observations about damage to the head leading to physical impairments. The Edwin Smith papyrus (3000–2500 BCE) records 48 medical cases, which include cases involving head and brain injury. Here is an example from case 8:

> If thou examinest a man having a smash of his skull . . . thou shouldst palpate his wound. Shouldst thou find that there is a swelling protruding on the outside of that smash which is in his skull . . . on the side of him having that injury which is in his skull; (and) he walks shuffling with his sole, on the side of him having that injury which is in his skull. . . . (Wilkins, 1964)

In this example, the writer is identifying paralysis of one side of the body (i.e., **hemiplegia**) due to head injury.

Like the Egyptians, the Greeks were cardio-centrists, but the brain did not go completely unnoticed. Hippocrates (460–370 BCE) observed that damage to one side of the brain resulted in problems with the opposite side of the body (**FIGURE 1-11**). Aristotle (384–322 BCE) correctly theorized localization, the idea that a certain part of the body is responsible for certain mental functions, but he attributed these to the wrong organ, the heart instead of the brain (**FIGURE 1-12**). What did he believe about the brain? He thought it was a radiator meant to cool the blood, which had been heated up by the heart.

Later History

Moving into the Common Era (CE), thinkers shifted their attention from the heart to the head. Two

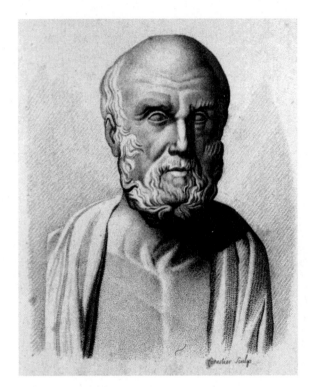

FIGURE 1-11 Hippocrates.
Courtesy of the National Library of Medicine.

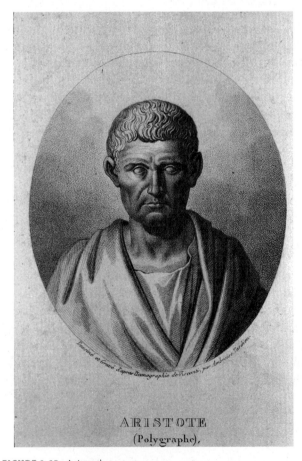

ARISTOTE
(Polygraphe),

FIGURE 1-12 Aristotle.
Courtesy of the National Library of Medicine.

famous Romans, Galen (CE 130–200) and Augustine (CE 354–430), postulated that mental functions were localized in the brain (**FIGURE 1-13**). Specifically, they believed these functions were localized in the

open spaces of the brain known as the **ventricles**. This belief gave rise to what is known as the **cell doctrine**, that the cells or ventricles of the brain had psychic gases called humors in them responsible for mental functions. This theory persisted for approximately 1,000 years until the time of the Renaissance, when people like Andreas Vesalius (1514–1564) began to conduct careful studies of brain anatomy and construct detailed drawings, which future scientists would use to more thoroughly study the brain (**FIGURE 1-14**).

Modern History

In the 18th and 19th centuries, focus shifted from the brain ventricles to the brain tissue itself. Phrenologists, like Franz Josef Gall (1758–1828), believed that bumps on people's scalps were due to raised portions of brain tissue (**FIGURE 1-15**). These raised portions represented mental strengths, such as memory, math ability, and color perceptions, and personality traits such as agreeableness or combativeness (**FIGURE 1-16**). This belief led to the development of the profession of **phrenology**, whose practitioners examined and analyzed people's skulls in a procedure called cranioscopy (**FIGURE 1-17**). Phrenologists are examples of radical

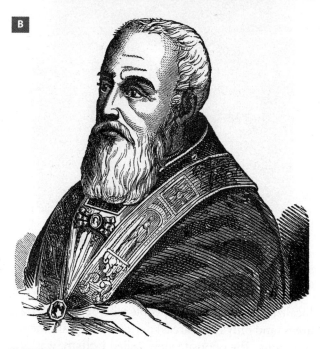

FIGURE 1-13 **A.** Galen. **B.** Augustine.

A. Courtesy of the National Library of Medicine.
B. © ilbusca/iStockphoto.

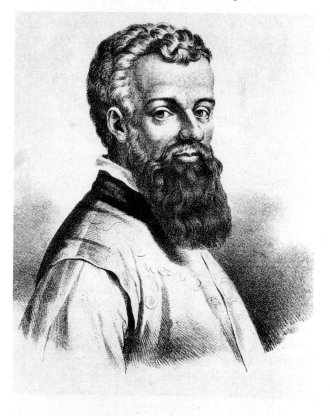

ANDRE VESALI.
1514–1564 A.D.

FIGURE 1-14 Andreas Vesalius.

Courtesy of the National Library of Medicine.

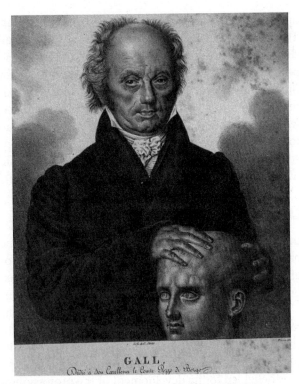

FIGURE 1-15 Franz Josef Gall performing a cranioscopy.
Courtesy of the National Library of Medicine.

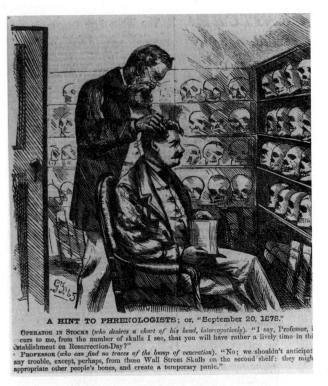

FIGURE 1-17 Phrenologist performing a cranioscopy.
Courtesy of the National Library of Medicine.

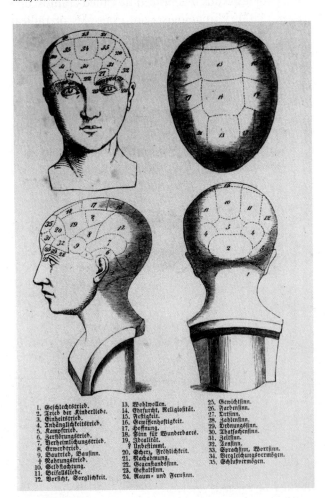

FIGURE 1-16 Phrenology charts.
Courtesy of the National Library of Medicine.

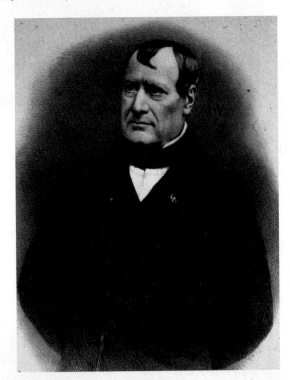

FIGURE 1-18 Marie-Jean-Pierre Flourens.
Courtesy of the National Library of Medicine.

localizationists, meaning people who believed certain areas (and only those areas) performed certain mental functions. The opposite view, called **holism**, was presented by Marie-Jean-Pierre Flourens (1794–1867), who asserted that brain function was not so neatly organized. Flourens (**FIGURE 1-18**) argued that the whole brain, not just a discrete part of the brain, was involved in a mental function.

In the latter half of the 19th century, a mediating position between localists and holists known as **connectionism** developed. In 1861, Paul Broca (1824–1880) presented a patient nicknamed Tan (because "tan" was the only word he could say intelligibly) to his peers (**FIGURE 1-19**). Tan demonstrated loss of speech and a right hemiplegia. Tan died shortly after Broca's presentation and his brain was examined, revealing damage to the left frontal portion of the brain known today as Broca's area (**FIGURE 1-20** and **BOX 1-2**). We know from Broca's work that Broca's area is a key area in human speech production. Later, Karl Wernicke (1848–1904) built on Broca's work by identifying an area in the left posterior portion of the brain responsible for understanding language (**FIGURE 1-21** and **BOX 1-3**). This area eventually was named Wernicke's area. Both Broca and Wernicke contributed to the idea of connectionism, the belief that there are centers in the brain responsible for certain functions and that these areas are connected and work cooperatively (**BOX 1-4**).

Connectionism of one form or another has dominated neuroscience ever since thanks to scientists such as Roman Jakobson (1896–1982), A. R. Luria (1902–1977), Norman Geschwind (1926–1984), and Harold

particular area was crucial for speech production, and over the course of 2 years he found 12 more cases to substantiate his original findings. This area is known today as Broca's area, and the type of language problem associated with damage to it is known as Broca's aphasia.

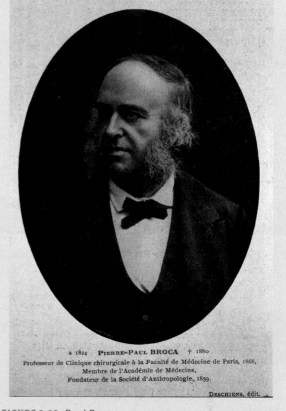

FIGURE 1-19 Paul Broca.
Courtesy of the National Library of Medicine.

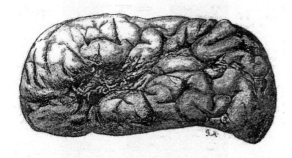

FIGURE 1-20 The brain of Leborgne (Tan).
Courtesy of the National Library of Medicine.

BOX 1-2 Paul Broca

The French physician Paul Broca lived in a time of tension in neuroscience. Franz Josef Gall, a phrenologist, and Marie-Jean-Pierre Flourens, a holist, were disputing how the brain worked and where mental faculties were located. Broca helped to bring the controversy to rest through a patient named Leborgne, more famously known as "Tan" because this was the only understandable word he said. When Tan died, Broca did an autopsy and discovered that Tan had a lesion on the third frontal convolution of the left hemisphere. Broca concluded that this

BOX 1-3 Karl Wernicke

Karl Wernicke was born in Germany in 1848 and studied both neurology and psychiatry. Wernicke, spurred on by Broca's work in France, began his own investigation on the effects of neuropathologies on speech and language. In his research, he observed that language disturbances occurred when other areas of the brain were damaged, but Broca's area was left intact. He found an area on the posterior part of the superior temporal gyrus that, when damaged, left patients with difficulty understanding other people's speech and language. From this, Wernicke postulated that this area, known today as Wernicke's area, is crucial for language comprehension. This area of the brain carries his name, as does the form of aphasia associated with damage to it: Wernicke's aphasia.

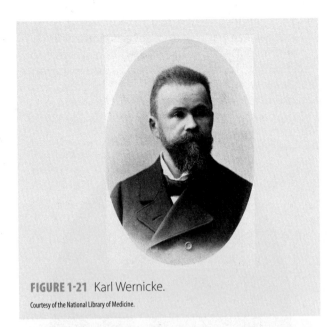

FIGURE 1-21 Karl Wernicke.
Courtesy of the National Library of Medicine.

BOX 1-4 The Duel

It is easy to think that earlier neuroscientists, like Broca and Wernicke, worked calmly and cooperatively on how the brain works. This was not always the case, however. Joseph Jules Dejerine (1849–1917) is remembered for being one of the first to describe a sudden loss of reading ability, known as alexia. He was a localist in the tradition of Broca and Wernicke. Pierre Marie (1853–1940) was a bitter opponent of Dejerine, accusing Dejerine of poor and substandard work. In response, Dejerine challenged Marie to a duel, thinking his honor had been attacked. The duel never happened. Instead, Marie defused the situation by publishing a letter stating that neither Dejerine's honor nor work was in question. In 1906, the bold Marie even challenged Broca's work from 30 years previously, arguing that Tan's speech loss was due to damage to both Broca's and Wernicke's areas, rather than just Broca's area. Marie's opinion held sway for over 70 years until 1979, when Tan's brain was scanned using computed tomography technology. The findings supported Broca's conclusions and showed that Marie was wrong.

BOX 1-5 Where Are the Famous Neurologists of Today?

Oliver Sacks (1933–2015) was probably the most famous neurologist in recent memory because of his popular writing (**FIGURE 1-22**) FreightBig Pro. He was born in Great Britain but immigrated to the United States in the 1960s. In 1966 he began work at Beth Abraham Hospital, where he treated survivors of encephalitis lethargica, also known as the "sleeping sickness," which is a disease that became an epidemic in the 1920s. The disease attacks the brain and leaves its victims unable to move or speak. Sacks developed a drug treatment that "unfroze" these patients who had not moved in decades. Sacks wrote a book called *Awakenings* in which he documented his treatment as well as the patients' temporary recovery. The book was made into a movie of the same name, with Robin Williams playing the role of Sacks. Dr. Sacks published many books of neurological tales, including *The Man Who Mistook His Wife for a Hat* and *An Anthropologist on Mars*. Sacks himself suffered from a neurological disorder known as prosopagnosia, or face blindness.

Antonio Damasio (b. 1944) is one of the most famous living neurologists (**FIGURE 1-23**). He was born in Portugal and studied medicine at the University of Lisbon. He moved to Boston, Massachusetts, and studied under Harold Goodglass at the Aphasia Research Center. One of his main research interests has been the neurobiology of emotions. Two of Damasio's most famous books are *Descartes' Error: Emotion, Reason and the Human Brain* and *The Feeling of What Happens: Body and Emotion in the Making of Consciousness*. His wife, Hanna, is also a well-known neuroscientist. Both of the Damasios currently work at the University of Southern California, and they often publish together.

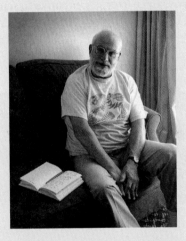

FIGURE 1-22 Oliver Sacks.

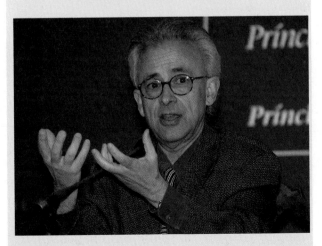

FIGURE 1-23 Antonio Damasio.

Goodglass (1920–2002). Of course, there have continued to be holists holding connectionists responsible to explain the complexities of brain function. Some of these scientists include John Hughlings Jackson (1835–1911), Pierre Marie (1853–1940), Henry Head (1861–1940), and Kurt Goldstein (1878–1965). More recent neurologists have continued to build upon the work of these scientists (**BOX 1-5**). Various theoretical perspectives discussed in this section are summarized in **FIGURE 1-24**. Of course, there is more to the debate than just whether the brain works through interconnected centers or as an integrated whole. **BOX 1-6** discusses another interesting debate called the mind–brain debate and **BOX 1-7** challenges a common myth about the brain's functioning.

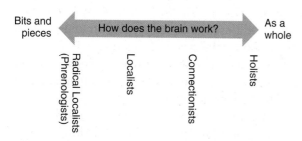

FIGURE 1-24 The range of theoretical perspectives on the brain.

BOX 1-6 The Mind–Brain Debate

Look again at the quote that began this chapter by Dr. Stephen Juan: "Every thought, every action, every deed relies upon this incredible organ [the brain]." What does Dr. Juan mean by "every thought . . . *relies*"? Is the mind that thinks the same as the brain, or is it different? In other words, can the mind be reduced to brain processes, or are the mind and the brain different substances that interact with one another? This question is known as the **mind–brain debate**. When it comes to this question, **dualists** believe that humans possess two entities, a material brain and an immaterial mind; in contrast, **monists** believe humans possess one entity only, a material brain/mind. For the majority of history, most people held to dualism and believed that humans consist of both a body and a soul and, thus, a brain and a mind. With the growing popularity of neuroscience, however, this view has been challenged by neuroscientists as well as some philosophers and theologians who are now opting for monistic explanations for human composition. It might appear from this discussion that there are only two options—dualism or monism—but there are a variety of views under each category (Green & Palmer, 2010; Huffman, 2013).

BOX 1-7 The 10% Myth

Every year, I quiz my neuroanatomy class about what percentage of their brain they think they use. Inevitably, a majority of the class picks "10%." Where did this myth come from and how does it stay in the public conscience? It probably originated with the American philosopher William James (1842–1910), who believed that humans used only a fraction of their mental potential (not brain), which is a plausible idea. He based this idea on cases of incredibly smart people, like William James Sidis (1898–1944). Named after his godfather, William James, Sidis was considered the smartest man who ever lived because of his remarkable language and mathematical skills. Lowell Thomas, in his 1936 introduction to *Dale Carnegie's How to Win Friends and Influence People*, added 10% to James' statement and said, "Professor William James of Harvard used to say that the average man develops only 10% of his latent mental ability." In time, "latent mental ability" morphed into "brain" in popular belief, and this myth has been propagated over time through popular media. One recent example is the 2014 movie *Lucy*, which tells the story of a woman named Lucy who, as the result of experiments, is able to access 100% of her brain's potential. Thanks to unlocking the use her entire brain, Lucy becomes both omnipresent and omniscient. The message of the movie is that we only use 10% of our brains leaving 90% unused, and that if we could harness that 90%, we could become Lucy.

The truth is that we use 100% of our brains every day. Brain imaging has shown this. In addition, we know that damage to a very small part of the brain can lead to catastrophic problems in communication and thinking, like in Alzheimer disease and stroke. Lastly, our brains make up about 2% of our body weight but consume about 20% of the body's oxygen. Why would only 10% of our brains need this much energy? The 10% myth is just that: a myth that makes a good Hollywood story.

▶ Neuroscience Today

Humans have long desired to see the brain, but early attempts involved opening the cranial vault and removing the brain. Early investigators, like Broca and Wernicke, spent years making careful behavioral observations and then waiting for their subjects to die in order to examine their brains. Postmortem dissection is still the gold standard for some diseases, like Alzheimer disease and chronic traumatic encephalopathy (CTE). CTE is a condition many former professional football players have suffered that can be reliably diagnosed only postmortem. Generally, however, advances beginning in the middle of the 20th century have allowed researchers to examine subjects while they are still alive.

Electrostimulation, or brain mapping, was the first technique that mapped the responses of the living brain to specific behaviors. Brain mapping was typically done as patients with conditions such as severe epilepsy underwent brain surgery to sever the connection between the two cerebral hemispheres. Two major observations from brain mapping were made. First, there is *some* relationship between a specific area of the brain and a specific experience or behavior. For example, if a certain part of the primary motor cortex is stimulated, then a body part might move. Similarly, if a certain area in the primary sensory cortex is stimulated, the patient might feel something in a part of the body. Second, there is a high degree of individual variation in people's brains. For example, language is localized in the left hemisphere for most people, but there is a certain subset of people with language in either the right hemisphere or spread between the two hemispheres.

The next important event was the development of the **computed tomography (CT)** scan in the 1970s. From the 1980s through the present day, there has been a technological explosion of neuroimaging techniques. In the 1990s, techniques were refined, and in the early 2000s, techniques have been combined and further refined.

Even with the technological explosion, there are still two basic imaging techniques, structural imaging and functional imaging. **Structural imaging** shows the brain's anatomy. In contrast, **functional imaging** shows the brain's activity (i.e., brain physiology)—that is, which brain areas are active under certain circumstances. There is no longer a firm divide between these two types of imaging because structural and functional imaging are being combined to form new, powerful imaging tools.

Structural Imaging Techniques

The standard in neuroimaging before CT was plain x-ray films (i.e., radiography). This technology was used to see dense structures, like bones, but worked poorly for viewing soft tissues like the brain. X-ray films are still used today to see skull fractures or craniofacial abnormalities, but this method needs to be used with caution because it involves exposure to radiation, which can lead to cancer if the patient is overexposed to it (Imbesi, 2009).

Computed tomography (*tomo is Greek for* "a cutting or section"; *graphy* is Greek for "a writing") refined the use of x-ray technology (**FIGURE 1-25**). CT passes

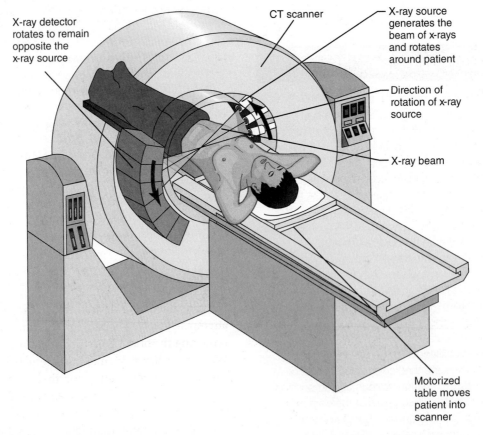

X-ray detector rotates to remain opposite the x-ray source

CT scanner

X-ray source generates the beam of x-rays and rotates around patient

Direction of rotation of x-ray source

X-ray beam

Motorized table moves patient into scanner

FIGURE 1-25 A patient in a CT scanner.

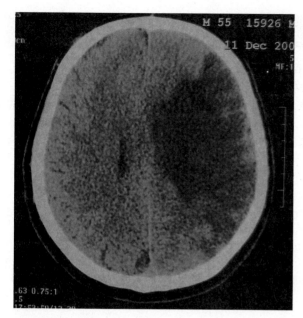

FIGURE 1-26 Example of a CT scan.

Courtesy of Constantin Potagas.

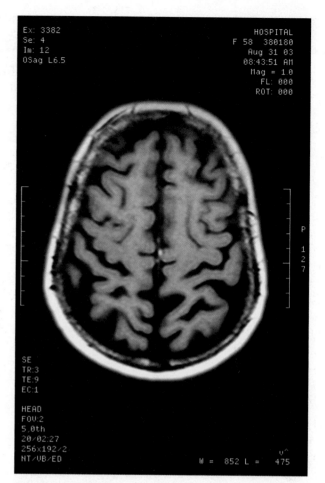

FIGURE 1-27 Example of an MRI scan.

© lucato/iStock/Thinkstock.

x-rays through the human body that reflect off of different densities of tissue, bone, and fluid in different ways, producing an image (**FIGURE 1-26**). Structures with higher densities (e.g., bone) show up better than structures with lower densities (e.g., brain tissue). The result is a two-dimensional image, which can be digitally processed into three-dimensional images. The advantages of this technique are that it is commonly used and thus easily accessible, making it a relatively inexpensive procedure. There are at least four disadvantages to using CT technology. First is the reality that the technique uses x-rays, posing a small risk of causing cancer. Second, CT shows anatomy only and not physiology. Third, the clarity of images is an issue when viewing soft tissues of the body because images are sharpest when of dense structures. Fourth, CTs sometimes do not pick up new damage to soft tissues. A CT taken at the time of patient admittance might be negative but when repeated the next day might be positive for tissue changes.

Magnetic resonance imaging (MRI) uses a magnetic current to flip protons within the body's water molecules. The signal that is produced is picked up by the MRI's receiver coils and the data are then formed into three-dimensional images (**FIGURE 1-27**). There are different ways to view tissue using MRI, T1-weighted images and T2-weighted images. A T1-weighted image is helpful in examining the structure of the cerebral cortex, whereas a T2-weighted image is useful in detecting swelling, inflammation, and white matter lesions. The main way to tell if you are looking at a T1-weighted versus a T2-weighted image is the color

of the brain ventricles. In the former, the ventricles will appear black; in the latter, they will appear white.

The advantages of MRI include a much sharper image (especially of soft tissues) compared to CT. In addition, harmful x-rays are not used, thus eliminating the risk of cancer. Disadvantages include the expense of the test compared to CT, claustrophobic reactions due to the narrow tube the patient enters, and the presence of MRI-unsafe metals in the patient's body (e.g., cochlear implants, vascular stents, brain-aneurysm clips, shrapnel). A sample MRI report can be viewed in **BOX 1-8**.

As mentioned previously, soft tissues are notoriously difficult to see through imaging techniques. Blood vessels, which are made up of soft tissue (endothelial, connective, and smooth muscular tissue) are difficult to image. However, **angiography** is an invasive technique that uses iodine as a contrast and x-rays to give excellent pictures of the blood vessels (**FIGURE 1-28**). It makes possible the diagnosis of conditions, like aneurysms and ischemic strokes, that previously were very difficult to diagnose through neuroimaging. The technique is invasive, meaning

BOX 1-8 Sample MRI Report

AMERICAN IMAGING CENTER

Patient Name: H. R.   Date of Birth: 7/11/1927   MRN: 10247583
At the request of: Charles Smith, MD   Age: 86   Sex: M   Exam Date: 8/8/2013

MRI BRAIN & SELLA W/WO CONTRAST

CLINICAL HISTORY: The patient complains of bilateral blurred vision with dizziness and unsteadiness for 2 months.

TECHNIQUE: A complete diagnostic set of multiplanar images was acquired using an open-ended, wide-aperture 1.5-Tesla MRI system equipped with high-performance gradients. Turbo parallel processing was employed for enhanced speed. Proprietary sound suppression was provided for patient comfort. Sequence selections, image planes, and slice parameters were adjusted for optimal visualization of regional anatomy and pathology anticipated by the patient's history.

Additional sets of T1-weighted images were obtained following uneventful intravenous injection of 10-cc gradlinium contrast material.

FINDINGS: The sella turcica is normal in size and shows a normal-size pituitary gland with uniform enhancement. The carotid siphon segment of both internal carotid arteries shows mild ectasia and tortuosity with a slight medial coursing on the right creating a lateral defect on the pituitary gland. The pituitary stalk is slightly angled to the left as a result. Optic chiasm is normal. There is no upward convexity at the diaphragm sellae nor is there a suprasellar component.

There is relatively contiguous increase in signal in periventricular white matter adjacent to the lateral ventricles bilaterally with FLAIR and T2 technique nonenhancing with multiple small foci more peripherally situated in the cerebral hemispheres bilaterally with similar signal characteristics. These are all nonenhancing and represent chronic small vessel ischemic changes. There is no mass lesion demonstrated with no shift in midline structures. The ventricles and cortical sulci are within normal limits for age, and there is no extracerebral fluid collection. There is no evidence of acute or chronic lobar or lacunar infarction.

Cranial nerve complex 7 and 8 is normal bilaterally with no evidence of cerebellopontine angle mass lesion.

The paranasal sinuses are well aerated without membrane thickening demonstrated. There has been cataract surgery in the right lobe.

IMPRESSION:

1. There are relatively severe periventricular white matter changes in both cerebral hemispheres representing chronic small vessel ischemic change.
2. There is mild deformity on the pituitary gland due to impression by slightly tortuous carotid siphon segment of right internal carotid artery without gland enlargement or focal lesion within the gland with normal appearance of optic chiasm.
3. There is no intraparenchymal focal mass or active process demonstrated with no abnormal enhancement noted.

Thank you kindly for referring your patient to our office.
Gregory G. Stump, MD
Board Certified Radiologist

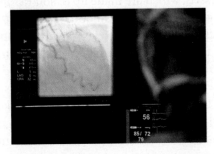

FIGURE 1-28 A physician observing an angiography.

there is a risk for bleeding, bruising, clotting, or swelling at the injection site. It also uses x-rays and thus exposes the patient to radiation (Imbesi, 2009).

Functional Imaging Techniques

Functional imaging techniques fall into two categories: spatial resolution and temporal resolution. **Spatial resolution** identifies the location of brain activity, whereas **temporal resolution** techniques deal with the time between a stimulus being introduced and the brain's response to it. Examples from both of these functional imaging categories will be discussed along with their advantages and disadvantages (**TABLE 1-1**).

Positron emission tomography (PET) is a spatial resolution technology that shows brain activity based on the brain's glucose metabolism (**FIGURE 1-29**). The underlying assumption of the technique is that active areas require more energy; thus they consume more glucose. A radioactive isotope, which is chemically attached to a glucose molecule, is injected into a patient's bloodstream. As the isotope decays, it emits photons, which are picked up by the scanner and formed into a three-dimensional image. The advantage of this technique is

TABLE 1-1 Comparison of Spatial and Temporal Resolution Techniques

Spatial Resolution: From Best to Worst	Temporal Resolution: From Best to Worst
Functional magnetic resonance imaging (fMRI)	EEG
Positron emission tomography (PET)	fMRI
Electroencephalography (EEG)	PET

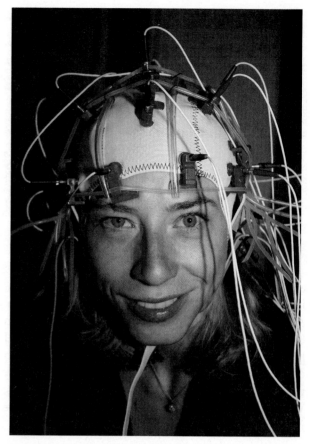

FIGURE 1-30 Patient undergoing EEG.
© Daniela Schraml/ShutterStock, Inc.

that it gives very useful data on brain activity, but there are disadvantages, including the invasive nature of the technique (i.e., it requires an injection into the bloodstream) and the fact that a radioactive material is used.

Electroencephalography (EEG) is a temporal resolution technique that measures the neuronal electrical activity through electrodes placed on the scalp (**FIGURE 1-30**). As a stimulus is presented to a subject's senses, the EEG monitors the brain's electrical responses to that stimulus. The result is a graph that compares electrical activity from each electrode over time (**FIGURE 1-31**). Advantages of this technique include its relatively low cost, the wide availability of the machines, and the good temporal resolution data the technology delivers. Its disadvantages include the limited spatial resolution EEG provides and its limitations in providing information on activity in deeper layers of the brain.

Combined Structural and Functional Imaging Techniques

As we entered the new millennium, many of the techniques described previously have been combined. For example, **functional magnetic resonance imaging (fMRI)** combines the advantages of MRI with the

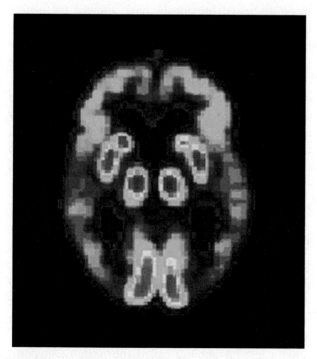

FIGURE 1-29 Example of PET.
Courtesy of the Alzheimer's Disease Education and Referral Center, a service of the National Institute on Aging.

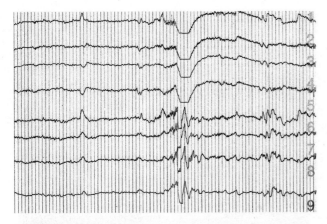

FIGURE 1-31 An EEG graph.
© iStockphoto/Thinkstock.

advantages of PET, showing both the anatomy and physiology of the brain by measuring blood oxygenation. Advantages include that it does not require the injection of a contrast like PET scans require. In addition, fMRI provides both spatial and temporal resolution data in one test. The main disadvantage is that fMRI is mainly used in research facilities and rarely in clinical settings. With this technology's advantages, it will likely move more into the mainstream in the near future.

Which Test When?

When a person arrives in the hospital's emergency department presenting with neurological signs and symptoms, CT is usually the first neuroimaging technique used. Typically, CT is followed up with MRI. Other neuroimaging studies, such as angiography or PET, are ordered if needed. Given the number of neuroimaging techniques available today, how does a neurologist determine which test to order?

The answer is that it depends on what condition is suspected. Remember that a careful neurological exam can tell much about which neurological condition a person may be suffering from. Often, neuroimaging studies are ordered to confirm a preliminary diagnosis already arrived at by the neurologist. If a neurologist suspects a stroke, the best studies to order are CT, MRI, and perhaps angiography. For conditions like aneurysms or arteriovenous malformations, cerebral angiography remains the gold standard, though CT or MRI may also be ordered. Neoplasms (e.g., brain tumors) are best evaluated through CT and MRI, as are central nervous system infections like meningitis. White matter diseases, like multiple sclerosis, are best evaluated through MRI or fMRI. CT and MRI are typically the choice for situations involving trauma to the head. EEG is an excellent tool for evaluating patients with epilepsy, brain tumors, and sleep disorders (Weiner & Goetz, 2004).

You can see that one neuroimaging technique is not necessarily better than another. Each technique is a tool in the neurologist's tool belt that should be used in just the right situation to give medical professionals the best information possible to diagnose and treat the patient with a neurological problem.

A Caution Regarding Imaging Techniques

Just because we can now "*see*" into the brain, we are tempted to correlate every possible thought or action with some specific area of the brain that might light up on an image. It must be remembered that because one area of the brain lights up does not mean that it is the sole area responsible for a function. The brain is a highly complicated organ and will probably never be fully understood in all its wonderful complexity.

Neuroimaging techniques (**TABLE 1-2**) are exciting, continuously developing tools that help us understand the power of the brain. These techniques are very useful in understanding the relationships among the brain, language, and other cognitive functions. It is important for SLPs and audiologists to be familiar with neuroimaging techniques so that they can be good consumers of current research and clinical information. They should also remember Hippocrates' sage advice about the power of observation and the wisdom of completing a careful, systematic examination of the communication system.

In terms of brain functioning, what was once thought to be a serial and linear process is now thought to be a nonserial, parallel, and highly complicated process. Neuroradiological techniques, like those discussed previously, have allowed us to peer into the brain and glimpse this complexity. This ability has led to various subfields emerging in neuroscience today, including fields such as molecular neuroscience (i.e., the study of important neurological molecules), cellular neuroscience (i.e., the study of neurons and other brain cells), systems neuroscience (i.e., the study of the motor system), behavioral neuroscience (i.e., the study of behaviors such as types of memory), and cognitive neuroscience (i.e., the study of higher level cognitive functions such as language).

▶ Conclusion

Why is it important to know about theoretical perspectives of brain function like connectionism and holism? The reason is that theoretical perspectives lead to the invention of diagnostic and therapeutic methods. For example, Harold Goodglass (a connectionist) developed a test for aphasia called the *Boston Diagnostic Aphasia Examination*. This test is based on connectionist ideas and ties types of aphasia to damaged areas

TABLE 1-2 Summary of Select Neuroimaging Techniques

Name	Structural or Functional	Positives	Negatives
Computed tomography (CT)	Structural	Inexpensive; commonly used; readily accessible	Danger of x-rays; structural only; clarity with soft tissues; sometimes do not pick up new damage
Magnetic resonance imaging (MRI)	Structural	Sharp, clear image (of soft tissues); no x-rays used	More expensive than CT; claustrophobic reactions; danger if metals in person's body
Angiography	Structural	Excellent pictures of vascular system; can diagnose conditions previously difficult to diagnose	Invasive (requires injection); uses x-rays (radiation)
Positron emission tomography (PET)	Functional	Good data on brain physiology (spatial resolution)	Invasive (requires injection); radioactive material used in injection
Electroencephalography (EEG)	Functional	Low cost; readily available; good temporal resolution	Limited spatial resolution; lack of information on deep brain structure function
Functional magnetic resonance imaging (fMRI)	Both	Provides both structural and functional data; no injection needed; no x-rays used	Rarely found in clinical settings

in the brain. However, Hildred Schuell developed the *Minnesota Test for the Differential Diagnosis of Aphasia* from a holist's perspective. Her test is not concerned with damaged brain areas, but rather with giving basic descriptions of patient strengths and weaknesses in order to plan therapy. As your professors teach you about different theories, always remember that *theory matters*! In other words, it has real-world implications for tests and therapy procedures and materials.

SLPs and audiologists also need to know about neurology because they will be working with people who have communication disorders that have a neurological origin. For example, people with autism make up a large percentage of many SLPs' caseloads, and this condition has neurological dimensions. It is important to learn and understand the normal nervous system in order to have a baseline for understanding an abnormal nervous system and the various communication disorders that can result (**FIGURE 1-32**). For example, there are several types of classic aphasias (i.e., an acquired multimodality language loss). It is widely known that damage to the anterior part of the cerebrum can result in certain aphasia types, and damage to the posterior cerebrum results in other types. It is important to understand how the anterior and posterior portions of the cerebrum work in order to understand the signs and symptoms our patients are experiencing. Another example is dysarthria (i.e., slurred and/or discoordinated speech). There are six different types

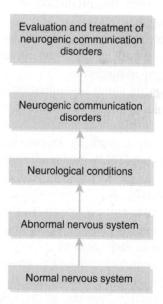

FIGURE 1-32 The importance of neurology to communication disorders.

of dysarthria that result from damage to different parts of the nervous system, and the characteristics of these types of dysarthria are different depending on where the damage is in the nervous system.

This is your opportunity to dive in and learn as much as you can about the nervous system so you will be an effective professional in understanding and treating your future patients. In addition, neurology is fun and interesting in its own right!

SUMMARY OF LEARNING OBJECTIVES

The following were the main learning objectives of this chapter. The information that should have been learned is below each learning objective.

1. The learner will define the following terms: *neurology, anatomy, physiology,* and *pathology.*
   - *Neurology* is the study of the anatomy, physiology, and pathology of the nervous system.
   - *Neuroanatomy* is the study of the nervous system's structure.
   - *Neurophysiology* is the study of the nervous system's function.
   - *Neuropathology* is the study of disease processes that affect both anatomy and physiology of the nervous system.

2. The learner will be able to create an argument as to why speech-language pathologists and audiologists need neurological training.
   - Knowing the terminology and abbreviations neurologists use will help SLPs and audiologists decode their language.
   - Knowing about the location of brain damage can help with the planning of assessment.
   - Knowing about neurological etiologies can help with the prediction of likely patient problems.
   - Knowing neurology helps in the documentation of patient improvement and efficacy of treatment methods.
   - Knowing about neuroplasticity helps in the careful planning of treatment to take advantage of this phenomenon.
   - Having a working knowledge of neurology helps SLPs and audiologists gain the respect of neurologists and other medical professionals.

3. The learner will be able to list various categories of neurological disorders and provide one example in each category.
   - *Inflammatory diseases:* encephalitis and meningitis
   - *Systematic atrophies of the central nervous system:* Huntington disease
   - *Extrapyramidal and movement disorders:* Parkinson disease
   - *Other degenerative diseases of the nervous system:* Alzheimer disease
   - *Demyelinating diseases of the central nervous system:* multiple sclerosis
   - *Episodic and paroxysmal disorders:* epilepsy
   - *Nerve, nerve root, and plexus disorders:* Bell palsy
   - *Polyneuropathies and other disorders of the peripheral nervous system:* Guillain-Barré syndrome
   - *Diseases of the myoneural junction and muscle:* myasthenia gravis
   - *Cerebral palsy and other paralytic conditions:* cerebral palsy and spinal cord injury
   - *Other disorders of the nervous system:* anoxia

4. The learner will be able to draw and explain the spectrum of belief as to how the brain works.
   - The brain works in bits and pieces: phrenology.
   - The brain is a series of interconnected centers: connectionism.
   - The brain works as an integrated whole: holism.

5. The learner will list and define structural and functional imaging techniques and list at least one reason why communication disorders professionals should know about neuroimaging techniques.
   - Structural imaging techniques
     - *X-ray imaging (radiography):* technique that uses x-rays to view skull fractures and craniofacial abnormalities
     - *Computed tomography (CT):* use of a computer to convert x-ray images into two- and three-dimensional images
     - *Magnetic resonance imaging (MRI):* use of magnets to flip protons in the body, which is picked up by a computer and converted into an image clearer than CT
     - *Angiography:* technique that uses injected dye to view the vascular system
   - Functional imaging techniques
     - *Positron emission tomography (PET):* a spatial resolution technology that shows brain activity based on the brain's glucose metabolism
     - *Electroencephalography (EEG):* a temporal resolution technique that measures the neuronal electrical activity through electrodes placed on the scalp
   - SLPs and audiologists are consumers of the reports generated from these technologies. These reports can be found in journal articles and in patient charts.

KEY TERMS

Activity barriers
Alzheimer disease
Anatomy
Angiography
Cell doctrine
Computed
 tomography (CT)
Connectionism
Dualists
Electroencephalography (EEG)
Functional imaging
Functional magnetic
 resonance imaging (fMRI)
Function barriers

Hemiplegia
Holism
Incidence
Magnetic resonance
 imaging (MRI)
Mind–brain debate
Monists
Nervous system
Neuroanatomy
Neurological disorder
Neurology
Neuropathology
Neurophysiology
Parkinson disease

Participation
 barriers
Pathology
Phrenology
Physiology
Positron emission
 technology (PET)
Prevalence
Spatial resolution
Structural imaging
Temporal resolution
Trephination
Trephines
Ventricles

DRAW IT TO KNOW IT

1. Sketch a person and include a simple picture of the brain, spinal cord, and nerves (see Figure 1-1). Label these three structures.

2. Draw WHO's model of health and disability (see Figure 1-4), and apply a medical case you are familiar with to it.

3. Draw the spectrum of views regarding how the brain works (see Figure 1-24).

QUESTIONS FOR DEEPER REFLECTION

1. Why are our neurological systems precious resources?
2. Why is theory important?
3. Why should SLPs and audiologists know about the nervous system?

4. Compare and contrast the strengths and weaknesses of each neuroimaging technique.
5. Why should communication disorders professionals be knowledgeable of neuroimaging techniques?

CASE STUDY

A 63-year-old female was admitted to the hospital with sudden right-sided weakness and loss of speech. Her neurologist diagnosed her with a (L) CVA, (R) hemiplegia, and global aphasia.

1. As a speech-language pathologist, why would it be important for you to know the following terms provided by the neurologist: CVA, hemiplegia, global aphasia?

2. Apply the World Health Organization's International Classification of Functioning, Disability and Health (ICF; Figures 1-4 and 1-5) to this case and answer the following questions:

a. What is this patient's *health condition*?
b. How might it affect her *function*?
c. How might it affect her *activities*?
d. How might it affect her *participation*?
e. What might be one *environmental factor* involved in her case?
f. What might be one *personal factor* involved in her case?

3. Using the WHO's ICD-10 section on diseases of the nervous system, which of the 11 categories might this patient's diagnosis best fit under?

SUGGESTED PROJECTS

1. Think about someone you know who has a neurological disorder (see the section on Classification of Neurological Disorders for ideas). Research this disease and write an essay that includes a description of the disease; its signs, symptoms, and cause(s); the methods by which it is evaluated and treated; and any speech, language, or hearing issues that may be associated with it.

2. Choose a famous person with a neurological disorder and write a case history (i.e., the story of how his or her disease began and has progressed) on the person.

3. Pick one of the historical figures mentioned in this chapter and write an essay describing the contribution that person made to the field of neuroscience.

4. Read the sample MRI report (Box 1-8), make a list of unfamiliar terms, and look them up in a medical dictionary.

REFERENCES

Baio, J., Wiggins, L., Christensen, D. L., Maenner, M. J., Daniels, J., & Warren, Z., . . . Durkin, M. S. (2018). Prevalence of autism spectrum disorder among children aged 8 years—Autism and developmental disabilities monitoring network, 11 sites, United States, 2014. *MMWR Surveillance Summaries, 67*(6), 1.

Bertolote, J. M. (2007). *Neurological disorders affect millions globally: WHO report.* Geneva, Switzerland: World Health Organization. Retrieved from http://www.who.int/mediacentre /news/releases/2007/pr04/en/index.html

Centers for Disease Control and Prevention (CDC). (2018). *Autism spectrum disorder (ASD): Data and statistics.* Atlanta, GA: CDC. Retrieved from http://www.cdc.gov/ncbddd /autism/data.html

Gooch, C. L. , Pracht, E., & Borenstein, A. R. (2017). The burden of neurological disease in the United States: A summary report and call to action. *Annals of Neurology, 81*(4), 479–484.

Green, J. B., & Palmer, S. L. (2010). *In search of the soul: Four views of the mind-body problem.* Eugene: OR: Wipf & Stock.

Hirtz, D., Thurman, D. J., Gwinn-Hardy, K., Mohamed, M., Chaudhuri, A. R., & Zalutsky, R. (2007). How common are the "common" neurologic disorders? *Neurology, 68,* 326–337.

Huffman, D. S. (2013). *An overview of the monism-dualism debate on human composition.* La Mirada, CA: Biola University Center for Christian Thought. Retrieved from https://cct.biola .edu/overview-monism-dualism-debate-human-composition/

Imbesi, S. G. (2009). Neuroradiology: Diagnostic imaging strategies. In J. Corey-Bloom & R. David (Eds.), *Clinical adult neurology* (pp. 53–77). New York, NY: Demos Medical.

Juan, S. (1998). *The odd brain: Mysteries of our weird and wonderful brains explained.* New York, NY: Angus & Robertson.

LaPointe, L. L. (1977). What the speech pathologist expects from the neurologist. In R. H. Brookshire (Ed.), *Clinical aphasiology: Proceedings of the conference 1977* (pp. 5–9). Minneapolis, MN: BRK Publishing.

Manasco, M. H. (2017). *Introduction to neurogenic communication disorders* (2nd ed.). Burlington, MA: Jones & Bartlett Learning.

Rubens, A. B. (1977). What the neurologist expects from the clinical aphasiologist. In R. H. Brookshire (Ed.), *Clinical aphasiology: Proceedings of the conference 1977* (pp. 1-4). Minneapolis, MN: BRK Publishing.

Weiner, W. J., & Goetz, C. G. (2004). *Neurology for the non-neurologist.* Baltimore, MD: Lippincott Williams & Wilkins.

Wilkins, R. H. (1964). Neurosurgical classic—XVII. *Journal of Neurosurgery, 21,* 240–244.

World Health Organization (WHO). (2010). *International classification of diseases (ICD).* Retrieved from http://www .who.int/classifications/icd/en/

World Health Organization. (2011). *World report on disability.* Retrieved from http://whqlibdoc.who.int/publications/2011 /9789240685215_eng.pdf

World Health Organization. (2014). *International classification of functioning, disability and health (ICF).* Retrieved from http:// www.who.int/classifications/icf/icf_more/en/

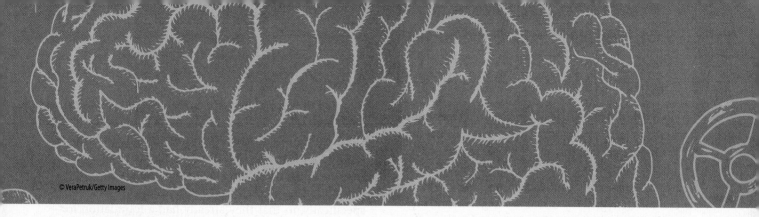

CHAPTER 2

Navigation and Organization of the Nervous System

CHAPTER PREVIEW

As we journey into the nervous system, we need language to navigate quickly around and through nervous system structures. To prepare for this journey, we will learn about the various planes of space, directional terms, and muscle actions relevant to neuroanatomy. In addition, we will survey how various neuroscientists have organized the nervous system, which allows for the better conceptualization of this complex system.

IN THIS CHAPTER

In this chapter, we will …
- Learn how to navigate around the nervous system using anatomical orientation terms
- Explore three approaches to organizing the nervous system
- Identify which of the three approaches this text will take

LEARNING OBJECTIVES

1. The learner will be able to list and define anatomical orientation terms to navigate nervous system structures.
2. The learner will list and briefly describe the three approaches to organizing the nervous system.

▶ Introduction

The journalist William F. Allman (1990) has described the brain as "a beautiful, monstrous mess." What he is referring to is the fact that the nervous system is a very complex system. How can one ever grasp and understand its complexity? Neuroscientists have developed several different grids by which to categorize and begin to understand this daunting system. In this chapter, various terms and concepts will be introduced to help in navigating through the nervous system system and its structures. In addition, three organizational approaches will be surveyed: the anatomical, functional, and developmental approaches.

▶ Navigation of the Nervous System

In looking at a nervous system structure like the brain, how does one navigate around it quickly and using only language? A picture is worth a thousand words, but sometimes pictures are not available and clinicians need to describe structures verbally. To help in this task, this section introduces key anatomical terms and concepts, including the anatomical position, anatomical versus clinical orientation, body planes, directional terms, and muscle actions.

Anatomical Terms

Many of the terms used in neuroanatomy have Greek and Latin origins. Education in these languages was a standard part of American and British education but fell into disfavor in the 1960s. Students prior to the 1960s who learned these languages had an advantage when learning anatomy in general, and neuroanatomy specifically, in that they already had a foundation for the Latin and Greek roots, prefixes, and suffixes used in these fields. Today, students report that unfamiliarity with these terms is sometimes a barrier to their learning and a disadvantage when taking standardized tests, like the SAT or GRE. For those without a background in Greek or Latin, **TABLE 2-1** is a valuable tool for navigating the terms that will be encountered in this text.

The Anatomical Position

The **anatomical position** is pictured in **FIGURE 2-1**. It serves as the starting position to describe anatomical features and positions. In this position, the body is erect, the palms face out, and the arms and face are forward. Why has this position become standard and not some other configuration? The anatomical position grew out of the world of human dissection and represents the position a cadaver lying on the dissection table.

TABLE 2-1 Summary of Some Prefixes and Suffixes Used in Neuroanatomy

Prefix or Suffix	Definition	Example
a-	Without	Aphasia—without speech
ab-	Away from	Abduction—to move structures away from each other
ad-	Toward	Adduction—to move structures toward each other
-algia	Pain	Neuralgia—nerve pain
an-	Without	Anoxia—without oxygen
angio-	Related to blood vessels	Angiography—neuroimaging technique for blood vessels
ante-/antero-	Before	Anterograde amnesia—not remembering what happened before
bi-	Two	Bilateral—occurs on both sides
brachy-	Short	Brachycephaly—having a flat or short head
brady-	Slow	Bradykinesia—slow movements

cephalo-	The head	Cephalocaudal—growth from head to tail
contra-	Opposite	Contralateral—opposite sided
cranio-	Skull	Cranium—the skull
-culus	Small	Homunculus—little man
de-	Cessation	Denervation—nerve supply loss
di-	Two	Diplopia—double vision
dys-	Impaired	Dysarthria—impaired articulation
ecto-	Outer	Ectoderm—an embryo's outermost layer of tissue
-ectomy	Removal	Craniectomy—surgical removal of part of the cranium
endo-	Inner	Endoderm—an embryo's innermost layer of tissue
ep-/epi-	Above	Epidural—above the dura mater
extra-	In addition to	Extrapyramidal tract—a nerve tract in addition to (or that complements) the pyramidal tract
-gen/-genic	Origin or beginning	Neurogenic—of a neurological origin
hemi-	One-sided or half	Hemiplegia—one-sided paralysis
hyper-	Too much	Hypertonia—too much muscle tone
hypo-	Too little	Hypotonia—too little muscle tone
infra-	Below	Infrahyoid muscles—muscles found below the hyoid bone
inter-	Between	Interhemispheric communication—communication between the left and right hemispheres
intra-	Within	Intracranial—within the cranium
ipsi-	Same	Ipsilateral—same sided
itis	Inflammation	Meningitis—inflammation in the meninges
kine-	Movement	Kinesiology—the study of movement
latero-	Side	Lateroversion—turning to one side
medio-	Middle	Mediopontine—the middle portion of the pons
micro-	Small	Microcephaly—abnormally small head
my-/myo-	Muscle	Myotrophy—nutrition of a muscle

(continues)

TABLE 2-1 Summary of Some Prefixes and Suffixes Used in Neuroanatomy *(continued)*

Prefix or Suffix	Definition	Example
neo-	New	Neoplasm—new growth (i.e., tumor)
neuro-	Nerve	Neurology—the study of the nervous system
oculo-	Eye	Oculomotor nerve—a cranial nerve that controls the eye muscles
-oma	Tumor	Neuroma—a tumor on a nerve
-osis	A condition	Neurosis—a mild mental illness
patho-	Abnormal	Pathology—the study of disease states
-pathy	Disease	Neuropathy—disease of the nervous system
peri-	Around	Periventricular—around the cerebral ventricles
-phage/-phagia	Eating	Dysphagia—swallowing disorder
-plasia	Growth	Hyperplasia—excessive growth
-plasty	Mold or repair	Cranioplasty—surgical repair of a skull defect
pseudo-	Not genuine	Pseudoscience—beliefs mistakenly thought to be based in science
quadra-/quadri-	Four	Quadriplegia—paralysis in all four limbs
re-	Again, repeat	Recurrent laryngeal nerve—a branch of the vagus nerve that descends to the chest then back up to larynx
sclerosis	Scarring, hardening	Multiple sclerosis—chronic disease of the brain due to patchy demyelination of the central nervous system
semi-	Half	Semicircular canals—part of the vestibular or balance system; three half-circle structures in the inner ear
soma-/somato-	Body	Somatosensory—the part of the nervous system that conveys sensory information to the brain for interpretation
tetra-	Four	Tetraplegia—same as quadriplegia (paralysis in four limbs)
-tomy	Cutting	Craniotomy—surgical removal of part of the skull
-trophic	Nourishment	Amyotrophic lateral sclerosis—a progressive motor neuron disease
-trophy	Growth	Atrophy—muscle wasting
uni-	One	Unilateral—on one side

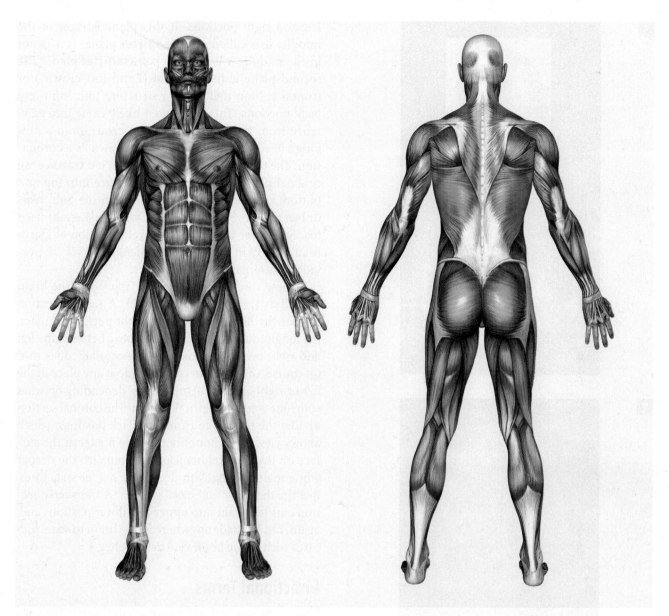

FIGURE 2-1 The anatomical position.

© Linda Bucklin/ShutterStock.

Anatomical Versus Clinical Orientation

There are two orientations to be aware of as you navigate images in neuroanatomy. The first is anatomical orientation, in which you view the brain as if you were standing looking at the top of someone's head (**FIGURE 2-2A**). In this view, the left side of the brain is on your left, and the right side of the brain is on your right. This is the view used in drawings and photos of the brain. The opposite of anatomical orientation is clinical orientation, in which you are looking at the brain from the person's feet rather than the top of the head (**FIGURE 2-2B**). The right side of the brain is on your left, and the left side is on your right. This is the orientation to use when viewing magnetic resonance

imaging (MRI) or computed tomography (CT) scans of the brain. As you navigate images in this text, keep these two orientations in mind.

Body Planes

There are three different ways to cut up the body, which grew out of the world of dissection (**FIGURE 2-3A** and **B**). The first is the **sagittal** (Latin for "arrow") section or plane. This term likely takes its name from the world of warfare, where an arrow or sword could cut or divide things into left and right portions (e.g., think of the legend of William Tell shooting an apple from the top of his son's head). The sagittal section cuts the body or a specific anatomical structure into

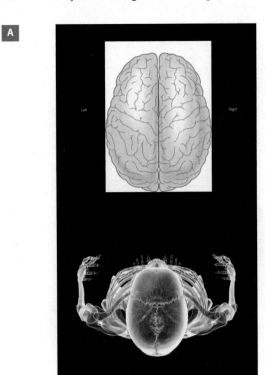

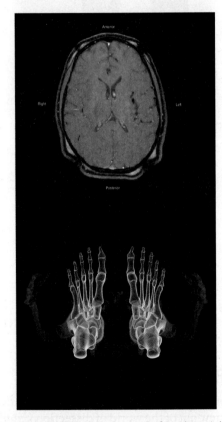

FIGURE 2-2 **A.** Anatomical orientation. If a subject's body was lying in the supine position, the observer would be viewing the brain from a superior angle. The observer's and subject's left and right sides would be aligned. **B.** Clinical orientation. If a subject's body was lying in the supine position, the observer would be viewing the brain from an inferior angle. The observer's and subject's left and right sides would be reversed.

© VisibleBody; MRI courtesy of Tia K. Hein.

left and right portions. If this plane is right in the middle, it is called a **midsagittal** plane. If it is not in the middle, it is called a **parasagittal** plane. The second plane is the **coronal** (Latin for "crown") or frontal section that splits a structure into front and back portions. This term most likely came into existence from the act of lowering a crown onto a new king's head through a ceremony known as a coronation. The third and final body section is a **transverse** or axial plane, which splits a structure into top and bottom portions. Those familiar with the *Star Wars* universe will remember that Obi-Wan Kenobi used his light saber to make a transverse section of Darth Maul's body in *The Phantom Menace*. **TABLE 2-2** provides a summary of these planes.

These three sections can be applied to the brain as well as the body (**FIGURE 2-3C**). A sagittal section divides the brain into left and right portions. In fact, the longitudinal fissure, a deep groove between the left and right cerebral hemispheres, essentially does this. Of course, this division can be made at any place in the left or right cerebral hemispheres, depending on what someone wants to see in the brain. The coronal section divides the brain into front and back portions, which allows viewing of not only the gray matter at the surface on the cerebral hemispheres, but also the deeper white matter along with deep gray matter structures, like the thalamus and basal ganglia. A transverse section cuts the brain into upper and lower portions and, again, can be made anywhere in the brain to see structures such as the brain ventricles better.

Directional Terms

How does one quickly move around an anatomical structure using language only? Directional terms are very useful tools for accomplishing this task and will be used heavily in this text. Some of these terms are useful for navigating around the body in general, and others are useful for navigating around the nervous system specifically.

The first set of these terms is superior and inferior. **Superior** means from a high position, whereas **inferior** means the opposite—from a low position. The second set is anterior and posterior. **Anterior** (**FIGURE 2-4A**) means toward the stomach and **posterior** toward the back (**FIGURE 2-4B**). The term **ventral** is sometimes used as a synonym for anterior and **dorsal** for posterior (think of a dolphin's dorsal fin). A third set is lateral and medial. Think of an imaginary line that runs through the center of the body (i.e., a midline); **lateral** would mean away from midline, whereas **medial** would refer to toward midline (or the middle of the body). Proximal and distal

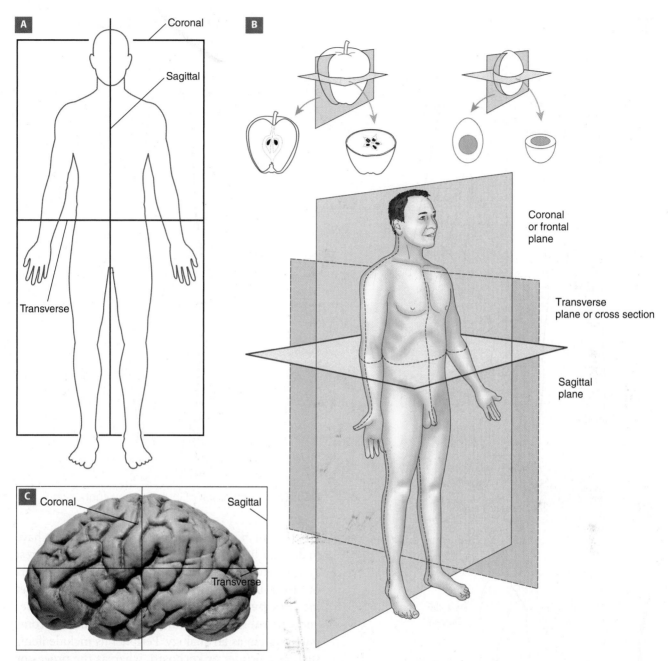

FIGURE 2-3 **A.** Sections applied to the body. **B.** Planes in three-dimensional view. **C.** Sections applied to the brain. Note that the body in parts A and B is facing anteriorly, and the brain in part C is a lateral view.
© Brand X Pictures/Thinkstock.

TABLE 2-2 Summary of the Three Body Planes

Plane Name	Alternative Name	Definition	Example
Sagittal	Lateral	Splits structure into right and left portions	The halves of an apple
Coronal	Frontal	Splits structure into front and back portions	Slices of bread
Transverse	Horizontal	Splits structure into upper and lower portions	The layers of a hamburger

A

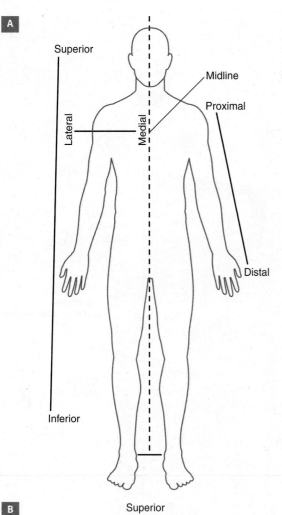

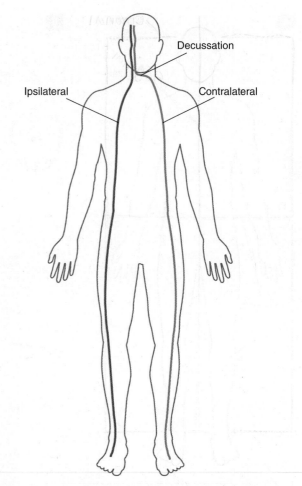

FIGURE 2-5 Comparison of ipsilateral and contralateral.

B

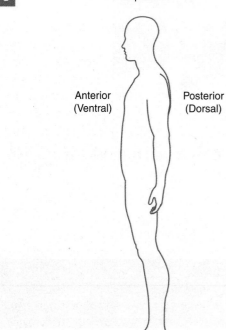

FIGURE 2-4 **A.** Directional terms applied to the body in an anterior view. **B.** Directional terms applied to the body in a lateral view.

are the fourth set of directional terms, and these have to do with limbs. **Proximal** refers to the point nearest a limb's attachment, whereas **distal** refers to the part of the limb farthest from its attachment. The fifth set includes **peripheral** (i.e., toward the outer surface) and **central** (i.e., toward the center). Think of a computer system as an analogy. Peripherals include items such as a printer or keyboard, whereas the processor is central and is appropriately termed the central processing unit. A sixth set is ipsilateral and contralateral. **Ipsilateral** means same sided, whereas **contralateral** means opposite sided (**FIGURE 2-5**). For example, your right arm and your right leg are on the same side of the body and thus are ipsilateral to each other. However, your right arm is contralateral to your left arm. Some nerve pathways are ipsilateral tracts, whereas others are contralateral. The point where a contralateral tract crosses from left to right (or right to left) is called the point of **decussation** or crossing. These sets of directional terms are summarized in **TABLE 2-3**.

We have been discussing how these directional terms apply to the body, but now it is time to explore how they apply to the brain. It is helpful to first consider how some of these terms would be applied to a four-legged

TABLE 2-3 Summary of Directional Terms

Term	Definition	Example
Superior (or cranial)	From a high position	The brain is superior to the heart.
Inferior (or caudal)	From a low position	The heart is inferior to the brain.
Anterior (or ventral)	Toward the stomach	The sternum is anterior to the heart.
Posterior (or dorsal)	Toward the back	The spine is posterior to the stomach.
Medial	Toward the body's midline	The heart is medial to the ribs.
Lateral	Away from the body's midline	The ribs are lateral to the heart.
Proximal	Point nearest limb's attachment	The shoulder is proximal to the elbow.
Distal	Point farthest from limb's attachment	The ankle is distal to the knee.
Peripheral	Toward the outer surface	The cell's wall is peripheral.
Central	Toward the center	The cell's nucleus is central.
Ipsilateral	Same side	Canadians drive ipsilateral as Americans.
Contralateral	Opposite side	Brits drive contralateral to Americans.

animal, like a dog, whose brain and spinal cord are organized in a horizontal direction (**FIGURE 2-6A**). Dorsal refers to the dog's back as well as the top of its brain, whereas ventral directs us to the dog's belly and the bottom of its brain. The term rostral (Latin for "beak" or "nose") helps us orient to the front of the dog as well as the front of the brain. The term **caudal** (Latin for "tail") directs us to the tail end of the dog and the back of the brain. **FIGURE 2-6B** applies these terms—dorsal, ventral, rostral, and caudal—to the brain, and **FIGURE 2-6C** applies them to the brainstem. In comparing these terms to the brain versus the brainstem, they may seem to be at odds; however, remember that the brainstem and spinal cord are oriented in a vertical direction in humans who are bipedal in comparison to a dog whose brain stem and spinal cord are oriented in a horizontal direction because they are quadrupedal.

Muscle Actions

Three sets of muscle actions will be addressed here (**TABLE 2-4**). The first is adduct and abduct. **Adduct** refers to bringing structures together (e.g., the vocal cords adduct when we talk), and **abduct** is the opposite—moving structures apart. These actions are pictured in **FIGURE 2-7** using the hands as an example. When we flare our fingers out, we are abducting or opening up the hand; when we bring the fingers together, we are adducting them. These actions are illustrated with the legs in **FIGURE 2-8A** and with the vocal cords in **FIGURE 2-9**. Some people find remembering the *add* in adduction helpful because it reminds them of addition in which you bring numbers together mathematically.

Second, **flexion** refers to bending a joint, whereas **extension** denotes straightening a joint (**FIGURE 2-8B**). These terms are applied to the hand in **FIGURE 2-8C** and the foot in **FIGURE 2-8D**. In his earlier days, Arnold Schwarzenegger did a lot of flexion and extension in bodybuilding competitions.

The third and final set is supine and pronate. **Supine** refers to lying faceup (i.e., ventral surface up). **Pronate** is the opposite and refers to lying facedown (i.e., ventral surface down). Think about sleeping as an example. Some people sleep on their stomachs (pronate position), whereas others sleep on their backs (supine position). The pronate position is also the preferred position of prayer in some religions.

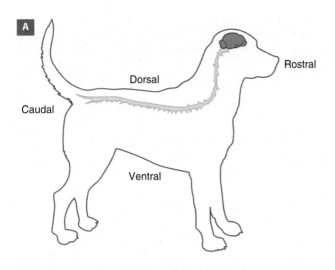

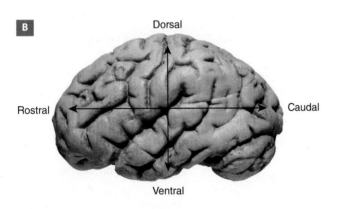

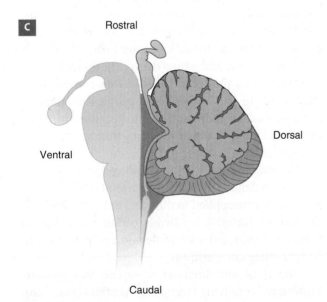

FIGURE 2-6 The directional terms ventral, dorsal, rostral, and caudal applied to **A.** a dog, **B.** the brain, and **C.** the brainstem.

© Brand X Pictures/Thinkstock.

TABLE 2-4 Summary of Muscle Actions		
Term	**Definition**	**Example**
Adduct	To bring structures together	The vocal folds are together during phonation.
Abduct	To move structures apart	The vocal folds are apart during breathing.
Flexion	To bend a joint	You bend your elbow to brush your teeth.
Extension	To straighten a joint	You straighten your elbow to reach into the refrigerator.
Supine	Lying with ventral surface up	John sleeps in the supine position (on his back).
Pronate	Lying with ventral surface down	Maria sleeps in the pronate position (on her stomach).

▶ Organizational Approaches to the Nervous System

An Anatomical Approach

An anatomical approach involves those structures that can be seen with the human eye (i.e., gross anatomy). This approach divides the nervous system into two basic sections, the **central nervous system (CNS)** and the **peripheral nervous system (PNS)** (FIGURE 2-10). At a basic level, the CNS is made up of the brain and spinal cord, and the PNS consists of the cranial and spinal nerves (FIGURE 2-11). These basic descriptions will be fleshed out in the following paragraphs.

The Central Nervous System

As mentioned previously, the CNS consists of the brain and spinal cord. Anatomically, the brain is made up of four structures: the brainstem, cerebellum,

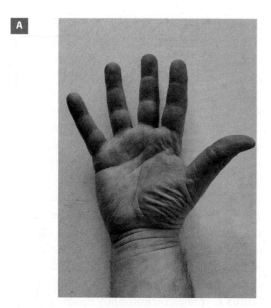
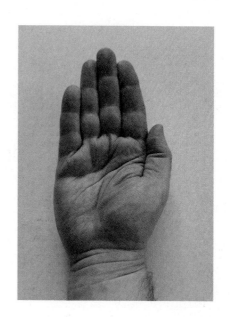

FIGURE 2-7 **A.** Abduct. **B.** Adduct.

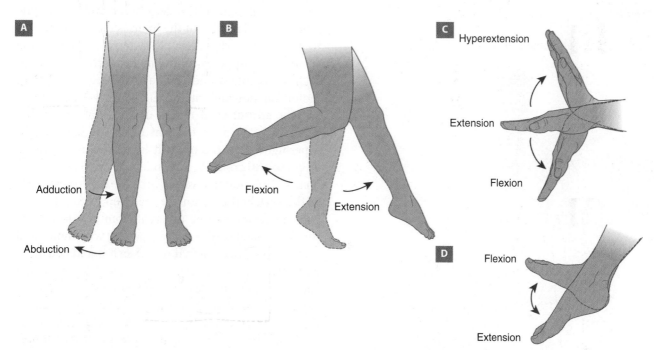

FIGURE 2-8 **A.** Adduction versus abduction. **B.** Flexion versus extension. **C.** Flexion versus extension with the hand. **D.** Flexion versus extension with the foot.

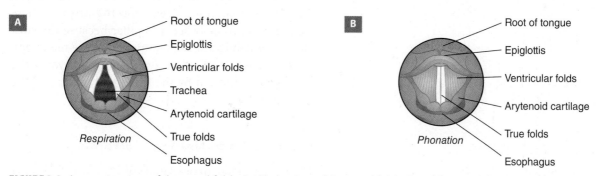

FIGURE 2-9 A superior view of the vocal folds. **A.** Abduction of the vocal folds. **B.** Adduction of the vocal folds.

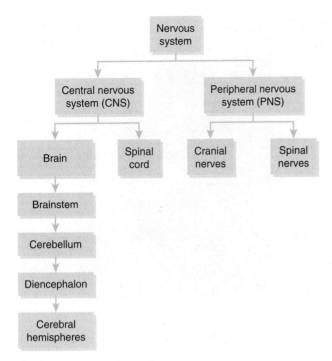

FIGURE 2-10 An anatomical approach.

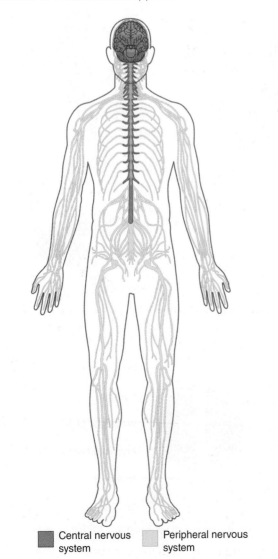

Central nervous system

Peripheral nervous system

FIGURE 2-11 The central and peripheral nervous systems.

diencephalon, and cerebral hemispheres (**FIGURE 2-12**). The **brainstem**, which consists of the medulla, pons, and midbrain, is continuous with the spinal cord and lies inferiorly to the cerebral hemispheres. (See, we are already using directional terms.) It controls many basic life functions and reflexes, including heartbeat and breathing. The brainstem also has many motor and sensory pathways that run between the brain and spinal cord. The **cerebellum**, which lies just posterior to the pons, is involved in the coordination and precision of fine motor movement. The thalamus, subthalamus, hypothalamus, and epithalamus make up the **diencephalon**, a term that will come up again in discussion of the developmental approach. The **thalamus** acts as a relay station for sensory fibers, the **subthalamus** regulates and coordinates motor function, the **hypothalamus** regulates various body functions (e.g., body temperature), and the **epithalamus** regulates genital development, the sleep–wake cycle, and optic reflexes. The last part of the brain is the two **cerebral hemispheres** with their characteristic grooves. The cerebral hemispheres control higher cortical functions such as cognition and language, as well as planning motor function and interpreting sensory experiences.

The **spinal cord** makes up the final part of the CNS, and it can be thought of as the information superhighway of the body. It is housed in the spinal or **vertebral column**, a cylinder of 32 to 34 bony segments. This number varies because the lowest parts of the vertebral column are made up of fused bones and this fusion can be different from person to person. The spinal cord is densely packed with motor and sensory fibers, and spinal nerves exit it and course to body structures, like muscles. Damage to the spinal cord can result in weakness or paralysis in different parts of the body depending on the level of damage. For example, damage to the cervical region (i.e., neck) can result in weakness or paralysis in all four limbs; damage lower in the lumbar region (i.e., lower back region) can impair only the legs.

Both the brain and spinal cord are wrapped in a three-layer membrane called the **meninges**. These membranes probably seem familiar because the condition **meningitis**, an inflammation of the meninges, is well known. The outermost meningeal layer is the dura mater, followed by the arachnoid mater and the pia mater.

The Peripheral Nervous System

The PNS is made up of 12 pairs of cranial and 31 pairs of spinal nerves. Most cranial nerves originate off the brainstem (except I and II) and transfer motor, sensory, special sensory, and parasympathetic

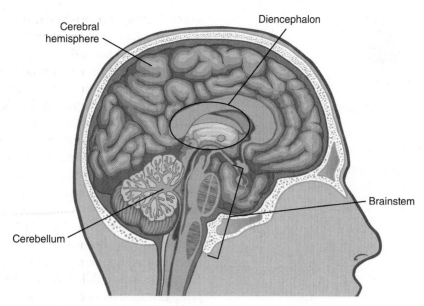

FIGURE 2-12 A sagittal section of the brain showing major brain structures.

© Oguz Aral/Shutterstock

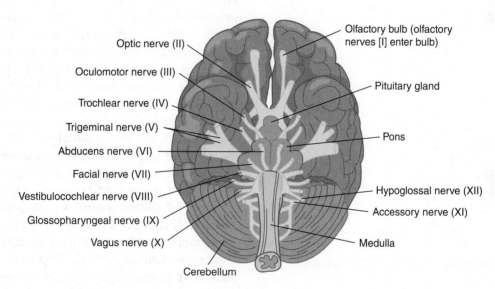

FIGURE 2-13 Ventral view of the brain and brainstem showing the 12 cranial nerves.

information back and forth between the brain and structures in the head and neck (**FIGURE 2-13**). Motor function involves information flowing from the brain to the muscles and other structures, leading to body movement and other functions. Sensory information, like temperature and touch, flows in the opposite direction, from the body to the brain. In addition to motor and sensory experiences, we also have special sensory experiences. Special senses have specialized organs devoted to them, and include vision, hearing, taste, and smell. Parasympathetic functions involve the regulation of organs and glands. Salivary glands are important parasympathetic structures in communication because they lubricate speech structures like the oral cavity and vocal cords.

In addition to our 12 cranial nerves, we have 31 pairs of spinal nerves that begin at the spinal cord and course out to the rest of the body (**FIGURE 2-14**). They are organized into different levels as follows: 8 cervical, 12 thoracic, 5 lumbar, 5 sacral, and 1 coccygeal. They send motor information from the brain to the body's muscles and sensory information from the body back to the brain. Reflexes are also mediated along both cranial and spinal nerves.

A Functional Approach

Using a functional approach, two major nervous system divisions are made: the sensory (or afferent) system and the motor (or efferent) system (**FIGURE 2-15**). The sensory system can be further broken down into the

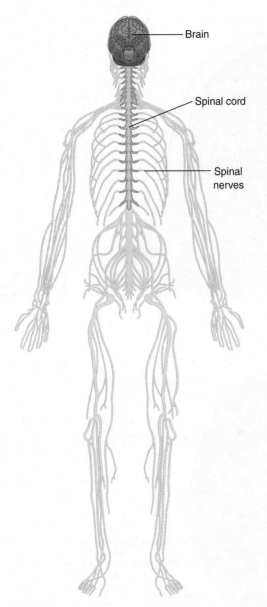

Brain

Spinal cord

Spinal nerves

FIGURE 2-14 Spinal nerves in relation to the brain and spinal cord.

somatosensory and the visceral sensory systems. The somatosensory system involves general sense information such as touch, pain, pressure, vibration, temperature, and proprioception in the skin and muscles as well as special senses like hearing, vision, and equilibrium. The **visceral sensory system** entails general sensory information like stretch, pain, temperature, and irritation in the internal organs, as well as sensations like nausea and hunger. It also conveys the special senses of taste and smell.

Like the sensory system, the motor system has two major divisions, the autonomic nervous system and the somatic nervous system. The **autonomic nervous system** involves body functions that happen automatically and without conscious control. There are three main divisions of this system—the sympathetic, parasympathetic, and enteric systems. The **sympathetic nervous system** (FIGURE 2-16) triggers what is known as our "fight-or-flight" response. For example, if you were out for a walk and stumbled across a rattlesnake, you would probably want to flee without thinking about it. How does the sympathetic nervous system achieve this survival response? It excites the body for action by increasing heart rate, blood pressure, and adrenaline. The **parasympathetic nervous system** (FIGURE 2-17) complements the sympathetic nervous system by doing the opposite. It is sometimes referred to as the "rest-and-digest" system. It calms and relaxes the body through slowing the heart and lowering blood pressure. The final part of the autonomic nervous system is the **enteric nervous system**, which manages the gastrointestinal system. Some neuroscientists have called this system a second brain because it can function independently of the brain. Normally it does communicate with the CNS through the sympathetic and parasympathetic nervous systems via the

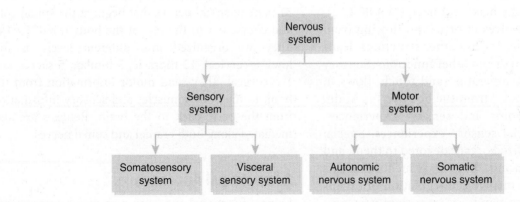

FIGURE 2-15 A functional approach.

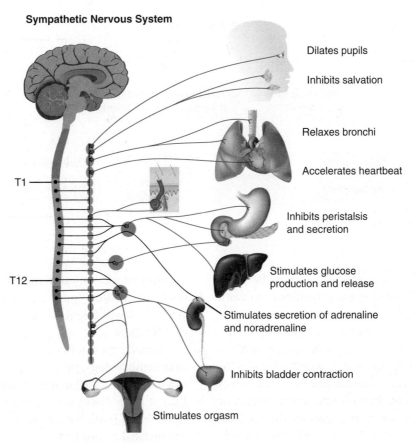

FIGURE 2-16 The sympathetic ("fight or flight") nervous system.
© Alila Sao Mai/Shutterstock.

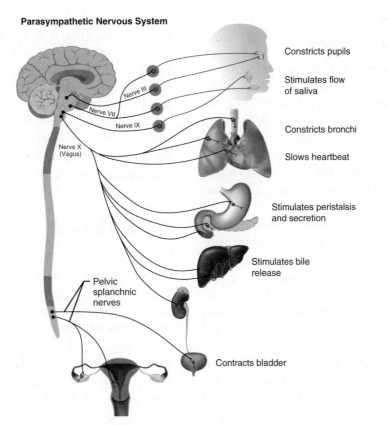

FIGURE 2-17 The parasympathetic ("rest and digest") nervous system.
© Alila Sao Mai/Shutterstock.

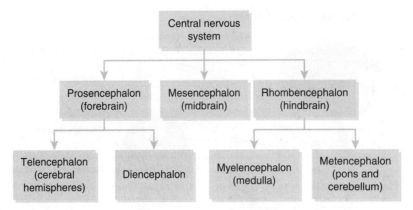

FIGURE 2-18 A developmental approach.

vagus nerve, but when connections between the vagus nerve and the CNS are severed, it continues to work (Li & Owyang, 2003).

In contrast to the autonomic nervous system, the **somatic nervous system** is a voluntary, conscious system that coordinates the body's skeletal muscles for movement. The 12 cranial nerves and 31 spinal nerves are part of this system. In addition, interneurons, or association neurons, are also a part of this system. These small neurons typically play an inhibitory role in motor function at the local level. In other words, they influence the functioning of other neurons called motor neurons.

A Developmental Approach

The developmental approach is focused more on the CNS, specifically the organization of the brain, rather than the nervous system as a whole (**FIGURE 2-18**). The names involved in this approach are Greek in nature and come from embryonic development. The Greek name for the CNS is encephalon (Greek *enkephalos*), which literally means "within the head." When a prefix is added, you have a reference to a certain nervous system structure.

During the fourth week of fetal development, the prosencephalon (*pros-* = "in the front"), **mesencephalon** (*mes-* = "in the middle"), and rhombencephalon (*rhomb-* = "diamond shaped") develop out of a precursor structure, the neural tube. These three structures can also be called the forebrain, midbrain, and hindbrain, respectively. The cerebral hemispheres and the diencephalon (*dia-* = through; thalamic structures) will begin to develop out of the **prosencephalon**, or forebrain. The mesencephalon will develop into the midbrain, and the rhombencephalon will

develop into the **myelencephalon** (medulla) and the **metencephalon** (pons and cerebellum). All of these structures will begin to emerge in the fifth week of development.

Usually these terms are used only in the context of neuroembryology, but *diencephalon* has been retained as a more general term referring to thalamic structures. Except for a discussion of neurological development, these terms (with the exception of diencephalon) will not be used in this text.

The Approach of This Text

This text mainly follows the anatomical approach for two reasons. First, it is the simplest and most concrete method of the three presented. It is a "what you see is what you get" approach. Second, the anatomical approach does not necessitate the use of as many unfamiliar Greek terms (e.g., rhombencephalon) with the exception of *diencephalon*. Using the anatomical approach, this text will move from bottom to top, from the spinal cord to brainstem, from the cerebellum to the diencephalon, and finally to the cerebral hemispheres.

▶ Conclusion

The organization of the nervous system was surveyed in this chapter, as well as various anatomical terms useful for navigating this system. Navigation around nervous system structures is aided by the concepts of anatomical position, anatomical versus clinical orientation, body sections, directional terms, and muscle actions. In the organization of the nervous system, anatomical, functional, and developmental approaches were briefly reviewed.

SUMMARY OF LEARNING OBJECTIVES

The following were the main learning objectives of this chapter. The information that should have been learned is below each learning objective.

1. The learner will be able to list and define anatomical orientation terms to navigate nervous system structures.
   - *Sagittal plane:* a section or plane that cuts the body or a specific anatomical structure into left and right portions
   - *Coronal plane:* a section or plane that cuts the body or a specific anatomical structure into front and back portions
   - *Transverse plane:* a section or plane that cuts the body or a specific anatomical structure into top and bottom portions
   - *Superior (cranial):* toward the head or from a high position
   - *Inferior (caudal):* toward the feet or from a low position
   - *Anterior (ventral):* toward the belly
   - *Posterior (dorsal):* toward the back
   - *Medial:* toward the midline of the body
   - *Lateral:* away from the midline of the body
   - *Proximal:* the point nearest a limb's attachment
   - *Distal:* the point farthest from a limb's attachment
   - *Peripheral:* toward the outer surface
   - *Central:* toward the center
   - *Ipsilateral:* same sided
   - *Contralateral:* opposite sided
   - *Adduct:* bringing structures together
   - *Abduct:* moving structures apart
   - *Flexion:* bending of a joint
   - *Extension:* straightening of a joint
   - *Supine:* lying on the back
   - *Pronate:* lying on the belly

2. The learner will list and briefly describe the three approaches to organizing the nervous system.
   - *Anatomical approach:* Focuses on those structures that can be seen with the human eye and divides the nervous system into two basic divisions, the central nervous system (CNS) and the peripheral nervous system (PNS).
   - *Functional approach:* Focuses on two major nervous system divisions—the sensory (or afferent) system and the motor (or efferent) system.
   - *Developmental approach:* Focuses on neurological development of the embryo, fetus, and newborn.

KEY TERMS

Abduct
Adduct
Anatomical position
Anterior
Autonomic nervous system
Brainstem
Caudal
Central
Central nervous system (CNS)
Cerebellum
Cerebral hemispheres
Contralateral
Coronal
Decussation
Diencephalon
Distal
Dorsal
Enteric nervous system

Epithalamus
Extension
Flexion
Hypothalamus
Inferior
Ipsilateral
Lateral
Medial
Meninges
Meningitis
Mesencephalon
Metencephalon
Midsagittal
Myelencephalon
Parasagittal
Parasympathetic nervous system
Peripheral

Peripheral nervous system (PNS)
Posterior
Pronate
Prosencephalon
Proximal
Sagittal
Somatic nervous system
Spinal cord
Subthalamus
Superior
Supine
Sympathetic nervous system
Thalamus
Transverse
Ventral
Vertebral column
Visceral sensory system

DRAW IT TO KNOW IT

1. Draw a picture of a man or woman and label the following: coronal, transverse, sagittal, superior, inferior, anterior, posterior, lateral, medial, proximal, and distal.

2. Draw a simple picture of the brain (FIGURE 2-19) and label the following: coronal, transverse, sagittal, dorsal, ventral, caudal, and rostral.

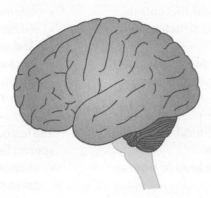

FIGURE 2-19 Simple drawing of the brain.

QUESTIONS FOR DEEPER REFLECTION

1. Explain why learning anatomical orientation terms is so important to neuroanatomy.

2. What approach to organizing the nervous system is most appealing? Why?

CASE STUDY

A speech-pathology graduate student has just begun the first day of her hospital externship. While doing rounds with the lead speech-language pathologist and the neurologist, the neurologist showed an MRI of a patient demonstrating a cerebral vascular accident (CVA) in the left frontal lobe. This student thought the neurologist had made a mistake because the area she had shown was clearly on the right side of the MRI image. Explain why there is confusion reading this MRI.

SUGGESTED PROJECTS

1. Make a *Jeopardy*-type game with the various navigational terms presented in this chapter. Create categories (directional terms, muscle actions, etc.) and cards with descriptions like in Table 2-3. Students then pick a category, and a card with a description is read from that category. The student responds with "What is _____."

2. As a class or in groups, have students play charades with the various navigational terms presented in the chapter.

REFERENCES

Allman, W. F. (1990). *Apprentices of wonder: Inside the neural network revolution.* New York, NY: Bantam Books.

Li, Y., & Owyang, C. (2003). Musings on the wanderer: What's new in our understanding of vago-vagal reflexes? V. Remodeling of vagus and enteric neural circuitry after vagal injury. *American Journal of Physiology–Gastrointestinal and Liver Physiology, 285*(3), G461–G469.

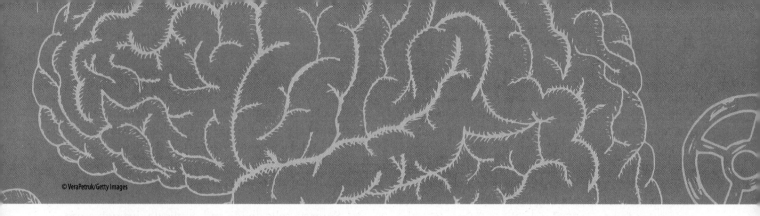

CHAPTER 3

Development of the Nervous System

CHAPTER PREVIEW

How did we get the complex nervous system that we have? This chapter will try to answer this question by exploring the development of the brain from the early weeks of development after fertilization through adolescence to old age. This process is complex, and we will find that when it does not go as planned, the result can be a neurodevelopmental disorder.

IN THIS CHAPTER

In this chapter, we will …

- Define neuroembryonic terms
- Briefly describe the development of the nervous system
- Describe common birth defects
- Discuss the development of the child's and adolescent's brain
- Survey how the neurological system changes with aging

LEARNING OBJECTIVES

1. The learner will define important neuroembryonic terms.
2. The learner will list and briefly describe the structural development of the nervous system from conception to old age.
3. The learner will list and describe common birth defects.

▶ Introduction

A human being begins as a single fertilized egg and develops into the complex organism we see walking around every day. Usually, this developmental process occurs without error, but about 3% of babies (1 in 33) born in the United States have a birth defect. These defects are the leading cause of death in babies, accounting for about 20% of deaths in infants (Centers for Disease Control and Prevention, 2018). In this chapter, we will survey the neurological development of babies, children, adolescents, and adults and will discuss some common birth defects.

▶ Genes, Chromosomes, and Cells

Genes reside on chromosomes, and chromosomes reside in the nucleus of a cell. Human somatic cells are diploid, meaning they have pairs of chromosomes. (*Somatic* comes from the Greek word *soma*, which means "body.") Overall, there are 23 pairs of chromosomes in humans, 46 individual chromosomes in all. Each person's unique collection of chromosomes is called a karyotype (**FIGURE 3-1**). Of these

46 chromosomes, 44 are autosomes (or nonsex chromosomes) and 2 are sex chromosomes, either XX (female) or XY (male). In contrast, sex cells or gametes (either an egg or a sperm) are haploid, meaning they have 23 total chromosomes. A female gamete, or egg, carries only the X sex chromosome, whereas the male gamete, or sperm, can carry either the X or the Y sex chromosome.

Somatic cells divide and duplicate through a process known as mitosis (**FIGURE 3-2**). In this four-stage process, a mother cell divides and forms two genetically identical daughter cells, each of which has 46 total chromosomes like the mother cell. In comparison, gametes are created through a different process, called meiosis. In this process, cell division occurs twice instead of once like in mitosis. The result of this double division process is four gametes (eggs or sperm); each gamete has 23 total chromosomes. When an egg (23 chromosomes) is fertilized by a sperm (23 chromosomes), a zygote is formed, which is diploid (46 total chromosomes). This zygote will then undergo mitosis and develop into a morula and then into an embryo and finally into a fetus.

Errors can occur during mitosis. One possible error is a whole chromosome deletion, known as monosomy. One example of this error is Turner

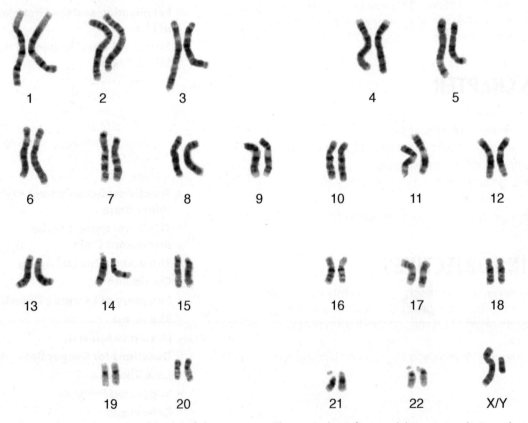

FIGURE 3-1 A karyotype is a person's collection of chromosomes. The term also refers to a laboratory technique that produces an image of a person's chromosomes. The karyotype is used to look for abnormal numbers or structures of chromosomes.

Chromosome distribution during mitosis and meiosis

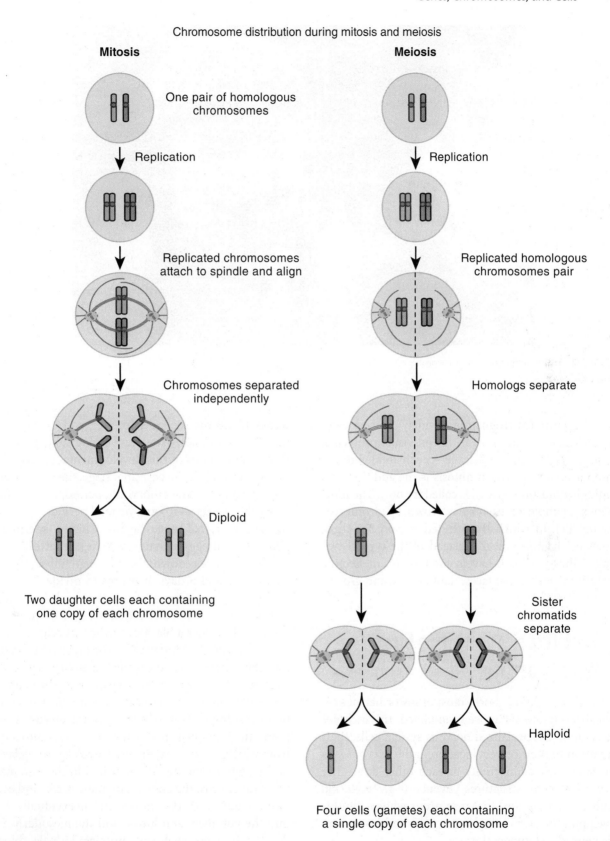

FIGURE 3-2 Comparison of mitosis and meiosis.

syndrome, in which a female has only one sex chromosome, an X. People with this disorder who survive birth have a small stature and a webbed neck and are unable to reproduce. Sometimes deletions do not involve whole chromosomes, but rather partial chromosome deletion like in cri du chat syndrome. In this condition, children have a weak cat-like cry, small head (microcephaly), high palate, round face, small

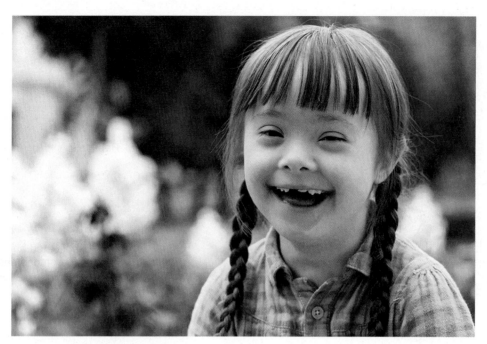

FIGURE 3-3 A girl with Down syndrome.
© DenKuvaiev/Getty Images.

receding chin (micrognathia), widely spaced eyes, low muscle tone, minor hearing and visual problems, mental retardation, and delayed speech and language. Another possible error in mitosis is the addition of a whole chromosome, which is called trisomy. The most famous example of trisomy is Down syndrome (or trisomy 21), in which the affected person has three copies of chromosome 21 instead of the typical two copies. These children have some level of intellectual disability as well as flat faces, slanted eyes, and growth failure (**FIGURE 3-3**).

▶ Fertilization and the First Weeks of Life

By the time a child is born, most of his or her neurological development has been completed. This includes the creation of specialized nervous system cells, their migration to their correct location in the nervous system, and their connectivity to each other and other nervous system structures. Events (e.g., maternal alcohol consumption) that may occur while a child is developing in utero may have a profound impact on this neurodevelopmental process (**TABLE 3-1**).

Pregnancy is often talked about in terms of menstrual or gestational age (GA), which begins at the date of a woman's last menstrual period. GA is dated this way because it is difficult to discern when fertilization has occurred. GA is conceptualized in terms of trimesters, with the first 12 weeks being the first trimester,

weeks 13–28 the second trimester, and weeks 29–40 the third trimester. However, biologically, there are three main phases of this developmental process. The first week is called the germinal stage, the next 7 weeks of pregnancy are the embryonic period, and the final 32 weeks (weeks 9–40) are the fetal period.

The germinal stage begins when a sperm cell penetrates an egg or ovum cell. As the fertilized cell or zygote travels down the fallopian tube over the course of about 5 days, it begins to divide. This process is known as cleavage, and the result is a ball of cells known as a morula. When the morula enters the uterus, it becomes a blastocyst when its cells differentiate into outer and inner cells. The outer cells develop into the support structures for the embryo (placenta, etc.), and the inner cells develop into the embryo. The embryonic stage officially commences once the blastocyst implants into the wall of the uterus. At this point, the inner cells rearrange themselves into a disc from which the embryo forms. Three beginning layers of the embryo can be distinguished in the disc made up of inner cells: the endoderm, mesoderm, and ectoderm (**FIGURE 3-4**). The endoderm will eventually form into the gut, liver, and lungs, and the mesoderm will develop into the skeleton, muscles, kidneys, blood, and heart. The **ectoderm**, which will be the focus of what follows, turns into the skin and nervous system (Howard Hughes Medical Institute, 2014).

du Plessis (2013) gives a helpful framing to the structural development of the central nervous system. She includes the following six phases: dorsal

TABLE 3-1 Timetable of Major Neurodevelopmental Events

Neurodevelopmental Event	Peak Activity (Gestational Age)	Example Abnormalities
Dorsal Induction		
Neural tube formation	3–4 weeks	Spina bifida, encephaloceles
Caudal eminence development	4–7 weeks	Caudal regression syndromes
Ventral Induction		
Prosencephalic development	2–3 months	
Cleavage		Holoprosencephaly
Midline formation		Agenesis of the corpus callosum
Neural proliferation	3–4 months	Microcephaly
Neuronal migration	3–5 months	Schizencephaly, lissencephaly
Cortical organization	5 months to years postnatal	Polymicrogyria
Myelination	Birth to years postnatal	Hypomyelination
Cerebellar and Brainstem Development	2 months to postnatal	(Ponto) cerebellar hypoplasia; Joubert syndrome; Dandy-Walker malformation

Data from: du Plessis, A. J. (2013). Fetal development. In M. L. Batshaw, N. J. Roizen, & G. R. Lotrecchiano (Eds.), *Children with disabilities* (7th ed., pp. 25–35). Baltimore, MD: Paul H. Brookes Publishing Company.

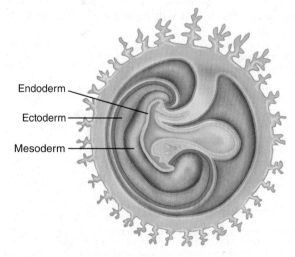

FIGURE 3-4 Layers of the embryo.

Endoderm

Ectoderm

Mesoderm

induction, ventral induction, neural proliferation, neuronal migration, cortical organization and synapse formation, and myelination. These phases do not occur in a strict sequential manner, but rather overlap each other.

▶ Structural Development of the Infant Brain

Dorsal Induction (GA: 3–7 Weeks)

Dorsal induction is a neurodevelopmental period in which the neural tube is formed. At around the third week of development, the dorsal ectoderm thickens to form the **neural plate**. By the fourth week of development, this plate bends and wraps around itself to form a tube (i.e., the **neural tube**) from which the brain and spinal cord will develop (**FIGURE 3-5**). The process of forming the neural tube is called **neurulation**. Both ends of the neural tube are initially open (openings are called **neuropores**) but close at around 6 weeks' GA (du Plessis, 2013).

The dorsal induction phase is a critical period of neurological development for the embryo (**FIGURE 3-6**). During this phase, the embryo is susceptible to what are called **neural tube defects (NTDs)**, which involve failure of the neuropores to close properly. This defect can happen to either the anterior neuropore or posterior neuropore. The three major types of NTDs are encephalocele, anencephaly, and spina bifida.

Failure in anterior neuropore closure can result in encephalocele or anencephaly. **Encephalocele** is a

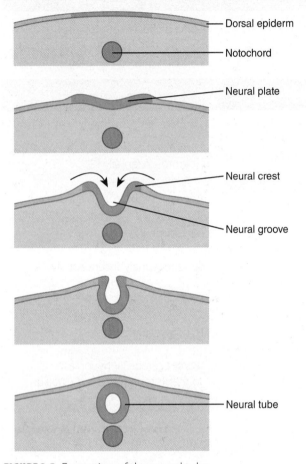

FIGURE 3-5 Formation of the neural tube.

rare malformation of the skull in which a malformed portion of the brain, usually the occipital lobe, protrudes from the skull in a sac (**FIGURE 3-7**). Children with this condition typically have hydrocephalus (i.e., excessive fluid in the brain), intellectual disability, craniofacial abnormalities, and motor issues such as ataxia (Liptak, 2013). Treatment involves surgery to remove the sac and place the protruding brain tissue back into the skull. Craniofacial abnormalities will also be corrected, and a shunt may be placed to reduce hydrocephalus. The prognosis for these children varies depending on a number of factors (National Institute of Neurological Disorders and Stroke [NINDS], 2018b). A better prognosis is associated with no hydrocephalus, frontal encephalocele rather than posterior, and minimal brain tissue in the sac (Liptak, 2013).

Anencephaly is a more severe NTD in which neurological development ceases at the brainstem, leaving the infant without cerebral hemispheres and thus without higher cortical functions (**FIGURE 3-8**). Half of these children are naturally aborted, and the other half die shortly after birth. Anencephaly occurs 2 to 3 times per 1,000 live births. There is no treatment for the condition (Kemp, Burns, & Brown, 2008; Liptak, 2013; NINDS, 2018a).

When an NTD affects the posterior neuropore, the result is one of the more well-known NTDs—**spina bifida (SB)** (**FIGURE 3-9**). SB occurs in both severe and less severe forms (**FIGURE 3-10**). The most severe form is called *myelomeningocele*, in which the spinal cord, spinal fluid, and meninges protrude from the spine. The infant will have a large cyst on his or

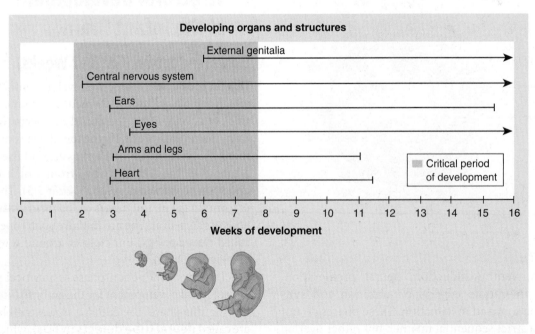

FIGURE 3-6 Embryonic development showing the critical period of development. During the embryonic stage—week 2 through week 8—all the major organ systems are forming. During this critical period of development, the embryo is highly vulnerable.

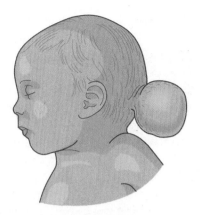

FIGURE 3-7 Encephalocele.

Courtesy of Centers for Disease Control and Prevention, National Center on Birth Defects and Developmental Disabilities.

her back that is reddish in color. The next type, which is less severe, is *meningocele*, in which the same cyst is present, but the spinal cord is intact and not wrapped inside the cyst. The final, and mildest, form is *occulta*, in which vertebrae are malformed. The infant will have a depression in his or her back, often with a tuft of hair on and around it (Kemp, Burns, & Brown 2008; NINDS, 2018g). Children with SB occulta are often asymptomatic, but children with SB myelomeningocele and meningocele may have motor and sensory issues, especially with the lower extremities. They may also have bowel and bladder incontinence (Kemp, Burns, & Brown 2008). Children with SB myelomeningocele sometimes have learning disabilities due to disruptions in neuron migration (Liptak, 2013).

Ventral Induction (GA: 2–3 Months)

Ventral induction is a neurodevelopmental period when the face and brain develop out of the superior end of the neural tube. After the neural tube closes, it will

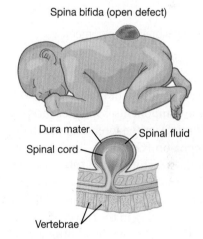

FIGURE 3-9 Spina bifida.

Courtesy of Centers for Disease Control and Prevention, National Center on Birth Defects and Developmental Disabilities.

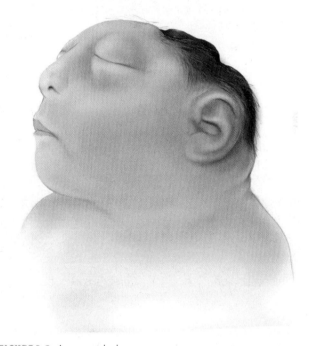

FIGURE 3-8 Anencephaly.

Courtesy of Centers for Disease Control and Prevention, National Center on Birth Defects and Developmental Disabilities.

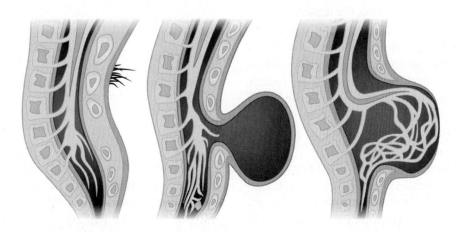

Spina bifida occulta   Meningocele   Myelomeningocele

FIGURE 3-10 Forms of spina bifida.

Courtesy of Centers for Disease Control and Prevention, National Center on Birth Defects and Developmental Disabilities.

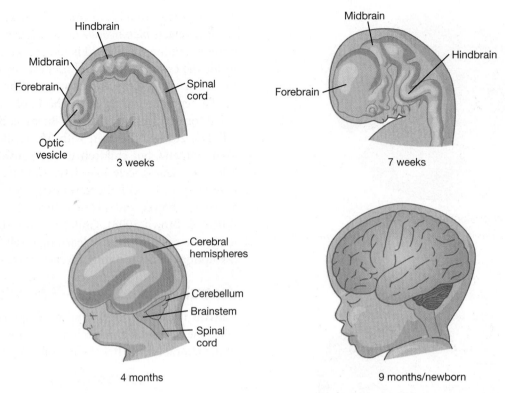

FIGURE 3-11 Fetal brain development.

bend ventrally, and the superior end goes on to form the major components of the brain (**FIGURE 3-11**). The first of these components is the prosencephalon (*Greek for "front brain"),* or the forebrain, which develops into the diencephalon (Greek for "back part of the front"; i.e., thalamic structures) and **telencephalon** (Greek for "front part of the front") or cerebral hemispheres. During ventral induction, cleavage of the prosencephalon occurs, resulting in the two cerebral hemispheres, a left one and a right one. In addition, midline formation occurs in what is called the corpus callosum. The corpus callosum is a band of fibers that connects the two cerebral hemispheres and allows them to communicate with each other. Second, the mesencephalon (Greek for "middle") becomes the midbrain. Third, the **rhombencephalon** (Greek for "diamond shape"), or hindbrain, develops into the myelencephalon (Greek for "the back of the back"; i.e., the medulla). Fourth, the metencephalon (Greek for "the front of the back") develops into the pons and cerebellum. A summary of these structures and what nervous system structures they turn into is found in **TABLE 3-2**.

These Greek terms are used by some neuroscientists as an organizational system for the central nervous system, but most of these terms have fallen out of use, except in neurodevelopmental contexts. In organizational systems based on gross or functional anatomy, the only term that is still typically used is diencephalon.

TABLE 3-2 Developmental Divisions and Mature Nervous System Structures

Division	Components
Telencephalon	Cerebral cortex, basal ganglia, olfactory bulbs
Diencephalon	Thalamus, hypothalamus, epithalamus, subthalamus
Mesencephalon	Midbrain
Metencephalon	Pons, cerebellum
Myelencephalon	Medulla

Data from: Spence, S. A. (2009). *The actor's brain: Exploring the cognitive neuroscience of free will.* Oxford, UK: Oxford University Press, p. 157.

One condition involving errors in ventral induction is noteworthy. **Holoprosencephaly** is a failure in brain cleavage (**FIGURE 3-12**). The condition is rare, occurring in 1 in every 30,000 births. There are three forms of the disorder. *Alobar holoprosencephaly* involves no cleavage at all, leaving the infant with no hemispheric development. In other words, the brain is

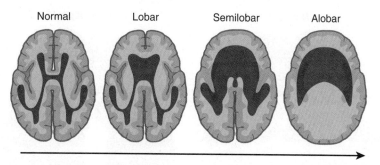

Normal   Lobar   Semilobar   Alobar

FIGURE 3-12 Different degrees of holoprosencephaly.
© University of Florida Department of Pediatrics.

just one mass with no hemispheric divisions or corpus callosum. Children also have craniofacial abnormalities, like cyclopia (having only one eye) or cleft lip. *Semilobar holoprosencephaly* is a milder form involving some development of the longitudinal fissure that divides the left and right hemispheres. Like the alobar form, the corpus callosum is absent. *In lobar holoprosencephaly*, the least severe form, the infant's brain looks nearly normal; however, there are some abnormal connections between the hemispheres and abnormal development of the corpus callosum (Kemp, Burns, & Brown 2008; NINDS, 2018c).

Neural Proliferation (GA: 3–4 Months)

Neurogenesis means the birth of new neurons; this process is at the heart of the neural proliferation stage. Not only neurons proliferate but also glial cells. These cells will eventually form the gray and white matter of the cerebral hemispheres. They are initially born out of the spinal cord and brainstem, but later the whole periventricular area (i.e., the area around the future brain ventricles) is involved in their production. The dorsal part of this area, which will be important for cognition, becomes filled with excitatory neurons. These neurons use the neurotransmitter glutamate; the ventral area develops interneurons (neurons that connect neurons together) that use the inhibiting neurotransmitter gamma-aminobutyric acid (GABA). Interneurons are initially excitatory but later take on an inhibitory role (du Plessis, 2013).

In this stage, if something happens that affects the normal proliferation of nervous system cells, the brain's mass will be abnormally small because it lacks the correct number of these cells (**FIGURE 3-13**). This condition is known as **microcephaly**, and it is most often caused by viruses or alcohol exposure (du Plessis, 2013). The effects of microcephaly vary from child to child. Some have normal intelligence, whereas others have intellectual disability as well as motor and sensory issues. Speech issues are common in those with the more severe form (NINDS, 2018e).

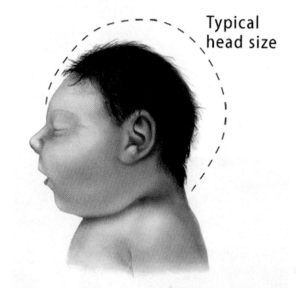

Typical head size

FIGURE 3-13 A baby with microcephaly.
© Centers for Disease Control and Prevention.

Neuronal Migration (GA: 3–5 Months)

After the proliferation of nervous system cells, these cells begin to migrate in waves from the inside of the brain where they were produced to the outer layers of the brain. A chemical called *reelin* signals these cells as to where they should stop in this migration. Eventually, by about a GA of 20 weeks, the migration ends and the six layers of the cerebral cortex are established. During the migratory process, some cells cluster together to form hills in the brain (gyri) while others form valleys (sulci), giving the brain its characteristic bumpy appearance. It is also during this period that the four lobes of the brain develop as well as their specific functions (e.g., occipital lobe and vision).

Two conditions associated with abnormal neuronal migration are schizencephaly (**FIGURE 3-14**) and lissencephaly (**FIGURE 3-15**). **Schizencephaly** is a rare condition characterized by abnormal openings or clefts in the cerebral hemispheres. These clefts are places where neurons failed to migrate. They can be bilateral, affecting both cerebral hemispheres, or

Normal   Schizencephaly

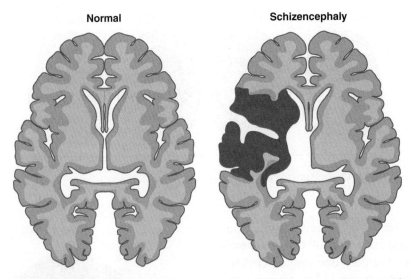

FIGURE 3-14 Transverse section of the brain showing schizencephaly. The darkened area (image on the right) illustrates where brain tissue would be missing resulting in a cleft.

© University of Florida Department of Pediatrics

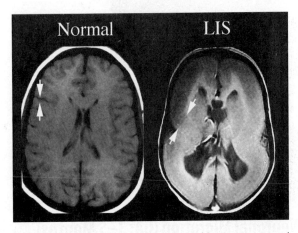

FIGURE 3-15 Neuroimaging of a normal brain compared to a lissencephalic brain. The lissencephalic brain is missing the folds of cortical tissue normally seen in the brain.

Courtesy of Dr. Joseph G. Gleeson, The Rockefeller University.

unilateral, affecting only one. The issues associated with the condition will be more severe in the bilateral form versus the unilateral form. Possible issues include speech and language problems, developmental delays, and intellectual disability (NINDS, 2018f). **Lissencephaly** is caused by a lack of reelin, resulting in the brain having a smooth appearance, absent of its characteristic hills and valleys (gyri and sulci) (du Plessis, 2013; Kemp, Burns, & Brown, 2008). Symptoms of this condition include intellectual disability, seizures, and failure to thrive (NINDS, 2018d). Supportive care is the only form of treatment for schizencephaly and lissencephaly.

Cortical Organization and Synapse Formation (GA: 5 Months to Years Postnatal)

Once neurons form and migrate to their intended location in the central nervous system, they begin to sprout projections called dendrites and axons. These projections begin to form connections (i.e., synapses) between neurons, leading to the saying, "Neurons that fire together, wire together; those that don't, won't." This process is known as **synaptogenesis**. Once these connections are made, the neurons begin to communicate with each other. At first there are more connections than are needed. A process called **synaptic pruning** will take place later and last into the teen years (and perhaps the whole life span), during which these extra connections are eliminated.

One condition associated with errors in cortical organization is **polymicrogyria**, a condition in which children have too many folds (gyri) in the cerebral hemispheres (Kemp, Burns, & Brown 2008). This can occur in one hemisphere or both or just in one focal hemispheric area. When the condition affects a small part of the brain, the symptoms are mild, with the most common symptom being seizures. The more extensive the polymicrogyria is, the more severe the symptoms are. These symptoms can include epilepsy, developmental delay, intellectual disability, and speech and swallowing problems (National Institutes of Health [NIH], 2009b).

Myelination (GA: Birth to Years Postnatal)

Myelin is a white, fatty substance produced by specialized glial cells called oligodendroglia. This substance coats axons to speed up the transmission of electrical impulses. The myelination process begins at a GA of about 6 months, but only up through the spinal cord and brainstem. The process will continue into the cerebral hemispheres and reach its peak during the first year of postnatal life. This first year of postnatal life is when infants gain greater control of their body and progress from lifting their heads to rolling to crawling and eventually begin to stand and walk. This maturing motor control is due to greater myelination. The myelination process continues into the adult years.

Some children suffer from a recessive genetic disorder called **hypomyelination**. In this condition, children have a reduced ability to produce myelin. Developmentally, these children are normal up to about 1 year of age, but then development slows. As they continue to age, they experience paresis, muscle atrophy, neuropathy, cataracts, dysarthria, and mild to moderate intellectual disability (NIH, 2009a).

▶ Functional Development of the Infant Brain

Ultrasound technology has provided a window into prenatal development, allowing detailed observations of fetal behavior over the course of pregnancy. Fetal movements involving flexion and extension of the trunk begin in the first trimester (0–12 weeks) at around 10 to 12 weeks of gestation. Reflexes, such as the startle reflex, begin to be evident as early as 10 weeks. At 12 weeks, the fetus displays isolated movements of the head and limbs. Head movements include head rotation and flexion. Facial behaviors such as eye blinking, mouthing, yawning, tongue protrusion, smiling, grimacing, sucking, swallowing, and hiccupping emerge in the second trimester (13–28 weeks). Head behaviors (e.g., rotation) become more frequent as well as moving the hands to the head, mouth, eye, face, and ear. The frequency of these second trimester movements becomes more numerous in the third trimester (29–40 weeks). At 36 weeks, these movements become more highly coordinated (Du Plessis, 2013; Kurjak et al., 2005).

As can be seen, the structural growth of the nervous system corresponds to the functional developmental of the fetus. Neuron proliferation, migration, and organization lead to greater connections between the brain and the body and thus more coordinated movements of the head, trunk, and limbs.

▶ The Development of the Adolescent Brain

The beginning of adolescence is marked by the beginning puberty, which typically begins at 10 to 11 years of age in girls and 11 to 12 years in boys. Parents often note this change from childhood to adolescence through a change of behavior. For example, a family friend reported the following regarding her teenage daughter: "She gets mad really easily. I wonder if it's because she stays up so late and sleeps so long in the morning. The warm, funny, affectionate child I knew seems to be gone, replaced by a moody stranger." Though this change is shocking for parents, those familiar with neurodevelopment at this age will say that this behavior is typical for adolescence. For the teen in this example, her body as well as her brain are changing, and much of the moody behavior is tied to these changes. The good news for parents is that it will get better as the teen moves through adolescence and enters adulthood.

Adolescence is a period of profound brain development. Previously it was thought that brain development was complete by adolescence, but now we know that this development is not complete until about the age of 25 years. What is the nature of this profound brain development? Synapses are overproduced until just before puberty and then are pruned in adolescence, which increases the responsiveness of neural networks. In addition, gray matter thins as these excess synaptic connections that are not used are eliminated. During this pruning process, the brain is not functioning optimally, and adolescents will typically struggle with tracking multiple thoughts and focusing their attention. Overall, this brain development through synaptic pruning begins in the back of the brain and moves forward to the front of the brain to the prefrontal cortex (**FIGURE 3-16**). We know that the prefrontal cortex is crucial for three main functions: restraint, organization, and initiative—three functions with which teens struggle. If teens are not relying fully on their prefrontal cortex, then the question is, what are they relying on? The answer would be their emotional processing system (i.e., amygdala), which explains why teens react emotionally and misinterpret emotional cues from others (Giedd, 2004; Powell, 2006).

All of this discussion leads to the conclusion that (1) the adolescent brain is very plastic (i.e., malleable and changeable), and (2) an understanding of adolescent brain development helps to explain much of adolescent behavior. Adolescents rely more on their feelings and impulses rather than logic and planning because

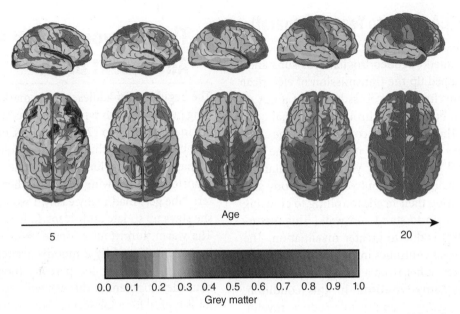

FIGURE 3-16 Back to front development of the adolescent brain. Red shows more gray matter, and blue shows less gray matter. Gray matter wanes as the brain matures and neurons are pruned. Areas for basic function mature early, higher executive functions later.

the prefrontal cortex has not fully developed. This leads to less-than-ideal planning and judgment and potentially to risky, impulsive behavior. Laurence Steinberg, a professor of psychology, summarizes the teen brain this way: "It's like turning on the engine of a car without a skilled driver at the wheel" (Wallis & Dell, 2004).

▶ The Brain in Normal Aging

In normal aging, the brain experiences both structural and chemical changes. Structurally, the brain loses neural circuits and, thus, loses plasticity. In addition, the cortex thins due to a decrease in both gray and white matter. Even neurons show structural change as dendrites thin and decrease in numbers. Chemically, there are decreases in neurotransmitter levels (e.g., glutamate, dopamine, serotonin) and a decrease in the number of receptor sites available for these chemical messengers. Behaviorally, these brain changes can be seen in older, healthy adults as deficits in some

memory skills (e.g., working memory), attention, learning, and language (Burda, 2011).

▶ Conclusion

The development of the nervous system is a complex process. About 3 weeks after fertilization, the neural tube develops. The superior end of the neural tube develops into the face and brain. As the brain develops, neurons proliferate and migrate to their proper spots in the nervous system. Synapses form as the cerebral cortex further organizes itself. Neuron axons are then myelinated, leading to more efficient neural firing, as shown by an infant's motor development. Synapses continue to be developed during childhood but are significantly pruned back during adolescence. As a person ages, the cerebral cortex thins due to a decrease in both gray and white matter. These changes, along with chemical changes in the brain, lead to the types of cognitive decline we see in normal, healthy aging.

SUMMARY OF LEARNING OBJECTIVES

The following were the main learning objectives of this chapter. The information that should have been learned is below each learning objective.

1. The learner will define important neuroembryonic terms.
    - *Gestational age (GA):* the age of a baby measured against the mother's last menstrual period

- *Germinal stage:* when an egg is fertilized by a sperm and becomes a morula
- *Morula:* an early stage of the embryo when it is a solid ball of cells

- *Neural tube:* a tube that forms from an embryo's ectoderm, which will become the nervous system
- *Neural tube defect (NTD):* a defect in the formation of the neural tube

2. The learner will list and briefly describe the structural development of the nervous system.
   - *Dorsal induction:* Occurs at a GA between 3 and 7 weeks and is when the neural tube is formed.
   - *Ventral induction:* Occurs at a GA between 2 and 3 months and is when the face and brain begin to develop.
   - *Neural proliferation:* Occurs at a GA between 3 and 4 months and is when nervous system cells are created.
   - *Neuronal migration:* Occurs at a GA between 3 and 5 months and is when nervous system cells begin to migrate in waves from the inside of the brain where they were produced to the outer layers of the brain.
   - *Cortical organization and synapse formation:* Occurs at a GA between 4 months and years postnatal and is when neurons sprout projections and make connections.
   - *Myelination:* Occurs between birth and years postnatal and is when axons receive their coating of myelin.

3. The learner will list and describe common birth defects.

- *Encephalocele:* a neural tube defect in which a malformed portion of the brain protrudes through the skull
- *Anencephaly:* a neural tube defect in which neurological development ceases with the development of the brainstem, leaving the infant without cerebral hemispheres
- *Spina bifida:* a neural tube defect that leaves a cyst on an infant's back, which sometimes has spinal cord fibers in it, leading to possible motor and sensory issues
- *Holoprosencephaly:* a condition in which the brain fails to cleave, leaving the infant with little to no hemispheric development
- *Microcephaly:* a failure in neuron proliferation, leaving an infant with a small brain and a small skull
- *Schizencephaly:* a condition that involves clefts in the cerebral hemispheres
- *Lissencephaly:* a condition in which the brain does not have its normal convolutions and appears smooth in appearance
- *Polymicrogyria:* a condition involving insufficient cortical organization, leaving infants with too many gyri in their cerebral hemispheres
- *Hypomyelination:* a genetic condition in which children do not produce enough myelin, leading to serious motor and sensory issues

KEY TERMS

Anencephaly
Dorsal induction
Ectoderm
Encephalocele
Holoprosencephaly
Hypomyelination
Lissencephaly
Microcephaly

Neural plate
Neural tube
Neural tube defects (NTDs)
Neurogenesis
Neuropores
Neurulation
Polymicrogyria
Rhombencephalon

Schizencephaly
Spina bifida (SB)
Synaptic pruning
Synaptogenesis
Telencephalon
Ventral induction

DRAW IT TO KNOW IT

1. Draw your own flowchart illustrating the processes of mitosis and meiosis.

2. Look at Figure 3-5 and draw the formation of the neural tube.

QUESTIONS FOR DEEPER REFLECTION

1. Compare and contrast the processes of mitosis and meiosis.
2. How are chromosomes different than genes?
3. Explain the six stages of nervous system development.

4. Given the six stages of nervous system development, discuss what disorders can occur in each stage.

CASE STUDY

Michelle is a pregnant mother just about at full term at almost 40 weeks. During a routine obstetrician visit, the physician measured around her belly and remarked, "This baby is small for being 37 weeks." Michelle responded that she is not 37 weeks pregnant, but rather almost 40 weeks pregnant. The obstetrician looked quickly at the medical chart, realized her error, and stated, "The baby shouldn't be this small at almost 40 weeks. We need to admit you to the hospital and induce labor." Labor was induced, and Michael was born weighing just 3 pounds, 7 ounces (1.7 kilograms).

It was observed at birth that Michael was missing fingers on his left hand, displayed webbing between his fingers and toes, and had microcephaly. Later, Michael was diagnosed with Cornelia de Lange syndrome (CdLS), a rare genetic condition caused by a sporadic gene mutation.

1. What is microcephaly?
2. At what stage of development does microcephaly occur?
3. How does microcephaly relate to neurogenesis?

SUGGESTED PROJECTS

1. Pick one of the developmental neurological disorders mentioned in this chapter and write a two- to three-page paper with the following: (a) a description of the disorder, (b) the cause, and (c) long-term effects.
2. Do further research on the adolescent brain and write a two- to three-page paper on your findings. In the paper, reflect on your own teenage years and how some of your behavior during those years might be explained by brain development.
3. Find a senior citizen (someone older than 65 years) and interview him or her about any changes he or she has noticed in cognition and/or language. Write a summary of the interview in a two-page paper.

REFERENCES

Burda, A. N. (2011). *Communication and swallowing changes in healthy aging adults.* Burlington, MA: Jones & Bartlett Learning.

Centers for Disease Control and Prevention (CDC). (2018). *Birth defects: Data and statistics.* Division of Birth Defects and Developmental Disabiliities, National Center on Birth Defects and Developmental Disabiliities. Retrieved from https://www.cdc.gov/ncbddd/birthdefects/data.html

du Plessis, A. J. (2013). Fetal development. In M. L. Batshaw, N. J. Roizen, & G. R. Lotrecchiano (Eds.), *Children with disabilities* (7th ed., pp. 25–35). Baltimore, MD: Paul H. Brookes Publishing Company.

Giedd, J. N. (2004). Structural magnetic resonance imaging of the adolescent brain. *Annals of the New York Academy of Sciences, 1021*(1), 77-85.

Howard Hughes Medical Institute. (2014). *Human embryonic development.* Retrieved from http://www.hhmi.org/biointeractive/human-embryonic-development

Kemp, W. L., Burns, D. K., & Brown, T. G. (2008). *Pathology: The big picture.* New York, NY: McGraw-Hill Medical.

Kurjak, A., Stanojevic, M., Andonotopo, W., Scazzocchio-Duenas, E., Azumendi, G., & Carrera, J. M. (2005). Fetal behavior assessed in all three trimesters of normal pregnancy by four-dimensional ultrasonography. *Croatian Medical Journal, 46*(5), 772–780.

Liptak, G. S. (2013). Neural tube defects. In M. L. Batshaw, N. J. Roizen, & G. R. Lotrecchiano (Eds.), *Children with disabilities* (7th ed., pp. 451–472). Baltimore, MD: Paul H. Brookes Publishing Company.

National Institute of Neurological Disorders and Stroke (NINDS). (2018a). *Anencephaly information page.* Retrieved from https://www.ninds.nih.gov/disorders/all-disorders/anencephaly-information-page

National Institute of Neurological Disorders and Stroke. (2018b). *Encephaloceles information page.* Retrieved from https://www.ninds.nih.gov/Disorders/All-Disorders/Encephaloceles-Information-Page/2926/organizations/1012

National Institute of Neurological Disorders and Stroke. (2018c). *Holoprosencephaly information page.* Retrieved from https://www.ninds.nih.gov/Disorders/All-Disorders/Holoprosencephaly-Information-Page/2947/organizations/1062

National Institute of Neurological Disorders and Stroke. (2018d). *Lissencephaly information page.* Retrieved from https://www.ninds.nih.gov/Disorders/All-Disorders/Lissencephaly-Information-Page

National Institute of Neurological Disorders and Stroke. (2018e). *Microcephaly information page.* Retrieved from https://www.ninds.nih.gov/disorders/all-disorders/microcephaly-information-page

National Institute of Neurological Disorders and Stroke. (2018f). *Schizencephaly information page.* Retrieved from https://www.ninds.nih.gov/Disorders/All-Disorders/Schizencephaly-Information-Page

National Institute of Neurological Disorders and Stroke. (2018g). *Spina bifida information page.* Retrieved from https://www.ninds.nih.gov/disorders/all-disorders/spina-bifida-information-page

National Institutes of Health (NIH). (2009a). *Hypomyelination and congenital cataract.* Retrieved from http://ghr.nlm.nih.gov/condition/hypomyelination-and-congenital-cataract

National Institutes of Health. (2009b). *Polymicrogyria.* Retrieved from http://ghr.nlm.nih.gov/condition/polymicrogyria

Powell, K. (2006). Neurodevelopment: How does the teenage brain work? *Nature, 442*, 865-867.

Wallis, C., & Dell, K. (2004). What makes teens tick. *Time Magazine, 163*(19), 56–65.

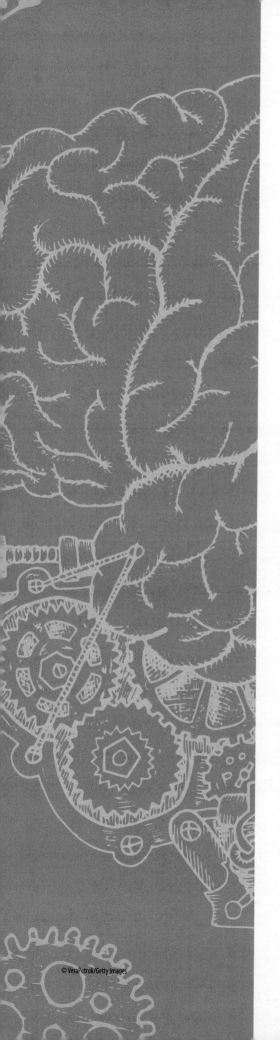

PART II

General Neuroanatomy

© VeraPetruk/Getty Images

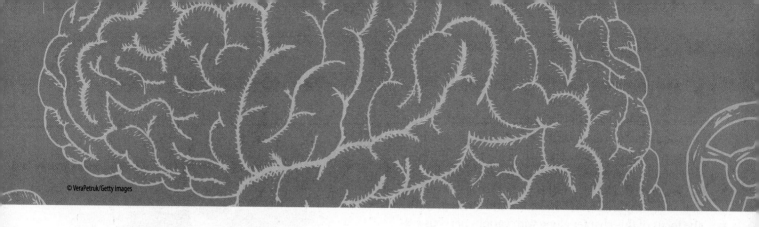

© VeraPetruk/Getty Images

CHAPTER 4

The Cells of the Nervous System

CHAPTER PREVIEW

Now it is time to dig into the nervous system and explore the cells that make up the nervous system, including their form and function. In addition, we will explore diseases related to these cells.

IN THIS CHAPTER

In this chapter, we will . . .

- Review the history of research regarding cells and neurons
- Discuss the structure of molecules, cells, tissues, organs, and systems
- Survey the different cells that make up the nervous system
- Examine the form and function of neurons
- Explore nervous system disorders that involve nervous system cells

LEARNING OBJECTIVES

- The learner will define the following: *molecule, cell, tissue, organ, and system*.
- The learner will list and briefly describe each nervous system cell.
- The learner will accurately label the parts of a neuron and synapse.
- The learner will list and briefly describe the steps in neuron function.
- The learner will list and briefly describe select nervous system disorders involving nervous system cells.

▶ Introduction

Neurons and glial cells form the foundation for the nervous system. Historically, neuroscientists have been more interested in neurons than glial cells; however, a newfound respect has been found for glial cells through the work of R. Douglas Fields and others. Neurons are still vitally important, and their form and function will be the focus of this chapter along with various nervous system disorders that arise from neuron dysfunction. Before discussing neurons, we will briefly survey how we have come to know what we do about neurons. In addition, we will set the context for talking about neurons by talking about the structure and function of cells in general.

▶ Historical Considerations

The 18th and 19th centuries led to many advances in understanding the nervous system. The same is true about biology in general. Many of these advances were made possible by the invention of the microscope. Although microscopes had been around since the 16th century, Anton van Leeuwenhoek (1632–1723) is considered the father of microscopy. He made many biological discoveries through the use of microscopes, such as the detection of bacteria.

In the 1830s, Matthias Schleiden (a botanist) and Theodor Schwann (a zoologist) made observations using microscopy; from their conclusions, they proposed the **cell theory**. This theory states that all organic beings (humans, animals, and plants) are composed of individual cells (Wallace, King, & Sanders, 1986). As microscopists continued to examine cells, they found this theory to be true of all cells except one type—nervous system cells. These cells looked strange, with all the odd-looking projections around them. It seemed that the nervous system was the exception to the cell theory in that the fundamental building blocks were cells plus these projections. Because of limited techniques, scientists in the first half of the 19th century did not know that these projections were an actual part of nervous system cells.

In 1873, an Italian scientist named Camillo Golgi (1843–1926) developed a way to stain a whole neuron using silver nitrate (**FIGURE 4-1**). This method, the Golgi method, is still in use today. Through this method, Golgi could see the entire neuron, which included the cell body, dendrites, and axon (**FIGURE 4-2**). He also noticed something else—the neurons appeared connected to each other. This observation was problematic at first because it violated the cell theory, which stated that cells were individual units and not dependent on each other. Neurons appeared connected and dependent on each other, which Golgi described in his reticular theory.

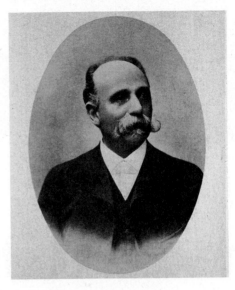

FIGURE 4-1 Camillo Golgi.

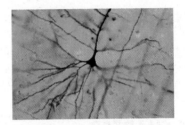

FIGURE 4-2 A pyramidal neuron stained using the Golgi method.

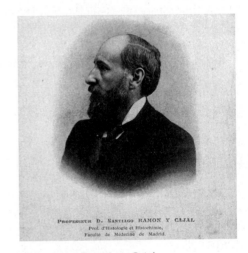

PROFESSEUR D. SANTIAGO RAMON Y CAJAL
Prof. d'Histologie et Histochimie,
Faculté de Médecine de Madrid.

FIGURE 4-3 Santiago Ramón y Cajal.

Around Golgi's time, a Spanish physician and scientist named Santiago Ramón y Cajal (1852–1934) further refined Golgi's method and discovered that neurons did not actually physically touch each other (**FIGURE 4-3**). There was a space between them, which modern microscopy has since confirmed. Cajal had upheld the cell theory, and his discovery gave rise to the **neuron doctrine**, the belief that each neuron is a separate cell and the fundamental building block of the nervous system.

During the latter half of the 19th century, other important discoveries were made about the nervous system. Motor and sensory neurons were discovered. Motor neurons take movement information from the brain to the body, and sensory neurons take sensory information from the body to the brain. In addition, in terms of the spinal cord and spinal nerves, it was found that sensory neurons enter the spinal cord dorsally through a dorsal nerve root and that motor neurons leave the spinal cord through a ventral nerve root.

In 1833, Johannes Müller (1801–1858) put forth the **law of specific nerve energies**. The law revolves around our sensory experience. It states that the origin of the sensation (e.g., visual or tactile) does not determine our sensory experience, but rather the pathway it is carried on. For example, whether you see the night sky or mechanically press your finger against your eye, your sensory experience is visual (i.e., seeing stars). This occurs because the optic tracts are visual tracts and connect to the visual centers of the brain. The whole system is visual, so sensory experience, no matter the stimulus (e.g., gently pressing the eye), is visual.

Cajal built further on the law of specific nerve energies and proposed that connections between neurons were not random, but rather were specific and predetermined. Cajal also proposed another law on the **dynamic polarization of neurons**. He theorized that information flows only one way through a neuron, beginning with dendrites, then through the cell body, and finally through the axon. In other words, dendrites always send information to the cell body, and axons always send information away from the cell body. This theory has been found to be generally true, but there are exceptions. For example, sometimes synapses are bidirectional (Jessell & Kandel, 1993).

A few final pieces of the nervous system picture need to be mentioned. Both involve Sir Charles Sherrington (1857–1952), an English scientist and Nobel Prize winner. In 1897, he described how the spaces between neurons functioned and called them synapses. He also described how our reflexes work.

This walk through history has given us the pieces we need to discuss the form and function of neurons. Before we do that, we will survey molecules and cells in general to give a context for neurons and other nervous system cells.

▶ Cell Structure and Function

Molecules

Molecules consist of two or more atoms held together by a chemical bond (McQuarrie & Rock, 1984). Cells are mostly composed of four families of molecules: simple sugars, fatty acids, amino acids, and nucleotides

(Alberts et al., 1983). We will briefly look at each of these molecules.

First, simple sugars are also known as carbohydrates. They can be small molecules (like table sugar) or chains of small sugar molecules (like glycogen). Sugars are stored until they are needed as energy to power cellular functions of small sugar molecules. Second, fatty acids, or lipids, are more commonly known as fats. These molecules are important in the cell's architecture, making up the cell membrane. In the nervous system, lipids make up a large percentage of myelin, a substance that coats axons and speeds transmission of signals. Third, amino acids are organic compounds made up of amine (–NH2) and carboxylic acid (–COOH). In the brain, two amino acids—glutamate and gamma-aminobutyric acid (GABA)—are important excitatory and inhibitory neurotransmitters. Proteins consist of chains of amino acids. Some are structural in nature (globular proteins), whereas others act as enzymes, which facilitate chemical reactions. Structural proteins can be found in the cell membrane; they act as gates, allowing some materials in and out of the cell. Proteins that are enzymes perform a variety of chemical reactions, one being the breakdown of unneeded neurotransmitters in synapses. Finally, nucleotides (or nucleic acids) are large molecular chains in the cell's nucleus. Two nucleotides of note are deoxyribonucleic acid (DNA), the genetic code for our bodies (**FIGURE 4-4**), and ribonucleic acid (RNA), the mechanism for building our body's structure, including our nervous systems (Alberts et al., 1983).

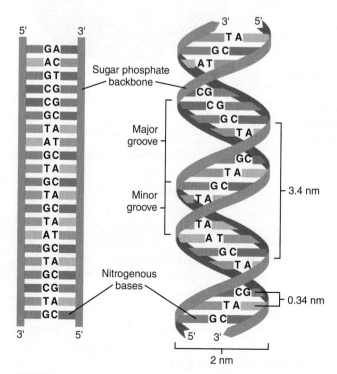

FIGURE 4-4 Diagram of a DNA molecule.

The Cell

Cells are the fundamental units of an organism. The analogy of a city is helpful in understanding the different components of a cell (**FIGURE 4-5**). In ancient times, cities had walls for protection, and the cell membrane acts as a protective wall for the cell. The cell **membrane** is a double-walled structure (bilipid membrane) made up of lipids and proteins that when bonded together are called lipoproteins (**FIGURE 4-6**). Proteins form the innermost and outermost walls of the membrane, and lipids fill the center. Globular proteins act as gates in the membrane that allow substances, like ions (small molecules with electric charges), into and out of the cell. The cell's **nucleus** acts like the mayor of the cell. It contains DNA, which is the genetic code that regulates the maintenance of the cell and production of new cells. Inside the nucleus is the **nucleolus**, which contains RNA. The nucleolus can be thought of as the general contractor of the cell that directs the creation of proteins needed to build and repair the cell. The **endoplasmic reticulum** with its **ribosomes** then acts as a production plant for proteins needed by the cell. The **mitochondria** are the cell's energy factories, where oxygen and sugars are metabolized by enzymes, and their energy powers the cell. The **Golgi apparatus** (named after Camillo Golgi) is the cell's mail office that packages and sends sugars and proteins out of the cell. **Lysosomes** are the garbage collectors of the cell and use enzymes to break down and recycle used molecules. The **centrosome** is like the city planning department, directing the growth of the cell through cell division. Lastly, the **cytoskeleton** is like a city's transportation system. It is made up of **microtubules** that transport molecules around the cell. These cell components are summarized in **TABLE 4-1**.

Cells, Tissues, and Systems

In our bodies, cells are only one level of organization. When groups of similar cells come together to carry out certain functions, we call the product a **tissue** (e.g., muscle tissue, nervous tissue). When various tissues are brought together to carry out certain functions, we are now at the level of **organs** (e.g., heart, brain). As organs are grouped together to carry out certain functions, we have now reached the **systems** level. There are numerous systems in the human body (e.g., circulatory, digestive, reproductive), including the one under discussion in this text, the nervous system.

▶ An Overview of Nervous System Cells

There are two basic types of nervous system cells in the human body, neurons and glial (or neuroglial) cells. **TABLE 4-2** displays examples of different nervous system cells and their functions (**FIGURE 4-7**). No one

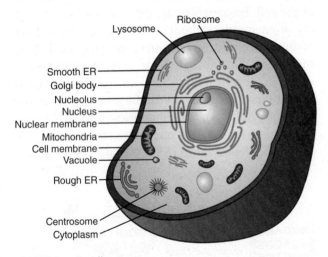

FIGURE 4-5 A cell.

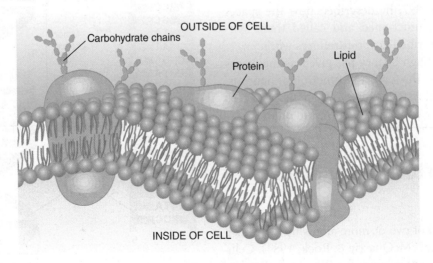

FIGURE 4-6 A bilipid membrane.

TABLE 4-1 Summary of Cell Components

Cell Structure	Cell Function	City Analogy
Membrane	Serves as selectively permeable barrier/protector	City walls
Golgi apparatus	Stores and delivers proteins	Post office
Cytoplasm	Contents of cell (except nucleus)	The city itself
Mitochondria	Produce energy for the cell	Energy factory
Nucleus	Acts as genetic control center	Mayor's office
Nucleolus	Produces ribosomes	Construction (builds factories)
Ribosomes	Produce proteins	Factory
Centrioles	Assist in cell division and microtubule formation	Planning department
Lysosomes	Digest cell debris and bacteria	Sanitation
Microtubules	Contribute to cell framework and movement of cell parts	Infrastructure
Endoplasmic reticulum (ER)	Rough ER produces proteins; smooth ER produces fatty acids, calcium, and enzymes	Factory

TABLE 4-2 Some Cells of the Nervous System

Category	Cell Types	Location	Examples of Functions
Neuronal cells	Neurons	CNS and PNS	Communicate within nervous system and with organs, muscles, and glands
Glial cells	Astrocytes	CNS	Maintain neural environment, repair/feed neurons, modulate neural transmission, modulate breathing
	Oligodendroglia	CNS	Produce myelin
	Microglia	CNS	Scavenge debris and defend against foreign substances
	Schwann cells	PNS	Produce myelin
	Satellite cells	PNS	Maintain neuronal environment

Abbreviations:
CNS, central nervous system; PNS, peripheral nervous system.
Data from Brodal, P. (2010). *The central nervous system* (4th ed.). New York, NY: Oxford University Press, pp. 19–27; Snell, R. S. (2001). *Clinical neuroanatomy for medical students* (5th ed.). Baltimore, MD: Lippincott Williams & Wilkins, pp. 34–66.

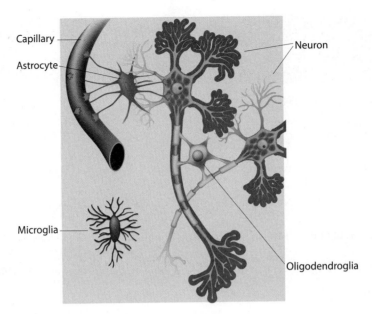

FIGURE 4-7 Cells of the central nervous system.

© Alila Medical Images/Shutterstock.

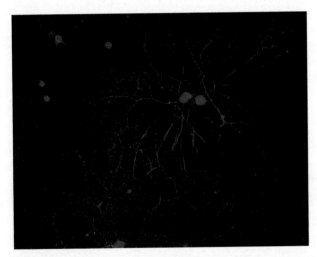

FIGURE 4-8 A fluorescent micrograph of a neuron in culture, showing neuronal cell body and the dendritic extensions.

really knows how many total cells (neurons and glial cells) make up the human nervous system. Many sources report that humans have 100 billion neurons and 1 trillion glial cells (Allen & Barres, 2009; Kandel, Schwartz, Jessell, Siegelbaum, & Hudspeth, 2013) but do so without reference to a source (Herculano-Houzel, 2009).

Neurons

The most well-known nervous system cell is the neuron. A **neuron** (Greek for "nerve") is a cell with specialized projections that transfers information throughout the body via an electrochemical process (**FIGURE 4-8**). Neurons are found in both the peripheral nervous system (PNS) and the central nervous system (CNS).

There are approximately 85 billion to 100 billion neurons in the human brain that range in size between 4 and 100 microns (1 micron is one-thousandth of a millimeter) (Herculano-Houzel, 2009).

Glial Cells

Glial (Greek for "glue") **cells** were once thought to be simple support cells to neurons that anchored, nourished, insulated, and protected them. These cells were thought to play no role in the transmission of information throughout the nervous system. Research has challenged this assumption, showing that glial cells do modulate neurotransmission (Fields, 2009) and may even play a role in regulating basic life functions, like breathing (Gourine et al., 2010).

Astrocytes

Astrocytes (Greek for "star-shaped cell") are star-shaped cells that nourish neurons and help to maintain the neuronal environment (Kandel et al., 2013). Fields (2009) reports that astrocytes do more than first thought. In fact, they work with neurons to control the activity that occurs in synapses by regulating ions, neurotransmitters, and other molecules. Astrocytes also secrete substances that stimulate the formation of new synapses.

Oligodendroglia and Schwann Cells

Oligodendroglia (Greek for "few tree glue") and **Schwann cells** (named after physiologist Theodor Schwann) both produce and coat axons with myelin. Oligodendroglia perform this function in the CNS;

Schwann cells are the PNS equivalent. Both coat only segments of the axon because the axon is not continuously coated. The uncoated areas, called nodes of Ranvier, help to facilitate the propagation of electrical signals down the axon due to the signal jumping from one node to the next. The thickness of the myelin coating is proportional to the thickness of the axon. Myelin is 70% lipid and 30% protein. Lipids act as insulators that keep the signal in the axon, and proteins provide structural stability for the myelin sheath (Kandel et al., 2013).

Microglia

Microglia (Greek for "small glue") are CNS cells that are produced in the bone marrow. Their function is not well understood, but they are thought to defend nervous system structures by warding off foreign invaders. This role means that microglia are part of the immune system (Kandel et al., 2013). In addition, they rally to areas of damage in the brain or spinal cord, producing a scar tissue–like substance on injuries. This process is known as gliosis (Webster, 1999).

Satellite Cells

Satellite (Latin for "attendant") **cells** are the astrocytes of the PNS that surround neurons, helping to nourish them. They also maintain the neuronal environment by taking up neurotransmitters, like GABA. Satellite cells also appear to respond to neuron injury, a similar function to astrocytes in the CNS (Hanani, 2010).

▶ Neuron Form and Function

Now that we have surveyed different nervous system cells, we will focus on neurons because they are important in neural transmission. We will first learn the form or structure of neurons and then turn our attention to how they work.

Neuron Form

Discussing neuron form involves two structures, the neuron itself and something called a synapse. We will look at the structure and types of neurons first and then explore the structure of a synapse. This will prepare us to consider neuron function since both structures are crucial to the sending of neural messages.

The Neuron

Neurons are unique cells in the human body, with their specialized projections and electrochemical communication process (**FIGURE 4-9**). Unlike other cells in the human body, neurons have projections

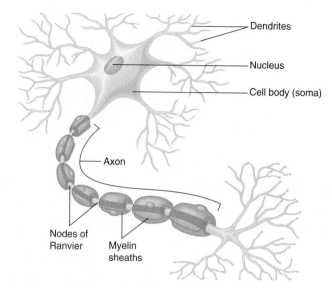

FIGURE 4-9 A neuron.

BOX 4-1 What Is the Longest Axon in the World?

The longest axon in the world belongs to the giant squid (**FIGURE 4-10**). This sea creature's axons run down the sides of its mantle and power its jet propulsion mechanism. The axons can be as long as 16 feet and as thick as a dime (about 16 mm). What about humans? What is the longest axon? This honor goes to the sciatic nerve, which runs from the end of the spinal cord in the lower back to the big toe. If pressure is applied to this nerve through a herniated vertebral disc or a narrowing of the vertebral column, a person may experience a condition called sciatica, in which pain radiates down the leg.

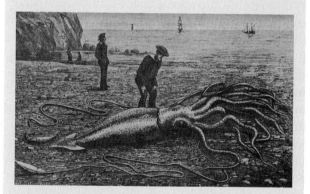

FIGURE 4-10 A giant squid.

(e.g., axons) that can be quite long, sometimes up to several feet (see **BOX 4-1**) and also Nissl bodies where protein synthesis occurs. Neurons contain two basic parts—a cell body or **soma** (Greek for "body") and projections called **neurites**. Neurites can be further divided into two main types—**dendrites** (Greek for "tree"), which receive signals and pass them toward the cell body, and **axons** (Greek for "axis"), which

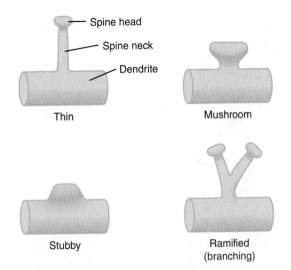

Spine head
Spine neck
Dendrite

Thin

Mushroom

Stubby

Ramified
(branching)

FIGURE 4-11 Types of dendritic spines.

conduct these signals away from the cell body. Dendrites and axons are also known as nerve fibers. Some dendrites have spines on them that are involved in chemical transmission of signals (Bear, Connors, & Paradiso, 2007). These spines come in different shapes and sizes and are critical pieces to forming cortical circuits (Arellano, Benavides, DeFelipe, & Yuste, 2007) (**FIGURE 4-11**). Their shape also appears to isolate connections from each other, so there is no interference (Araya, Eisenthal, & Yuste, 2006; Araya, Jiang, Eisenthal, & Yuste, 2006).

Axons also have unique features. As mentioned earlier, a fatty, white coating called **myelin** coats axons. This coating is made up of water, proteins, and lipids. Functionally, myelin not only keeps electrical signals in the axon but also speeds up the transmission of signals. An analogy for myelin is the rubber coating on electrical cords in our homes. Myelin is essential to a properly working nervous system; demyelinating diseases, like multiple sclerosis, can result in severe neurological deficits. The production of myelin is called **myelination**. In humans, this process begins during the 14th week of development and continues into adolescence. It can be observed behaviorally through the improved motor skills of babies. Oligodendroglia cells produce myelin in the CNS, whereas Schwann cells produce it in the PNS (Snell, 2001).

Neurons can be classified in several different ways; one of the most common ways is by the number of neurites the neuron has. Using this system, there are three basic types of neurons: unipolar, bipolar, and multipolar (**FIGURE 4-12**). Unipolar (or pseudopolar) neurons have a single projection that functions as an axon and comes off the cell body. These neurons are typically sensory in nature (e.g., touch, pain). Bipolar neurons have two projections, one dendritic and the other axonic. These neurons are located in structures devoted to special senses, like hearing, smell, and vision. Lastly, multipolar neurons are motor in nature and have multiple projections coming off the cell body, most of which are dendrites along with a single axon.

Neurons can also be classified based on their connections. **Sensory neurons** connect to sensory structures in the body. In contrast, **motor neurons** connect to body structures involved with movement, like muscles. **Interneurons** connect neurons together and transmit signals between them. Other classification schemes include classifying neurons based on dendrite shape, axon length, and neurotransmitter chemistry (Bear, Connors, & Paradiso, 2007).

The Synapse

Neurons connect with each other in order to pass signals to each other; these places of connection are called **synapses** (Greek, "to join together") (**FIGURE 4-13**). The ends of axons house terminal buttons (or *boutons*). Within these buttons are vesicles or sacs that hold chemicals called neurotransmitters; when stimulated, the presynaptic membrane vesicles release the neurotransmitters, which pass through the synaptic space or cleft and connect to receptor sites on the postsynaptic membrane. The result is that the signal is passed from one neuron to the other neuron through this chemical process. After the signal is passed from one neuron to another, some of the neurotransmitters are reabsorbed by the presynaptic membrane (or a neighboring glial cell) and returned to the vesicles. Other neurotransmitters may be broken down by enzymes in the synaptic cleft.

There are three types of synapses (**FIGURE 4-14**). An **axodendritic synapse** involves the axon of one neuron connecting and sending a chemical signal to the dendrite of another neuron. These connections are usually excitatory in nature. Axons can also connect directly to the soma of the neuron. These connections are called **axosomatic synapses**, and they are usually inhibitory. The last type of synapse involves one axon connecting with another axon. This is called an **axoaxonic synapse**, and it is typically modulatory, meaning it regulates a signal (Seikel, King, & Drumright, 2010).

Neurotransmitters

As mentioned earlier, **neurotransmitters** are chemical messengers that transmit messages from a presynaptic membrane to a postsynaptic membrane through the synaptic cleft. There are over 100 known neurotransmitters, and many of these chemicals are crucial to functions that speech-language pathologists (SLPs) and audiologists care about, including speech, language, hearing, and swallowing.

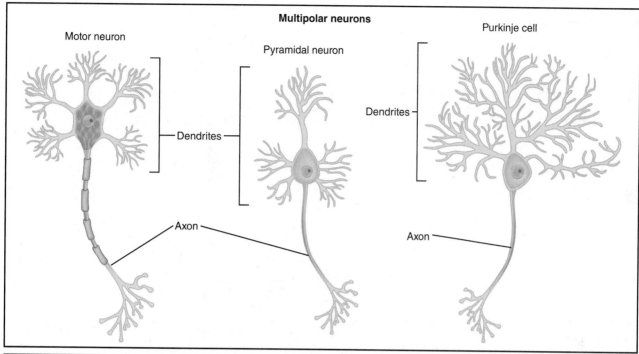

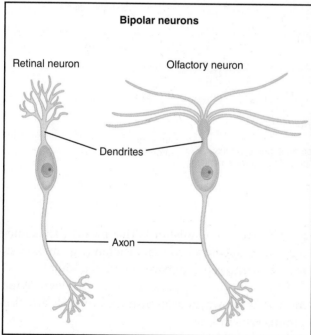

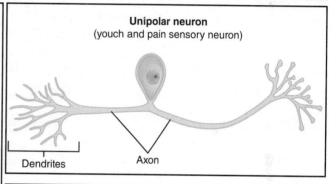

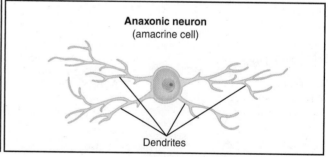

FIGURE 4-12 Types of neurons.

© Alila Medical Images/Shutterstock.

In order to be a neurotransmitter, Purves (2004) states three conditions must be met:

- It must be present in the presynaptic membrane.
- It must be released in response to presynaptic depolarization.
- There must be specific postsynaptic receptors to receive it.

In terms of structure, there are two basic categories of neurotransmitters: large molecule and small molecule. Large molecule neurotransmitters (neuropeptides) are considered large because they consist of 3 to 36 amino acids. In terms of effect, they are long lasting. Small molecule neurotransmitters (amines and amino acids) consist of single amino acids and are short lasting. It was once thought that each neuron held only one specific neurotransmitter, but now we know that a neuron can hold multiple types. Small molecules are held in synaptic vesicles on the presynaptic membrane, and large molecules are stored in secretory granules on the axon terminals.

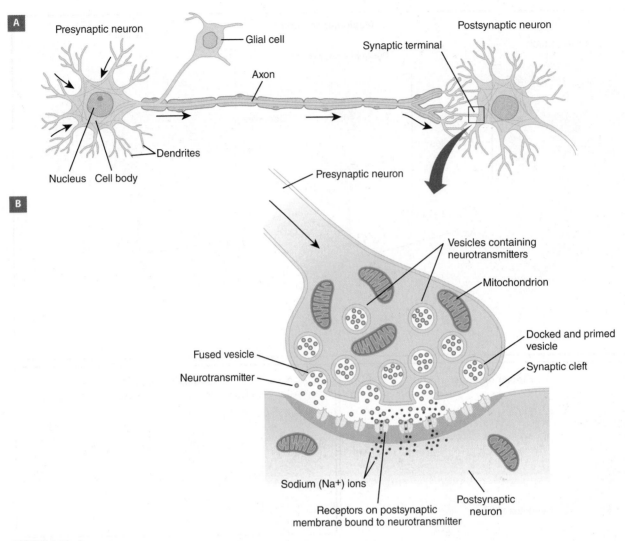

 A

Presynaptic neuron

Glial cell

Postsynaptic neuron

Synaptic terminal

Axon

Dendrites

Nucleus   Cell body

B

Presynaptic neuron

Vesicles containing neurotransmitters

Mitochondrion

Docked and primed vesicle

Synaptic cleft

Fused vesicle

Neurotransmitter

Sodium (Na+) ions

Receptors on postsynaptic membrane bound to neurotransmitter

Postsynaptic neuron

FIGURE 4-13 A synapse.

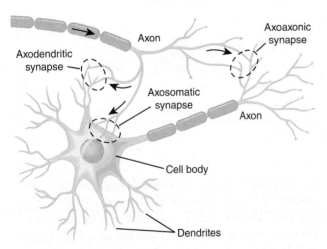

Axon

Axoaxonic synapse

Axodendritic synapse

Axosomatic synapse

Axon

Cell body

Dendrites

FIGURE 4-14 Three types of synapses.

Functionally, neurotransmitters mediate transmission between neurons by exciting (starting), inhibiting (stopping), or modulating (regulating a signal) postsynaptic action potentials. Second, neurotransmitters modulate synaptic communication in small groups of neurons (neuromodulation). This means they sometimes help to control communication (e.g., make fast, make slower, keep going over a period of time).

The following list presents a brief overview of the most well-known neurotransmitters, which are also summarized in **TABLE 4-3**.

- ***Acetylcholine (ACh)***: ACh was the first neurotransmitter to be discovered. It was first identified in 1951 by Henry Hallett Dale through his work on the nervous system's relationship to the heart. It is a rapid-fire neurotransmitter of the PNS neuromuscular junction that causes muscle tissue to contract. It is also released at the neuromuscular junction between the vagus nerve and cardiac tissue. Neurons that release ACh are called cholinergic neurons. After being released at the neuromuscular junction, ACh's action is stopped by an enzyme called acetylcholinesterase (AChE) that breaks it down so it can be reused. ACh has a restricted role in the CNS, being found only in the brainstem,

TABLE 4-3 Some Important Neurotransmitters and Their Characteristics

Name	Abbreviation	Group	Function	Storage	Surplus Effect	Deficit Effect	Agonist Drug	Antagonist Drug
Acetylcholine	ACh	Acetylcholine	Excitatory: stimulates skeletal muscle contraction; involved in memory and learning	Axon terminal	Severe muscle spasms; difficulty in thinking and learning	Cognitive issues, like memory loss; associated with dementia and Alzheimer disease	Nicotine	Curare
			Inhibitory: cardiac tissue					
Glutamate	Glu	Amino acid	Excitatory: memory, learning, movement	Axon terminal	Possible epileptic seizures (with low GABA levels)	Fatigue, cognitive impairment	Theanine	Alcohol
Gamma-aminobutyric acid	GABA	Amino acid	Inhibitory: blocks action of excitatory neurotransmitters; sleep–wake cycle	Axon terminal	Sleeping problems, impaired thinking	Anxiety and other mood disorders	Diazepam, alprazolam	Benzodiazepines
Dopamine	DA	Monoamine	Inhibitory: indirect motor pathway	Axon terminal	Psychosis, bipolar disorder (manic stage), schizophrenia, addictions	Parkinson disease	L-dopa, cocaine	Chlorpromazine
			Excitatory: direct motor pathway, heart rate, blood pressure, reward/pleasure					
Epinephrine (adrenaline)	E, Ad	Monoamine	Excitatory: fight-or-flight response (increases blood flow, heart rate, and blood sugar; dilates pupils)	Axon terminal	Anxiety	Fatigue, poor concentration	Ephedrine	Alpha and beta blockers

(continues)

TABLE 4-3 Some Important Neurotransmitters and Their Characteristics (continued)

Name	Abbreviation	Group	Function	Storage	Surplus Effect	Deficit Effect	Agonist Drug	Antagonist Drug
Norepinephrine (noradrenaline)	NE, NAd	Monoamine	Excitatory: fight-or-flight response (increases arousal; focuses attention; enhances memory; increases blood flow, heart rate, blood pressure, and blood sugar)	Axon terminal	Anxiety, panic attacks	Depression, low energy levels, attention-deficit/hyperactivity disorder	Caffeine, amphetamines	Lithium
Serotonin	5-HT	Monoamine	Regulatory: mood, sleep, appetite	Axon terminal	Agitation, autism	Depression, mood disorders	Selective serotonin reuptake inhibitors	Clozapine
Substance P	SP	Peptide	Excitatory: stimulates perception of pain; stimulates inflammation in response to injury	Soma	Inflammatory disorders (e.g, skin conditions like eczema, psoriasis)	Decreased levels associated with Alzheimer disease, type 1 diabetes	Hemokinin 1	Aprepitant

Data from: Blumenfeld, H. (2010). *Neuroanatomy through clinical cases*. Sunderland, MA: Sinauer Associates; Kandel, E. R., Schwartz, J. H., Jessell, T. M., Siegelbaum, S. A., & Hudspeth, A. J. (2013). *Principles of neural science* (5th ed.). New York, NY: McGraw-Hill; Guyton, A. C., & Hall, J. E. (2006). *Textbook of medical physiology* (11th ed.). Philadelphia, PA: Elsevier Saunders.

the base of the forebrain, and the basal ganglia. It is thought to regulate CNS neuronal activity, especially alertness, attention, memory, and learning. The degeneration of cholinergic neurons in the CNS is thought to be behind the memory issues in Alzheimer disease (Bear, Connors, & Paradiso, 2007; Blumenfeld, 2010; Nolte, 2002; Purves, 2004).

- *Glutamate*: Glutamate is the ACh of the CNS. It is the major excitatory chemical of synaptic activity in the CNS and plays a role in synaptic plasticity. It is involved in both learning and memory. There is some evidence that imbalances in glutamate play a role in schizophrenia (Kandel et al., 2013). High levels of the chemical can lead to epileptic seizures in combination with low GABA levels.

- *Gamma-aminobutyric acid (GABA)*: GABA is the main inhibitory neurotransmitter of the CNS. It acts by binding to postsynaptic receptor sites, blocking the action of other neurotransmitters. Neurons that contain GABA are called GABAergic neurons. In addition to controlling information flow in the nervous system, GABA plays a role in the sleep–wake cycle (Blumenfeld, 2010). Low levels of GABA have been linked to depression and other mood disorders, and high levels are associated with insomnia.

- *Dopamine*: Dopamine plays a role in motor control as well as our reward system. It is involved in three CNS pathways (**FIGURE 4-15**). The first is the *mesostriatal pathway* that begins in the substantia nigra and projects to the basal ganglia. Damage to

this pathway can lead to movement disorders such as Parkinson disease. The second pathway is the *mesolimbic pathway* that originates from an area in the brainstem called the tegmentum and projects to the limbic system, which is our emotional system. This pathway is important in reward and addiction. Dysfunction in this pathway can lead to positive schizophrenic symptoms such as delusions or hallucinations. The third pathway is the *mesocortical pathway*, which also arises from the tegmentum (area of the brainstem), but projects to the prefrontal cortex. Impairment to this pathway leads to the negative symptoms of schizophrenia, like flat affect and emotion, lack of speech, and lack of motivation (Blumenfeld, 2010).

- *Epinephrine*: Also known as adrenaline, epinephrine is involved in regulating heart rate, blood pressure, and breathing and in the fight-or-flight response. Epinephrine-containing neurons originate in the brainstem and project to the thalamus and hypothalamus (Purves, 2004). High levels are associated with anxiety; low levels are associated with fatigue and poor concentration.

- *Norepinephrine*: Norepinephrine is also known as noradrenaline. Neurons containing this neurotransmitter arise out of the brainstem and project to the entire forebrain. Norepinephrine modulates attention, sleep–wake cycle, and mood and is involved in our fight-or-flight response. Impaired levels of it have been linked to attention-deficit/hyperactivity disorder, narcolepsy (sleep

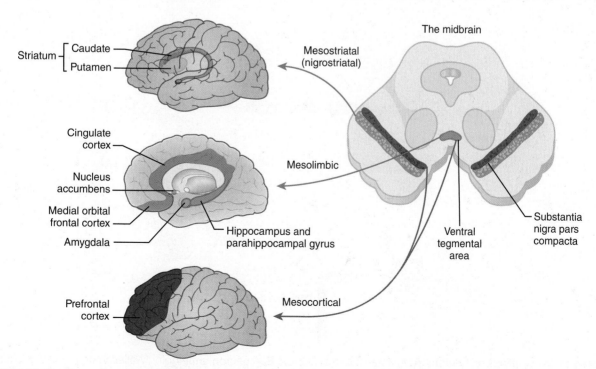

FIGURE 4-15 The three dopaminergic projection systems.

attacks), and mood disorders like depression, manic-depressive disorder, and anxiety (Blumenfeld, 2010).

- ■ *Serotonin*: Serotonergic neurons (i.e., neurons that contain serotonin) originate in the brainstem and project to the entire forebrain. They have both excitatory and inhibitory effects on the nervous system and regulate functions such as mood, sleep, and appetite. Low levels of this neurotransmitter relate to depression, anxiety, obsessive-compulsive disorders, and eating disorders. Serotonin also plays a role in arousal in the sleep–wake cycle, and thus a surplus can disrupt this cycle (Blumenfeld, 2010).

- ■ *Substance P*: The perception of pain is an important protective biological mechanism. For example, imagine how much damage we could do to our hand around a hot burner if we did not perceive pain. Substance P sensitizes us to pain and also causes inflammation at an injury site, which leads to healing (Kandel et al., 2013). Chronically increased levels of substance P can lead to inflammatory skin disorders, such as eczema, whereas low levels have been associated with Alzheimer disease and type 1 diabetes.

Neuron Damage and Repair

Neurons in the CNS or PNS are sometimes damaged through injury. This damage can occur through cutting or crushing an axon, a phenomenon known as an *axotomy*. When an axotomy occurs, the neuron enters an active degeneration process called **Wallerian degeneration** (FIGURE 4-16), named after British physiologist Augustus Waller (1856–1922). In this process, that part of the axon that is distal from the soma and anterograde from the injury degenerates and the axon terminal pulls away from the synapse. Microglia scavenge the debris left by the Wallerian degeneration. Axons in the CNS regenerate poorly because of a buildup of glial cells as scar tissue at the end of the damaged axon; axons in the PNS, in contrast, retain some ability to regenerate (FIGURE 4-17). Why is there a difference in regeneration properties between the two parts of the nervous system? It may be because the CNS needs stability once the brain is fully developed in order to be precise in its functioning, and to do so means giving up regeneration abilities (Kandel et al., 2013).

Important Aspects of Neuron Function

As stated earlier, neurons and glial cells are the primary cells of the nervous system, but we will be considering only neurons here. The main job of neurons is communication, which they do through tracts, or neural pathways. A neural pathway consists of a series of neurons connected together to make communication between the brain and the body possible. We will discuss specific neural pathways when we discuss the internal organization of the spinal cord as well as the motor speech system.

The communication between the brain and the body takes two basic forms. First there is **efferent communication**, which is top-down or descending

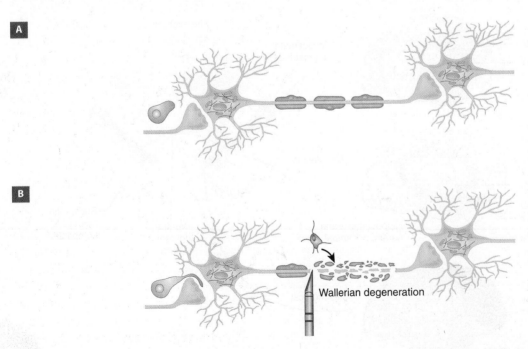

FIGURE 4-16 Injury effects on neurons. **A.** An intact, normal neuron. **B.** A neuron undergoing Wallerian degeneration after axonal damage.

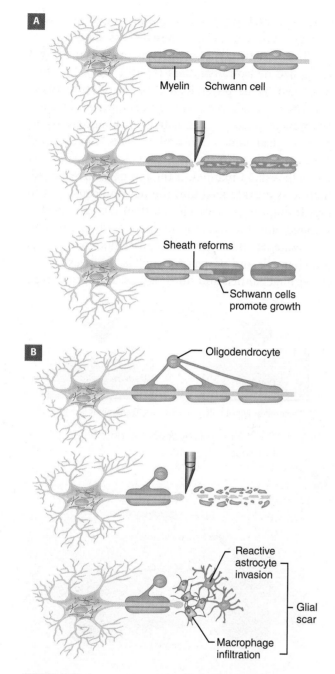

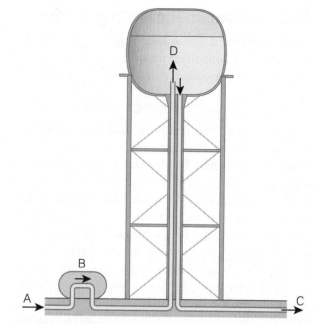

FIGURE 4-18 Water tower illustration of gradients and transport (see text for details).

FIGURE 4-17 Axon regeneration in the nervous system. **A.** Axon regeneration occurs in the peripheral nervous system. **B.** Axons in the central nervous system are more likely to undergo Wallerian degeneration.

communication through neural pathways from the brain to the body. Second there is **afferent communication**, which is bottom-up or ascending communication through neural pathways from the body to the brain. Overall, the communication of neurons in these pathways involves two phases: an electrical phase involving the dendrites, soma, and axon of the neuron and a chemical phase involving the synaptic cleft and neurotransmitters. Thus, the communication of neurons is said to be *electrochemical* in nature, a word that captures both of these phases. This being said, how does a neuron work?

Neuron function is complicated, but we will briefly describe neuron function in enough detail for SLPs and audiologists to understand the basics of it. We will also explore how neuron dysfunction can lead to various neurological conditions, many of which affect speech and hearing.

Two concepts are important to understanding how a neuron works: **transport** and **gradient** (i.e., an imbalance). In regard to the first concept, transport, there are two types: (1) *active transport*, in which energy is used to move something from point A to point B, and (2) *passive transport*, in which no energy is used to move something from point A to point B. Both of these ideas can be illustrated in the example of a water tower (**FIGURE 4-18**). To get water from point A to point D, energy has to be expended (i.e., active transport) using a pump B because of gravity. However, to get the water in D to point C, one only has to open a valve and allow gravity to push the water down through the pipes. No energy is used in this second process (i.e., passive transport) (Seikel, King, & Drumright, 2010).

The second concept to understand is a gradient. A gradient is a sloping or imbalance of some sort. For example, a mountain road has a grade (or gradient) to it. Membranes, like the ones found in neurons, are semipermeable, meaning they allow some substances (in this case, ions) in and keep others out. Because of the neuron membrane's semipermeable nature, gradients or imbalances of two types occur—concentration gradients and charge (or electrical) gradients (Seikel, King, & Drumright, 2010). These will be further explained in the next section.

The Firing Neuron: The Analogy of a Gun

Neuron function is like a gun. First, the gun must be loaded. Second, something must trigger the gun to fire. Third, the gun is reloaded in order to be used again.

Step 1: The Loaded Neuron (Polarization)

In a state of rest, the neuron is said to be polarized, meaning there are two imbalances. First, there is an imbalance of sodium (Na^+), with a large concentration of it on the outside of the neuron membrane and a small concentration on the inside. The + following the symbol for sodium (Na) indicates we are talking about a sodium ion. Ions are atoms that have either gained or lost an electron, causing them to gain either a positive or a negative charge. Like a magnet, positive charges will repel other positive charges but will be attracted to negative charges. In addition to the Na^+ imbalance, there is a large concentration of potassium (K^+) on the inside of the membrane and a smaller amount on the outside. Again, the neuron's semipermeable membrane is responsible for maintaining these imbalances. Second, there is an electrical or charge gradient, with the interior of the neuron being more negative (–70 mV) than outside the neuron. **FIGURE 4-19** illustrates these two imbalances. The concentration and charge gradients put the neuron in a position of being ready to fire. All that is needed is the right circumstance for the trigger to be pulled and the neuron to fire.

Step 2a: The Chemical Firing of the Neuron (Chemical Transmission)

Chemical transmission occurs at the synapse between a neuron and another neuron's dendrites, soma, or axon (or a muscle or gland). Neurotransmitters are released from the synaptic vesicles from the presynaptic membrane. From here, they venture into the synaptic cleft and attach to receptors on the postsynaptic membrane. The neurotransmitter acts like a key and the receptor on the postsynaptic membrane is like a lock. When the key unlocks the lock, the action signal is transmitted to the receiving neuron, as illustrated in **FIGURE 4-20**. Common neurotransmitters include ACh

(muscle contraction) and dopamine (smoothness of muscle movement), which were discussed earlier.

There are two types of postsynaptic receptors that recognize neurotransmitters (**FIGURE 4-21**). The first is known by its physiological name of **ionotropic receptors**. These receptors are also known by their anatomical name, ligand-gated ion channels. Their physiological name (ionotropic) means "ion feeding." These receptors directly open and close ion gates and do so in a rapid manner. If the ion gates are opened, then ions quickly feed into the neuron, causing it to fire. If the ion gates are closed, then ions are quickly stopped, and the signal is stopped. Both GABA and glutamate use this type of receptor; glutamate opens ion channels and propagates signals, whereas GABA closes ion channels and stops signals. The second type

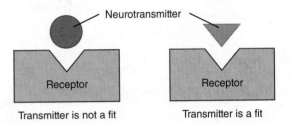

FIGURE 4-20 The lock and key system of postsynaptic receptors and neurotransmitters.

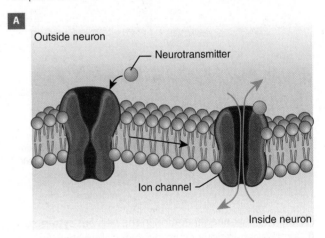

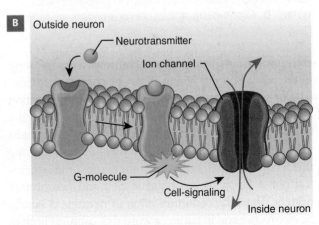

FIGURE 4-21 Two types of postsynaptic receptors. **A.** An ionotropic receptor. **B.** A metabotropic receptor.

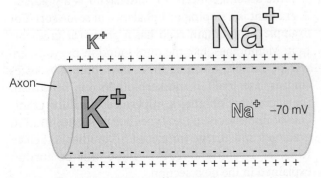

FIGURE 4-19 Two imbalances in a polarized neuron.

of postsynaptic receptors is **metabotropic receptors** (physiological name meaning "feeding" or "nourishing" through metabolization), or G protein–linked receptors (anatomical name). When a neurotransmitter connects to one of these receptors, a molecule (G protein) in the postsynaptic cell is mobilized and either directly or indirectly, through a series of reactions, opens and closes ion channels. These receptors are slower than ionotropic receptors because they are less direct. Overall, the sending of a signal down the neuron is slower and can last anywhere from milliseconds to days. Dopamine is an example of a neurotransmitter that uses these kinds of receptors.

Step 2b: The Electrical Firing of the Neuron (Depolarization)

When neurotransmitters attach to receptor sites on the postsynaptic membrane, small molecular ion gates at the nodes of Ranvier open. (Note: The nodes of Ranvier are unmyelinated sections of neuron.) The opening of these gates causes sodium to rapidly and passively transport into the neuron. Previous gradients are equalized. This sudden change in polarity from the influx of positive sodium ions triggers an **action potential**, a rapid change in membrane polarity, which moves or propagates like a wave down the axon (Guyton & Hall, 2006). This process is called **depolarization**. Zemlin (1998) states that "every sensation we experience, every thought we have, every movement we execute is dependent upon the generation and transmission of electrical energy called an action potential" (p. 385). **FIGURE 4-22** illustrates this process. It is at the nodes of Ranvier where depolarization

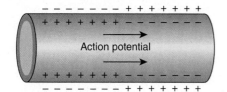

FIGURE 4-22 An action potential.

occurs. The signal that has been created jumps from node to node instead of the whole membrane (i.e., myelinated portions) depolarizing. This process of jumping speeds the transmission of the signal down the axon (Guyton & Hall, 2006).

Step 3: The Reloading of the Neuron (Repolarization)

At this point, sodium gates close and a different set of molecular gates open that allow potassium ions to rush out of the neuron. Because these ions are also positively charged, their absence causes the interior of the axon to become negative again, stopping the depolarization process. The sodium ions are pumped more slowly outside of the neuron membrane by the sodium–potassium (Na^+/K^+) pump, which uses the hydrolysis of ATP to provide the needed energy (**BOX 4-2**) and is thus a form of active transport (**FIGURE 4-23**). This pump exports three sodium ions

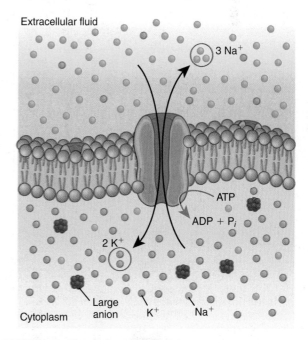

FIGURE 4-23 The sodium–potassium pump.
Modified from © Alila Medical Media/Shutterstock.

BOX 4-2 Adenosine Triphosphate and the Sodium–Potassium Pump

Adenosine triphosphate (ATP) releases energy when it is broken down by the enzyme adenosine triphosphatase (ATPase) (**FIGURE 4-24**). The by-product of this process is adenosine diphosphate (ADP) and a single phosphate, which recombine with an ADP molecule and form ATP again, making ATP a reusable molecule. ATPase is found in the plasma membrane of cells and is responsible for powering the sodium–potassium (NA^+/K^+) pump through this breakdown process, called ATP hydrolysis. This pump uses one ATP molecule for every three Na^+ ions sent out of the neuron and every two K^+ ions that are pumped into the neuron. By doing so, the NA^+/K^+ pump reestablishes the neuron's resting membrane potential. Because the NA^+/K^+ pump uses ATP as energy, this pumping process is considered active rather than passive. ATP is synthesized through three processes: glycolysis in the cytoplasm of cells (**FIGURE 4-25A**), the citric acid cycle in a cell's mitochondria (**FIGURE 4-25B**), and the electron transport chain that occurs through the inner mitochondrial membrane (**FIGURE 4-25C**).

(continues)

BOX 4-2 Adenosine Triphosphate and the Sodium–Potassium Pump *(continued)*

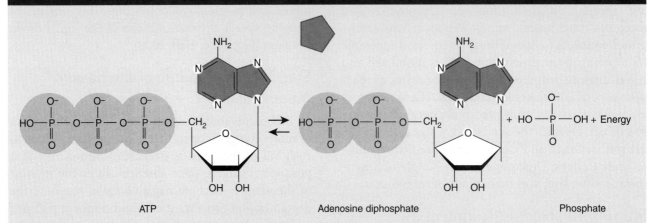

ATP   Adenosine diphosphate   Phosphate

FIGURE 4-24 Adenosine triphosphate (ATP). ATP is the primary high-energy molecule produced in human cells. Bonds between the phosphate groups are hydrolyzed to liberate energy, which is applied to cellular processes.

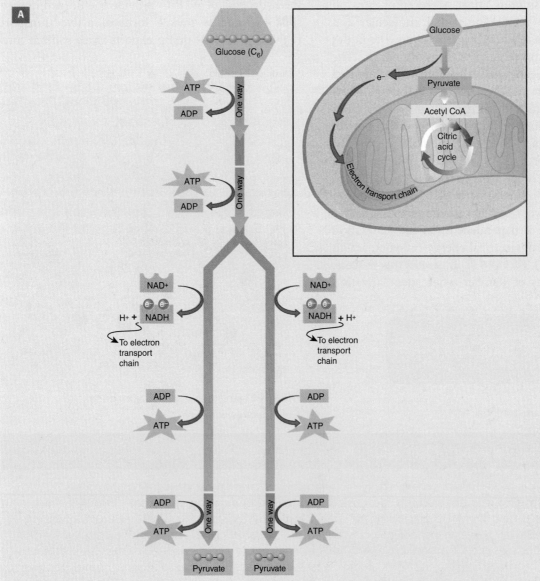

FIGURE 4-25A Glycolysis. The breakdown of one glucose molecule yields two pyruvate molecules, a net of two adenosine triphosphate (ATP) and two nicotinamide adenine dinucleotide (NADH) molecules. The two NADH molecules shuttle pairs of high-energy electrons to the electron transport chain for ATP production. Glycolytic reactions do not require oxygen, and some steps are irreversible.

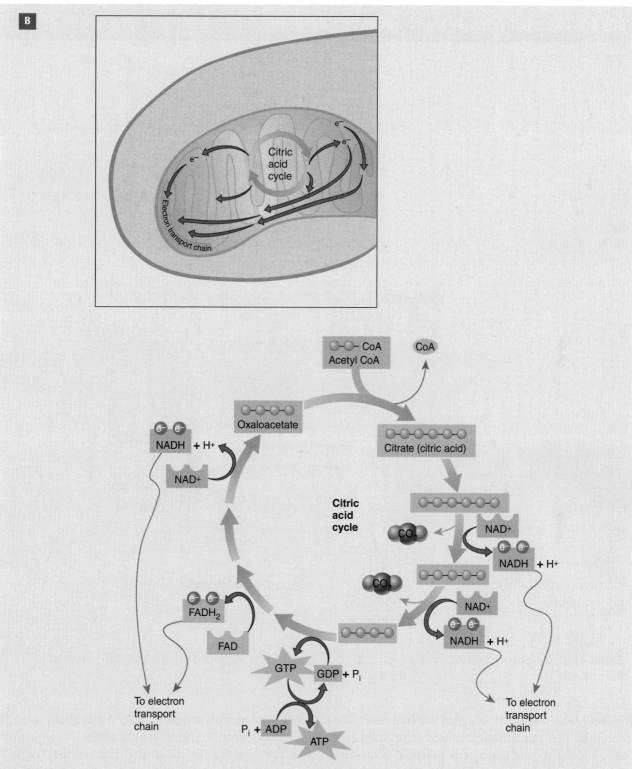

FIGURE 4-25B The citric acid cycle. This circular pathway accepts one acetyl coenzyme A (CoA) molecule and yields two carbon dioxide (CO_2), three nicotinamide adenine dinucleotide (NADH), one flavin adenine dinucleotide hydroquinone ($FADH_2$), and one guanosine triphosphate (GTP). (GTP is readily converted to adenosine triphosphate [ATP].) The electron shuttles NADH and $FADH_2$ to carry high-energy electrons to the electron transport chain for ATP production.

(continues)

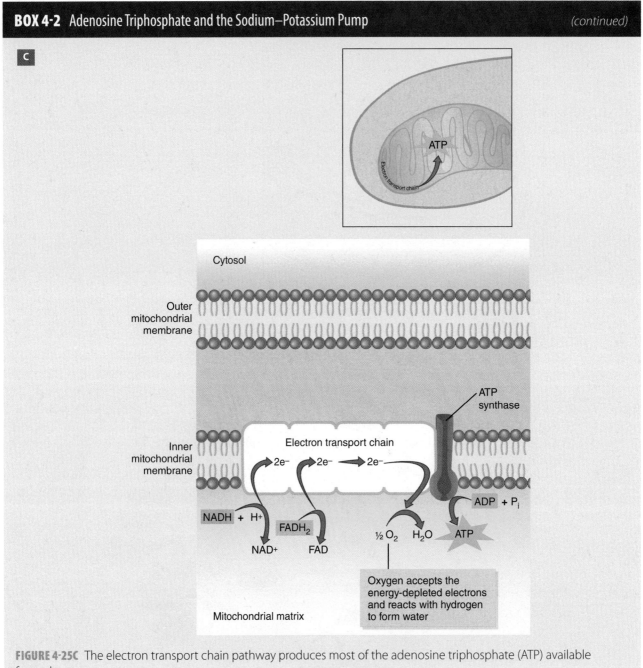

FIGURE 4-25C The electron transport chain pathway produces most of the adenosine triphosphate (ATP) available from glucose.

for every two potassium ions that are imported. The neuron is then put into a polarized state again (see Step 1) as the resting membrane potential is reestablished, and the neuron is ready to fire when needed.

The All-or-None Principle

For the visually minded, the graphs shown in **FIGURE 4-26** might help illustrate the whole process of neuron function in one picture. A threshold (around –55 mV) needs to be crossed in order for the neuron to fire (see the middle dotted line on the graph in Figure 4-26A[b]). When this threshold is reached, the neuron will depolarize and fire at a fixed strength. If the threshold is not met, the neuron will not fire. Thus, neurons function in an all-or-none manner, meaning either they fire or they do not, much like a light switch. This is called the **all-or-none principle**.

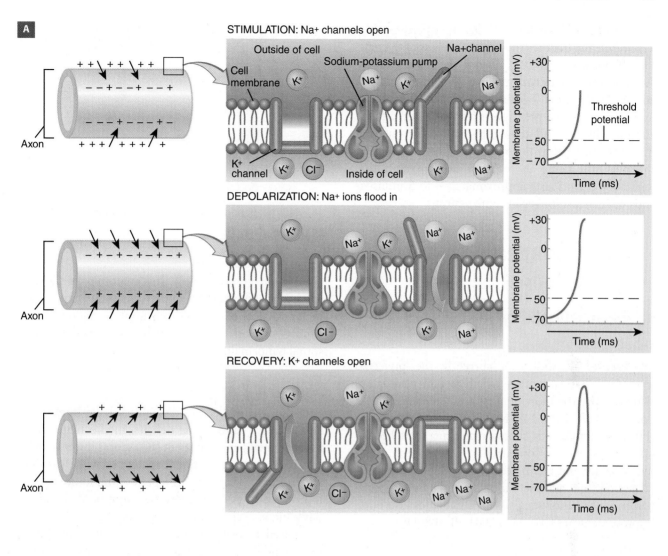

A. STIMULATION: Na+ channels open

Outside of cell

Cell membrane

Sodium-potassium pump

Na+channel

K+

Na+

K+

Na+

K+ channel

K+

Cl−

Inside of cell

K+

Na+

Threshold potential

DEPOLARIZATION: Na+ ions flood in

RECOVERY: K+ channels open

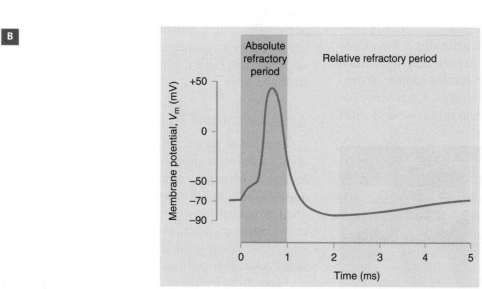

FIGURE 4-26 **A.** The development of the absolute and relative refractory periods. **B.** Summary graph showing the absolute and relative refractory periods.

In addition, there are two refractory periods. (The term *refractory* denotes the responsiveness of the neuron.) If another stimulus is given to the neuron during the **absolute refractory period** (1–2 milliseconds), nothing will happen because Na$^+$ channels are inactivated. During the **relative refractory period**, the neuron will respond to another stimulus, but that stimulus must be stronger than normal due to Na$^+$ channels still being in recovery mode. The whole refractory period lasts approximately 4 to 5 milliseconds but can last longer in some neurons.

▶ Select Disorders of Nervous System Cells

Intellectual Disability

What Is It?

Intellectual disability is currently the preferred term for what was once called mental retardation (**FIGURE 4-27**). The Individuals With Disabilities Education Act of 2004 (PL 108-446) defines intellectual disability as "significantly sub-average general intellectual functioning, existing concurrently with deficits in adaptive behavior and manifested during the developmental period, that adversely affects a child's educational performance" (Individuals With Disabilities Education Improvement Act [IDEA] of 2004, PL 108-446).

Causes

Neurologically, what causes this "significantly sub-average general intellectual functioning"? Bear, Connors, and Paradiso (2007) report that intellectual disability is associated with a smaller number of dendritic spines as well as morphological differences. Specifically, the spines are long and thin instead of short

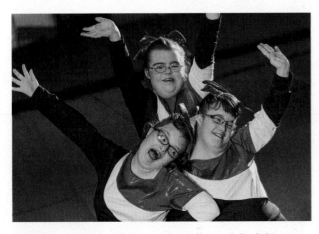

FIGURE 4-27 Three children with intellectual disabilities.
© kali9/Getty Images

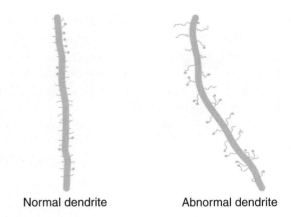

Normal dendrite   Abnormal dendrite

FIGURE 4-28 Normal and abnormal dendrites.

and rounded (**FIGURE 4-28**). This anatomical difference can be caused by external environmental factors (e.g., maternal alcohol or drug consumption, mercury poisoning) or internal factors such as gene and chromosomal abnormalities (Shapiro & Batshaw, 2013).

Signs and Symptoms

People with intellectual disabilities have intellectual and adaptive functioning deficits. Intellectual deficits involve intelligence quotient (IQ) scores lower than 70 and issues with reasoning, problem solving, learning, and abstract language. Adaptive functioning refers to how well a person meets the common demands of daily life as well as how independent he or she is as compared to peers. Deficits in adaptive functioning can include not meeting developmental or social milestones as well as difficulty functioning in two or more of the following: communication, self-care, home living, social skills/participation, use of the community, self-direction, health, safety, academics, leisure activities, and work.

Assessment and Treatment

Assessment of people with suspected intellectual disability involves a psychologist's assessment of intellectual functioning through an intelligence test. In addition, SLPs would assess both symbolic (e.g., words) and nonsymbolic (e.g., gestures) communication, play, social communication and interaction, receptive and expressive language skills, speech, and oral motor skills. An audiologist would assess hearing abilities.

Treatment by the SLP is indicated if a person's language abilities lags behind his or her cognitive abilities. For example, a 12-year-old child with the cognitive level of a 5 year old but language abilities of a 3 year old would be a prime candidate for speech language therapy because there is a gap between cognition and language. However, if the child's cognitive and language levels matched, then speech language treatment might not be indicated because the child would be doing as well as he or she could. For those who qualify for treatment, therapy would be individualized for each person, but could focus on treatment targets like turn-taking, social interaction through play, speech and language production, and/or literacy.

Brain Tumors

What Are They?

Brain tumors, also known as **neoplasms** (Greek for "new growth"), are abnormal growths of nervous system cells (**FIGURE 4-29**). Sometimes one of these cells will cease functioning as it should and will replicate

itself, forming a mass of abnormal cells. The names of brain tumors are taken from the type of cell from which they originate. For example, **astrocytomas** develop from astrocytes, and **neuromas** develop from nerve tissue (**TABLE 4-4**). As the mass grows, it can impair brain function in various ways, usually through putting pressure on normal neural tissue (**FIGURE 4-30**).

Tumors of the brain can be benign (approximately 46% of cases) or malignant (approximately 54% of cases) (Centers for Disease Control and Prevention, 2004). Malignant tumors tend to grow quickly and spread to other parts of the body, but benign tumors are slow growing and do not spread. Both are dangerous and potentially lethal because they create increased pressure inside the skull. Brain tumors can originate in the brain (**primary brain tumor**) or somewhere else in the body (**metastatic brain tumor**).

Causes

The cause of these masses is unknown, but it is thought that at least one factor is tumor suppressor genes being turned off, thus allowing cells to go haywire and form masses (Newton, 1994). There is a long list of possible environmental factors, but none, other than ionizing radiation exposure from situations like radiotherapy during childhood, has been definitively linked to brain tumor development. Although epidemiological

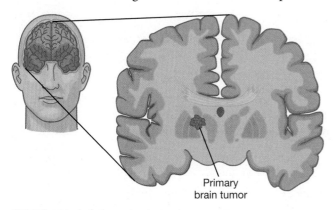

FIGURE 4-29 A primary brain tumor.
Courtesy of the National Library of Medicine.

TABLE 4-4 Select Examples of Brain Tumors		
Name	**Description**	**Where Arises From**
Schwannoma (or acoustic neuroma)	Slow-growing tumor, typically on the 8th cranial nerve, but can affect other cranial or spinal nerves	Sheath around nerve fibers
Astrocytoma	Fast- or slow-growing, invasive, cancerous tumor that rarely spreads outside the brain	Astrocytes
Chordoma	Rare cancerous tumor that occurs at lower spine or base of skull; can metastasize	Leftover cells from fetal development
Craniopharyngioma	Slow-growing tumor near base of skull and optic nerves	Leftover cells from fetal development
Ependymoma	Slow- or fast-growing tumor located near or in the brain ventricles	Ependymal cells that line areas with cerebrospinal fluid
Medulloblastoma	Cancerous tumor found in cerebellum or near brainstem; more common in children	Cells from embryonic stage of development
Meningioma	Benign or cancerous; slow- or fast-growing tumor that compresses brain tissue as it grows, causing neurological symptoms	Cells in the meninges
Oligodendroglioma	Benign or cancerous; slow- or fast-growing tumor found typically in frontal or temporal lobes	Oligodendroglia

Data from: Gould, D. J., & Brueckner-Collins, J. K. (2016). *Neuroanatomy* (5th ed.). Philadelphia, PA: Wolters Kluwer; Bhatnagar, S. C. (2013). *Neuroscience for the study of communicative disorders*. Philadelpia, PA: Lippincott Williams & Wilkins.

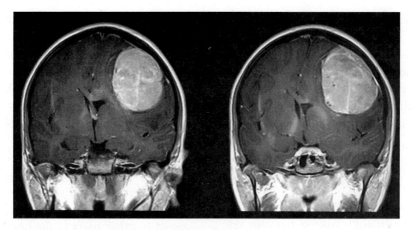

FIGURE 4-30 A magnetic resonance imaging (MRI) scan of the brain showing a large tumor.
© DeanAustinPhotography/iStock/Getty Images.

TABLE 4-5 The World Health Organization's Grading System for CNS Tumors

	Tumor Grade	Description
Low Grade	Grade I tumor	A benign, slow-growing tumor whose cells look almost normal under a microscope. Associated with long-term survival. Least likely to reoccur.
	Grade II tumor	A benign or malignant, slow-growing tumor whose cells look slightly abnormal under a microscope. Has some tendency to spread. Can reoccur as a higher grade tumor.
High Grade	Grade III tumor	A malignant, fast-growing tumor whose cells look abnormal under a microscope. Has a tendency to spread and a tendency to reoccur as a higher grade tumor.
	Grade IV tumor	A malignant, fast-growing tumor whose cells look very abnormal under a microscope. Tumor forms own vascular system to power its growth and invasiveness. Tumor has necrosis in its center.

Data from: Eckley, M., & Wargo, K. A. (2010). A review of glioblastoma multiforme. *U.S. Pharmacist, 35*(5), 3-10.

evidence suggests a connection between cell phone use and brain tumors, no definitive connection has been established at this time (Bondy et al., 2008; Khurana, Teo, Kundi, Hardell, & Carlberg, 2009; Peter, Linet, & Heineman, 1995).

Signs and Symptoms

Symptoms of brain tumors can include headache, seizures, personality changes, motor (e.g., paralysis) impairment, and sensory impairment (e.g., visual changes). Patients can also experience speech, language, hearing, and cognitive problems. Other problems include nausea, vomiting, fatigue, and drowsiness.

Diagnosis and Treatment

Tumors are diagnosed through consideration of the patient's signs and symptoms and through neuroimaging studies such as computed tomography and magnetic resonance imaging. Part of the diagnostic process is grading the tumor with the World Health Organization's grading system for CNS tumors (TABLE 4-5). Grading a tumor means determining how serious it is. Treatment typically involves tumor resection (i.e., surgery) for both benign and cancerous tumors and radiation, and/or chemotherapy for cancerous tumors (Weiner & Goetz, 2004). The treatment of choice depends on the tumor's grade.

Amyotrophic Lateral Sclerosis

What Is It?

Amyotrophic lateral sclerosis (ALS), also known as Lou Gehrig disease, is the most well-known type of motor neuron disease (MND). Other MNDs include pseudobulbar palsy, primary lateral sclerosis, progressive muscular atrophy, and progressive bulbar palsy (**TABLE 4-6**). As the name implies, MND is a problem with motor neurons. In ALS, both the upper and the lower motor neurons wither, whereas in other MNDs either the lower or the upper motor neurons are affected (**FIGURE 4-31**). ALS typically has an onset between the ages of 40 and 60 years and is more common in men than in women. The condition affects about 3.9 out of 100,000 people (Mehta et al., 2014).

Causes

About 10% of ALS cases occur due to familial inheritance, but the remaining 90% of cases occur for unknown reasons (National Institute of Neurological Disorders and Stroke [NINDS], 2018). One recent study has implicated prions (misfolded proteins) as a possible cause of familial ALS (Grad et al., 2011).

TABLE 4-6 Motor Neuron Disorders

Name	Description
Amyotrophic lateral sclerosis	Progressive neurological disease of the upper and lower motor neurons
Pseudobulbar palsy	Progressive neurological disease of the upper motor neurons that has many of the symptoms of progressive bulbar palsy, a condition affecting the lower motor neurons
Primary lateral sclerosis	Progressive neurological disease of the upper motor neurons
Primary muscular atrophy	Progressive neurological disease of the lower motor neurons in the spinal cord
Progressive bulbar palsy	Progressive neurological disease of the lowest motor neurons in the brainstem

Data from: National Institute of Neurological Disorders & Stroke. (2018). Motor neuron diseases fact sheet. Retrieved from https://www.ninds.nih.gov/Disorders/Patient-Caregiver-Education/Fact-Sheets/Motor-Neuron-Diseases-Fact-Sheet

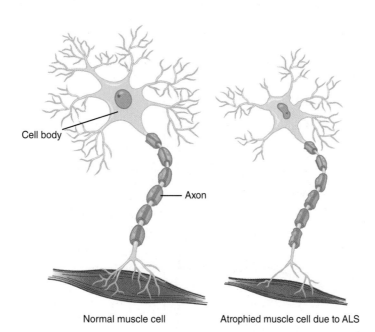

Cell body

Axon

Normal muscle cell   Atrophied muscle cell due to ALS

FIGURE 4-31 Healthy neuron versus neuron with amyotrophic lateral sclerosis (ALS). Note how the ALS neuron is withered and smaller than the normal neuron.

Signs and Symptoms

ALS is characterized by progressive weakness that often begins in the hands, feet, or mouth. Most patients die from respiratory failure within 3 to 5 years, but a small percentage may live 10 or more years. In addition to progressive weakness, patients experience dysarthria that progresses to speechlessness, dysphagia, and dyspnea (i.e., breathing difficulty).

Diagnosis and Treatment

ALS is diagnosed through a combination of clinical presentation and ruling out other MNDs. There is no cure or effective treatment at this time (NINDS, 2018), but a drug, riluzole, has been used successfully in some patients. The drug slows the progression of symptoms and delays the need for ventilator support. It may add a few months to a person's life, but not years (Carlesi et al., 2011).

Multiple Sclerosis

What Is It?

In **multiple sclerosis (MS**; "multiple scarring"), the myelin sheath around the axon is damaged, impairing the ability of neurons to communicate with other neurons and muscles. The condition has an onset between 20 and 50 years of age and affects 150 out of 100,000 people (Dilokthornsakul et al., 2016).

Causes

The cause of MS is the body's own immune system, which attacks the myelin, resulting in progressive scarring of the brain's white matter (**FIGURE 4-32**). Why does the body attack itself? The answer to that question is still unknown, though some have posited it has polygenic origins (i.e., from multiple genes) (Compston & Coles, 2002). MS is more common in women than in men, usually first appearing in the person's 30s. It can appear in one of four different forms (**FIGURE 4-33**). The first form is relapsing–remitting (RR) MS, in which the patient either has an

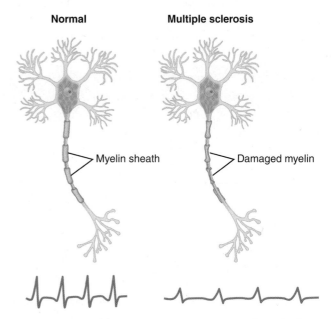

FIGURE 4-32 Healthy neuron versus neuron with multiple sclerosis (MS). Note how the myelin has been depleted on the axon. The jagged lines below the picture show the relative firing strength of each neuron.

Modified from © Alila Medical Media/Shutterstock.

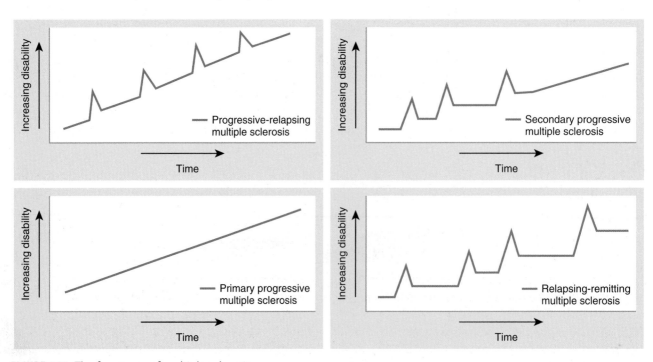

FIGURE 4-33 The four types of multiple sclerosis.

attack with full recovery or has a full attack with some residual deficits. Second, primary progressive (PP) MS progresses steadily without recovery or remission. Third, secondary progressive (SP) MS begins like RR MS, but over time transitions into the steady decline of PP MS. Fourth, progressive-relapsing (PR) MS shows steady progression with ongoing attacks (Lublin & Reingold, 1996).

Signs and Symptoms

Almost any symptom can be manifested because of MS. Patients report a "pins and needles" prickling sensation in the fingers and/or toes, numbness, and weakness. Both speech and swallowing problems can result. Patients also have issues with walking and balance. Once thought to be uncommon, hearing problems in patients with MS are now receiving greater attention. Lewis et al. (2010) reported that people with MS had poorer hearing thresholds than a control group (also see Saberi, Hatamian, Nemati, Banan, & Honarmand, 2012).

Diagnosis and Treatment

The diagnosis of MS is made through clinical presentation and neuroimaging. There is no cure for this disease, but there are medications, such as corticosteroids or interferon beta-1a, that can lessen inflammation and the symptoms of the condition (Compston & Coles, 2002). Rehabilitative therapy is also beneficial for speeding recovery after attacks.

Myasthenia Gravis

What Is It?

Myasthenia gravis (MG; "grave muscle weakness") is a progressive autoimmune disease of the neuromuscular junction that affects women in their 30s and men in their 50s (Weiner & Goetz, 2004). The body's antibodies block postsynaptic ACh receptors at the neuromuscular junction, resulting in muscle weakness and fatigue, which affects muscles involved with speaking and swallowing. One of the hallmark signs of the disorder is ptosis or droopy eyelids (Conti-Fine, Milani, & Kaminski, 2006).

Causes

In MG, the immune system malfunctions and sends antibodies that attack or block ACh receptors on the postsynaptic membrane. It is unknown why some people have an impaired immune system and what the specific antigen is, but genetics may play a role in developing the disease.

Signs and Symptoms

Two of the primary signs of MG are increasing weakness as muscles are used, but improvement of muscle function after rest, and drooping of both eyelids (ptosis). Patients may also complain of double vision (diplopia), dysarthria, and dysphagia.

Diagnosis and Treatment

MG is diagnosed through clinical presentation as well as the presence of ACh antibodies. Drug therapy, such as the use of steroids, can reduce the severity of symptoms. Thymectomy, which involves the removal of the thymus gland from the chest, has been a common surgical technique for the condition with mixed results (Weiner & Goetz, 2004).

Guillain–Barré Syndrome

What Is It?

Guillain–Barré syndrome (GBS), named after the French physicians who first described it, is a rapid, progressive demyelinating disease of the PNS. There are different types of GBS, but the most commonly occurring form involves the body having an autoimmune response to the Schwann cells. When damaged, these cells cannot lay down the myelin needed by the PNS. Paralysis usually begins in the feet and hands, and progresses to the trunk. The maximum impact of the disease happens at about 1 month and may affect the respiratory muscles. Patients will then experience partial or full recovery over the course of weeks to months.

Causes

The disease's cause is unknown, but it is thought to be caused by an autoimmune response, botulism poisoning, or a viral infection (Kemp, Burns, & Brown, 2008; Weiner & Goetz, 2004). The thought is that one of these conditions can trigger an autoimmune response that results in GBS.

Signs and Symptoms

The primary sign of GBS is progressive weakness that begins in the feet and progresses to the upper body or weakness that begins in the face and hands and progresses to the lower body. Sensory issues also often appear in the form of a pins and needles sensation. As the weakness progresses, patients will have trouble walking and controlling their bowel and bladder functions. When the disease is at its worst, the patient will struggle with breathing and will typically need ventilator support.

Diagnosis and Treatment

GBS is difficult to identify in its early stages and is typically diagnosed through clinical presentation as the condition worsens. Because of GBS's effect on the respiratory muscles, the disease is a medical emergency requiring prompt intervention to maintain respiratory support. The patient will rapidly lose the ability to speak and swallow, so the SLP must be involved to assess when the patient will need alternate means of communication and nutrition. The SLP should also be assessing the patient's readiness for oral hydration and nutrition as he or she recovers from GBS. There are drug treatments that can shorten recovery times, but there is no cure for GBS at this time (Weiner & Goetz, 2004).

▶ Conclusion

Neurons are tiny cells, and a powerful microscope is required to see them. Even though they are small, damage to neurons can lead to serious neurological disorders, such as intellectual disability. In this chapter, the form and function of neurons have been reviewed as well as some diseases involving neurons. Many people with communication disorders suffer from these disorders; having a foundational understanding of neurons will help the SLP and audiologist have a better appreciation of people and their struggles with disorders caused by diseases of nervous system cells.

SUMMARY OF LEARNING OBJECTIVES

The following were the main learning objectives of this chapter. The information that should have been learned is below each learning objective.

1. The learner will define the following: *molecule, cell, tissue, organ, and system.*
   - *Molecule:* two or more atoms held together by a chemical bond
   - *Cell:* the fundamental unit of an organism
   - *Tissue:* groups of similar cells that come together to carry out certain functions
   - *Organ:* various tissues brought together to carry out certain functions
   - *System:* organs grouped together to carry out certain functions
2. The learner will list and briefly describe each nervous system cell.
   - *Neuron:* a cell with specialized projections that transfers information throughout the body via an electrochemical process
   - *Astrocytes:* star-shaped cells that nourish neurons and help to maintain the neuronal environment
   - *Oligodendroglia:* cells that produce and coat CNS axons with myelin
   - *Schwann cells:* cells that produce and coat PNS axons with myelin
   - *Microglia:* cells that defend nervous system structures by warding off foreign invaders
   - *Satellite cells:* the astrocytes of the PNS that surround neurons, helping to nourish them; also function in neurotransmitter uptake
3. The learner will accurately label the parts of a neuron and synapse.
   - Refer to Figures 4-9 and 4-13.
4. The learner will list and briefly describe the steps in neuron function.
   - *The loaded neuron (polarization):* The neuron is in a polarized state due to chemical and electrical imbalances.
   - *The firing neuron (depolarization):* Neurotransmitters are released into the synaptic cleft and fit into postsynaptic receptors. As a result, molecular gates open, allowing Na^+ in and erasing the former imbalances. These actions cause an action potential to run down the neuron.
   - *The reloading of the neuron (repolarization):* The molecular gates close, and through the sodium–potassium pump, polarization is reestablished.
   - *The all-or-none principle:* Neurons function in an all-or-none manner, meaning they either fire or they do not.
5. The learner will list and briefly describe select nervous system disorders involving nervous system cells.
   - *Intellectual disability:* significantly subaverage general intellectual functioning, existing concurrently with deficits in adaptive behavior and manifested during the developmental period, that adversely affects a child's educational performance
   - *Brain tumors:* abnormal growths of nervous system cells
   - *Amyotrophic lateral sclerosis:* a disease of the motor neurons leading to increasing weakness leading to eventual paralysis

- *Multiple sclerosis:* when the myelin sheath around the axon is damaged due to an autoimmune response, impairing the ability of neurons to communicate with other neurons and muscles

- *Myasthenia gravis:* a progressive autoimmune disease of the neuromuscular junction that leads to increasing weakness
- *Guillain–Barré syndrome:* a rapid, progressive demyelinating disease of the PNS from which patients usually improve

KEY TERMS

Absolute refractory period
Acetylcholine (ACh)
Action potential
Afferent communication
All-or-none principle
Amyotrophic lateral sclerosis (ALS)
Astrocytes
Astrocytomas
Axoaxonic synapse
Axodendritic synapse
Axons
Axosomatic synapse
Cells
Cell theory
Centrosome
Cytoskeleton
Dendrites
Depolarization
Dopamine
Dynamic polarization of neurons
Efferent communication
Endoplasmic reticulum
Epinephrine

Gamma-aminobutyric acid (GABA)
Glial cells
Glutamate
Golgi apparatus
Gradient
Guillain–Barré syndrome (GBS)
Intellectual disability
Interneurons
Ionotropic receptors
Law of specific nerve energies
Lysosomes
Membrane
Metabotropic receptors
Metastatic brain tumor
Microglia
Microtubules
Mitochondria
Molecules
Motor neurons
Multiple sclerosis (MS)
Myasthenia gravis (MG)
Myelin
Myelination

Neoplasms
Neurites
Neuromas
Neuron
Neuron doctrine
Neurotransmitters
Norepinephrine
Nucleolus
Nucleus
Oligodendroglia
Organs
Primary brain tumor
Relative refractory period
Ribosomes
Satellite cells
Schwann cells
Sensory neurons
Serotonin
Soma
Substance P
Synapses
Systems
Tissue
Transport
Wallerian degeneration

DRAW IT TO KNOW IT

1. Draw a neuron (see Figure 4-9) and label the following parts: dendrite, cell body, axon, and axon terminals.

2. Draw a synapse (see Figure 4-13) and label the following parts: vesicles, presynaptic membrane, synaptic cleft, postsynaptic membrane, and receptors.

QUESTIONS FOR DEEPER REFLECTION

1. Write an essay describing neuron function.

2. Explain what the absolute and relative refractory periods are, and include graphs and other pictures to illustrate these concepts.

CASE STUDIES

Janet is a department secretary at a university. She has noticed over the last few months difficulty hearing faculty and students in her left ear. She compensates by turning her right ear to people when they speak to her. In addition to this left ear hearing loss, Janet has begun to experience a ringing in her left ear and some dizziness. Janet was referred to an audiologist by her primary care physician who diagnosed her with a high-frequency sensorineural hearing loss. The audiologist referred Janet to a neurologist who ordered an MRI. The MRI revealed a brain tumor on the eighth cranial nerve.

1. What type of brain tumor is the likely type in this case?
2. Is this type of brain tumor fast or slow growing?
3. What type of treatment might Janet receive for her brain tumor?

Mark is a 23-year-old graduate student who experienced flu-like symptoms for a week followed by a 1-month decline in his motor and sensory abilities. His respiratory function was even affected, requiring a ventilator. After this 1-month period, Mark began to recover his motor and sensory abilities. His physician believes he will make a full recovery. Which of the following conditions is the most likely? Explain why you chose this answer.

1. Multiple sclerosis
2. Guillain–Barré syndrome
3. Myasthenia gravis
4. Amyotrophic lateral sclerosis

SUGGESTED PROJECTS

1. Pick one of the neurotransmitters mentioned in this chapter and write a two- to three-page paper about what it is, what it does, and disorders associated with either too much or too little of it.
2. Search through scholarly journals and find a case study on one of the neurological disorders mentioned in this chapter. Present the case to your class.
3. Pick one of the neurological disorders mentioned in this chapter and write a two- to three-page paper with the following sections: cause, signs/symptoms, diagnosis, treatment, speech/language/hearing issues.

REFERENCES

Alberts, B., Bray, D., Lewis, J., Raff, M., Roberts, K., & Watson, J. D. (1983). *Molecular biology of the cell*. New York, NY: Garland Publishing.

Allen, N. J., & Barres, B. A. (2009). Glia—more than just brain glue. *Nature, 457*, 675–677.

Araya, R., Eisenthal, K. B., & Yuste, R. (2006). Dendritic spines linearize the summation of excitatory potentials. *Proceedings of the National Academy of Sciences, 103*(49), 18799–18804.

Araya, R., Jiang, J., Eisenthal, K. B., & Yuste, R. (2006). The spine neck filters membrane potentials. *Proceedings of the National Academy of Sciences, 103*(47), 17961–17966.

Arellano, J. I., Benavides, R., DeFelipe, J., & Yuste, R. (2007). Ultrastructure of dendritic spines: Correlation between synaptic and spine morphologies. *Frontiers in Neuroscience, 1*(1), 131–143.

Bear, M. F., Connors, B. W., & Paradiso, M. A. (2007). *Neuroscience: Exploring the brain*. Baltimore, MD: Lippincott Williams & Wilkins.

Blumenfeld, H. (2010). *Neuroanatomy through clinical cases*. Sunderland, MA: Sinauer Associates.

Bondy, M. L., Scheurer, M. E., Malmer, B., Barnholtz-Sloan, J. S., Davis, F. G., & Il'yasova, D., . . . Buffler, P. A. (2008). Brain tumor epidemiology: Consensus from the Brain Tumor Epidemiology Consortium. *Cancer, 113*(S7), 1953–1968.

Carlesi, C., Pasquali, L., Piazza, S., Lo Gerfo, A., Caldarazzo Ienco, E., & Alessi, R., . . . Siciliano, G. (2011). Strategies for clinical approach to neurodegeneration in amyotrophic lateral sclerosis. *Archives Italiennes de Biologie, 149*(1), 151–167.

Centers for Disease Control and Prevention (CDC). (2004). *Data collection of primary central nervous system tumors*. National Program of Cancer Registries Training Materials. Atlanta, GA: U.S. Department of Health and Human Services, Centers for Disease Control and Prevention.

Compston, A., & Coles, A. (2002). Multiple sclerosis. *The Lancet, 359*, 1221–1231.

Conti-Fine, B. M., Milani, M., & Kaminski, H. J. (2006). Myasthenia gravis: Past, present, and future. *Journal of Clinical Investigation, 116*(11), 2843.

Dilokthornsakul, P., Valuck, R., Nair, K., Corboy, J., Allen, R., & Campbell, J. (2016). Multiple sclerosis prevalence in the United States commercially insured population. *Neurology, 86*, 1014–1021.

Fields, R. D. (2009). *The other brain: From dementia to schizophrenia, how new discoveries about the brain are revolutionizing medicine and science*. New York, NY: Simon and Schuster.

Gourine, A. V., Kasymov, V., Marina, N., Tang, F., Figueiredo, M. F., & Lane, S., . . . Kasparov, S. (2010). Astrocytes control breathing through pH-dependent release of ATP. *Science, 329*(5991), 571–575.

Grad, L. I., Guest, W. C., Yanai, A., Pokrishevsky, E., O'Neill, M. A., & Gibbs, E., . . . Cashman, N. R. (2011). Intermolecular transmission of superoxide dismutase 1 misfolding in living cells. *Proceedings of the National Academy of Sciences, 108*(39), 16398–16403.

Guyton, A. C., & Hall, J. E. (2006). *Textbook of medical physiology* (11th ed.). Philadelphia, PA: Elsevier Saunders.

Hanani, M. (2010). Satellite glial cells in sympathetic and parasympathetic ganglia: In search of function. *Brain Research Reviews, 64*(2), 304–327.

Herculano-Houzel, S. (2009). The human brain in numbers: A linearly scaled-up primate brain. *Frontiers in Human Neuroscience, 3*(31), 1–11.

Individuals with Disabilities Education Improvement Act (IDEA) of 2004, PL 108-446, 20 U.S.C. § 1400 et seq.

Kandel, E. R., Schwartz, J. H., Jessell, T. M., Siegelbaum, S. A., & Hudspeth, A. J. (2013). *Principles of neural science* (5th ed.). New York, NY: McGraw-Hill.

Kemp, W. L., Burns, D. K., & Brown, T. G. (2008). *Pathology: The big picture.* New York, NY: McGraw-Hill Medical.

Khurana, V. G., Teo, C., Kundi, M., Hardell, L., & Carlberg, M. (2009). Cell phones and brain tumors: A review including the long-term epidemiologic data. *Surgical Neurology, 72*(3), 205–214.

Jessell, T. M., & Kandel, E. R. (1993). Synaptic transmission: A bidirectional and self-modifiable form of cell-cell communication. *Cell, 72*, 1–30.

Lewis, M. S., Lilly, D. J., Hutter, M. M., Bourdette, D. N., McMillan, G. P., Fitzpatrick, M. A., & Fausti, S. A. (2010). Audiometric hearing status of individuals with and without multiple sclerosis. *Journal of Rehabilitation Research and Development, 47*(7), 669–678.

Lublin, F. D., & Reingold, S. C. (1996). Defining the clinical course of multiple sclerosis: Results of an international survey. *Neurology, 46*(4), 907–911.

McQuarrie, D. A., & Rock, P. A. (1984). *General chemistry.* New York, NY: WH Freeman and Company.

Mehta, P., Antao, V., Kaye, W., Sanchez, M., Williamson, D., & Bryan, L., . . . Horton, K. (2014). Prevalence of amyotrophic lateral sclerosis—United States, 2010–2011. *Morbidity and Mortality Weekly Report: Surveillance Summaries, 63*(7), 1–13.

National Institute of Neurological Disorders and Stroke (NINDS). (2018). *Motor neuron diseases fact sheet.* Retrieved from https://www.ninds.nih.gov/Disorders/Patient-Caregiver-Education/Fact-Sheets/Motor-Neuron-Diseases-Fact-Sheet

Newton, H. B. (1994). Primary brain tumors: Review of etiology, diagnosis and treatment. *American Family Physician, 49*(4), 787.

Nolte, J. (2002). *The human brain: An introduction to its functional anatomy.* St. Louis, MO: Mosby.

Peter, I. D., Linet, M. S., & Heineman, E. F. (1995). Etiology of brain tumors in adults. *Epidemiologic Reviews, 17*(2), 382–414.

Purves, D. (2004). *Neuroscience.* Sunderland, MA: Sinauer Associates.

Saberi, A., Hatamian, H. R., Nemati, S., Banan, R., & Honarmand, H. (2012). Hearing statement in multiple sclerosis: A case control study using auditory brainstem responses and otoacoustic emissions. *Acta Medica Iranica, 50*(10), 679–683.

Seikel, J. A., King, D. W., & Drumright, D. G. (2010). *Anatomy and physiology for speech, language, and hearing.* Clifton Park, NY: Delmar.

Shapiro, B. K., & Batshaw, M. L. (2013). Developmental delay and intellectual disability. In M. L. Batshaw, N. J. Rosen, & G. R. Lotrecchiano (Eds.), *Children with disabilities* (pp. 291–306). Baltimore, MD: Paul H. Brookes Publishing Company.

Snell, R. S. (2001). *Clinical neuroanatomy for medical students* (5th ed.). Baltimore, MD: Lippincott Williams & Wilkins.

Wallace, R. A., King, J. L., & Sanders, G. P. (1986). *Biology: The science of life.* Glenview, IL: Scott Foresman.

Webster, D. B. (1999). *Neuroscience of communication* (2nd ed.). San Diego, CA: Singular Publishing.

Weiner, W. J., & Goetz, C. G. (2004). *Neurology for the non-neurologist.* Baltimore, MD: Lippincott Williams & Wilkins.

Zemlin, W. R. (1998). *Speech and hearing science: Anatomy and physiology.* Boston, MA: Allyn and Bacon.

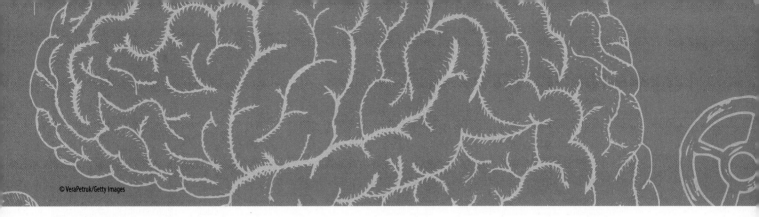

© VeraPetruk/Getty Images

CHAPTER 5

The Spinal Cord, Brainstem, Cranial Nerves, and Cerebellum

CHAPTER PREVIEW

It is now time to embark on a journey through macroscopic structures (i.e., structures that can be observed with the naked eye). We will begin this leg of the journey at the bottom, with the spinal cord, and make our way up to the spinal nerves, brainstem, cranial nerves, and cerebellum.

IN THIS CHAPTER

In this chapter, we will . . .
- Survey the form and function of the spinal cord and discuss spinal cord injury
- Explore the structure and function of the brainstem
- Review select disorders of the brainstem
- Study the cranial nerves and their relationship to speech, swallowing, and hearing
- Survey the form and function of the cerebellum

93

LEARNING OBJECTIVES

- The learner will label a diagram of a cross-section of the spinal cord.
- The learner will label a diagram of the brainstem.
- The learner will be able to list all the cranial nerves (Roman numeral and name).
- The learner will list important cranial nerves for articulation, voice, swallowing, and hearing.
- The learner will describe the form and function of the cerebellum.

▶ Introduction

The spinal cord serves as a sort of communications superhighway for motor or efferent communication from the brain to the body and sensory or afferent communication from the body to the brain. The spinal cord extends from the bottom of the vertebral column up to the brainstem's medulla. This chapter will begin by surveying the spinal cord's form and function as well as spinal cord injury. We will continue the journey through the brain by also studying spinal nerves, the brainstem, cranial nerves, and the cerebellum.

▶ The Spinal Cord

Ranging from 17 to 18 inches (43–46 cm) in length and ¼ to ½ inch (0.6–1.3 cm) in diameter, the spinal cord is a vital organ for interacting with our environment. Contained within it are both motor

and sensory fibers that transmit information regarding our movement and sense experiences as well as our reflexes. The spinal cord is surrounded by the bony vertebral column and a three-layered membrane called the meninges (**FIGURE 5-1**). Within these membranes, there is the arachnoid space filled with cerebrospinal fluid, essentially wrapping the spinal cord in a watery cushion.

Spinal Cord Form

External Organization

Like the vertebral column, the spinal cord is organized into five regions. The neck area is the cervical region, the chest is the thoracic region, the lower back is the lumbar region, the pelvis is the sacral region, and the tailbone area is the coccygeal region (**FIGURE 5-2**).

Spinal nerves emerge from the spinal cord and innervate the body below the neck (**FIGURE 5-3**). They are organized by neuroanatomists using the same

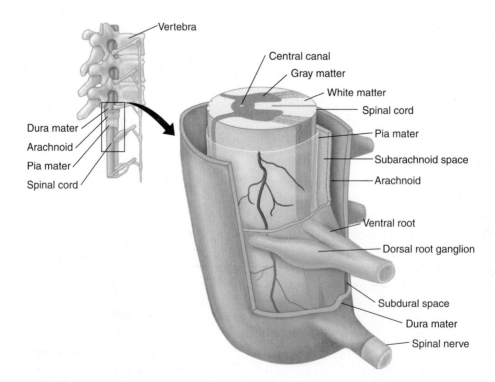

FIGURE 5-1 The vertebral column and spinal cord, which is surrounded by three layers: the dura mater, the arachnoid mater, and the pia mater.

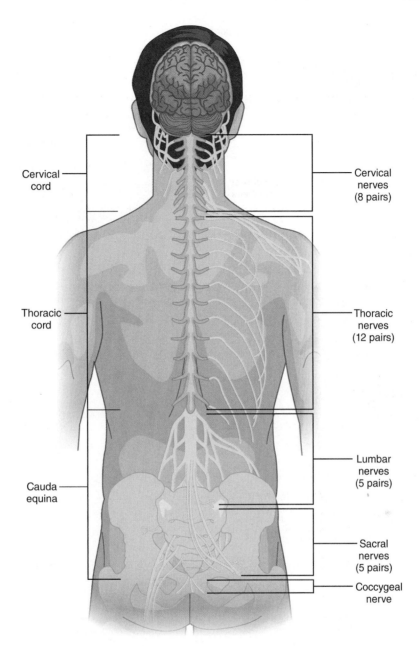

FIGURE 5-2 The five regions of the vertebral column and spinal cord.

divisions used to organize the spinal cord (e.g., cervical spinal nerves). The spinal nerves carry afferent (sensory) and/or efferent (motor) information. There are two types of nerve fibers in spinal nerves, general somatic and general visceral. **General somatic efferent (GSE) fibers** carry motor information to skeletal muscles and **general visceral efferent (GVE) fibers** carry motor information to smooth muscle, the heart, and glands. **General somatic afferent (GSA) fibers** carry sensory information from the skin, and **general visceral afferent (GVA) fibers** carry sensory information from the lungs and digestive tract (**FIGURE 5-4**).

As the ventral rami leave the spinal cord and vertebral column, some of them form a network (except for the thoracic region) called a **plexus**. These networks then branch out and innervate certain parts of the body. Because innervation of limbs comes out of these networks, damage to one spinal root will not result in a totally paralyzed limb. The general motor or efferent functions of each spinal nerve plexus are presented in **TABLE 5-1**. For an example of a plexus, see **FIGURE 5-5**, which is an illustration of the cervical plexus. This plexus (C1–C4) is responsible for innervating some muscles of the neck. For example, the following neck muscles function to lower the larynx:

- Sternohyoid (laryngeal depressor innervated by cervical spinal nerves 1, 2, and 3)
- Thyrohyoid (laryngeal depressor innervated by cervical spinal nerve 1 and cranial nerve XII)

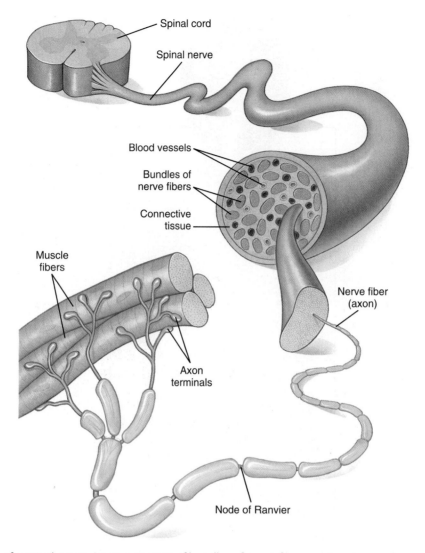

FIGURE 5-3 Structure of a spinal nerve. A nerve consists of bundles of nerve fibers, various layers of connective tissue, and blood vessels.

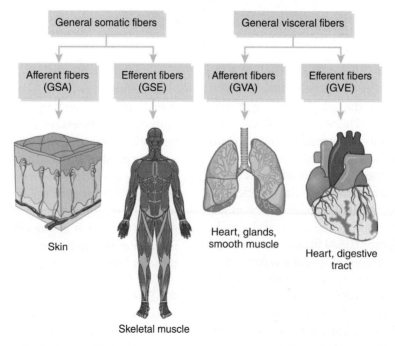

FIGURE 5-4 Different types of spinal nerve fibers.

TABLE 5-1 The Spinal Nerves, Their Plexuses, and Some of Their Motor Functions

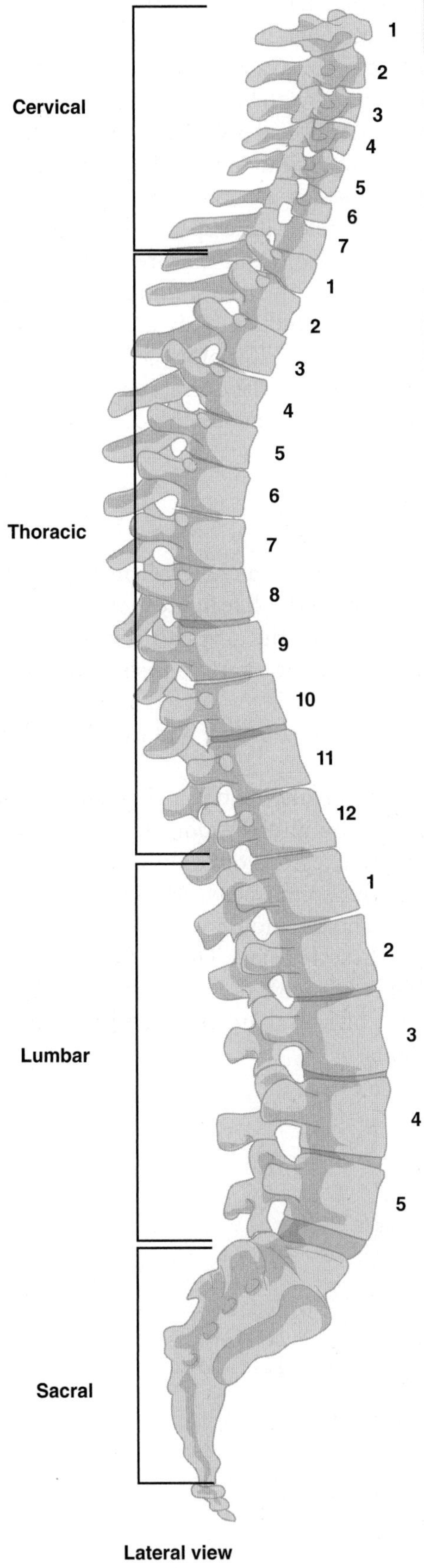

Lateral view

Cervical
Thoracic
Lumbar
Sacral

Spinal Nerve	Plexus	Motor Function
C1		
C2	Cervical plexus	Innervates muscles of neck and diaphragm
C3		
C4		
C5		
C6	Brachial plexus	Innervates pectoral girdle and upper limbs
C7		
T1		
T2		
T3		
T4		
T5		
T6	Intercostal spinal nerves (no plexus formation)	Innervate trunk muscle
T7		
T8		
T9		
T10		
T11		
T12		
L1		
L2		
L3		
L4	Lumbosacral plexus	Innervates pelvic girdle and lower limbs
L5		
Sacral		
Coccyx		

- Omohyoid (laryngeal depressor innervated by cervical spinal nerves 1, 2, and 3)
- Sternothyroid (laryngeal depressor innervated by cervical spinal nerves 1, 2, and 3)

The **phrenic nerve** originates mainly from the fourth cervical spinal nerve but receives some help from the third and fifth cervical spinal nerves. This nerve innervates the diaphragm, which, along with other muscles, is crucial for supplying the air power for speech.

Beginning laterally, each spinal nerve has a dorsal ramus (branch) and a ventral branch (**FIGURE 5-6A**). The dorsal ramus carries motor and sensory information (GSE and GSA) to and from the dorsal or posterior part of the body; the ventral ramus carries the same type of information to and from the ventral or anterior part. Moving medially, these two branches meet outside the vertebral column to form the spinal nerve. Still outside the vertebral column, another branch joins the spinal nerve. This branch is called the ramus communicantis, and it contains motor and sensory visceral nerve fibers (GVE and GVA).

Moving inside the vertebral column, the spinal nerve splits into a dorsal and a ventral root. The dorsal root is sensory, containing GVA and GSA fibers. In terms of general somatic sensation (GSA), each spinal nerve has an association with a specific skin region, known as a **dermatome** (from the Greek: *derma* = "skin"; *tome* comes from *temnein*, meaning "to cut"). The dermatomes of the human body are mapped in **FIGURE 5-7**. The ventral root is motor (GVE and GSE) (**FIGURE 5-6B**). Bulging from the dorsal root is the dorsal root ganglion, which contains the cell bodies of pseudounipolar neurons.

Internal Organization

A cross-section of the spinal cord is presented in Figure 5-6B. A gray butterfly-like figure in the midst of a white circle is apparent. The gray part is made up of neuron cell bodies, and the white consists of myelinated neuronal axons. We will examine the structure of the spinal cord's white matter first and then consider the gray matter.

The spinal cord's white matter is divided in half by the median fissure and the dorsal, lateral, and ventral white-matter regions or columns duplicated on each side of the spinal cord. Major ascending sensory and descending motor pathways or tracts course through these regions. These pathways are pictured in **FIGURE 5-8**, with the blue sections highlighting sensory pathways and red sections denoting motor systems.

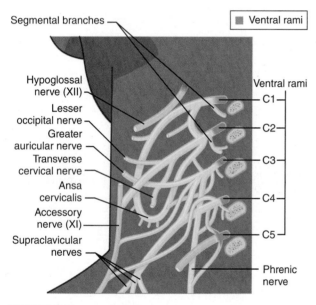

Segmental branches

Hypoglossal nerve (XII)
Lesser occipital nerve
Greater auricular nerve
Transverse cervical nerve
Ansa cervicalis
Accessory nerve (XI)
Supraclavicular nerves

■ Ventral rami

Ventral rami
C1
C2
C3
C4
C5
Phrenic nerve

FIGURE 5-5 The cervical plexus.

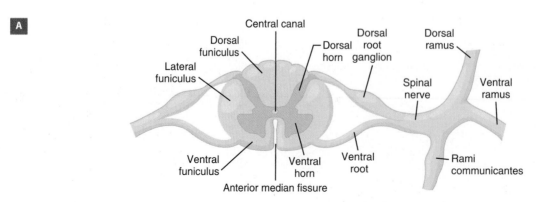

A

Central canal
Dorsal funiculus
Lateral funiculus
Dorsal root horn
Dorsal root ganglion
Dorsal ramus
Spinal nerve
Ventral ramus
Ventral funiculus
Ventral horn
Ventral root
Rami communicantes
Anterior median fissure

FIGURE 5-6A   A. Cross-section of the spinal cord showing spinal nerve connections.

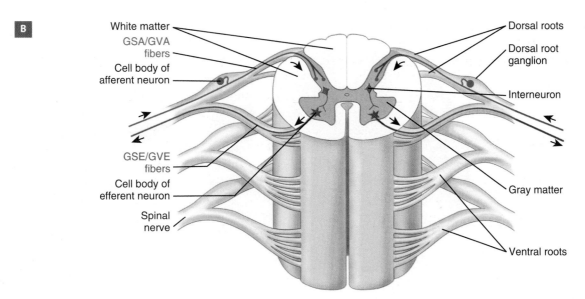

FIGURE 5-6B **B.** Cross-section of the spinal cord showing GSA/GVA and GSE/GVE fiber input and output.

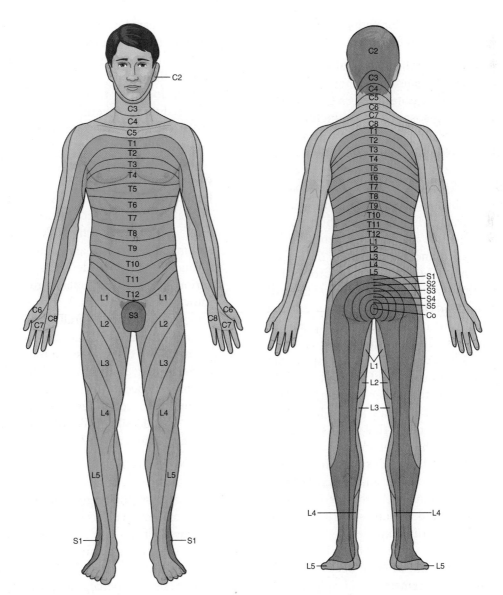

FIGURE 5-7 Dermatomes of the human body. Dermatomes are the sensory areas served by each of the spinal nerves.

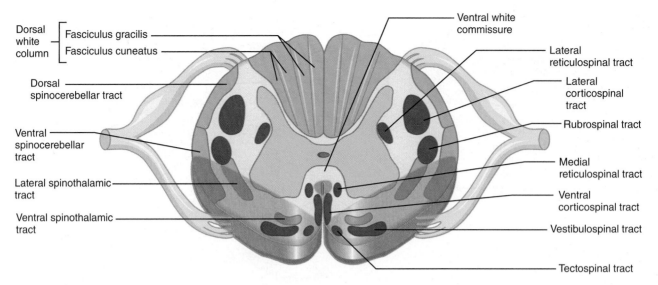

FIGURE 5-8 Cross-section of the spinal cord at the cervical levels showing motor (in red) and sensory pathways (in blue).

The major descending motor pathways in the spinal cord's white matter are as follows:

- **Lateral corticospinal/corticobulbar tract**: This nerve tract originates in the motor cortex of the frontal lobe, decussates (i.e., changes sides) at the lower medulla–spinal cord juncture, and then inputs along the spinal cord at the ventral horns (**FIGURE 5-9**). That part of the tract from the cortex to the brainstem is called the corticobulbar tract (*bulbar* refers to the brainstem because of its bulbus appearance). Motor neurons in this tract arise in the cerebral cortex input into brainstem nuclei or the ventral horn of the spinal cord and are known as the upper motor neurons (UMNs). Motor neurons that leave the brainstem nuclei or the ventral horn of the spinal cord and connect to muscles are called the lower motor neurons (LMNs). Symptoms of UMN damage are different than those of LMN damage (**BOX 5-1**). Functionally, it is responsible for contralateral movement of the body and, in the case of the corticobulbar portion, contralateral movement of muscles in the head and some muscles in the neck. This tract is of major importance to speech production.
- **Anterior (or ventral) corticospinal tract**: This tract originates in the motor and premotor areas of the frontal lobe and then courses ipsilateral down the spinal cord, inputting at the ventral horn. It controls the trunk muscles.
- **Rubrospinal tract**: The rubrospinal tract begins in the midbrain, where it decussates and courses down the brainstem and spinal cord until inputting in the ventral horn of the spinal cord. In terms of function, it modulates flexor tone in the upper extremities. Flexor tone is the amount of tension present in muscles when a joint is flexed.
- **Vestibulospinal tract**: This tract originates in the medulla and courses down the spinal cord ipsilateral until inputting into the ventral horn. Functionally, this tract controls extensor tone, which is the amount of tension present in muscles when a joint is extended.
- **Reticulospinal tract**: This tract is made of a medial (pontine) tract and a lateral (medullary) tract. It originates where the brainstem's pons and medulla meet, an area known as the reticular formation, and then descends and terminates at various levels of the spinal cord. It is involved in muscle tone in the trunk muscles as well as the proximal limbs and overall helps to control a person's posture and facilitate gait (walking).
- **Tectospinal tract**: Also known as the colliculospinal tract, the tectospinal tract connects the midbrain (specifically, the superior colliculus of the midbrain) to the cervical regions of the spinal cord. Functionally, it coordinates the movement of the head and neck with the eyes.

Sensory tracts are divided into parts by the neurons that make up the tract. For example, first-order neurons carry sensory signals from the sense receptors to the central nervous system. Second-order neurons decussate from one side of the central nervous system to the other side and input into the thalamus. Third-order neurons route sensory information to the appropriate sensory perception processing area in the cerebral cortex (fourth-order neurons).

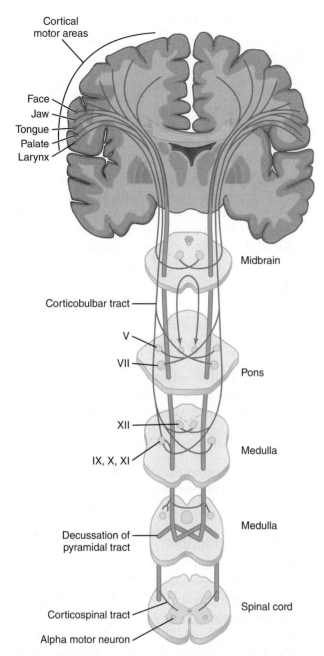

FIGURE 5-9 The lateral corticospinal/corticobulbar tract. This major descending motor pathway mediates volitional motor activity.

The major ascending sensory tracts are as follows:

- **Dorsal columns**: As their name implies, the dorsal columns reside in the dorsal area of the spinal cord. The first-order neuron begins in the sensory receptors and courses through the dorsal root ganglia and synapses with the dorsal horn of the spinal cord. The second-order neuron arises from the dorsal horn, decussates, and then travels to the thalamus, which projects a third-order neuron to the somatosensory cortex

---

BOX 5-1 Upper Motor Neuron Damage Versus Lower Motor Damage

The concept of upper motor neurons (UMNs) and lower motor neurons (LMNs) is not an anatomical notion; rather, it is a neuropathological concept that helps explain the symptoms of chronic UMN versus LMN damage. When the UMNs are initially damaged by a lesion via a stroke, the patient experiences flaccid paralysis, loss of muscle tone (hypotonia), and loss of reflexes (areflexia). As the condition becomes chronic, these symptoms change into the classic signs of UMN damage: spastic weakness (paresis), too much muscle tone (hypertonia), exaggerated reflexes (hyperreflexia), and involuntary muscular contractions and relaxations (clonus). LMN damage is the opposite of chronic UMN damage and resembles acute UMN damage with flaccid paralysis and areflexia. In addition, patients experience muscle wasting (atrophy) and muscle twitches (fasciculations).

(**FIGURE 5-10**). These columns consist of two bundles, the fasciculus gracilis (the slender bundle) and the fasciculus cuneatus (the wedge-shaped bundle). The dorsal columns relay fine and discriminative touch, pressure, and proprioceptive sensory information to the brainstem, then the thalamus, and finally the sensory cortex for final processing. **Proprioception** can be thought of as the body's eyes for itself. In other words, through various receptors throughout the body, the brain has a sense of where its various parts are in space at any given time.

- **Spinothalamic tracts**: There are two spinothalamic tracts, the ventral and the lateral. The lateral tract lies in the lateral portion of the spinal cord and the ventral tract in the ventral portion. Its first-order neuron begins at the sensory receptors and passes through the dorsal root ganglia and synapses with the dorsal horns of the spinal cord. Its second-order neuron then ascends from the dorsal horn to the thalamus. The tract's third-order neuron leaves the thalamus and projects to the somatosensory cortex. Functionally, this tract sends the following sensory information to the somatosensory cortex: pain, temperature, and crude touch. The ventral tract has the same basic route as the lateral tract but is responsible for light touch (e.g., touching the skin with a cotton ball).
- **Spinocerebellar tracts**: There are two spinocerebellar tracts, the ventral tract and the dorsal

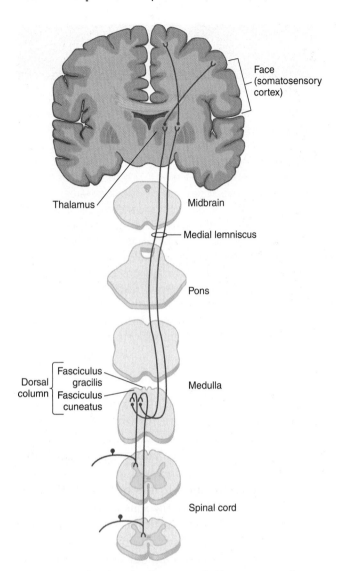

FIGURE 5-10 The dorsal column–medial lemniscus pathway.

tract. Both lie on the lateral edge of the spinal cord, but as the names imply, one is dorsal in location and the other is more ventral. They are two-neuron tracts that originate in peripheral sense receptors. They then course through the dorsal root ganglions and input into the dorsal horn. From there, the dorsal tract ipsilaterally ascends to input in the cerebellum, while the ventral tract decussates and inputs into the cerebellum (second-order neuron). The spinocerebellar tracts convey proprioceptive information about the body to the cerebellum.

The descending and ascending tracts of the spinal cord are summarized in **TABLE 5-2**.

Now we will consider the spinal cord's gray matter. The gray matter consists of the dorsal horn at the top of the butterfly's upper wing and the ventral horn at the bottom. It is at these horns that the spinal

nerve roots connect. Each spinal nerve passes through a notch between the vertebrae. Motor information leaves the spinal cord's ventral root and courses to skeletal muscles and viscera, whereas sensory information enters the spinal cord through the dorsal root via its spinal nerve. Beginning above the first cervical vertebra (C1), this arrangement of dorsal and ventral roots repeats itself 31 times down the length of the spinal cord.

As discussed earlier, the content of the spinal cord white matter is various ascending and descending neural tracts. The dorsal gray matter is divided into six layers and is involved in sensory information (e.g., touch), whereas the ventral gray matter is involved in motor information through different types of LMNs. These neurons are classified by the type of muscle they innervate:

- **Alpha motor neurons** innervate *extrafusal* muscle fibers. These muscle fibers are what contract a muscle.
- **Gamma motor neurons** innervate *intrafusal* muscle spindles. These muscle fibers, which involve both a motor and a sensory neuron, form stretch receptors called muscle spindles. This mechanism is important for proprioception and reflexes.

The motor neuron plus the muscle fiber it innervates are called a **motor unit**.

Spinal Cord Function

As mentioned in the introduction, motor and sensory information passes up and down the spinal cord between the body and the brain. The major motor and sensory tracts and their functions have already been outlined. There is one last important topic to cover—reflexes. Reflexes are lightning-quick responses to stimuli controlled at the level of the spinal cord and spinal nerves. Instead of sending a signal all the way to the cerebral cortex and back down the spinal cord, the signal is sent to the spinal cord, which in turn responds and sends a signal back to the muscle. This signaling process is called the **reflex arc**, but how does it work? Muscles contain spindles, structures that detect the amount of stretch in a muscle. When a muscle is stretched (e.g., the physician's reflex hammer hitting the patellar tendon), information is sent via sensory neurons to the dorsal roots of the spinal gray matter. This information is then sent to motor neurons via an intercalated neuron, a neuron that makes connections between two neurons. A motor message is then sent through the ventral root for the muscle to contract (or, in essence, oppose the

TABLE 5-2 Major Descending and Ascending Pathways in the Spinal Cord

Type	Tract	Origin	Decussation	Ending	Function
Descending Motor Tracts	Lateral corticobulbar	Primary motor cortex (BA4)	Medulla–spinal cord juncture	Brainstem	Movement of contralateral head region
	Lateral corticospinal	Primary motor cortex (BA4)	Medulla–spinal cord juncture	Spinal cord	Movement of contralateral limbs
	Rubrospinal	Midbrain	Midbrain	Cervical spinal cord	Flexor tone
	Anterior corticospinal	Primary (BA4) and premotor (BA6) cortex	None	Cervical and thoracic spinal cord	Trunk muscles
	Vestibulospinal	Pons and medulla	None	Throughout whole spinal cord	Extensor tone and spinal reflexes
	Reticulospinal	Pons and medulla	None	Throughout whole spinal cord	Posture and gait
	Tectospinal	Midbrain	Midbrain	Cervical spinal cord	Coordination of head and eye movements
Ascending Sensory Tracts	Dorsal column	Spinal cord	Medulla	Primary sensory cortex via thalamus	Fine touch, vibratory sense, proprioception
	Spinothalamic	Spinal cord	Spinal cord	Primary sensory cortex via thalamus	Crude touch, pain, pressure, temperature
	Spinocerebellar	Spinal cord	None	Cerebellum	Proprioception

stretching, which is called the stretch reflex). This process is illustrated in **FIGURE 5-11**. Reflex messages do eventually make it to the cerebral cortex for perceptual processing (e.g., pain). Damage along this pathway can cause reflexes to be diminished or completely absent.

Select Disorders of the Spinal Cord

Spinal Cord Injury

What Is It?

Spinal cord injury (SCI) involves traumatic damage to the spinal cord in which it is partially or completely severed or crushed (**BOX 5-2**). There are about 17,500 new cases of SCI each year and approximately 285,000 people currently living with SCI in the United States.

Causes

In the United States, vehicle crashes account for approximately 38% of SCIs, followed by falls (30%) and violence (13.5%). Males account for over 81% of SCIs, and 63% of cases involve non-Hispanic whites (National Spinal Cord Injury Statistical Center [NSCISC], 2017).

Signs and Symptoms

Damage from this type of injury can result in paresis (incomplete) or plegia (complete) depending on what level of the spinal cord is damaged (**FIGURE 5-12**).

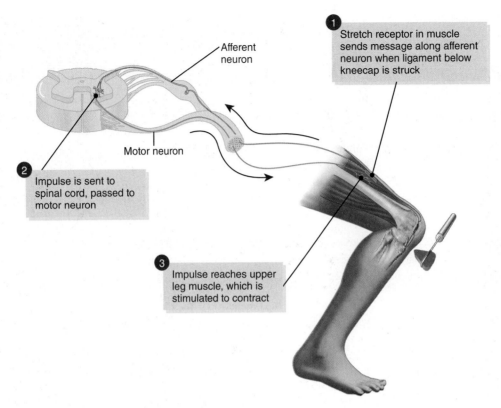

1 Stretch receptor in muscle sends message along afferent neuron when ligament below kneecap is struck

Afferent neuron

Motor neuron

2 Impulse is sent to spinal cord, passed to motor neuron

3 Impulse reaches upper leg muscle, which is stimulated to contract

FIGURE 5-11 The reflex arc.

BOX 5-2 Christopher Reeve and Spinal Cord Injury

Christopher Reeve (1952–2004) was an American actor best known for playing Superman in the *Superman* movies of the 1970s and 1980s. On May 27, 1995, he was thrown from a horse, and the injuries he sustained resulted in quadriplegia. He required a wheelchair and a portable ventilator to help him breathe. After his injury, Reeve became an activist for people with SCI. He also advocated for stem cell research, believing that a cure for SCI could result from this research. He died on October 10, 2004, due to cardiac arrest following an adverse reaction to an antibiotic he was taking to treat a pressure ulcer.

The term *complete* refers to complete loss of sensation or movement, and *incomplete* denotes partial loss of movement or sensation. Approximately 59% of cases are either complete or incomplete quadriplegia; the remaining 41% are complete or incomplete paraplegia (NSCISC, 2017).

Assessment and Treatment

Diagnosis of SCI is made through a neurological exam along with neuroimaging. Treatment can include surgery, steroid treatment, and rehabilitation. Treatment revolves around steroids to reduce swelling in and around the spinal cord, surgery to remove any bone fragments and to stabilize the spine, and rehabilitation (**FIGURE 5-13**). The prognosis varies from patient to patient, but the majority of cases involve some lasting impairment in movement and/or sensation.

Myelitis

What Is It?

Myelitis is a general term for inflammation of the spinal cord. If the inflammation is to only the gray matter of the spinal cord, the condition is called *poliomyelitis*. If it is confined to the white matter, it is called *leukomyelitis*. If the inflammation involves both the white and the gray matter, it is called *transverse myelitis*. If the inflammation extends to the meninges, it is called *meningomyelitis*. Poliomyelitis or polio is probably the most well-known form of myelitis because of the great epidemics of the 20th century that left many people paralyzed below the waist, including one of our presidents, Franklin D. Roosevelt (**BOX 5-3**).

Causes

Myelitis can be caused by a variety of factors, including immune system disorders, viruses, bacteria, fungi,

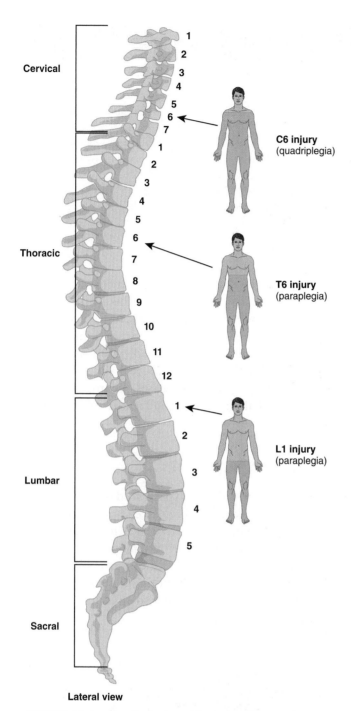

Cervical

1
2
3
4
5
6
7

C6 injury
(quadriplegia)

Thoracic

1
2
3
4
5
6
7
8
9
10
11
12

T6 injury
(paraplegia)

1
2

L1 injury
(paraplegia)

3
4
5

Lumbar

Sacral

Lateral view

FIGURE 5-12 Levels of spinal cord injury and the results.

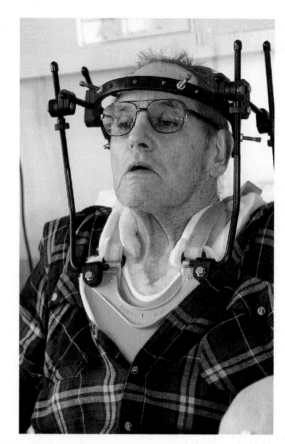

FIGURE 5-13 A spinal cord injury patient wearing a halo ring brace to stabilize the spinal cord.

BOX 5-3 Franklin Delano Roosevelt and Polio

Franklin D. Roosevelt (1882–1945) was the 32nd president of the United States, a position he held for an unprecedented 12 years. At about the age of 40, Roosevelt contracted polio while on vacation in Canada. Because of his illness, he was paralyzed from the waist down. Roosevelt was careful to hide his disability and was rarely photographed in a wheelchair. In fact, only two known photographs exist depicting him in one. Roosevelt served as president during a crucial time in our nation's history. He helped pull the country out of the Great Depression and guided the United States through World War II.

---

parasites, and toxic agents (e.g., lead). Sometimes the cause is unknown and is referred to as idiopathic myelitis.

Signs and Symptoms

The primary sign of the disease is rapid loss of motor and/or sensory abilities in the legs and possibly the loss of reflexes. If it is the poliomyelitis form, motor abilities will be affected, but not sensory. In the leukomyelitis variety, motor abilities are preserved but sensory abilities are impaired or lost. In the transverse form, both motor and sensory abilities are impaired. Some specific symptoms patients experience include weakness, pain, dysesthesia, and bowel and bladder issues.

Assessment and Treatment

Myelitis is usually diagnosed through a combination of blood tests and spinal tap to discern the cause of the inflammation. If the cause is bacterial or parasitic,

BOX 5-4 My Experience With Peripheral Neuropathy

When I was in my early 30s, I read a *Time* magazine article about diabetes. The article contained a list of diabetic symptoms, and as I scanned the list I realized that I had almost all the symptoms (e.g., dry mouth, frequent bathroom trips). My wife told my sister-in-law, who is a nurse, about this and she asked that I stop by her emergency department to have my blood checked. I did and she got a 600 reading on my blood sugar test (normal is around 100). I saw my physician shortly after, who diagnosed me with type 2 diabetes and immediately put me on medication. One of the symptoms I had been experiencing was strange sensation (dysesthesia; Greek for "impaired sensation") in my feet. There were times when my feet hurt or burned. Sometimes I could not wear socks or have the blankets on my feet. My doctor told me this was the beginning of peripheral neuropathy. Apparently, the extra sugar in my blood was breaking down small capillaries in my feet, which was affecting sensory nerve endings in my feet. He was unsure whether it would get better or not because it depended on how long I had had diabetes and the damage that had been done. Fortunately, most of the neuropathy has disappeared because my diabetes is now under control.

antibiotics will be employed. Fungal infections will be treated with antifungal medications. Viruses are difficult to treat after infection, but vaccines can prevent myelitis. Poliomyelitis has all but been eradicated in the United States due to a vaccine developed in the 1950s, but it does still unfortunately occur in other places around the world (Victor & Ropper, 2001).

Peripheral Neuropathy

What Is It?

Peripheral neuropathy is an inflammation of the peripheral nervous system that results in degeneration of the spinal nerves.

Causes

This condition can have a variety of causes, including toxic poisoning (e.g., alcohol abuse), infections, metabolic disorders (e.g., diabetes), and nutritional issues, such as the lack of vitamin B1 in beriberi. A good causal example is diabetes, a condition that causes excessive sugars in the blood. This excess sugar degenerates small capillaries in the extremities, causing nerve fibers to die. As nerve fibers die, people lose sensation in their fingers and hands, and with this loss of sensation are susceptible to wounds that will not heal because of the diabetes.

Signs and Symptoms

Sensory impairment or loss is the main symptom of peripheral neuropathy, but people can lose motor function as well. In the case of sensory impairment, patients might experience burning, prickling, and eventual numbness.

Assessment and Treatment

Peripheral neuropathy is diagnosed through clinical presentation and laboratory tests. For example, in diabetes, a blood test will determine the presence or absence of the disease, and sensory testing of the feet will tell the extent of the neuropathy if diabetes is indeed present. Treatment can consist of treating the underlying disease process. In the case of diabetes, the use of oral medications or insulin can control the disease and prevent the neuropathy from worsening. In some cases, neuropathies can be reversed if the disease is treated early enough (**BOX 5-4**).

▶ Brainstem

At the superior end of the spinal cord is the brainstem (**FIGURE 5-14**). It contains both ascending (sensory) and descending (motor) tracts as well as nuclei that make up major centers for sensory and motor function. Life functions, such as breathing, heart rate, blood pressure, and digestion, are found in it, as are centers for wakefulness and alertness. It also has nuclei for most of the cranial nerves.

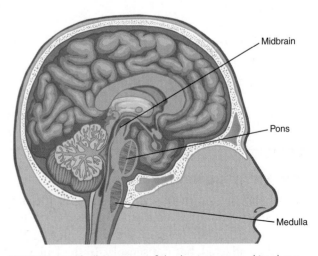

FIGURE 5-14 An illustration of the brainstem and its three main parts: the medulla, pons, and midbrain.

© Oguz Aral/ShutterStock.

External Organization of the Brainstem

The Medulla

The lowest part of the brainstem is a 1-inch-long (2.5-cm-long) structure called the **medulla**. The medulla's lower boundary is the spinal cord, and the pons forms the upper boundary (**FIGURE 5-15**). The medulla is ventral (or anterior) to the cerebellum and is connected to it by the inferior **cerebellar peduncle** (Latin for "stalk"). Between the upper medulla and the cerebellum is the bottom of the fourth ventricle. On the medulla's anterior surface are the pyramids, which contain descending motor tracts, and the olive. Inside the olive is the inferior olivary nucleus that integrates signals from

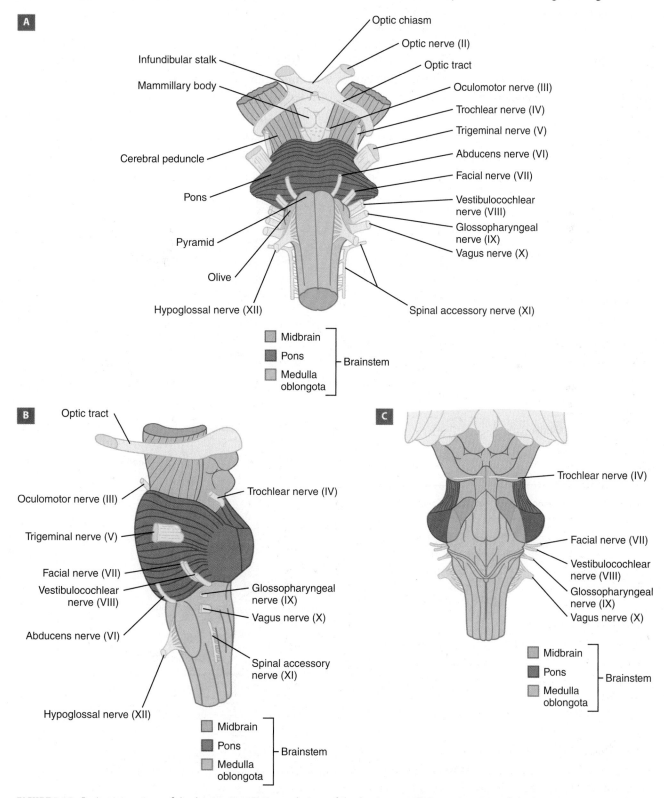

FIGURE 5-15 A. Anterior view of the brainstem. **B.** Lateral view of the brainstem. **C.** Posterior view of the brainstem.

the spinal cord and the cerebellum for the purpose of coordinating motor movements and learning. Many of the tracts discussed earlier this chapter run through the medulla, including the corticospinal, spinocerebellar, spinothalamic, and dorsal columns tracts. Roughly 80% of motor tracts cross, or decussate, at the level of the lower medulla (**FIGURE 5-16**).

In neuroanatomy, a nucleus is a cluster of specialized neurons that serve a specific purpose in the nervous system, and the medulla contains many such nuclei (Figure 5-16). For example, cranial nerve IX, X, XI, and XII nuclei arise from the medulla, while cranial nerve V and VIII nuclei dip down into the medulla

from the pons. Various autonomic nervous system nuclei are located in the medulla, including cardiac, vasoconstrictor, gastrointestinal motility, respiratory, and swallowing centers. In addition, several reflexes are mediated at this level, including coughing, vomiting, and gagging by the nucleus of solitarius and swallowing by the nucleus ambiguous.

The Pons

The **pons** (Latin for "bridge") lies superior to the medulla, anterior to the cerebellum, and inferior to the midbrain (Figure 5-15). It is about an inch (2.5 cm) in length and is bulbous in shape. The cerebellum is

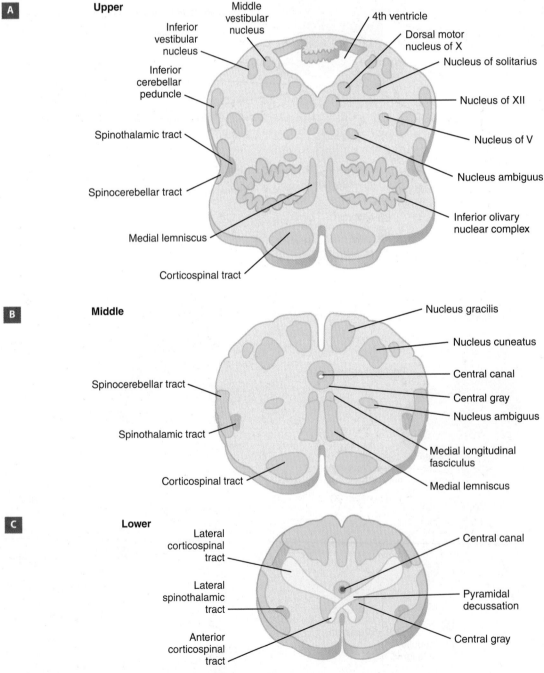

FIGURE 5-16 Cross-sections of the various levels of the medulla. **A.** The upper medulla. **B.** The middle medulla. **C.** The lower medulla.

connected to the pons by the middle cerebellar peduncles, and between the two structures lies the fourth ventricle (**FIGURE 5-17**).

Overall, the pons acts as a bridge, relaying neural tracts between the cerebral cortex, cerebellum, and lower structures like the medulla and spinal cord. Some of these tracts include corticobulbar and corticospinal tracts. The pons contains nuclei that help regulate respiration, swallowing, hearing, eye movements, and facial expression and sensation. There are also a number of cranial nerve nuclei in the pons, including nuclei for cranial nerves V, VI, VII, and VIII (Saladin, 2007; Zemlin, 1998). The superior olivary nucleus and lateral lemniscus (Greek for "ribbon") are found in the pons, both of which play an important relay function for auditory information.

The Midbrain

The **midbrain** lies inferior to the diencephalon and superior to the pons (Figure 5-15). Its ventral portion consists of two **cerebral peduncles**; the dorsal consists of the **tectum** (Latin for "roof-like"). Each peduncle has a dorsal part called the **tegmentum** (Latin for "covering") and a ventral piece called the **crus cerebri** (Latin for "leg of the brain"), which are fibers that link the pons with the cerebral hemispheres. Between these is a layer of dark gray matter called the **substantia nigra** (Latin for "black substance") where the neurotransmitter dopamine is produced (**FIGURE 5-18**). Dopamine plays an important role in addiction and movement. Destruction of dopamine-producing cells can cause progressive neurological movement disorders, like Parkinson disease. The tectum contains the paired superior and inferior colliculi (Latin for "little hills"). The **inferior colliculi** are the auditory center of the midbrain and are important in moving the eyes and/or head toward the source of a sound and our startle response to a loud noise. This area may play a role in disorders like posttraumatic stress disorder (PTSD) (Davis, Falls, & Gewirtz, 2000). The **superior colliculi** are the visual center of the midbrain, receiving input

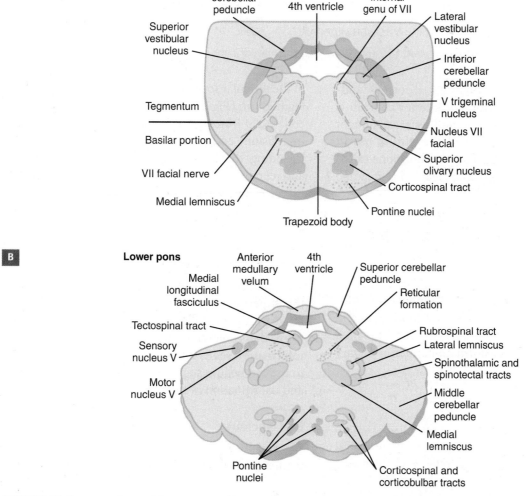

FIGURE 5-17 Cross-sections of the upper and lower pons. **A.** Upper pons. **B.** Lower pons.

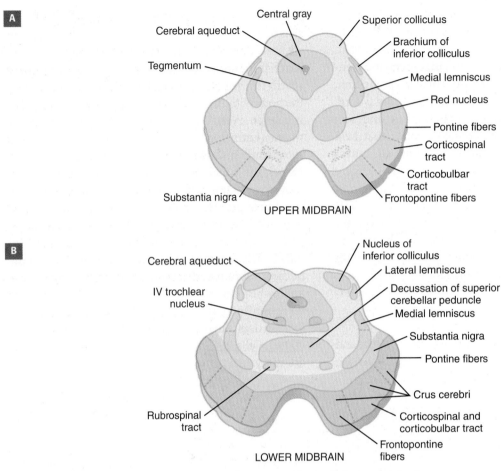

FIGURE 5-18 Cross-sections of the midbrain. **A.** Upper midbrain. **B.** Lower midbrain.

from the retinas and the primary visual cortex. Sandwiched between the superior and inferior colliculi is a small endocrine gland that René Descartes thought was the seat of the soul named the **pineal gland** (Latin for "pine cone"). It produces a hormone called melatonin, which helps regulate sleep and circadian rhythms.

Internal Organization of the Brainstem

Tegmental Regions

The tegmentum is the core of the brainstem, which is continuous throughout the medulla, pons, and midbrain. The nontegmental areas are not continuous and lie near the surface of the brainstem. The tegmental areas include the reticular formation, inferior olivary complex, and red nucleus.

Reticular Formation

As mentioned, in neuroanatomy, a nucleus is a group of neuron cell bodies that relay and integrate neural signals. It also plays a role in the reflex arc. The nuclei

of the reticular formation are scattered throughout the tegmentum (Figure 5-17B). These nuclei receive axon collaterals from special sensory systems (e.g., hearing, vision) and project axons throughout the brain, including the brainstem, cerebellum, diencephalon, and cerebral hemispheres. The reticular formation regulates many aspects of human experience, including consciousness, the sleep–wake cycle, cardiovascular functions, and respiration.

Inferior Olivary Nucleus

The inferior olivary nucleus (not to be confused with the superior olivary nuclei related to hearing) is a bulge on the medulla (Figure 5-16). It receives axons from the cerebral cortex and after processing the information sends it to the cerebellum. Its connection to the cerebellum suggests it plays a role in the control and coordination of motor movements.

Red Nucleus

The **red nucleus** is a paired structure located in the tegmentum of the midbrain next to the substantia nigra (Figure 5-18). Its name comes from the fact that it is pink due to the presence of iron. It receives connections from the cerebral cortex, and its axons give rise to the rubrospinal tract that descends the brainstem and inputs into the spinal cord's ventral horn cells. This tract modulates flexor tone in the upper extremities and probably participates in activities such as a baby's ability to crawl and arm swinging in walking.

Nontegmental Regions

As mentioned earlier, nontegmental areas of the brainstem are found at or near the brainstem's surface rather than deep in the tegmentum. Three nontegmental areas will be briefly discussed: the tectum, cerebral peduncles, and ventral pons.

Tectum

The tectum is the roof of the midbrain. Dorsally, it has two hills: the superior colliculi and the inferior colliculi. The superior colliculi are connected to vision and the inferior colliculi to hearing. The inferior colliculi's axons carry auditory information to the thalamus's auditory center, the medial geniculate body, which then is projected to the cerebral cortex's auditory areas.

Cerebral Peduncles

The cerebral peduncles, or crus cerebri, are bulges on the ventral side of the midbrain. The lateral corticospinal and corticobulbar tracts run through these bulges, the lateral corticobulbar tract being important for speech production. Between the peduncles and the tegmentum is the substantia nigra, which produces dopamine. The substantia nigra has a close connection to the basal ganglia, an important structure in speech production.

Ventral Pons

The corticopontine fibers originate from the motor cortex, pass through the cerebral peduncles, and input into ventral pons nuclei. Projections from the ventral pons then course to the cerebellum. Because of the pontine nuclei's close connection to the cerebellum, it is thought this connection plays a role in motor movement error correction. Error correction is an important aspect of learning new motor skills (think of learning tennis). This would be an important skill for learning to speak both a first and a second language.

Select Disorders of the Brainstem

The Medulla

One disorder that can result from medullar damage is **Wallenberg syndrome** (also called *lateral medullary syndrome*). It is typically caused by a stroke involving one of the arteries that supplies blood to the medulla. Patients with this condition experience contralateral loss of pain and temperature in the body, ipsilateral loss of pain and temperature in the face, vertigo, ataxia, paralysis of the ipsilateral palate and vocal cord, and dysphagia. One additional symptom is frequent and violent hiccups that can last for weeks and make speaking, eating, and sleeping difficult. Treatment for Wallenberg syndrome is generally centered on relieving symptoms, rehabilitation, and counseling patients in adjusting to life with the syndrome. The prognosis varies from patient to patient, with some making a complete recovery, whereas others may have ongoing disability and/or handicap.

The Pons

Damage to the ventral pons can result in coma and/or **locked-in syndrome (LIS)**. LIS is characterized by quadriplegia and cranial nerve paralysis except for eye movements. Basically, the person is locked inside his or her body, unable to move, but is cognitively intact. The person cannot speak or swallow, and somatosensory abilities may or may not remain intact. Treatment involves support and rehabilitation, especially establishing a system for communication. The prognosis is poor for patients with LIS; 90% of those with the condition die within 4 months of onset.

The memoir *The Diving Bell and the Butterfly* by Jean-Dominique Bauby (1998), as well as the film of the same title, familiarized the general public with this condition. Bauby did not recover from LIS and died about a year and a half after his stroke. Though extremely rare, there have been documented cases of people with LIS having spontaneous, full recoveries. A British woman named Kate Allatt suffered a brainstem stroke around the age of 40 years and was diagnosed with LIS, but made a complete recovery (British Broadcasting Corporation [BBC], 2012). Another British woman, Kerry Pink, also reportedly recovered from the syndrome (BBC, 2010).

The Midbrain

Midbrain damage can result in Weber or Benedikt syndrome. **Weber syndrome** is characterized by contralateral hemiplegia and ipsilateral oculomotor paralysis with ptosis. The hemiparesis affects the lower face muscles and tongue. **Benedikt syndrome** is similar to Weber syndrome but results in contralateral hemiparesis and ataxic tremor.

▶ The Cranial Nerves

When we were learning about spinal nerves, we learned that they carry four different kinds of fibers—general somatic afferent (GSA), general somatic efferent (GSE), general visceral afferent (GVA), or general visceral efferent (GVE). There are 12 cranial nerves that carry some of these same types of fibers. However, some cranial nerves also carry special somatic and special visceral fibers for a total of seven possible fibers. Special senses refer to our special sense organs, like the eyes or ears. More specifically, **special somatic afferent (SSA) fibers** conduct visual and auditory information from the eyes and inner ear to the appropriate cerebral cortex area. (*Note:* There are no special somatic efferent [SSE] fibers.) **Special visceral efferent (SVE) fibers** control glands in the head and neck, and **special visceral afferent (SVA) fibers** relay special sense information like smell and taste.

As mentioned, there are 12 pairs of cranial nerves that control sensory, special sensory, motor, and visceral (or parasympathetic) functions of the head and neck. Most, except cranial nerves I and II, originate from the brainstem (**FIGURE 5-19**). Not all the cranial nerves play a role in speech and hearing, so critical attention should be directed toward six cranial nerves: V, VII, VIII, IX, X, and XII. All the cranial nerves are presented in **TABLE 5-3**, along with a mnemonic that has helped many students remember them.

Cranial Nerve I: The Olfactory Nerve

The olfactory nerve (I) is an SVA that mediates our sense of olfaction (Latin for "to smell"). This nerve is not considered a true cranial nerve because it does not arise from the brainstem and because it does not interface with the thalamus. It is, however, included with the other cranial nerves, being the shortest of all of them.

Bipolar olfactory receptor cells (first-order neurons) imbedded in the nasal cavity's epithelium pass upward through the cribriform plate of the ethmoid bone and input into mitral cells (second-order neurons) in the olfactory bulb (**FIGURE 5-20**). The bulb then projects as the olfactory tract to third-order

neurons in the cerebral cortex. This tract divides into two branches, a lateral branch and a medial branch. The medial branch projects through the anterior commissure, a white matter tract connecting the temporal lobes, and connects to the olfactory bulb on the other side. The lateral branch projects to the olfactory cortex of the temporal lobe of cerebral cortex. This area then sends fibers to the limbic system (amygdala) as well as to the hippocampus. The fact that smell can have strong connections to both emotion and memory are explained by these two connections.

Trauma to the nose can lead to the cribriform plate shifting and shearing off olfactory neurons, leaving a person with **anosmia**, which is a loss of smell. Trauma to the nose can also lead to **cerebral spinal rhinorrhea** (Greek for "nose flow"), in which cerebrospinal fluid leaks through the nose. This rare condition can occur through a basal skull fracture (i.e., fracture to bones on the bottom of the skull) that leads to bone fragments puncturing the meninges, the three-layer membrane that surrounds the brain and spinal cord. This kind of damage can create a route for infection leading to a condition called meningitis, an infection in the meninges (Seikel, King, & Drumright, 2010). Lastly, temporal lobe epilepsy can lead to olfactory hallucinations, which often involve unpleasant smells (Monkhouse, 2006).

Cranial Nerve II: The Optic Nerve

Like the olfactory nerve, the optic nerve (II) does not originate off the brainstem, but unlike the olfactory nerve, it does connect with the thalamus. Overall, the optic nerve is an SSA fiber tract that conducts visual information to visual centers of the brain. Though not involved in speech and hearing, it is obviously involved in decoding the graphemes associated with written language.

This tract begins with the photoreceptor rod (night vision) and cone (daylight and color) cells of the retina (first-order neurons) and then projects to bipolar neurons (second-order neurons) that enhance visual contrast. These neurons then connect with an inner layer of ganglion cells whose axons form the optic nerve (third-order neurons) that projects to the lateral geniculate body of the thalamus (**FIGURE 5-21**). The projections from the nasal regions of the optic nerve cross (known as the optic chiasm), while the temporal regions remain uncrossed (**FIGURE 5-22**). Fourth-order neurons project from the thalamus via the geniculocalcarine tract (also known as the optic radiations) to the visual cortex in the occipital lobe.

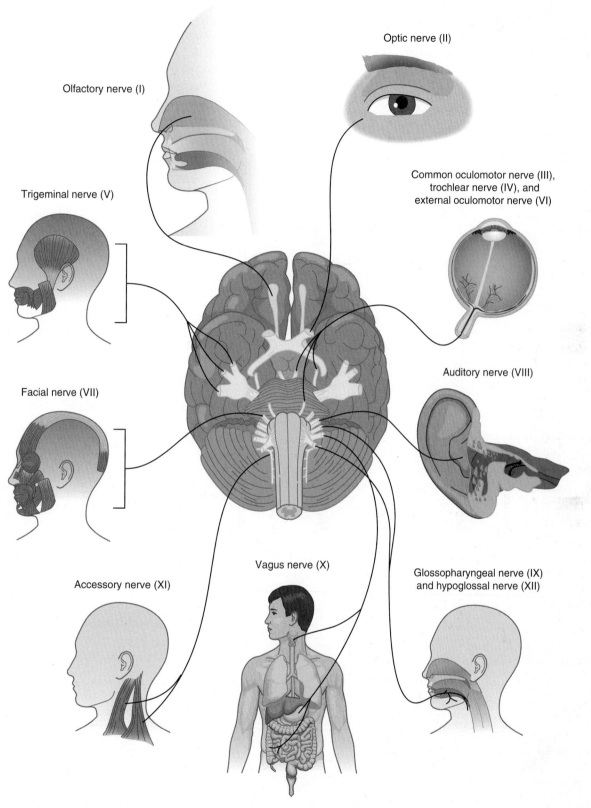

FIGURE 5-19 The cranial nerves.

TABLE 5-3 The Cranial Nerves

Mnemonic	Number	Name	Origination	Function	Dysfunction	Speech/Hearing Importance
On	I	Olfactory	Olfactory bulb	**Sensory** SVA: smell	Anosmia	None
Old	II	Optic	Thalamus	**Sensory** SSA: vision	Visual disturbances; visual loss	None (language in terms of reading/writing)
Olympus	III	Oculomotor	Midbrain	**Motor** GSE: eyeball movement; controls eyelids GVE: pupil constrictor	Loss of pupillary light reflex; papilledema; ptosis	None
Towering	IV	Trochlear	Midbrain	**Motor** GSE: eyeball movement	Diplopia; nystagmus	None
Tops	V	Trigeminal	Pons	**Motor** SVE: chewing muscles **Sensory** GSA: touch, pain, temperature, vibration for face, mouth, anterior two-thirds of tongue	Loss of sensations (see Function column); difficulty chewing, abnormal jaw-jerk reflex	Speech/chewing
A	VI	Abducens	Pons	**Motor** GSE: eyeball movement	Strabismus; nystagmus	None
Fin	VII	Facial	Pons	**Motor** SVE: face muscles GVE: salivary glands **Sensory** GSA: sense at auricle's concha; behind auricle SVA: taste in anterior two-thirds of tongue	Facial paresis or plegia; loss of taste	Speech
And	VIII	Auditory (vestibulocochlear)	Pons/medulla	**Sensory** SSA: hearing and balance	Hearing loss; balance issues	Hearing

Mnemonic	CN	Name	Location	Function	Signs	Communication
German	IX	Glossopharyngeal	Pons/medulla	**Motor** SVE: pharyngeal movement GVE: parotid gland **Sensory** GVA: middle ear; pharynx, posterior one-third of tongue SVA: taste on posterior one-third of tongue GSA: tactile sensation on external and middle ear	Absent gag; impaired or absent swallow; loss of taste; loss of pharyngeal movement	Speech
Viewed	X	Vagus	Medulla	**Motor** SVE: pharyngeal and laryngeal muscles GVE: viscera of the thoracic and abdominal cavities **Sensory** GSA: tactile sensation to external ear canal GVA: pain sense from mucous membranes of pharynx, larynx, esophagus, trachea, and thoracic and abdominal viscera SVA: taste from epiglottis/pharynx	Absent gag; impaired or absent swallow; loss of velar movement; loss of voice	Speech/voice/resonance
Some	XI	Spinal accessory	Medulla	**Motor** SVE: neck and shoulder muscles	Droopy shoulder, movement of neck	None
Hops	XII	Hypoglossal	Medulla	**Motor** GSE: tongue muscles	Loss of tongue movement; tongue fasciculation, tongue atrophy	Speech

Abbreviations:
GSA, general somatic afferent; GSE, general somatic efferent; GVA, general visceral afferent; GVE, general visceral efferent; SSA, special somatic afferent; SVA, special visceral afferent; SVE, special visceral efferent.
Data from Monkhouse, S. (2006). *High-yield neuroanatomy* (5th ed.). Philadelphia, PA: Wolters Kluwer; Bhatnagar, S. C. (2013). *Neuroscience for the study of communicative disorders* (4th ed.). Philadelphia, PA: Wolters Kluwer; Gould, D. J. & Brueckner-Collins, J. K. (2016). *Cranial nerves: Functional anatomy.* Cambridge, UK: Cambridge University Press.

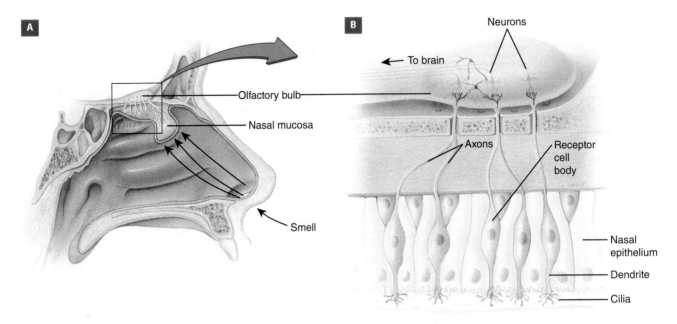

FIGURE 5-20 **A.** Olfactory receptor cells in the lining of the nasal cavity and the olfactory bulb. **B.** Enlarged view of the olfactory receptor cells.

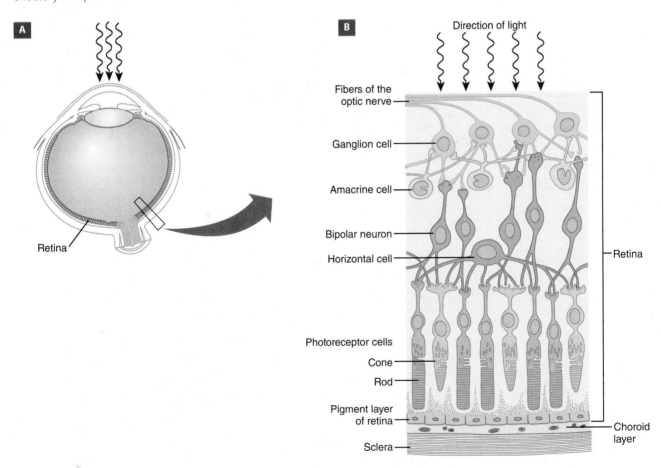

FIGURE 5-21 Neurons of the retina. **A.** The eye. **B.** Cellular components on the retina.

Damage to the optic system will result in different types of problems, depending on where the damage is in the system (**FIGURE 5-23**). Some level of blindness is one possibility, and hemianopsia (Greek for "half seeing") is another. For example, if the left

optic nerve is damaged, a person would suffer from monocular blindness. This condition would result not in a total loss of vision in the left visual field, but only a small fraction of this field outside the binocular field. If the lesion is further down the

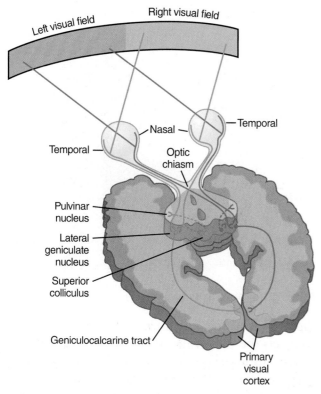

FIGURE 5-22 The visual pathway.

optic nerve at the optic chiasm, the subject would lose both temporal visual fields (bitemporal hemianopsia), whereas a lesion behind the optic chiasm but before the thalamus would result in loss of the left temporal and right nasal fields (homonymous hemianopsia).

Cranial Nerve III: The Oculomotor Nerve

The oculomotor nerve (III) is a motor nerve made up of GSE and GVE fibers. The nerve arises from the midbrain, courses through the red nucleus to the cerebral peduncles, and then exits as inferior and superior branches. The GSE component innervates the following muscles that control the eyeball's movement up and out, inward, and down and out (**FIGURE 5-24**):

- Superior levator palpebrae (elevates upper eyelids)—superior branch
- Superior rectus muscle (elevates, adducts, and rotates eyeballs inward)—superior branch
- Medial rectus muscle (adduction of the eyeballs)—inferior branch

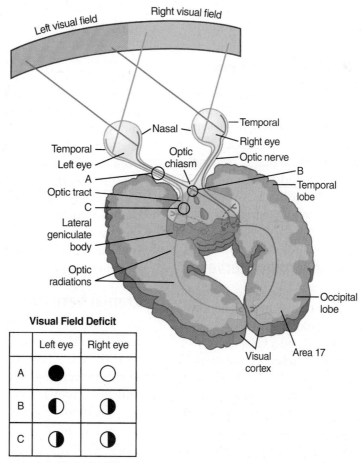

FIGURE 5-23 The visual pathway and the effect of lesions at different levels of the pathway. Damage at A would result in monocular blindness. Damage at B would result in heteronymous bitemporal hemianopsia. Damage at C would result in homonymous right hemianopsia.

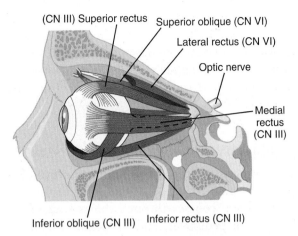

FIGURE 5-24 Muscles of the eye with their cranial nerve innervation.

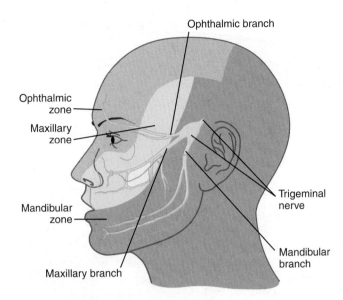

FIGURE 5-25 The trigeminal nerve (V).

■ Inferior rectus muscle (depresses, adducts, and rotates eyeballs inward)—inferior branch

The GVE fibers of the nerve constrict the pupils and also help to focus the eyes.

Damage to oculomotor nerve GVE fibers leaves the pupil dilated and unable to focus. Damage to the GSE fibers would result in **ptosis** (Greek for "falling") or droopy upper eyelids, **strabismus** (Greek for "to squint") or crossed vision, and **diplopia** (Greek for "double eyes") or double vision.

Cranial Nerve IV: The Trochlear Nerve

Cranial nerve IV is called the trochlear (Greek for "pulley") nerve, and it is another eyeball muscle nerve containing GSE fibers. It arises from a midbrain nucleus called the trochlear nucleus and innervates the superior oblique muscle that is responsible for turning the eyeball down and out (Figure 5-24). Damage to this nerve results in difficulty moving the eyes downward, which can make walking down stairs difficult, and diplopia.

Cranial Nerve V: The Trigeminal Nerve

The trigeminal nerve (V) originates from the lateral surface of the pons and it splits into three branches: the ophthalmic, maxillary, and mandibular (**FIGURE 5-25**). The trigeminal is both an SVE and a GSA nerve.

In terms of motor (SVE) function, the mandibular branch innervates muscles that lower the mandible (mylohyoid and anterior belly of the digastric), raise the mandible (temporalis, masseter, and medial pterygoid), and protrude the mandible (lateral pterygoid muscle). The opening and closing movements of the mandible are important in sound production and chewing. The trigeminal nerve controls

the tensor tympani, a muscle of the middle ear that connects the wall of the middle ear to the malleus. When this muscle contracts, it stiffens the ossicular chain of the middle ear. This protective reflex guards against intense low-frequency sounds, particularly the sound of one's own voice and chewing. The trigeminal also dilates the eustachian tube, thus helping to equalize pressure between the middle ear and the environment.

As far as sensory function, the ophthalmic branch relays sensation from the upper face back to the brainstem and cerebral cortex. The maxillary branch carries sensory information from the nose, mouth, lower face, auditory meatus, and meninges. Finally, the sensory portion of the mandibular branch relays sensation from the lateral side of the head and scalp, lower jaw, anterior two-thirds of the tongue, and mucous membranes of the mouth. This branch also carries proprioceptive information from the muscles of chewing to the brainstem. This sensory feedback information is important for jaw opening and closing during speech and chewing.

Cranial Nerve VI: The Abducens Nerve

So far, we have seen that the oculomotor (III) and trochlear (IV) nerves control movement of the eyeball. There is a final and third nerve that contributes to this movement called the abducens (Latin for "to pull away from") nerve (VI). This is a GSE nerve like the oculomotor nerve. Its nucleus is found in the dorsal part of the pons, which projects through the point where the pons and medulla meet. It courses to the orbit and innervates one muscle—the lateral rectus muscle, which moves the eyeballs laterally

(Figure 5-24). If injured, the eyeballs will deviate inward, leading to diplopia

Cranial Nerve VII: The Facial Nerve

The facial nerve (VII) has motor (SVE), sensory (GSA), special sensory (SVA), and parasympathetic (GVE) functions, but only the motor aspect has relevance for speech production. The facial nerves originate from the cerebellopontine angle and have two branches, the intracranial and extracranial (**FIGURE 5-26**). The intracranial branch is involved in sensory, special sensory, and parasympathetic functions. These functions include sensory information behind the auricle and in the auricle's concha (GSA), taste on the anterior two-thirds of the tongue (SVA), and gland secretion (GVE; lacrimal, sublingual, and submandibular glands). The extracranial branch (SVE) innervates all the facial muscles that are crucial in speech production and the oral preparatory and oral stages of swallowing. These muscles include the following:

- Orbicularis oris (constricts oral opening)
- Risorius (retracts lip corners)
- Buccinator (moves food onto molars for grinding)
- Levator labii superioris (elevates upper lip)
- Zygomatic minor (elevates upper lip)
- Levator labii superioris alaeque nasi (elevates upper lip)
- Levator anguli oris (draws mouth corner up)
- Zygomatic major (elevates and retracts mouth angle)
- Depressor labii inferioris (pulls lips down and out)
- Depressor anguli oris (depresses mouth corners)
- Mentalis (pulls lower lip out)
- Platysma (depresses mandible)

Additionally, the facial nerve innervates the posterior belly of the digastric muscle (depresses mandible and elevates the hyoid bone), the stylohyoid muscle (elevates the hyoid bone), and the stapedius muscle (dampens vibrations on the stapes) of the middle ear.

The SVE fibers originate out of the facial motor nucleus in the pons (**FIGURE 5-27**). This nucleus is divided in such a way that the lower face muscles (i.e., speech muscles) receive only contralateral innervation, whereas the upper face muscles receive bilateral innervation. If there is unilateral damage to the left cerebral cortex (i.e., a UMN lesion), then the result is deficits (e.g., weakness) in the right lower face muscles, with the upper right face muscles unaffected because they receive bilateral innervation. Thus, a person with this kind of damage could still wrinkle the right forehead and close the right eye, but the right side of the lower face would droop. If the damage is to the LMNs, then the whole ipsilateral side of the face is paralyzed (upper and lower face muscles). An example of an LMN disorder is Bell palsy (**FIGURE 5-28** and **BOX 5-5**).

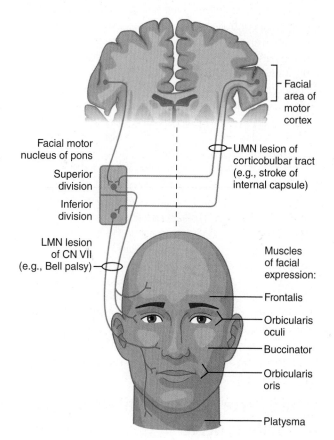

FIGURE 5-27 Effects of upper and lower motor neuron lesions on cranial nerve VII and its motor control of the upper and lower face muscles.

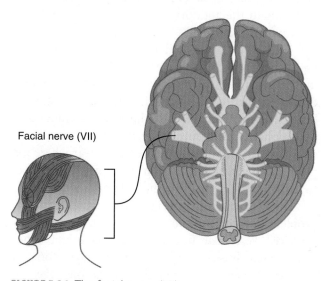

FIGURE 5-26 The facial nerve (VII).

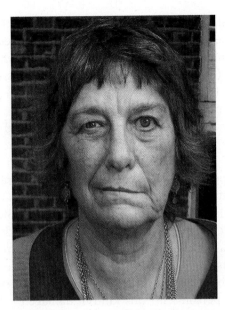

FIGURE 5-28 A woman with Bell's palsy, a lower motor neuron disorder that affects all the facial muscles on one side of the face. Note the drooping on the left side of her face.

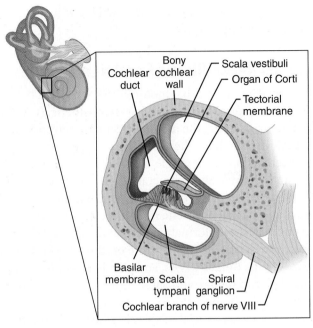

FIGURE 5-29 The spiral ganglion of the auditory pathway.

BOX 5-5 Bell's Palsy

The term **palsy** is a Middle English word that came from the Latin word *paralysis*. It refers to paralysis, weakness, or even uncontrolled movements (e.g., shaking). The condition known as Bell's palsy (also known as seventh nerve palsy or idiopathic facial paralysis) is named after the 19th-century Scottish surgeon Charles Bell, who first described the condition in which one side of the face is weakened or paralyzed due to dysfunction of cranial nerve VII, the facial nerve (Figure 5-28). The cause of the condition is unknown, but it might occur after a viral infection that leaves the facial nerve inflamed and swollen. Stress may be another trigger for the condition. The symptoms of the condition include rapid onset of facial weakness on one side of the face, facial drooping, drooling, hyperacusis (sensitivity to loud sounds), changes to taste, and headache. In most cases, these symptoms last 4 to 6 months and then resolve. A small number of people may have the symptoms for life. Assessment of the condition is made through the patient's clinical presentation and through ruling out other conditions, like stroke. Treatment revolves around corticosteroids to decrease swelling, antiviral drugs in cases where a viral cause is suspected, and physical therapy to prevent facial muscles from atrophying.

Cranial Nerve VIII: The Vestibulocochlear (or Auditory) Nerve

The main cranial nerve of hearing is the auditory nerve (VIII). It is also known as the vestibulocochlear nerve, a more accurate name that describes its SSA branches, one for hearing and one for balance.

The cochlear branch begins with the spiral ganglion, a collection of neuron somas that are first-order neurons. These neurons receive auditory information from the hair cells inside the organ of Corti (**FIGURE 5-29**). Their axons form the cochlear nerve, which joins the vestibular branch to become the vestibulocochlear nerve. The vestibulocochlear nerve courses to the border of the pons and medulla and inputs into the cochlear nucleus. Auditory information is then relayed via a second neuron to the superior olivary complex in the pons. A third neuron continues the relay from the superior olivary complex to the inferior colliculus of the midbrain and a fourth from the inferior colliculus to the medial geniculate body of the thalamus. A final neuron projects from the thalamus to the auditory cortex, where the auditory information is decoded.

The vestibular branch has a more complicated pathway that begins with the vestibular ganglion picking up vestibular information from the semicircular canals. The axons of this ganglion form the vestibular branch, which interfaces with the cochlear branch and becomes the vestibulocochlear nerve. The vestibular nerves input in the vestibular nucleus near where the pons and medulla meet. From there, neurons project to the spinal cord, cerebellum, thalamus, and cortex.

Damage to cranial nerve VIII is associated with problems in equilibrium and hearing. In terms of impaired vestibular function, patients might experience balance issues and/or dizziness. Symptoms of auditory impairment could include various levels of hearing loss in addition to ringing in the ear, which is called tinnitus.

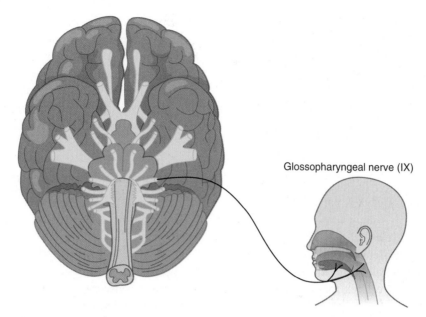

FIGURE 5-30 The glossopharyngeal nerve (IX).

Cranial Nerve IX: The Glossopharyngeal Nerve

The glossopharyngeal nerve originates at the medulla, and, like the facial nerve, it has both motor and sensory functions (**FIGURE 5-30**). In terms of motor function, it has GVE and SVE fibers, and for sensory it has GVA and SVA as well as GSA fibers. Only its SVE and GVA functions are notable for speech. Its SVE component innervates the stylopharyngeus muscle, a muscle that helps to elevate the pharynx and larynx. Elevation of the larynx is an important function in swallowing and may play a role in phonation. In terms of GVA function, the glossopharyngeal nerve relays touch, pain, and temperature information from the pharynx and tongue back to the brainstem and the sensory areas of the cerebral cortex. This function provides important feedback information for the motor function of these structures. This nerve mediates the gag reflex that involves a reflex contraction of the pharyngeal constrictor that helps to evacuate foreign materials in the throat and assists in vomiting.

Cranial Nerve X: The Vagus Nerve

The vagus nerve originates from the medulla and has three main branches: pharyngeal, superior laryngeal, and recurrent laryngeal. It has both motor (GVE, SVE) and sensory (GSA, GVA, and SVA) functions. Relevant for speech are its motor (SVE) functions (**FIGURE 5-31**).

The pharyngeal branch enters the pharynx, where it connects with branches from the glossopharyngeal and superior laryngeal nerves. From there, it distributes fibers

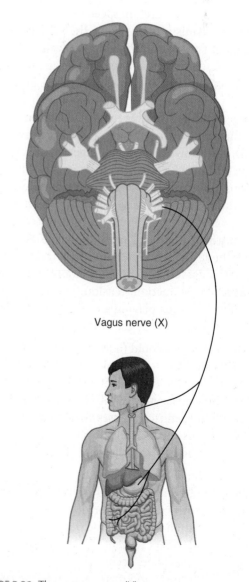

FIGURE 5-31 The vagus nerve (X).

to the pharyngeal and palatal muscles, with the exception of the stylopharyngeus (innervated by IX) and the tensor veli palatini (innervated by V). The muscles this branch innervates include the following:

- Superior pharyngeal constrictor (narrows pharyngeal diameter)
- Middle pharyngeal constrictor (narrows pharyngeal diameter)
- Inferior pharyngeal constrictor (narrows pharyngeal diameter)
- Salpingopharyngeus (elevates lateral pharyngeal wall)
- Levator veli palatini (elevates velum)
- Musculus uvulae (shortens velum)
- Palatoglossus (lowers velum)
- Palatopharyngeus (lowers velum)

These connections mean that the pharyngeal branch controls pharyngeal constriction as well as palatal elevation through its SVE fibers. Palatal elevation is a key feature in speech and swallowing, and this mechanism is known as the velopharyngeal mechanism. For speech, the palate elevates, allowing for the production of non-nasal sounds and lowers for the production of nasal sounds. Children born with cleft palate will commonly have trouble with the velopharyngeal mechanism due to musculature weakness. When the palate does not seal off the nasal cavity sufficiently, it is known as velopharyngeal insufficiency.

The larynx, which contains the vocal folds, is the voice-producing organ. As air passes upward during expiration, it vibrates the vocal folds, which in turn produce sound or voice. The vocal folds are controlled by the intrinsic laryngeal muscles, which are innervated by the superior and recurrent laryngeal branches of the vagus nerve. These muscles are responsible for the adduction, abduction, tension, and relaxation of the vocal cords, thus playing a critical role in speech production. They include the following:

- Lateral cricoarytenoid (adducts vocal folds)
- Transverse arytenoids (adduct vocal folds)
- Oblique arytenoids (adduct vocal folds)
- Posterior cricoarytenoid (abducts vocal folds)
- Cricothyroid muscle (tenses vocal folds)
- Thyrovocalis (tenses vocal folds)
- Thyromuscularis (relaxes vocal folds)

As mentioned, cranial nerve X contains two branches, the superior laryngeal nerve and the recurrent laryngeal nerve. The recurrent laryngeal nerve (RLN) controls all the intrinsic laryngeal muscles through its SVE fibers (except the cricothyroid muscle). This branch is called "recurrent" because it courses down under the aorta and then back up to the larynx. Damage to the RLN, especially bilateral damage, can be

catastrophic for voice production. The superior laryngeal nerve's external branch controls the cricothyroid muscle, which is crucial for pitch control. Its internal branch relays sensory information from the thyrohyoid membrane, a broad layer of tissue that runs from the hyoid bone down to the thyroid cartilage.

The vagus nerve's afferent functions include taste from the epiglottis and pharynx (SVA) and tactile sensation from the external ear canal (GSA). In addition, it conveys pain information from the mucous membranes of the following:

- Pharynx
- Larynx
- Trachea
- Esophagus
- Thoracic viscera
- Abdominal viscera

Cranial Nerve XI: The Spinal Accessory Nerve

The accessory nerve (XI), which begins at the medulla, is sometimes referred to as the spinal accessory nerve. It is motor in nature (SVE) and has two portions, the cranial and the spinal (**FIGURE 5-32**). The cranial portion joins the vagus nerve and becomes indistinguishable from it, thus possibly playing a role in pharyngeal and laryngeal function. It is debated whether this function is the work of the vagus nerve alone or a combination of the vagus and the accessory nerve; thus it is unknown whether the accessory nerve plays any role in speech. For the purposes of this text, we will assume it does not have a speech function. The spinal portion innervates the sternocleidomastoid and trapezius muscles of the neck.

Cranial Nerve XII: The Hypoglossal Nerve

Lastly, cranial nerve XII, the hypoglossal nerve (**FIGURE 5-33**), originates at the bottom of the medulla and controls the muscles of the tongue. It is a GSE nerve. The tongue is crucial for chewing, swallowing, and speech and damage to it can cause significant issues with these functions. It is the prime organ of articulation and consists of both intrinsic and extrinsic muscles.

Intrinsic tongue muscles enable precise tongue movements, like the ones needed for articulation. These include the following:

- Superior longitudinal (elevates, retracts, and deviates tongue tip)
- Inferior longitudinal (depresses tongue tip; retracts and deviates tongue)
- Transverse (narrows the tongue)
- Vertical (pulls tongue down to mouth floor)

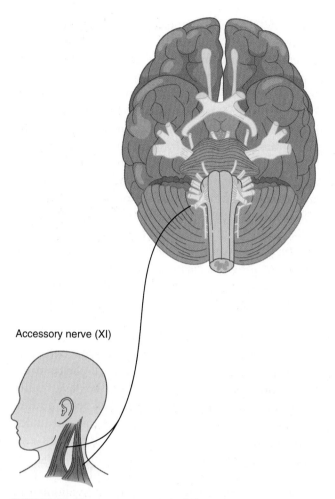

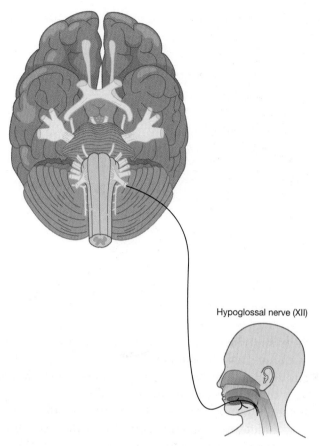

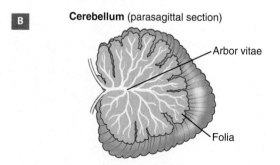

FIGURE 5-33 The hypoglossal nerve (XII).

FIGURE 5-32 The accessory nerve (XI).

The extrinsic tongue muscles work to move the tongue as a whole unit. This group of muscles includes the following:

- Genioglossus (retracts, protrudes, and depresses tongue)
- Hyoglossus (pulls tongue sides down)
- Styloglossus (draws tongue up and back)
- Chondroglossus (depresses tongue)

The palatoglossus is also an extrinsic tongue muscle but is controlled by cranial nerve X.

▶ The Cerebellum

Anatomy of the Cerebellum

Macroscopic Anatomy

The cerebellum (Latin for "little brain") lies inferior to the cerebral hemispheres and posterior to the pons (FIGURE 5-34). It looks like a piece of cauliflower in that it has numerous wrinkles, called folia, that give the cerebellum enormous surface area like the cerebral cortex. The cerebellum also has lobes similar to the cerebral cortex. The cerebellum's lobes include

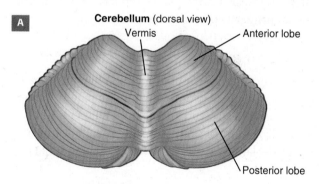

FIGURE 5-34 The cerebellum shown in isolation. **A.** Posterior view of the cerebellum. **B.** Sagittal section of the cerebellum.

the anterior, posterior, and flocculonodular (Latin for "small mass") lobes (FIGURE 5-35). It also has two hemispheres like the cerebral cortex, a right hemisphere and a left hemisphere. The two hemispheres are separated by a mound of tissue called the vermis.

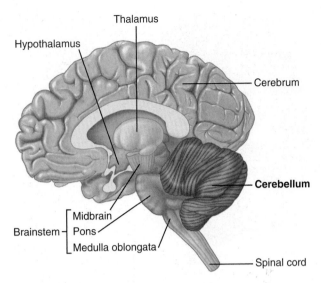

FIGURE 5-35 The cerebellum shown in relation to the rest of the brain.

Each hemisphere is made up of a central core of white matter and a surface of gray matter. Three large bundles of fibers called peduncles connect the cerebellum with the spinal cord, brainstem, and cerebral hemispheres. There are three of these bundles—the inferior, middle, and superior cerebellar peduncles. The inferior and middle cerebellar peduncles carry mainly afferent information, whereas the superior peduncle carries primarily motor information.

Microscopic Anatomy

The cerebellum has about 80% of the total neurons in the brain, some 69 billion neurons compared to about 18 billion in the cerebral cortex (Azevado et al., 2009). Cerebellar neurons are arranged in three layers: the molecular layer, the Purkinje cell layer, and the granular layer (**FIGURE 5-36**). The molecular layer consists of the dendrites from Purkinje neurons, a class of large GABA-ergic cells located only in the cerebellum. This layer also contains two other cells—stellate cells and basket cells—that provide inhibitory communication to Purkinje cells. The somas of Purkinje cells lie in the second Purkinje layer. The axons of these neurons project the neurotransmitter GABA to inhibit cerebellar nuclei deep in the cerebellum. This inhibitory control facilitates the cerebellum's motor coordination function. The granular layer contains the Purkinje cells' axons as well as granule cells, which use glutamate to excite the Purkinje, basket, stellate, and Golgi cells. Golgi cells have an inhibitory role on granule cells. This layer also has mossy fibers, which are one of the major afferent inputs into the cerebellum and are part of two tracts—the spinocerebellar and the pontocerebellar. They excite granule cells.

There are four major cerebellar pathways. The vestibulocerebellar pathway helps in overall body posture and balance as well as coordination of eye movements with body posture. The vermal spinocerebellar pathway maintains muscle tone and posture over trunk muscles and muscles in the pectoral and pelvic girdles. The paravermal spinocerebellar pathway maintains posture and muscle tone over distal limb muscles (e.g., hands, feet, lower arms and legs). Finally, the pontocerebellar pathway is responsible for planning, initiating, and timing motor activity that is volitional in nature. These pathways are summarized in **TABLE 5-4**.

Cerebellar Function
Motor Function

Functionally, the cerebellum is like a second brain, monitoring sensory input from a wide array of sensory

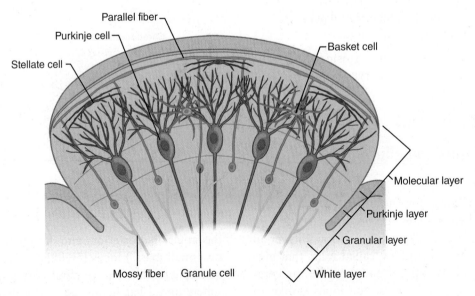

FIGURE 5-36 Cellular layers of the cerebellum.

TABLE 5-4 Major Cerebellar Pathways

Pathway Name	Function
Vestibulocerebellar	Overall body posture and balance; coordination of eye movements
Vermal spinocerebellar	Trunk and girdle muscle tone and posture
Paravermal spinocerebellar	Distal muscle group tone and posture
Pontocerebellar	Planning, initiating, and timing of volitional motor activity

TABLE 5-5 Symptoms of Cerebellar Damage

Symptom	Description
Ataxia	Discoordinated, clumsy movements
Dysmetria	Over- or undershooting touching a mark
Dysdiadochokinesia	Inability to perform rapid, alternating movements of hand or mouth
Nystagmus	Fast, involuntary eye movements either side to side or up and down
Ataxic dysarthria	Slurred or scanning (broken into syllables) speech
Hypotonia	Reduced muscle tone and reflexes; muscle tire

sources and integrating this feedback into motor movement. It monitors head and body position at rest as well as muscle tension and spinal cord activity. The cerebellum participates in the planning, monitoring, and correction of motor movement using all the sensory input it collects. This structure is also involved in our learning of motor skills. Cerebellar control is ipsilateral as compared to the cerebral cortex, where the majority of control is contralateral in nature.

Because speech is a motor process, it makes sense that the cerebellum would play an important role in speech production. It has long been known that a stroke in the cerebellum can lead to a type of dysarthria called ataxic dysarthria. Patients with this condition sound like they are intoxicated because their breathing and voice quality are irregular, articulation overshoots and undershoots place targets, and their speech rate is slow. In addition to this kind of motor coordination, the cerebellum may play a role in motor planning and a disorder of motor planning, apraxia of speech. This role is theorized because some of the symptoms of ataxic dysarthria and apraxia of speech overlap (e.g., speech timing, slowness of speech) (Mariën et al., 2014).

The motor functions of the cerebellum can be tested through a variety of methods. The finger–nose–finger method involves a person touching the examiner's finger, then his or her own nose, and then the examiner's finger again. The observer is looking for accuracy and smoothness of movement. Another test is diadochokinesia ability, which is a person's ability to make rapid, alternating movements with either the fingers or the mouth. For the mouth, the speech-language pathologist will ask the patient to say "pa-ta-ka" as fast as possible. Uncoordinated, sloppy movement may indicate cerebellar damage.

Linguistic Function

Growing evidence points to the cerebellum having an important modulating role in nonmotor, linguistic functions. Neuroimaging studies as well as cases of cerebellar-induced aphasia have contributed to the idea of a "linguistic cerebellum" (Mariën & Manto, 2015). Theorized language functions include assistance in the following: perception of speech/language, verbal working memory, verbal fluency, grammar processing, writing, and reading (Mariën et al., 2014).

Select Disorders of the Cerebellum

All cerebellar disorders are motor in nature (although, as mentioned, there are some cases of possible cerebellar-induced aphasia; see Mariën et al., 2014, for more information). The symptoms of these disorders are shown in **TABLE 5-5**. Four specific syndromes are discussed in the following sections.

Cerebellar Hemispheral Syndrome

Cerebellar hemispheral syndrome can be caused by stroke, tumor, and multiple sclerosis. The syndrome primarily affects the ipsilateral limbs, causing tremor, dysmetria, and dysdiadochokinesia. Patients also experience the **Holmes rebound phenomenon**, which can be elicited by the patient holding out one of his or her arms while the examiner tries to push down on it. The rebound phenomenon occurs when the examiner lets go of the patient's arm, which then bounces up significantly.

Vermal Syndrome

Vermal syndrome is due to damage to the vermis. Common causes include stroke, tumor, multiple sclerosis, and other degenerative disorders. The condition primarily affects the trunk muscles, causing unsteadiness, tremor, postural issues, and gait ataxia. **Gait ataxia** involves the patient walking with a wide base (i.e., the feet wide apart), which gives the sense of extra stability.

Friedreich Ataxia

Friedreich ataxia is an inherited, progressive neurological disorder that follows an autosomal recessive inheritance pattern. Symptoms begin between the ages of 8 and 14 years and can include progressive muscle weakness in the limbs, loss of coordination, dysmetria, dysarthria, curvature of the spine, and vision and hearing issues. Most patients have cardiac issues (chronic myocarditis); as a result, the median age of death is 35 years.

Cerebellar Agenesis

Can a person live without a cerebellum? The answer is *yes,* and the rare condition is known as **primary cerebellar agenesis.** Yu, Jiang, Sun, and Zhang (2014)

present a case of a 24-year-old woman who was admitted to the hospital with a 1-month history of dizziness and nausea. Her mother reported that she began to walk at age 7 years and speak at 6 years. Doctors at the hospital performed a computed tomography scan and discovered that she did not have a cerebellum. cerebrospinal fluid filled the space where the cerebellum should have been. The woman was remarkably functional despite this significant loss of 10% of the brain's volume and 50% of the brain's neurons, demonstrating how the brain rewires itself and compensates for losses. Though primary cerebellar agenesis is rare, other cases have been reported in the literature (Boyd, 2010; Glickstein, 1994).

▶ Conclusion

Following the course of this chapter is akin to tracing a tree up its trunk and through its branches. The spinal cord is the trunk that transitions into the brainstem and cerebellum. From the brainstem, branches called cranial nerves extend away from the brainstem and connect to head and neck structures. These nerves play a role in linking the cerebrum to the body by relaying either motor, sensory, special sensory, or parasympathetic information or some combination of the four. Many of these nerves are of concern to the speech-language pathologist and audiologist because they relay information related to articulation, voice, hearing, and swallowing.

SUMMARY OF LEARNING OBJECTIVES

The following were the main learning objectives of this chapter. The information that should have been learned is below each learning objective.

1. The learner will label a diagram of a cross-section of the spinal cord.

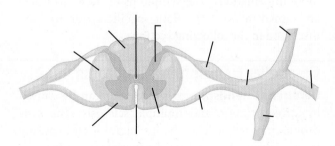

2. The learner will label a diagram of the brainstem.

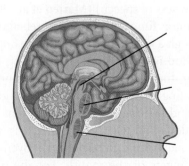

3. The learner will be able to list all the cranial nerves (Roman numeral and name).

On	I	Olfactory
Old	II	Optic
Olympus	III	Oculomotor
Towering	IV	Trochlear
Tops	V	Trigeminal
A	VI	Abducens
Fin	VII	Facial
And	VIII	Auditory
German	IX	Glossopharyngeal
Viewed	X	Vagus
Some	XI	Spinal accessory
Hops	XII	Hypoglossal

4. The learner will list important cranial nerves for articulation, voice, swallowing, and hearing.
   - *Articulation:* Cranial nerves involved in speaking include V, VII, X, XI, and XII.
   - *Voice:* Cranial nerves for voice include V, VII, X, and XII.
   - *Swallowing:* Cranial nerves V, VII, X, XI, and XII are used for the oral preparatory and oral phases of the normal swallow. The pharyngeal phase of the swallow depends on another set of muscles to move food and liquid through the pharynx. These muscles are controlled by cranial nerves IX, X, and XI.
   - *Hearing:* Cranial nerves V, VII, and VIII are involved in hearing.

5. The learner will describe the form and function of the cerebellum.
   - The cerebellum is located inferior to the cerebral hemispheres and posterior to the pons.
   - It has lobes similar to the cerebral cortex. The cerebellum's lobes are the anterior, posterior, and flocculonodular (Latin for "small mass") lobes.
   - The cerebellum also has two hemispheres like the cerebral cortex, a right hemisphere and a left hemisphere.
   - It monitors head and body position at rest as well as muscle tension and spinal cord activity.
   - It participates in the planning, monitoring, and correction of motor movement using all the sensory input it collects.
   - It is involved in our learning of motor skills.
   - The cerebellum may have an important role in assisting in language functions.

KEY TERMS

Alpha motor neurons
Anosmia
Anterior (ventral) corticospinal tract
Benedikt syndrome
Cerebellar hemispheral syndrome
Cerebellar peduncle
Cerebral peduncles
Cerebral spinal rhinorrhea
Crus cerebri
Dermatome
Diplopia
Dorsal columns
Friedreich ataxia
Gait ataxia

Gamma motor neurons
General somatic afferent (GSA) fibers
General somatic efferent (GSE) fibers
General visceral afferent (GVA) fibers
General visceral efferent (GVE) fibers
Holmes rebound phenomenon
Inferior colliculi
Lateral corticospinal/corticobulbar tract
Locked-in syndrome (LIS)
Medulla

Midbrain
Motor unit
Myelitis
Palsy
Peripheral neuropathy
Phrenic nerve
Pineal gland
Plexus
Pons
Primary cerebellar agenesis
Proprioception
Ptosis
Red nucleus
Reflex arc
Reticulospinal tract

Rubrospinal tract
Special somatic afferent (SSA) fibers
Special visceral afferent (SVA) fibers
Special visceral efferent (SVE) fibers

Spinal cord injury (SCI)
Spinocerebellar tracts
Spinothalamic tracts
Strabismus
Substantia nigra
Superior colliculi
Tectospinal tract

Tectum
Tegmentum
Vermal syndrome
Vestibulospinal tract
Wallenberg syndrome
Weber syndrome

DRAW IT TO KNOW IT

1. Sketch a cross-section of the spinal cord along with its spinal nerve (see Figure 5-6). Label all the important structures.

2. Sketch a cross-section of the spinal cord and label all the motor and sensory tracts (see Figure 5-8).

3. Sketch the brainstem and label the midbrain, pons, and medulla.

QUESTIONS FOR DEEPER REFLECTION

1. Describe the functions of the brainstem.
2. List and describe disorders that can occur in brainstem injury.

3. List the cranial nerves involved in each of the following: speech, voice, swallowing, hearing.
4. List the functions of the cerebellum.

CASE STUDIES

A 50-year-old man experienced a sudden loss of muscle function in the left side of his face. In addition, he experienced pain behind his left ear and some changes in taste. Stroke was ruled out as the remainder of his motor function was preserved, and he was diagnosed with Bell's palsy. Given his symptoms, please explain the following:

1. What cranial nerve VII muscle fibers are responsible for the loss of muscle function on the left side of his face, pain behind his ear, and the changes in his taste? Look at Table 5-3 if you need help.
2. Is this condition a lower motor neuron or upper motor neuron issue? Please explain why you think so.

Mary is a 47-year-old-female who was diagnosed with Stage IV breast cancer about a year ago. She is status post chemotherapy and bilateral mastectomy and is currently completing radiation therapy to the chest. Recently, she has been experiencing difficulty moving her tongue, which is affecting chewing, swallowing, and speech. Upon investigation, the left side of her tongue appears paralyzed. An MRI revealed a lesion at the base of her skull that appears to be affecting one of her cranial nerves. Which cranial nerve do you think is being affected and why?

SUGGESTED PROJECTS

1. Take one of the disorders in this chapter and write two to three pages about it including the following sections: cause, signs and symptoms, diagnosis, treatment, and speech/swallowing/hearing issues.

2. Create a digital movie using your smartphone, teaching the class about reflexes and the reflex arc. Include reflexes important in communication disorders.

REFERENCES

Azevedo, F. A., Carvalho, L. R., Grinberg, L. T., Farfel, J. M., Ferretti, R. E., & Leite, R. E., . . . Herculano-Houzel, S. (2009). Equal numbers of neuronal and nonneuronal cells make the human brain an isometrically scaled-up primate brain. *Journal of Comparative Neurology, 513*(5), 532–541.

Bauby, J. D. (1998). *The diving bell and the butterfly*. New York, NY: Vintage Books.
Boyd, C. A. (2010). Cerebellar agenesis revisited. *Brain, 133*, 941–944.

British Broadcasting Corporation. (2010). *"I recovered from locked-in syndrome."* Retrieved from http://www.bbc.com/news/health-10985836

British Broadcasting Corporation. (2012). *Woman's recovery from "locked-in" syndrome.* Retrieved from http://www.bbc.com/news/health-17363584

Davis, M., Falls, W. A., & Gewirtz, J. (2000). Neural systems involved in fear inhibition: Extinction and conditioned inhibition. In M. Myslobodsky & I. Weiner (Eds.), *Contemporary issues in modeling psychopathology* (pp. 113–142). Norwell, MA: Kluwer Academic.

Glickstein, M. (1994). Cerebellar agenesis. *Brain, 117*, 1209–1212.

Mariën, P., Ackermann, H., Adamaszek, M., Barwood, C. H., Beaton, A., & Desmond, J., . . . Leggio, M. (2014). Language and the cerebellum: An ongoing enigma. *The Cerebellum, 13*(3), 386–410.

Mariën, P., & Manto, M. (Eds.). (2015). *The linguistic cerebellum.* Waltham, MA: Academic Press.

Monkhouse, S. (2006). *Cranial nerves: Functional anatomy.* Cambridge, UK: Cambridge University Press.

National Spinal Cord Injury Statistical Center (NSCISC). (2017). *Spinal cord injury facts and figures at a glance.* Birmingham, AL: University of Alabama at Birmingham. Retrieved from https://www.nscisc.uab.edu/Public/Facts%20and%20Figures%20-%202017.pdf

Saladin, K. S. (2007). *Anatomy and physiology: The unity of form and function.* Dubuque, IA: McGraw-Hill.

Seikel, J. A., King, D. W., & Drumright, D. G. (2010). *Anatomy and physiology for speech, language, and hearing.* Clifton Park, NY: Delmar.

Victor, M., & Ropper, A. H. (2001). *Principles of neurology* (7th ed.). New York, NY: McGraw-Hill.

Yu, F., Jiang, Q.-J., Sun, X.-Y., Zhang, R.-W. (2014). A new case of complete primary cerebellar agenesis: Clinical and imaging findings in a living patient. *Brain, 138*(6), e353. https://doi.org/10.1093/brain/awu239

Zemlin, W. R. (1998). *Speech and hearing science: Anatomy and physiology.* Boston, MA: Allyn and Bacon.

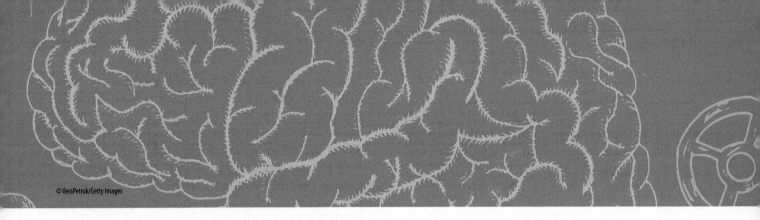
© VeraPetruk/Getty Images

CHAPTER 6

Diencephalon, Basal Ganglia, and Brain Ventricles

CHAPTER PREVIEW

In this chapter we will explore what sits above the brainstem and inside the brain—the diencephalon and surrounding structures. More specifically, we will learn about the thalamus, basal ganglia, and brain ventricles. We will also survey a few select disorders associated with these structures.

IN THIS CHAPTER

In this chapter, we will . . .

- Learn about the four parts of the diencephalon
- Survey the form and function of the basal ganglia
- Describe the brain ventricles
- Discuss the role of cerebrospinal fluid
- Survey disorders related to damage to the structures listed here

LEARNING OBJECTIVES

- The learner will list the four parts of the diencephalon and briefly describe the function of each.
- The learner will draw the basal ganglia and describe the function of these nuclei.
- The learner will list the names of the four brain ventricles.
- The learner will describe cerebrospinal fluid's composition and its function.
- The learner will list and briefly describe disorders associated with the diencephalon, basal ganglia, and brain ventricles.

▶ Introduction

In this chapter, the diencephalon, basal ganglia, and brain ventricles will be explored. Special attention will be paid to what these structures might contribute to speech, language, and hearing.

▶ The Diencephalon

The diencephalon is located between the cerebrum and the brainstem, resting above the midbrain of the brainstem. Its location makes it a prime area for connecting the cerebral cortex to the rest of the body. It also connects the nervous system to the endocrine system, our hormone system. The diencephalon consists of four parts: the thalamus, subthalamus, hypothalamus, and epithalamus (**FIGURE 6-1**).

Thalamus

Thalamus is a Greek term meaning "inner chamber" or "bedroom." The thalamus sits on top of the midbrain and consists of two halves, or hemispheres, each being about the size of a walnut (**FIGURE 6-2**). In terms of

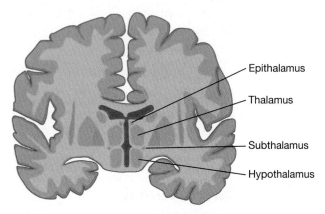

FIGURE 6-1 Coronal section of the brain showing the epithalamus, thalamus, subthalamus, and hypothalamus.

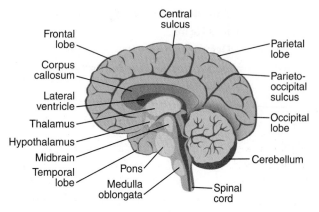

FIGURE 6-2 Medial view of the brain illustrating the location of the thalamus.
© Alila Medical Images/Shutterstock.

function, the thalamus has been traditionally viewed as a sensory fiber relay station or switchboard between the cerebral cortex and subcortical areas. Perhaps a more modern-day analogy for the thalamus's function would be an Internet router, but instead of routing a very general signal, it routes specific information to specific cortical areas. More specifically, the thalamus processes all sensory information (except olfaction), routing it to specialization cerebral cortex locations, which in turn process the particular type of sensory information (e.g., vision). The thalamus is involved in motor function, but only indirectly through directing some extrapyramidal fibers, which control more autonomic functions, to the basal ganglia (Sherman, 2006; Webster, 1999).

Structure and Function of the Thalamus

The thalamus is made up of several different nuclei. (See **TABLE 6-1** for a list of all thalamic nuclei and **FIGURE 6-3** for a picture of thalamic nuclei.) These nuclei are specialized in the sense that they have specific functions. We will now survey the thalamic nuclei, paying close attention to those involved with speech, language, or hearing.

Medial Nuclei

The dorsomedial nuclei (DMs) receive information from the hypothalamus, amygdala, and other thalamic nuclei. After processing this information, they project it to the prefrontal cortex and septal area (i.e., the septum pellucidum—a membrane that separates the right and left ventricles) (Webster, 1999). The DMs function in attention and eye–head control. They also are involved in emotion and autonomic control (Castro, Merchut, Neafsey, & Wurster, 2002).

Lateral Dorsal Nuclei

This group contains three nuclei. Information inputs into the lateral dorsal nucleus (LD) from the hypothalamus and other thalamic nuclei and then projects to the septal area, cingulate gyrus, and parahippocampal gyrus. These structures are involved in the limbic system, where emotional processing takes place (Webster, 1999). The lateral posterior nucleus (LP) receives information from two ventral thalamic nuclei and the superior colliculus and then projects to the parietal association cortex (areas 5 and 7). Its functions include eye control and vision. The pulvinar nucleus (P), the largest nucleus in the thalamus, receives input from the superior colliculus and projects to the secondary visual cortex (areas 18 and 19). Like the LP, the P is involved in vision and eye control.

TABLE 6-1 Thalamic Nuclei

Group	Thalamic Nucleus	Afferent Inputs	Efferent Outputs
Medial	Dorsomedial (DM)	Hypothalamus, amygdala, other thalamic nuclei	Prefrontal cortex, septal area
Lateral dorsal	Lateral dorsal (LD)	Hypothalamus; other thalamic nuclei	Septal area, cingulate gyrus, parahippocampal gyrus
	Lateral posterior (LP)	Ventral posterior medial and lateral nuclei	Superior and inferior parietal lobe
	Pulvinar (P)	Superior colliculus, visual association cortices, frontal eye cortex	Superior colliculus, visual association cortices, frontal eye cortex
Lateral ventral	Ventral anterior (VA)	Basal ganglia, cerebellum	Motor cortices
	Ventral lateral (VL)	Basal ganglia, cerebellum	Motor cortices
	Ventral posterior lateral (VPL)	Medial lemniscus, spinothalamic tract	Postcentral gyrus
	Ventral posterior medial (VPM)	Trigeminothalamic tract	Postcentral gyrus
	Medial geniculate body (MGB)	Inferior colliculus	Primary auditory cortex
	Lateral geniculate body (LGB)	Optic tract	Primary visual cortex
Anterior	Anterior nucleus (AN)	Mammillary body	Cingulate cortex
Intralaminar	Centromedian Parafascicular	Reticular formation Other thalamic nuclei	Cerebral cortex Basal ganglia
Reticular	Reticular	Cerebral cortex, basal ganglia, other thalamic nuclei	Other thalamic nuclei, basal ganglia
Midline	Midline	Amygdala, cingulate gyrus, hypothalamus	Amygdala, cingulate gyrus, hypothalamus

Data from: Webster, D. B. (1999). *Neuroscience of communication* (2nd ed.). San Diego, CA: Singular Publishing.

Lateral Ventral Nuclei

This grouping contains six nuclei. The ventral posterior lateral nucleus (VPL) and ventral posterior medial nucleus (VPM) are often grouped together as the ventral posterior (VP) nuclei because they have the same projections and functions. The VPL receives input from the medial lemniscus and spinothalamic tract. The spinothalamic tract transmits pain, temperature, and crude touch information from the body to the thalamus. The VPM receives its inputs from the trigeminothalamic tract, which has the same sensory function as the spinothalamic tract, but from the several cranial nerves associated with the face (V, VII, IX, X) instead of the body in general. The VPL

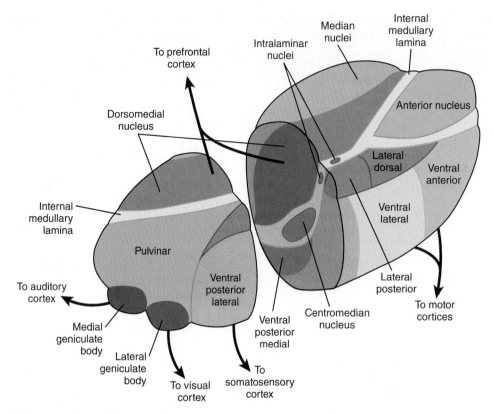

FIGURE 6-3 The thalamic nuclei and their projections.

and VPM both project from the thalamus to the sensory cortex (areas 3, 2, 1) and are thus involved in somatosensory function. The VPM is the more crucial nucleus to remember for speech because it relays sensory information from the speech structures as they move and make articulatory contact.

The ventral lateral nucleus (VL) and ventral anterior nucleus (VA) also are grouped because they have the same inputs and projections. Both receive input from the basal ganglia and the cerebellum and then project to motor cortices, the VL to the primary motor cortex (area 4) and the VA to the premotor cortex (area 6) and supplementary motor area. The VL functions in executing movements, whereas the VA is involved in motor planning; both are involved in speech production.

The final two nuclei in this grouping are sometimes classified under lateral ventral nuclei, as we have done here, or sometimes grouped together under the metathalamus (*meta* is Greek for "after"). The **medial geniculate body (MGB)** relays auditory information from subcortical midbrain structures (i.e., inferior colliculus) to the primary auditory cortex of the temporal lobe, and thus is important for our sense of hearing. Visual information is sent via the optic nerve to the **lateral geniculate body (LGB)** of the thalamus, which then projects to the primary visual cortex of the occipital lobe. The MGB is the auditory center

of the thalamus, whereas the LGB is the visual center. Many confuse the functions of the MGB and LGB, but a helpful mnemonic is medial = music (hearing) and lateral = light (vision).

Anterior Nucleus

The anterior nucleus (AN) is involved in emotional processing due to its connection to the limbic system. The mammillary bodies receive input from the amygdala and hippocampus, which are part of the limbic system, and then project to another limbic structure, the cingulate cortex. Because of these connections, the AN is intimately involved in our emotional processing system.

Intralaminar Nuclei

There are two intralaminar nuclei of the thalamus, the centromedian intralaminar nucleus and the parafascicular intralaminar nucleus. These nuclei receive input from the reticular formation and other thalamic nuclei and project to the basal ganglia and numerous places in the cerebral cortex. Their connections would suggest a role in arousal and motor function.

Reticular Nuclei

The reticular nuclei receive input from the cerebral cortex, basal ganglia, and other thalamic nuclei but do not project information to the cerebral cortex. Rather, they make connections to other thalamic nuclei and the basal ganglia (Webster, 1999). Kandel, Schwartz, Jessell, Siegelbaum, and Hudspeth (2013) report that the reticular nuclei monitor all the information between the cerebral cortex and the thalamus and act as a filter for information ascending to the cortex.

Midline Nuclei

These nuclei are interconnected with the amygdala, cingulate gyrus, and hypothalamus. Their function is not well understood, but they may facilitate emotional processing.

Blood Supply to the Thalamus

The anterior portion of the thalamus (VA, VL, and anterior DM) is supplied by the tuberothalamic arteries that branch off of the internal carotid artery's (ICA's) posterior communicating artery (P-com) (**FIGURE 6-4**). The paramedial thalamus is supplied by the paramedian thalamic artery that arises from the posterior cerebral artery (PCA). The inferior lateral portion of the thalamus is supplied by PCA's inferolateral arteries, which are also known as the thalamogeniculate arteries. The posterior thalamus's blood supply is provided by the PCA's posterior choroidal arteries (Li et al., 2018).

Thalamic Disorders

In addition to being a relay station, the thalamus also plays a role in the perception of pain, regulation of cortical arousal, and control of the sleep–wake cycle

(Sherman, 2006). The thalamus receives projections from multiple ascending sensory pathways, including pathways for pain (Ab Aziz & Ahmad, 2006). Damage to the thalamus can result in **thalamic pain syndrome**, which is also known as Dejerine-Roussy syndrome. This condition involves burning or tingling sensations and possibly hypersensitivity to stimuli that would not normally be painful, such as light touch or temperature change. The condition can be both severe and debilitating.

The thalamus relays important fibers related to cortical arousal from the brainstem's reticular formation to the cerebral cortex. Damage to specific thalamic regions associated with these fibers can result in disorders of consciousness, such as coma, excessive daytime sleepiness (i.e., **hypersomnia**), and patients who are passive and do not move or talk (i.e., **akinetic mutism**) (Castaigne et al., 1981).

What role does the thalamus play in speech and language? Johnson and Ojemann (2000) have proposed that the dominant ventrolateral thalamus (the left ventrolateral thalamus in most people) plays an important role in language and coordinating the cognitive and motor aspects of language. Using electrical stimulation to this area, they were able to induce misnaming and perseverations as well as articulation errors.

Crosson (1984) described what is now called **thalamic aphasia**, a type of aphasia noted to have three main characteristics. The first is fluent verbal output with semantic paraphasias that often results in jargon. The second characteristic is auditory comprehension that is less severe than one would expect for the severity

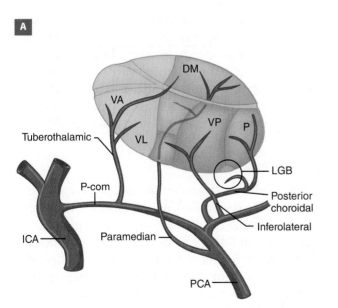
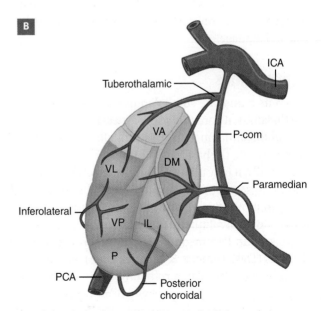

FIGURE 6-4 Blood supply to the thalamus showing four main arteries and the thalamic nuclei they supply. **A.** Lateral view of the thalamus and its blood supply. **B.** Dorsal view of the thalamus and its blood supply. *Abbreviations*: DM, dorsomedial; ICA, internal carotid artery; IL, intralaminar nucleus; LGB, lateral geniculate body; P, pulvinar nucleus; PCA, poster cerebral artery; VA, ventral anterior; VL, ventral lateral; VP, ventral posterior.

TABLE 6-2 Fluent Aphasic Conditions Compared

	Wernicke	Transcortical Sensory	Conduction	Thalamic	Anomic
Fluency	+	+	+	+	+
Auditory comprehension	−	−	+	=	+
Repetition	−	+	−	=	+

+, preserved; −, significantly impaired; =, minimally impaired.

of verbal output. The third characteristic is minimally impaired or even intact repetition. These symptoms are consistent in cases of damage to the dominant thalamic hemisphere (Crosson, 1992), which is consistent with Johnson and Ojemann's (2000) findings.

Thalamic aphasia defies classical definitions of fluent aphasia (TABLE 6-2). It is obviously different from Wernicke aphasia, in which patients are fluent with paraphasias but have significantly impaired auditory comprehension and repetition. It is also different from transcortical sensory aphasia, which involves significantly impaired auditory comprehension with fluent, neologism-filled speech and preserved but echolalic repetition. Thalamic aphasia is also different from conduction aphasia due to thalamic aphasia's relatively intact repetition (Papathanasiou, Coppens, & Potagas, 2013). The occurrence of thalamic aphasia suggests that subcortical structures, such as the thalamus, along with the cerebral cortex play an important role in language.

Subthalamus

Given its name, the subthalamus obviously lies below the thalamus; it contains a set of specialized cells called the subthalamic nucleus. Functionally, it has more in common with the basal ganglia than with the thalamus. Specifically, it may play a role in the selection of actions and impulse control. Damage to the subthalamus can result in motor problems like hemiballismus, which is a one-sided involuntary flinging of the limbs sometimes seen in Parkinson disease or other neurological diseases (Das, Romero, & Mandel, 2005). Subthalamic damage may also play a role in obsessive-compulsive disorder and general impulsivity (Carter, 2009; Frank, Samanta, Moustafa, & Sherman, 2007; Mallet et al., 2008). Deep brain stimulation of the subthalamus has been shown to relieve some types of tremors and other

involuntary movements (Kitagawa et al., 2000), which demonstrates the subthalamus's close connection to the basal ganglia (**BOX 6-1**).

Hypothalamus

The term *hypothalamus* means "under chamber." It is about the size of an almond and lies just under the anterior ventral surface of the thalamus (**FIGURE 6-6**). In terms of function, it can be thought of as a linker and a regulator. It is a linker because it connects the nervous system to the endocrine system (i.e., hormonal system) via the hypothalamus's **pituitary gland**. In addition, the hypothalamus is a regulator because it controls aspects of metabolism, body temperature, food intake, circadian rhythms, emotion, and secondary sex characteristics, among other functions (**FIGURE 6-7**). These functions could all be said to revolve around the idea of **homeostasis** or maintaining the body's status quo (Fauci, 2008). The hypothalamus does not appear to play any direct role in speech, language, or hearing, but it may play an indirect role in regulating some substances that be involved in neurotransmitter function, which in turn may affect disorders such as dyslexia, aphasia, and developmental speech delay (Kurup & Kurup, 2003).

Epithalamus

The epithalamus lies superior and posterior to the thalamus. It consists of the pineal gland, habenula, and stria medullaris. The **pineal** ("pine cone") **gland** is an endocrine gland that gets its name from its pinecone shape (Figure 6-6). It is about the size and shape of a grain of rice, being about 5 to 8 millimeters in size. It produces a hormone known as melatonin, which is involved in regulating the sleep–wake cycle, as well as our circadian rhythms, and in gonad development. After puberty, this gland hardens due to a buildup of

BOX 6-1 Deep Brain Stimulation

Deep brain stimulation is like a pacemaker for the brain. It has been shown to be effective for treating chronic pain as well as tremors and other involuntary movements. Deep brain stimulation is enabled through a neurosurgical procedure to open the skull and place a device that provides a continuous electrical signal to specific areas of the brain (**FIGURE 6-5**). For treating chronic pain, the target would be specific thalamic nuclei. For treating tremor and other involuntary movements, the internal part of the globus pallidus (GPi) and the subthalamic nucleus could be targets. The procedure has brought relief to patients with many different diagnoses, including Parkinson disease and Huntington disease. Some advantages of the procedure are (1) it can be done on both sides of the brain to control symptoms affecting both sides of the body, (2) its effects are reversible, and (3) it can control symptoms on a continuous 24-hour basis. There are risks for the procedure as there are for any medical procedure. Some risks include cerebral hemorrhage, cerebrospinal fluid leaking, or an infection at the surgical site.

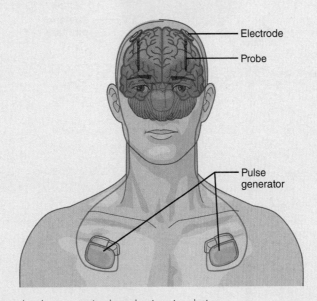

FIGURE 6-5 Illustration of electrode placement in deep brain stimulation.

National Institute of Mental Health (NIMH), National Institutes of Health (NIH,). *Brain stimulation therapies*. Retrieved from https://www.nimh.nih.gov/health/topics/brain-stimulation-therapies/brain-stimulation-therapies.shtml

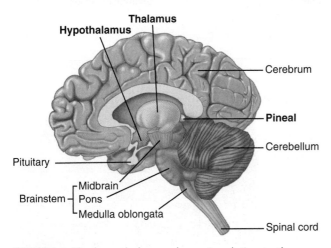

FIGURE 6-6 The hypothalamus shown in relation to the thalamus.

calcium (i.e., calcification) and becomes a useful landmark in neuroimaging because of its dense structure. The famous philosopher René Descartes believed the pineal gland was the seat of the soul.

The habenula ("rein") is a group of nuclei that lies anterior to the pineal gland. It is involved in olfactory reflexes, such as when we salivate at the smell of food (i.e., parotid salivary reflex) or gag in response to a noxious odor. The habenula is also involved in stress responses due to connections to the limbic system as well as our reward processing system (Andres, Düring, & Veh, 1999; Matsumoto & Hikosaka, 2008). The stria medullaris, a white matter tract, connects the habenular nuclei to the limbic system (Swenson, 2006).

▶ The Basal Ganglia

Structure and Function of the Basal Ganglia

The **basal ganglia** are a group of structures that make up most of the remaining subcortical gray matter regions of the brain. They consist of three large

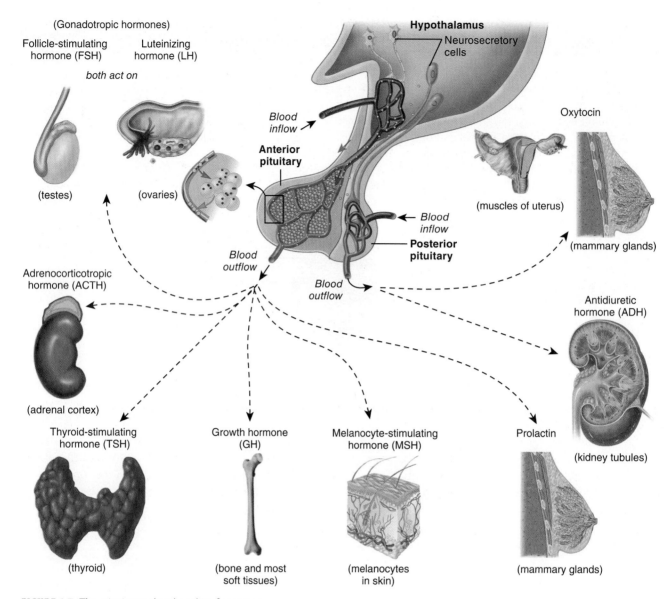

FIGURE 6-7 The pituitary gland and its functions.

nuclei, the **caudate nucleus**, **globus pallidus**, and **putamen** (FIGURE 6-8). The globus pallidus (Latin for "pale globe") and putamen (Latin for "shell") reside together but are separate from the caudate nucleus. Along with the midbrain's substantia nigra and sub-thalamic nuclei, these structures are key components of the basal ganglia and the extrapyramidal motor system. Damage to this motor system results in dyskinesias or movement disorders.

The caudate nucleus (Latin for "having a tail") is in the shape of an arch (FIGURE 6-9). It has a bulbous head anteriorly and a thin tail that leads into a second bulge, the **amygdala** (part of the limbic system). The caudate is separated from the globus pallidus and putamen by the internal capsule. Functionally, the caudate and putamen

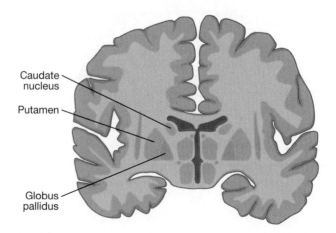

FIGURE 6-8 Coronal view of main structures of the basal ganglia.

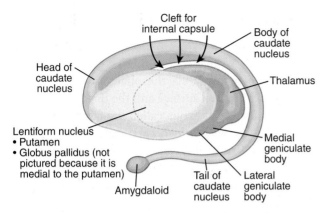

FIGURE 6-9 Lateral view of the basal ganglia in isolation.

are one nucleus called the **striatum**, a term that means "striped." Anatomically, the putamen and the globus pallidus are lumped together under the name **lenticular** (Latin for "lens") **nucleus**. The globus pallidus has two nuclei, an external (GPe) and an internal (GPi).

Functionally, the basal ganglia have two major pathways that run through them (**FIGURE 6-10**). There is a *direct pathway* from the striatum to the medial globus pallidus to the VA and VL thalamic nuclei, which facilitates movement. In addition, an *indirect pathway* runs from the striatum to the lateral globus pallidus to subthalamic nuclei back to the medial globus pallidus and finally back to the VA and VL thalamic nuclei. This indirect pathway functions to inhibit movement (Castro et al., 2002).

The basal ganglia also have many connections to the cerebral cortex, but their connections to cortical

motor areas are the most significant. Using the neurotransmitter dopamine, which is produced in the midbrain's substantia nigra, the basal ganglia regulate important extrapyramidal motor functions such as posture, balance, arm swinging, and other body movements (e.g., walking). This regulation includes activating, sustaining, and inhibiting motor movements.

Damage to the basal ganglia can be classified in different ways. LaPointe and Murdoch (2014) suggest two categories: **dyskinesias**, which are involuntary movements, and **akinesias**, which are involuntary postures. The category of dyskinesias include tremors (rhythmic shaking), athetosis (slow, writhing movements of the head and hands), chorea (quick, abrupt fidgeting of the hands and/or feet), ballismus (quick flinging of a limb), and **tics** (quick, stereotyped motor or vocal behaviors). In contrast, akinesias include rigidity (limb resistance to passive movement), dystonia (simultaneous agonist and antagonist muscle contraction resulting in distorted movements and postures), and bradykinesia (slow movements).

Patients with basal ganglia damage can have both dyskinesias and akinesias at the same time. For example, the three hallmark characteristics of Parkinson disease include two akinesias (bradykinesia and rigidity) and one dyskinesia (tremor). Another example is Huntington disease, which typically has one dyskinesia (chorea) and one akinesia (dystonia). There are also basal ganglia disorders that have just one category, like Tourette syndrome and its motor and vocal tics (**BOX 6-2**).

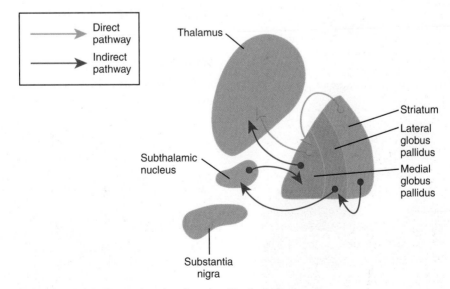

FIGURE 6-10 The basal ganglia circuit illustrating the direct and indirect pathways.

BOX 6-2 Tourette Syndrome

Tourette syndrome (TS) is a neurological disorder characterized by involuntary motor and/or vocal tics. A tic is a repetitive, involuntary behavior. TS is named after a French neurologist named Georges Gilles de la Tourette (1857–1904), who first described the condition in 1885. The exact etiology of the condition is unknown, but there is evidence through twin studies that it may be inherited. The symptoms of TS emerge in early childhood (age 3 to 9 years), and the condition affects males three to four times more often than it does females. About 200,000 people in the United States suffer from TS, and another 1 in 100 may have a mild **FIGURE 6-11**, undiagnosed form of the condition. The symptoms of the disease are sometimes the worst in adolescence and improve as the person ages. As mentioned earlier, the primary symptom is tics. Motor tics can involve behaviors like eye blinking, facial grimacing, or sudden jerks of the head. Vocal tics can include grunting or barking sounds, throat clearing, or sniffing. TS is diagnosed through clinical presentation and ruling out other neurological disorders. There is no cure for the condition, but neuroleptic drugs (i.e., antipsychotic drugs like aripiprazole [Abilify]) do bring some relief to some people with TS, although patients may complain that the drugs' side effects are worse than the symptoms of TS.

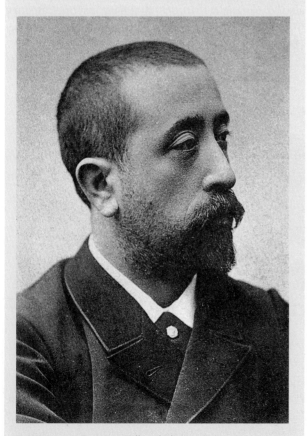

FIGURE 6-11 Georges Gilles de la Tourette.

Internal Capsule and Corona Radiata

Almost all sensory information is relayed through the thalamus with the exception of olfaction, which has its own pathway via the olfactory bulbs. Fibers between the cortical surface and the thalamus create a fan-shaped sheet of axons called the **corona radiata** ("radiating crown"), which carries nearly all neuron traffic to and from the cerebral cortex (**FIGURE 6-12**). Much cerebral activity takes place in this dense white matter area because disorders involving it result in significant deficits in cognitive, social, and emotional abilities. Multiple sclerosis is a disorder in which the myelin-producing oligodendroglia are lost, resulting in the white myelin sheath that surrounds axons being either thinned or lost altogether. This leads to multiple scars in places like the corona radiata, and thus the name multiple sclerosis or "multiple scarring" (Reich et al., 2007). The neurons involved can no longer effectively transfer signals, and patients suffer motor, cognitive, and sometimes even psychiatric problems (Daroff, Fenichel, Jankovic, & Mazziotta, 2012).

As the fibers of the corona radiata course down, they taper as they enter the **internal capsule**, a narrow space between the caudate nucleus and the lenticular nucleus (Catani & de Schotten, 2012). The internal capsule is illustrated in Figure 6-11. The internal capsule bends as it passes between the thalamus and the basal ganglia; the bend is called the **genu** (Latin for "knee") of the internal capsule. Lesions to the genu can affect the corticobulbar tract, an important motor pathway for voluntary motor function in the head and neck (e.g., speech), and lead to either hemiplegia or hemiparesis.

Basal Ganglia Disorders

Parkinson Disease

What Is It?

Parkinson disease (PD) is a progressive extrapyramidal movement disorder involving degeneration of the

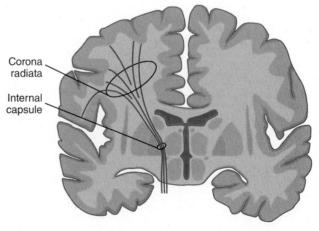

FIGURE 6-12 The internal capsule and corona radiata.

substantia nigra and thus the loss of dopaminergic innervation of the striatum. Dopamine has a dampening effect on motor movement; thus, with a loss of dopamine, the dampening effect is lost and muscles become too rigid (**FIGURE 6-13**). As a result, the direct pathway no longer functions correctly and the indirect pathway dominates function, resulting in overinhibition of movement.

Cause

The cause of PD is unknown, though both environmental toxins and genetics have been suggested etiologies. The disease typically begins around 60 years of age, usually with increasing tremors being the first symptom. In about 10% to 15% of cases, disease onset occurs before age 50 years, as in the case of Michael J. Fox (**BOX 6-3**).

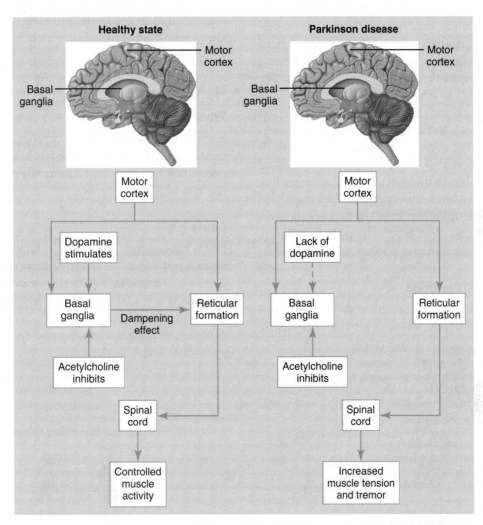

FIGURE 6-13 The brain in a healthy state versus in a Parkinsonian state. Note the loss of the dampening effect in Parkinson disease.

BOX 6-3 Michael J. Fox and Parkinson Disease

Michael J. Fox is a Canadian American actor best known for his roles in the television show *Family Ties* and the *Back to the Future* movies. In 1991 he was diagnosed with early-onset PD, but he kept his condition private until 1998 when his symptoms became more pronounced. As his symptoms worsened, **FIGURE 6-14** he reduced his on-screen activities and began to do voice-over work on films like *Stuart Little*. In 2000, Fox established the Michael J. Fox Foundation, an institution dedicated to finding a cure for PD. He has managed his condition through the use of the drug carbidopa-levodopa (Sinemet), a drug that reduces the symptoms of PD, and through a surgery called thalamotomy, during which select portions of the thalamus are destroyed. Fox continues to appear in television and film, often playing characters who display PD characteristics.

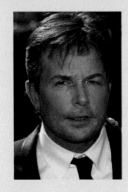

FIGURE 6-14 Michael J. Fox.

Kemp, Burns, and Brown (2008) report that about 20% of patients with PD will also develop dementia.

Signs and Symptoms

The three main signs of PD are bradykinesia, tremor, and rigidity (**FIGURE 6-15**). Bradykinesia (Greek for "slow movements") is the most significant of the three, robbing the patient of the ability to make timely, smooth movements. Bradykinesia is seen most easily in the Parkinsonian gait, which is characterized by short, shuffling steps and pedestal turning (a slow turning of direction through many small steps). The PD tremor is visible when the hands are at rest (i.e., a resting tremor) and disappears when the person intentionally uses his or her hand. The tremor vibrates at about 3 to 5 Hz. Rigidity in those with PD is most obvious in the face. They display what is called masked facies, which is impairment in the facial muscles that leaves the face looking expressionless. Rigidity is also present in the respiratory muscles, leaving the person with less-than-ideal breath support for speech. Patients often complain of hypophonia, or weak voice.

Diagnosis and Treatment

Diagnosis of PD is made through a neurological exam. At this time, there is no test that clearly identifies the disease. In addition, there is no cure for PD. Dopamine-based drugs can alleviate the symptoms for a time but do nothing to treat the underlying disease process. Pallidotomy, a surgical procedure in which lesions are made on the medial globus pallidus, has had mixed success in reducing akinesia and increasing movement. In another surgical method, deep brain stimulation, an electrode is implanted in the brain and electrically stimulates the medial globus pallidus, which disrupts its inhibiting effect.

Huntington Disease
What Is It?

Huntington disease (HD) is a progressive hereditary neurological disorder (**FIGURE 6-16**). It affects 12 out of every 100,000 people and commonly presents between the ages of 35 and 42 years.

Cause?

HD is caused by a mutation on chromosome 4. This mutation is passed to offspring through an autosomal dominant inheritance pattern, meaning that parents with HD have a 50% chance of having children who eventually develop the disease. When HD appears, it degenerates the basal ganglia and enlarges the brain's ventricles (**FIGURE 6-17**).

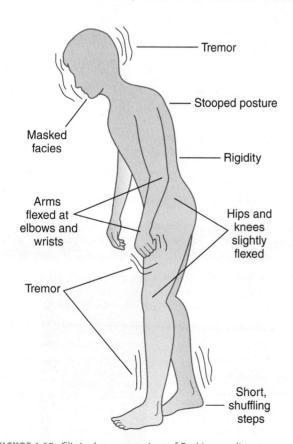

FIGURE 6-15 Clinical presentation of Parkinson disease.

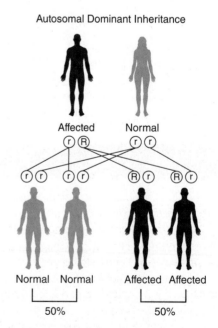

FIGURE 6-16 The autosomal dominant pattern of inheritance. Note the 50% chance of parents passing the Huntington gene onto their offspring.

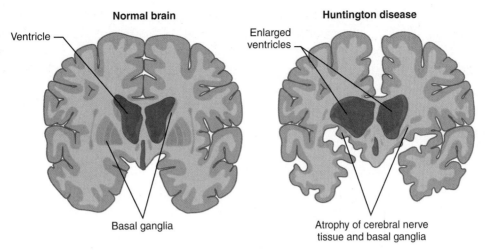

Normal brain

Ventricle

Basal ganglia

Huntington disease

Enlarged ventricles

Atrophy of cerebral nerve tissue and basal ganglia

FIGURE 6-17 A coronal section of a normal brain versus a brain with Huntington disease.
© Blamb/Shutterstock.

BOX 6-4 A Case of Huntington Disease

Joe was diagnosed with HD when he was 36 years old. His first symptoms were mood problems and a decrease in cognitive abilities. These symptoms worsened over time and were joined by involuntary writhing movements called chorea. In addition, Joe developed obsessive-compulsive behaviors. One of these was an obsession with collecting train paraphernalia, which quickly cluttered his house and frustrated his wife Marilyn. As Joe continued to deteriorate, he became a safety risk for wandering and falls. Eventually Marilyn had to put Joe in assistive care. Joe grew increasingly unstable and, during a home visit, he took a gun from his gun safe and shot himself. Joe's two children have both been tested for HD and, fortunately, neither child has the gene.

Signs and Symptoms

The first signs are being fidgety and clumsy. In many ways, HD is the opposite of PD. In HD, the loss of neurons in the striatum results in impairment to the indirect, inhibiting pathway, resulting in increased movement (hyperkinesia) in the form of involuntary writhing movements (chorea). Worsening depression and dementia also occur in this population. Some patients, because of their diagnosis and prognosis, opt to commit suicide (**BOX 6-4**).

Diagnosis and Treatment

HD is hypothesized through a person's clinical presentation and then confirmed through a genetic test. Computed tomography and magnetic resonance imaging scans may be ordered, but sometimes changes in the basal ganglia are not apparent. Like PD, there is no cure for HD. Medications are available to reduce symptoms such as chorea. Psychiatric medications can be prescribed to treat depression, psychosis, and behavior problems. There also are medications that improve the memory issues characteristic of dementia. As the person's condition worsens, it usually becomes more and more difficult for the family to care for him or her, and care in a long-term nursing home may eventually be needed.

Basal Ganglia and Aphasia

It is unclear whether damage to the basal ganglia causes aphasia. Two aphasic syndromes have been suggested. Damasio, Damasio, Rizzo, Varney, and Gersh (1982) reported Wernicke-type aphasia; Wallesch and colleagues (Brunner, Kornhuber, Seemüller, Suger, & Wallesch, 1982; Wallesch, 1985; Wallesch et al., 1983; Wallesch & Wyke, 1985) described transcortical motor aphasia (**TABLE 6-3**). More recently, Radanovic and Scaff (2003) reported three patients with motor-articulatory issues (not aphasia) and one patient with transcortical motor aphasia. It appears that damage to the basal ganglia can lead to a variety of deficits, including dysarthria, dysphonia, and comprehension, naming, and repetition problems (Radanovic & Scaff, 2003).

TABLE 6-3 Nonfluent Aphasic Conditions Compared

	Broca	Transcortical Motor	Mixed Transcortical	Global
Fluency	–	–	–	–
Auditory comprehension	+	+	–	–
Repetition	–	+	+	–

+, preserved; –, significantly impaired.

▸ The Brain Ventricles

Structure and Function

In addition to white and gray matter, the brain contains spaces called *ventricles*. There are four ventricles in the brain: a right and left lateral ventricle (also called first and second ventricles), a third ventricle, and a fourth ventricle (**FIGURES 6-18** and **6-19**). The right and left ventricles look like horseshoes, the third ventricle like a misshapen donut, and the fourth ventricle like a diamond. The left and right ventricles each have three horns (i.e., projections). The anterior horn is located in the cerebral hemisphere's frontal lobes, and the posterior horn is in the parietal lobe. The inferior ventricle horn is located in the temporal lobe. The body of the lateral ventricle connects the anterior and posterior horns. The third ventricle is located at midline in the diencephalon. It articulates with the two lateral ventricles via the intraventricular foramen. The third ventricle narrows near the midbrain to form the long cerebral aqueduct, which leads to the fourth ventricle located posterior to the pons and anterior to the cerebellum. A pair of lateral recesses course under the cerebellum and connect with the subarachnoid space of the meninges at the cerebellomedullary cistern. This connection means that the ventricular system and the subarachnoid space are continuous.

All the brain's ventricles are filled with **cerebrospinal fluid (CSF)**, a clear and colorless fluid that looks like plasma. CSF is also found in the subarachnoid space of the meninges (**FIGURE 6-20**). The **choroid plexus** (Latin for "the delicate knot") is a structure located in each ventricle that produces CSF at a rate of 400 to 500 milliliters (mL) each day. CSF moves between the ventricles via the

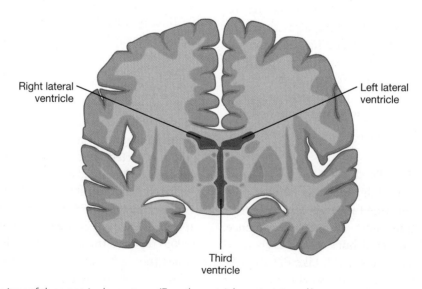

Right lateral ventricle   Left lateral ventricle

Third ventricle

FIGURE 6-18 Coronal view of the ventricular system. (Fourth ventricle not pictured.)

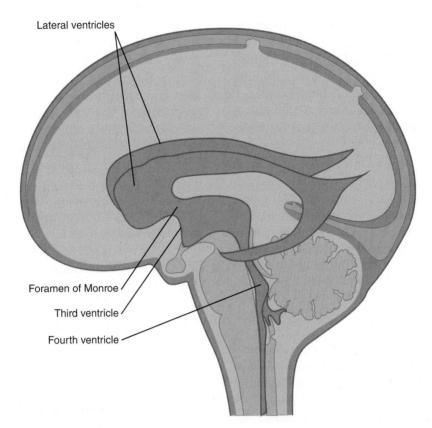

FIGURE 6-19 Lateral view of the ventricular system.

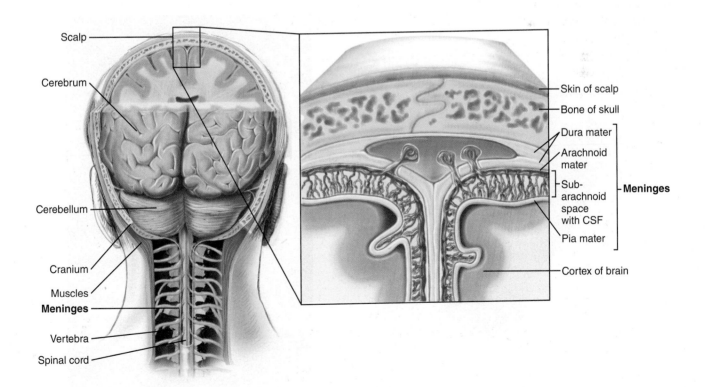

FIGURE 6-20 Cerebrospinal fluid (CSF) shown residing in the meninges.

interventricular foramen and the cerebral aqueduct. Overall, there is approximately 125 mL of CSF in the nervous system, which is replenished every 7 hours. Old CSF is absorbed into the venous system through the arachnoid villi, which are small bumps that protrude into the brain's venous system. This allows CSF to exit the subarachnoid space and enter the bloodstream.

CSF has four basic functions. First, it *protects* brain tissue by acting as a water cushion. Second, it lightens the weight of the brain from 1,400 grams to about 25 grams through *buoyancy* (think of how much lighter you seem in a pool). Third, it *reduces waste* by removing metabolic waste from the nervous system. Fourth, CSF helps to *transport* nutrients and hormones to the brain.

Disorders of the Ventricles

The most well-known condition involving the ventricles and CSF is **hydrocephalus** (Latin for "water brain"), in which CSF accumulates in the brain ventricles causing brain tissue to be compressed against the skull (**FIGURE 6-21**). There are two forms of hydrocephalus, obstructive and nonobstructive. In obstructive

hydrocephalus, a narrowing (stenosis) of the passageways that connect the ventricles can lead to CSF buildup because CSF cannot freely move through the system. Nonobstructive hydrocephalus involves problems in the absorption of CSF (and in rare cases, the production of CSF). For example, a person may not reabsorb old CSF, resulting in swollen brain ventricles.

Hydrocephalus can be congenital or acquired through brain injury, meningitis, or tumor. It is a very dangerous condition in that, if not treated, it can result in increased intracranial pressure leading to severe brain damage and even death. It is probably a more serious condition for adults than for infants because adult skulls are fused. Infant skulls do not completely fuse until about 18 months of age, and thus, less pressure is put on the brain.

Most cases of hydrocephalus are treated with surgically inserted shunts, which act as drainage pipes for excess CSF (**FIGURE 6-22**). Typically, a small incision is made in the scalp and skull, and the shunt is placed through the brain into one of the ventricles. The line is then run down the skin and into the peritoneal cavity, the tissues of which can absorb the incoming CSF. Potential problems can arise with a hydrocephalic shunt. When the scalp is cut and a hole is made in

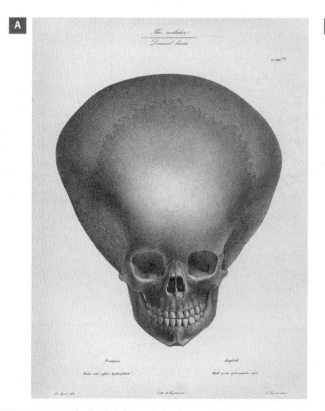

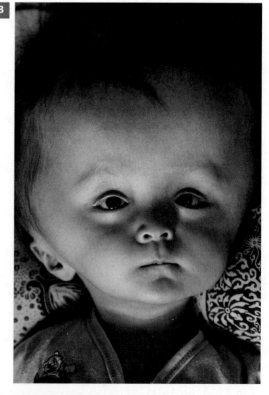

FIGURE 6-21 **A.** Skull of child with hydrocephalus. **B.** Photo of a child with hydrocephalus.

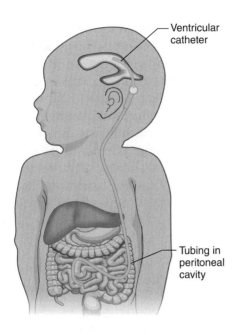

Ventricular
catheter

Tubing in
peritoneal
cavity

FIGURE 6-22 Illustration of a ventricular-peritoneal shunt.

the skull, a hemorrhage between the skull and brain can occur. In addition, a hemorrhage can occur in the brain itself, resulting in damaged brain tissue and further neurological problems. Patients may also experience bleeding in the ventricles. There is also a risk of introducing a bacterial infection into the CSF. Lastly, sometimes shunts become plugged and need to be redone (Shipley, 2012).

▶ Conclusion

When we think of the brain, we usually think of a bumpy, spherical mass. This chapter has attempted to open the brain up and see the interesting structures inside. Who knew that we had not one, but four holes in our head! Much attention has been given to the cerebral hemispheres, but as this chapter has attempted to demonstrate, there is much going on below the surface.

SUMMARY OF LEARNING OBJECTIVES

The following were the main learning objectives of this chapter. The information that should have been learned is below each learning objective.

1. The learner will list the four parts of the diencephalon and briefly describe the function of each.
    - *Thalamus:* a sensory fiber relay station or switchboard between the cerebral cortex and subcortical areas that processes all sensory (except olfaction) information flowing to and from the cerebral cortex.
    - *Subthalamus:* a part of the diencephalon that may play a role in the selection of actions and impulse control.
    - *Hypothalamus:* a linkage that connects the nervous system to the endocrine system (i.e., hormonal system) via the hypothalamus's pituitary gland. In addition, the hypothalamus is a regulator because it controls aspects of homeostasis (e.g., metabolism, body temperature, food intake).
    - *Epithalamus:* a part of the diencephalon that has functions related to the sleep–wake cycle, circadian rhythms, olfaction, and stress responses.
2. The learner will draw the basal ganglia and describe the function of these nuclei.
    - The three nuclei are the caudate nucleus, globus pallidus, and putamen.
    - These nuclei function via direct and indirect pathways to facilitate and inhibit movement.
3. The learner will list the names of the four brain ventricles.
    - We have four ventricles: a right, left, third, and fourth ventricle.
4. The learner will describe cerebrospinal fluid's composition and its function.
    - It consists of a clear and colorless fluid that looks like plasma.
    - It has four functions: protection, buoyancy, waste reduction, and transport.
5. The learner will list and briefly describe disorders associated with the diencephalon, basal ganglia, and brain ventricles.
    - *Thalamic pain syndrome (Dejerine-Roussy syndrome):* a condition involving burning or tingling sensations and possibly hypersensitivity to stimuli that would not normally be painful, such as a light touch or a temperature change.
    - *Thalamic aphasia:* a type of aphasia characterized by fluent verbal output, semantic paraphasias, jargon, mildly impaired auditory comprehension, and minimally impaired repetition.

- *Parkinson disease:* a progressive extrapyramidal movement disorder involving degeneration of the substantia nigra and thus the loss of dopaminergic innervation of the striatum.
- *Huntington disease:* a progressive hereditary neurological disorder that leads to increased movement (hyperkinesia) in the form of involuntary writhing movements (chorea). Worsening depression and dementia also occur in this condition.

- *Aphasia associated with the basal ganglia:* Findings are unclear. Damage to the basal ganglia can lead to a variety of deficits, including dysarthria, dysphonia, and comprehension, naming, and repetition problems. Transcortical motor aphasia and Wernicke aphasia are possibilities, according to the literature.
- *Hydrocephalus:* a condition that occurs when cerebrospinal fluid accumulates in the brain ventricles, causing brain tissue to be compressed against the skull.

KEY TERMS

Akinesia
Akinetic mutism
Amygdala
Basal ganglia
Caudate nucleus
Cerebrospinal fluid (CSF)
Choroid plexus
Corona radiata

Dyskinesia
Genu
Globus pallidus
Homeostasis
Hydrocephalus
Hypersomnia
Internal capsule
Lateral geniculate body (LGB)

Lenticular nucleus
Medial geniculate body (MGB)
Pineal gland
Pituitary gland
Putamen
Striatum
Thalamic aphasia
Thalamic pain syndrome tic

DRAW IT TO KNOW IT

1. Draw a coronal section of the brain (see Figures 6-1 and 6-8) and label the following: epithalamus, thalamus, subthalamus, hypothalamus, caudate nucleus, putamen, globus pallidus, right lateral ventricle, left lateral ventricle, third ventricle, and fourth ventricle.

2. Draw a sagittal (or medial) section of the brain (see Figure 6-2) and label the following: medulla, pons, midbrain, thalamus, hypothalamus, cerebellum, lateral ventricle, corpus callosum, and cerebral hemispheres.

QUESTIONS FOR DEEPER REFLECTION

1. Compare and contrast thalamic aphasia to other types of aphasia.
2. What role does the basal ganglia play in speech?

3. Predict what the speech of people with Parkinson disease and people with Huntington disease is like.

CASE STUDY

Ellie is a 41-year-old female who has become progressively ill in the last few years. More specifically, her movements have become increasingly erratic with chorea, her speech slurred, and she has developed severe depression. Ellie has fallen several times and her husband is thinking of putting her into a long-term care facility because it is becoming more and more difficult to care for his wife. Ellie's brother Doug (age 45) is developing symptoms similar to Ellie.

1. Which of the following conditions do you think Ellie and Doug have?
   a. Parkinson disease
   b. Thalamic pain syndrome
   c. Huntington disease
   d. Myasthenia gravis
2. Why did you pick the answer you did?
3. What brain structure is most likely involved in this condition?
4. What is the long-term outlook for Ellie and Doug?

SUGGESTED PROJECTS

1. Write a two- to three-page paper on the topic of thalamic aphasia.
2. Find a case study about thalamic aphasia in the scholarly literature and present the case to the class.
3. Write a two- to three-page paper on the role of the basal ganglia in speech production.
4. Find someone with either Parkinson disease or Huntington disease and interview the patient and/or his or her family.

REFERENCES

Ab Aziz, C. B., & Ahmad, A. H. (2006). The role of the thalamus in modulating pain. *Malaysian Journal of Medical Sciences, 13*(2), 11.

Andres, K. H., Düring, M. V., & Veh, R. W. (1999). Subnuclear organization of the rat habenular complexes. *Journal of Comparative Neurology, 407*(1), 130–150.

Brunner, R. J., Kornhuber, H. H., Seemüller, E., Suger, G., & Wallesch, C. W. (1982). Basal ganglia participation in language pathology. *Brain and Language, 16*(2), 281–299.

Carter, R. (2009). *The human brain book.* New York, NY: DK Publishing.

Castaigne, P., Lhermitte, F., Buge, A., Escourolle, R., Hauw, J. J., & Lyon-Caen, O. (1981). Paramedian thalamic and midbrain infarcts: Clinical and neuropathological study. *Annals of Neurology, 10*(2), 127–148.

Castro, A. J., Merchut, M. P., Neafsey, E. J., & Wurster, R. D. (2002). *Neuroscience: An outline approach.* St. Louis, MO: Mosby.

Catani, M., & de Schotten, M. T. (2012). *Atlas of human brain connections.* Oxford, UK: Oxford University Press.

Crosson, B. (1984). Role of the dominant thalamus in language: A review. *Psychological Bulletin, 96*(3), 491–517.

Crosson, B. (1992). *Subcortical functions in language and memory.* New York, NY: Guilford Press.

Damasio, A. R., Damasio, H., Rizzo, M., Varney, N., & Gersh, F. (1982). Aphasia with nonhemorrhagic lesions in the basal ganglia and internal capsule. *Archives of Neurology, 39*(1), 15–20.

Daroff, R. B., Fenichel, G. M., Jankovic, J., & Mazziotta, J. C. (2012). *Bradley's neurology in clinical practice* (6th ed.). Philadelphia, PA: Saunders.

Das, R. R., Romero, J. R., & Mandel, A. (2005). Hemiballismus in a patient with contralateral carotid artery occlusion. *Journal of Neurological Sciences, 238,* S392.

Fauci, A. S. (2008). *Harrison's principles of internal medicine.* New York, NY: McGraw-Hill Medical.

Frank, M. J., Samanta, J., Moustafa, A. A., & Sherman, S. J. (2007). Hold your horses: Impulsivity, deep brain stimulation, and medication in Parkinsonism. *Science, 318,* 1309–1312.

Johnson, M. D., & Ojemann, G. A. (2000). The role of the human thalamus in language and memory: Evidence from electrophysiological studies. *Brain and Cognition, 42,* 218–230.

Kandel, E. R., Schwartz, J. H., Jessell, T. M., Siegelbaum, S. A., & Hudspeth, A. J. (2013). *Principles of neural science* (5th ed.). New York, NY: McGraw-Hill.

Kemp, W. L., Burns, D. K., & Brown, T. G. (2008). *Pathology: The big picture.* New York, NY: McGraw-Hill Medical.

Kitagawa, M., Murata, J., Kikuchi, S., Sawamura, Y., Saito, H., Sasaki, H., & Tashiro, K. (2000). Deep brain stimulation of subthalamic area for severe proximal tremor. *Neurology, 55*(1), 114–116.

Kurup, R. K., & Kurup, P. A. (2003). Hypothalamic digoxin and hemispheric chemical dominance: Relation to speech and language dysfunction. *International Journal of Neuroscience, 113*(6), 797–814.

LaPointe, L. L., & Murdoch, B. E. (2014). *Movement disorders in neurologic disease: Effects on communication and swallowing.* San Diego, CA: Plural Publishing.

Li, S., Kumar, Y., Gupta, N., Abdelbaki, A., Sahwney, H., & Kumar, A., . . . Mangla, R. (2018). Clinical and neuroimaging findings in thalamic territory infarctions: A review. *Journal of Neuroimaging, 28*(4), 343–349.

Mallet, L., Polosan, M., Jaafari, N., Baup, N., Welter, M. L., & Fontaine, D., . . . Pelissolo, A. (2008). Subthalamic nucleus stimulation in severe obsessive-compulsive disorder. *New England Journal of Medicine, 359*(20), 2121–2134.

Matsumoto, M., & Hikosaka, O. (2008). Representation of negative motivational value in the primate lateral habenula. *Nature Neuroscience, 12*(1), 77–84.

Papathanasiou, I., Coppens, P., & Potagas, C. (2013). *Aphasia and related neurogenic communication disorders.* Burlington, MA: Jones & Bartlett Learning.

Radanovic, M., & Scaff, M. (2003). Speech and language disturbances due to subcortical lesions. *Brain and Language, 84*(3), 337–352.

Reich, D. S., Smith, S. A., Zackowski, K. M., Gordon-Lipkin, E. M., Jones, C. K., & Farrell, J. A., . . . Calabresi, P. A. (2007). Multiparametric magnetic resonance imaging analysis of the corticospinal tract in multiple sclerosis. *Neuroimage, 38*(2), 271–279.

Sherman, S. M. (2006). Thalamus. *Scholarpedia, 1*(9), 1583.

Shipley, C. (2012). *Hydrocephalus shunt video* [Video file]. Retrieved from https://www.youtube.com/watch?v=Yb9dSjDykpI

Swenson, R. (2006). Thalamic organization. In R. Swenson (Ed.), *Review of clinical and functional neuroscience.* Hanover, NH: Dartmouth Medical School. Retrieved from http://www.dartmouth.edu/~rswenson/NeuroSci/chapter_10.html

Wallesch, C. W. (1985). Two syndromes of aphasia occurring with ischemic lesions involving the left basal ganglia. *Brain and Language, 25*(2), 357–361.

Wallesch, C. W., Kornhuber, H. H., Brunner, R. J., Kunz, T., Hollerbach, B., & Suger, G. (1983). Lesions of the basal ganglia, thalamus, and deep white matter: Differential effects on language functions. *Brain and Language, 20*(2), 286–304.

Wallesch, C. W., & Wyke, M. A. (1985). Language and the subcortical nuclei. In S. P. Newman & R. Epstein (Eds.), *Current perspectives in dysphasia* (pp. 182–197). Edinburgh, Scotland: Churchill Livingstone.

Webster, D. B. (1999). *Neuroscience of communication* (2nd ed.). San Diego, CA: Singular Publishing.

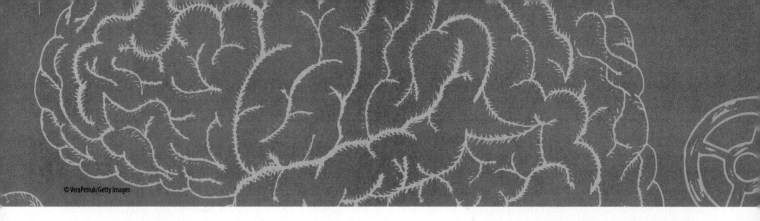
© VeraPetruk/Getty Images

CHAPTER 7

The Cerebrum: A Survey

CHAPTER PREVIEW

As we ascend the central nervous system, we get to what most people think of when they think of the brain—the cerebral hemispheres. In this chapter, we will broadly survey the cerebral hemispheres as well as common disorders associated with their damage.

IN THIS CHAPTER

In this chapter, we will . . .
- Survey how the brain is protected and nourished
- Describe the anatomical features of the cerebral hemispheres
- Survey the lobes of the brain and their function
- Explain the phenomenon of hemispheric specialization
- Survey some examples of disorders associated with cerebral hemisphere damage

LEARNING OBJECTIVES

- The learner will list four structures/systems that nourish and protect the brain.
- The learner will identify important features of the cerebral hemispheres, including the lobes of the brain.
- The learner will describe the phenomenon of hemispheric specialization, especially how it relates to language.
- The learner will list and briefly describe causes of damage to the cerebral hemispheres.
- The learner will describe the phenomenon of brain plasticity and its principles.

▶ Introduction

The human brain weighs approximately 3 pounds, which is about 2% of a human's body weight, yet it consumes about 20% of the body's energy. We humans certainly do not have the largest brains on earth in terms of size (think of a whale or elephant brain), but in comparison to our body size, our brains are quite large. Is this the reason for our superior cognitive skills compared to apes, whales, and elephants? Currently, researchers believe it is not brain size that makes a difference in our cognitive abilities, but rather the number and organization of neurons (Herculano-Houzel, 2009).

Our brains really consist of two brains. We have a left hemisphere and a right hemisphere that together account for 82% of the brain's mass (Herculano-Houzel, 2009). The surface of the brain consists of what is called the cerebral cortex (*cortex* is Latin for "bark"), which is made up of neuron cell bodies. These cell bodies produce a gray color, hence the term *gray matter*. Under this layer lies a layer of *white matter* that consists of neuronal axons. This tissue is white because of the myelin coating on the axons. The purpose of this chapter is to survey the cerebral hemispheres, especially their gray matter, as well as structures that protect and nourish the hemispheres. We will end this chapter by reviewing various disorders associated with them.

▶ The Protection and Nourishment of the Cerebrum

Protection: The Meninges

The cerebral tissues have a gelatinous consistency and are made of delicate cells and connections. The meninges, a three-layered membrane that surrounds both the brain and the spinal cord, provides a measure of protection for these central nervous system (CNS) structures (**FIGURE 7-1**). Our skull protects the brain against things that might penetrate brain tissue, but the meninges is an added layer of protection against blows and shocks to the head as well as against bony protrusions on the inside of the skull. A person need only look at the inside of the skull to realize it is not an especially hospitable place for the delicate tissues of the brain (**FIGURE 7-2**). In addition to providing protection, the meninges also support the brain, as will be seen.

The three layers of the meninges are as follows: dura mater, arachnoid mater, and pia mater. The **dura mater** (Latin for "tough mother") is a membrane that adheres to the inside of the skull. It is made of two dense layers of fibrous connective tissue, an external periosteal lining the inside of the skull (absent in the spinal meninges) and an inner meningeal layer. (Note: Periosteum is a membrane that covers the surface of bones.) Under normal circumstances, these two layers are always pressed together, except where they form

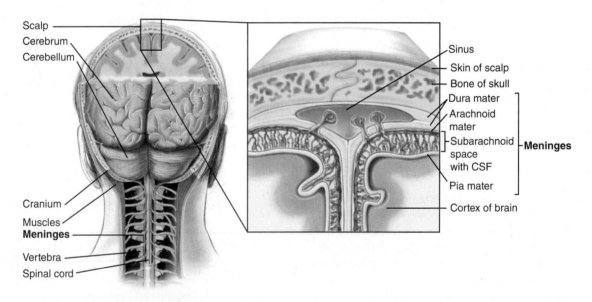

FIGURE 7-1 The three layers of the meninges are connective tissue covering the brain. The outermost layer is the dura mater, followed by the arachnoid mater and subarachnoid space, and finally the pia mater.

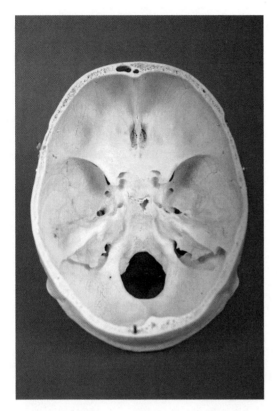

FIGURE 7-2 The inside of the cranial vault. Note the rough inner surface.

© Jones and Bartlett Learning. Specimen courtesy of the Biology Department, Northeastern University.

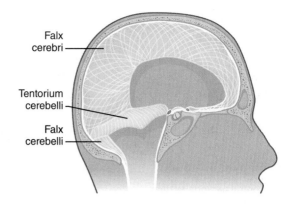

FIGURE 7-3 The falx cerebri, tentorium cerebelli, and falx cerebelli.

sinuses. The dura not only surrounds the brain, but it also creates compartments for the cerebral hemispheres and the cerebellum. For example, it plunges down the longitudinal fissure, a deep groove that separates the right and left hemispheres, to form the falx cerebri (*falx* is Latin for "curved blade"). Additionally, the dura mater separates the occipital lobes of the brain from the cerebellum to form a structure known as the tentorium cerebelli (Latin for "tent of the cerebellum"). It also descends between the hemispheres of the cerebellum to form the falx cerebelli (Latin for "curved blade of the cerebellum") (**FIGURE 7-3**).

There is a potential space between the skull and the dura mater called the **epidural space** and another potential space under the dura called the **subdural space**. (Note: A potential space refers to a space that could occur between two structures that are normally pressed together.) The epidural space is an actual space at the level of the spinal cord. During childbirth, some mothers receive an epidural, which is a shot of painkillers that temporarily blocks spinal nerve transmission of pain signals. These potential spaces can become actual spaces when a pathology occurs. For example, if a blood vessel is breached, blood can get into the spaces, a condition known as a **hematoma**. Patients

who experience a hematoma often report headache as a main symptom. This pain results because dura is well supplied with sensory nerves from the trigeminal nerve (cranial nerve V).

Under the dura mater is the next layer, the **arachnoid mater** (Latin for "spider mother"). The arachnoid consists of thin and delicate connective tissue (collagen plus elastic fibers). It gets its name from the actual space below it, called the **subarachnoid space**. Blood vessels and lacey, spider-web-like support structures (i.e., trabeculae) occupy this space as well as cerebrospinal fluid (CSF). The brain is essentially wrapped in a waterbed, and this fluid protects and supports the brain. Floating on this cushion also reduces the weight of the brain on itself.

The final and innermost meningeal layer is the **pia mater** (Latin for "faithful mother"). It adheres tightly to the hills (gyri) and valleys (sulci) of the brain. It consists of thin, delicate connective tissue made of collagen and elastic fibers. Blood vessels that run on the surface of the brain actually are located on top of the pia mater in the subarachnoid space.

The arachnoid mater and the pia mater are sometimes grouped together and called the *leptomeninges,* or "thin meninges." The dura mater is sometimes referred to as the *pachymeninx,* or "thick meninges."

Protection: The Blood–Brain Barrier

Over a century ago, early pioneers in neuroscience discovered that if blue dye were injected into the vascular system, it would stain all the tissues in the body blue with two exceptions—the brain and the spinal cord. To explain this finding, neuroscientists theorized that some sort of barrier must prevent the blue dye from reaching the CNS. Today, this barrier is called the **blood–brain barrier (BBB)**.

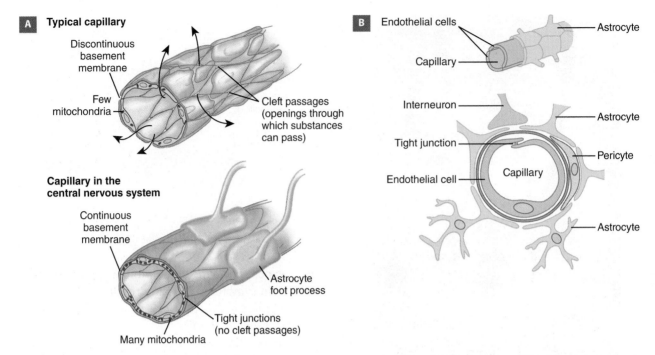

FIGURE 7-4 **A.** The structure of a typical capillary versus a nervous system capillary. **B.** The structure of the blood–brain barrier.

The BBB is located in the walls of CNS blood vessels (**FIGURE 7-4**). Endothelial cells are tightly packed together and thus are semipermeable, meaning they let smaller molecules from the bloodstream (e.g., oxygen molecules) in but keep larger substances (e.g., bacteria) out (**FIGURE 7-5**). Large molecules, such as glucose, that are needed by the brain are actively transported through the vascular walls. Tight junctions hold cells together and tightly regulate which substances can pass through. The BBB protects the brain from foreign invaders, hormones, antibodies, and other substances that might adversely affect it. By doing this, the BBB maintains a constant environment for the brain and makes infections of the brain very rare, but when they do occur, they are very hard to treat. There is an exception: The BBB of fetuses and infants is not fully developed; thus, they are susceptible to drugs and other substances. This is why substance abuse (e.g.,

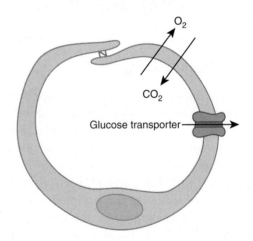

FIGURE 7-5 Transport of substances through the blood–brain barrier.

alcohol) during pregnancy can be so devastating to fetal brains (**BOX 7-1**).

BOX 7-1 Fetal Alcohol Spectrum Disorder

Fetal alcohol spectrum disorder (FASD) is a spectrum of disorders that occur due to maternal alcohol consumption during pregnancy. Neither the placenta nor the fetus's BBB are impediments to alcohol. The fetal liver cannot metabolize alcohol, and once the fetal brain is exposed to it, the central nervous, peripheral nervous, and autonomic nervous systems can all be affected. More specifically, if the brain is exposed to alcohol during the first trimester, it can interfere with migration and organization of neurons within the nervous system. Microcephaly and intellectual disability are possible outcomes (Clarren, Alvord, Sumi, Streissguth, & Smith, 1978). Other outcomes include learning disabilities and other cognitive deficits (e.g., attention deficit). Some children with FASD also have common facial characteristics, such as a smooth philtrum, a thin upper lip, and small eye openings. Children may be below average in height and weight. The Centers for Disease Control and Prevention (CDC) and other organizations have undertaken public awareness campaigns to warn potential parents of the dangers of alcohol consumption during pregnancy (**FIGURE 7-6**).

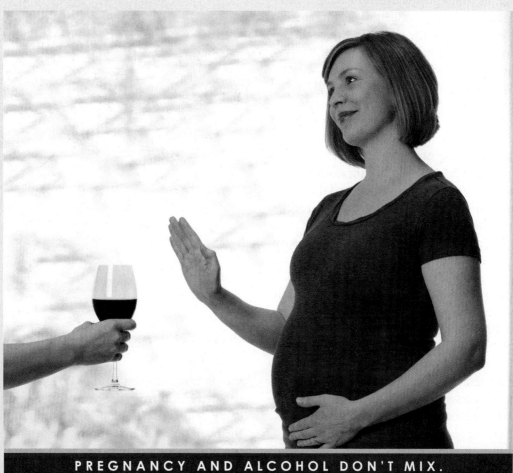

PREGNANCY AND ALCOHOL DON'T MIX.

What we know:

· There's no known safe amount of alcohol use during pregnancy or while trying to get pregnant.

· All types of alcohol are equally harmful, including all wines and beer.

· Alcohol can cause problems for a developing baby throughout pregnancy, including before a woman knows she's pregnant.

What can happen:

· Drinking alcohol during pregnancy can cause miscarriage, stillbirth, and a range of lifelong physical, behavioral and intellectual disabilities. These disabilities are known as fetal alcohol spectrum disorders (FASDs).

What you can do:

· FASDs are completely preventable if a woman does not drink alcohol during pregnancy.

· For more information, visit **www.cdc.gov/fasd** or call **800–CDC–INFO**.

When a pregnant woman drinks alcohol, so does her baby. Why take the risk?

FIGURE 7-6 A poster from the CDC campaign to raise aware about the connection between maternal alcohol consumption and fetal alcohol spectrum disorder.

There are, of course, challenges to having a BBB. Specifically, it is sometimes difficult to get therapeutic drugs (e.g., antibiotics) to the brain. To overcome the protective function of the BBB, special delivery systems have been developed. On a more negative note, many substances can compromise the BBB and lead to unfavorable effects on the brain, including conditions like meningitis, epilepsy, stroke, and brain tumors.

The body does have its own way around the BBB with **circumventricular organs (CVOs)**. These brain structures are highly vascular and lack the normal BBB. CVOs link the CNS, the vascular system, and the endocrine system, creating an alternative route for neuropeptides and hormones. Microglia stand as guards at CVOs, monitoring for pathogens. Some CVOs are sensory organs that monitor for the presence of salt and toxic substances. For example, the *subfornical organ*, which is located at the roof of the third ventricle, monitors salt concentration in the blood and relays data to the hypothalamus. Another example is the *area postrema* located at the posterior end of the fourth ventricle. It monitors the blood for toxins and initiates the vomit response if any are present. Other CVOs are secretory organs that secrete hormones into the bloodstream. Examples of these CVOs include the pituitary and pineal glands.

Nourishment: The Cerebral Arteries

As mentioned in the introduction, the brain is an energy hog, consuming approximately 20% of the oxygen in the body. Oxygen nourishes the brain; without it, the brain starves and quickly begins to die. Because of its oxygen dependency, the brain is less tolerant of ischemia (i.e., a lack of blood flow) than other tissues and organs in the body. In fact, only minutes of reduced blood flow and accompanying oxygen deprivation can lead to brain tissue damage (**TABLE 7-1**). To avoid oxygen deprivation, the brain has a rich blood supply. Oxygen enters the brain through two routes—the internal carotid arteries and

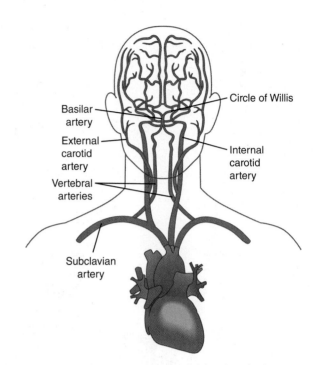

FIGURE 7-7 Major arteries supplying blood to the brain.

the vertebral arteries (**FIGURE 7-7**). Arteries bring oxygenated blood from the heart to the brain, and veins carry deoxygenated blood from brain tissues back to the heart. We will first survey the arterial system and then the venous system.

The carotid artery system includes the external carotid artery and the internal carotid artery. Both arise from the common carotid arteries (**FIGURE 7-8**). The external carotid artery supplies blood to the face muscles and to the oral, nasal, and eye (orbital) cavities. The internal **carotid artery** system is a major supplier of blood to the cerebral hemispheres. This artery, which runs up the anterolateral sides of the neck, bifurcates (i.e., splits) to form the anterior cerebral artery and the middle cerebral artery. The anterior cerebral artery supplies blood to the medial surface of the frontal and parietal lobes as well as the corpus callosum (**FIGURE 7-9**). The middle cerebral

TABLE 7-1 Cerebral Blood Flow and Function	
Functional Status	**Cerebral Blood Flow**
Normal function	40–55 mL/min per 100 grams brain tissue
Reduced brain function	20–40 mL/min per 100 grams brain tissue
Temporary loss of function	15–20 mL/min per 100 grams brain tissue
Brain tissue damage	<20 mL/min per 100 grams brain tissue over several minutes

Data from: Castro, A. J., Merchut, M. P., Neafsey, E. J., & Wurster, R. D. (2002). *Neuroscience: An outline approach.* St. Louis, MO: Mosby.

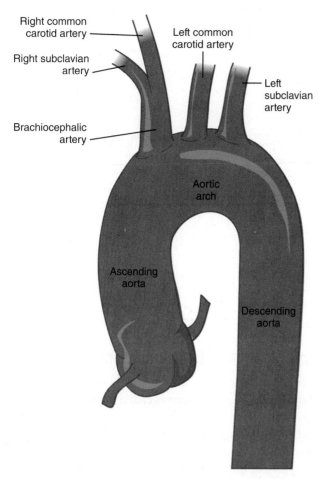

FIGURE 7-8 The internal and external carotid arteries arise from the common carotid artery. The right common carotid artery arises from the brachiocephalic artery, and the left common artery arises from aortic arch.

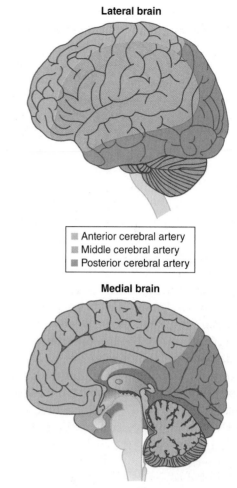

FIGURE 7-9 The cerebral cortex territory covered by the anterior, middle, and posterior cerebral arteries.

artery supplies the lateral portions of the hemispheres and has branches that supply internal structures, like the basal ganglia and internal capsule. Because many language areas in the brain are in this lateral region, strokes involving the middle cerebral artery can be devastating to language function. Before the anterior and middle cerebral arteries bifurcate, collateral branches course out to supply the following structures: the pituitary gland, the eye and optic tract, the hippocampus, and the globus pallidus.

The **vertebral artery** system arises from the subclavian arteries and supplies the brainstem, cerebellum, occipital lobe, and temporal lobe. The vertebral arteries course up the spinal column and the back of the neck to join and form the basilar artery. Several arteries branch off the basilar artery and supply brainstem and cerebellar structures. The basilar artery bifurcates into the posterior cerebral artery, which supplies the occipital lobe and the inferior portion of the temporal lobe.

The vertebral-basilar system, along with the carotid arteries, feeds a circular array of blood vessels called the **circle of Willis** (**FIGURE 7-10**). The ingenious

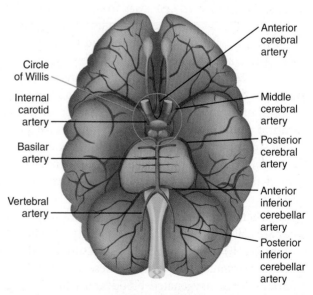

FIGURE 7-10 A ventral view of the brain showing the blood supply to the brain via the internal carotid arteries and the vertebral arteries to the circle of Willis.

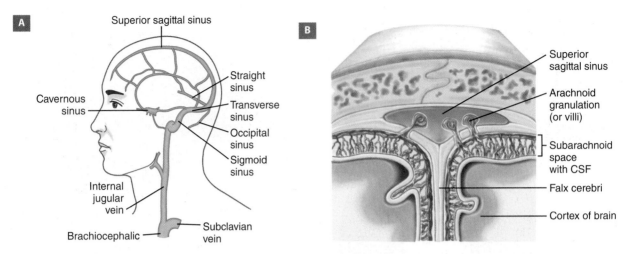

FIGURE 7-11 **A.** The venous system of the brain. **B.** The superior sagittal sinus.

design of the circle of Willis helps promote equal blood pressure and blood flow to all areas of the brain. For example, if one of the carotid arteries becomes occluded, blood will continue to supply the circle of Willis from the remaining carotid and basilar arteries. As people grow older, plaque deposits sometimes form on the carotid arteries, which can become almost completely or completely occluded. Even if this happens, blood will still feed the circle of Willis from the vertebral arteries.

Waste Removal: The Venous System

The arterial system brings oxygenated blood to brain tissue, whereas the **venous system** (Figure 7-11A in **FIGURE 7-11**) acts as a waste disposal system, moving deoxygenated blood away from the brain and moving used CSF away from the ventricular system. Small veins called venules collect deoxygenated blood from capillaries in the brain and dump it into veins. There are two main sets of cerebral veins: the superficial cerebral veins and the deep cerebral veins. The **superficial cerebral veins** collect blood from the cerebral cortex and subcortical white matter; the **deep cerebral veins** collect blood from subcortical gray matter structures, like the thalamus and hippocampus.

As mentioned in the section on the meninges, the dura mater has two layers. These two layers are tightly fused through most of the brain; however, there are areas where they are separated. These separated areas are called sinuses; a sinus is a cavity or channel (Figure 7-11B). Inside a sinus is a structure called the arachnoid granulation (or villi). These structures act as drains for deoxygenated blood and CSF, routing these fluids into the brain's venous system. From there, these fluids drain into the internal jugular veins and return to the heart.

▶ The Cerebrum

Important Cerebral Landmarks

The cerebral cortex has several notable landmarks. First, there are deep grooves called **fissures**, shallower grooves called **sulci** (singular = sulcus), and hills called **gyri** (singular = gyrus) (**FIGURE 7-12**). This hill and valley structure is a simple way to increase the surface area of the brain as well as the number of neurons, but also a way to keep the size of the brain relatively small and compact. The surface area of the human brain differs based on sex but generally is around 2.5 square feet (Bhatnagar, 2008; Jones & Peters, 1984), or the size of an unfolded newspaper, which is obviously too large to fit in the skull without crumpling. Cortical surface area and the high degree of folding in the human brain distinguish it from the brains of other primates (Toro et al., 2008).

There are a number of prominent gyri, sulci, and fissures in the human brain (**FIGURE 7-13**). The frontal lobe has four prominent gyri—the superior frontal

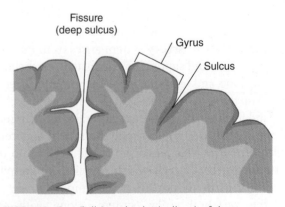

FIGURE 7-12 Gyri (hills) and sulci (valleys) of the cerebral cortex.

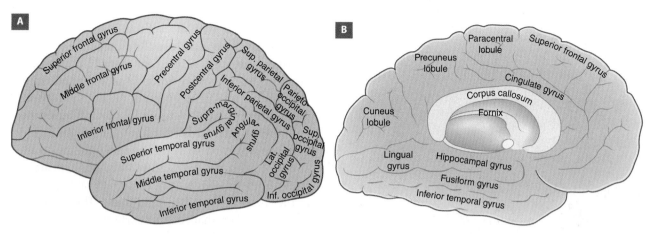

FIGURE 7-13 **A.** Prominent gyri of the lateral left hemisphere. **B.** Prominent gyri of the medial left hemisphere.

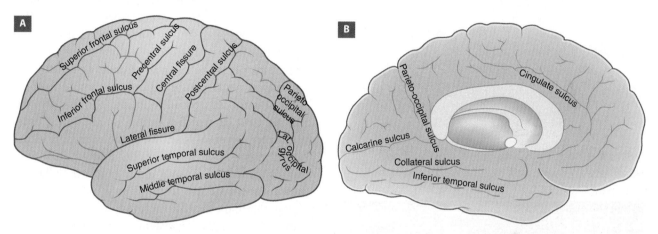

FIGURE 7-14 **A.** Prominent sulci of the lateral left hemisphere. **B.** Prominent sulci of the medial left hemisphere.

gyrus, the middle frontal gyrus, the inferior frontal gyrus, and the precentral gyrus. The parietal lobe also contains four gyri, named the postcentral gyrus, superior parietal gyrus, supramarginal gyrus, and angular gyrus. The temporal and occipital lobes each contain three large gyri. The occipital lobe contains the lateral, superior, and inferior occipital gyri, and the temporal lobe is made up of the superior, middle, and inferior temporal gyri. If the two cerebral hemispheres are pulled apart and the medial portions of the cerebral hemisphere are brought into view, additional gyri can be seen (Figure 7-13B). These include the cingulate, hippocampal, lingual, and fusiform gyri.

Where there are hills, there are valleys, and various sulci mark the boundaries between the gyri just noted (**FIGURE 7-14**). The prominent sulci of the lateral frontal lobe include the superior frontal, inferior frontal, and precentral sulci. The parietal lobe contains two notable sulci: the postcentral and the intraparietal sulci. The parieto-occipital sulcus separates the parietal lobe from the occipital lobe. The occipital lobe itself has one major sulcus, the lateral occipital sulcus. The superior and middle temporal sulci are found in

the temporal lobe. Again, if the two hemispheres are pulled apart, additional sulci can be observed in the medial portion of the hemispheres (Figure 7-14B). The cingulate sulcus separates the frontal and parietal lobes from the cingulate gyrus. The collateral sulcus separates the hippocampal gyrus from the fusiform gyrus, and the inferior temporal sulcus separates the fusiform gyrus from the inferior temporal lobe. The parieto-occipital and calcarine sulci run through the occipital lobe and eventually meet, separating the cingulate and lingual gyri.

In terms of deep brain valleys, there are three prominent fissures in the human brain. The **longitudinal fissure** runs from front to back and separates the two hemispheres (**FIGURE 7-15**). The **central fissure**, also known as the Rolandic fissure, separates the frontal lobe from the parietal lobe. Finally, the **lateral fissure**, or Sylvian fissure, separates the frontal and parietal lobes from the temporal lobe (see Figure 7-14A).

All healthy human brains have these hills and valleys; however, in some people, the cerebral cortex is smooth in appearance (**FIGURE 7-16**). This condition, known as **agyria** (a = "without"; gyria = gyri) or **lissencephaly**

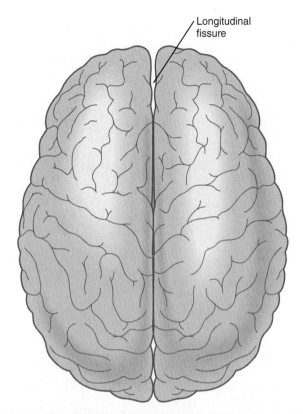

FIGURE 7-15 The longitudinal fissure is a deep groove that separates the left and right hemispheres.

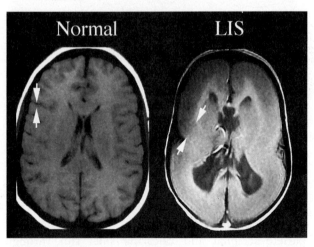

FIGURE 7-16 Imaging scan of a normal brain compared to a lissencephalic (LIS) brain.

Courtesy of Dr. Joseph G. Gleeson, University of California, San Diego.

("smooth brain"), causes severe motor, intellectual, and psychological disability (National Institute of Neurological Disorders and Stroke, 2018). Most people with this condition die before the age of 10 years, though there is at least one case of a person living into adulthood (Hooper, 2013).

Layers of the Cerebral Cortex

In addition to these hill and valley landmarks, the cerebral cortex consists of six distinguishable layers of tissue made up of pyramidal and nonpyramidal neuron cells (**FIGURE 7-17**). Pyramidal cells take their name from their pyramid shape and are motor in nature. Nonpyramidal cells are smaller, often star shaped ("stellate"), and are involved in sensory function as well as communication between different parts of the brain. In terms of this communication, there are four basic fiber connections in the cerebral hemispheres (Figure 7-17). First, there are *projection fibers* that project from the cerebral cortex to subcortical structures. Second, there are *callosal fibers* that connect the cortex of one hemisphere to the cortex of the other hemisphere. Third, there are *association fibers* that connect cortical structures in the same hemisphere. Fourth, there are *thalamocortical fibers* that connect the cerebral cortex to the thalamus.

In terms of cerebral cortex layers, layer I is called the molecular layer, and it consists of glial cells and axons. This layer of cortext is just underneath the pia mater. Layer II is the external granular layer, which is made up of small pyramidal cells and other neurons called granule cells. Small to medium pyramidal cells make up layer III, which is known as the external pyramidal layer. Layer IV is known as the internal granular layer. It consists of nonpyramidal cells (stellate neurons) and receives sensory input from the thalamus. The internal pyramidal layer (layer V) has medium to large pyramidal cells that project to motor areas such as the basal ganglia, brainstem, and spinal cord. This layer is where the primary motor cortex has its pyramidal cells known as Betz cells, which are the largest type of pyramidal neurons. These neurons send their long axons directly down the spinal cord through the corticobulbar and corticospinal tracts, where they synapse with cranial nerve nuclei or spinal cord ventral horn cells that, in turn, directly synapse to their intended muscle. The final layer, layer VI, is called the multiform layer, and it sends excitatory and inhibitory motor fibers to the thalamus. Layer IV and VI form a nice interconnection between the cerebral cortex and the thalamus. Below layer VI is the white matter of the brain (i.e., myelin-coated axons).

The Lobes of the Brain

As mentioned previously, there are four brain lobes (lobe = roundish projection) (**FIGURE 7-18** and **TABLE 7-2**). The **frontal lobe** lies at the front of the brain, just above the eyes. The posterior border of this lobe is the central fissure. Overall, its main functions include reasoning, planning, and voluntary motor movement. The frontal lobe is important for expressive language and the planning and execution of speech. Lying just posterior to the central fissure and superior to the lateral fissure is the **parietal lobe**, which functions in touch sensory perception,

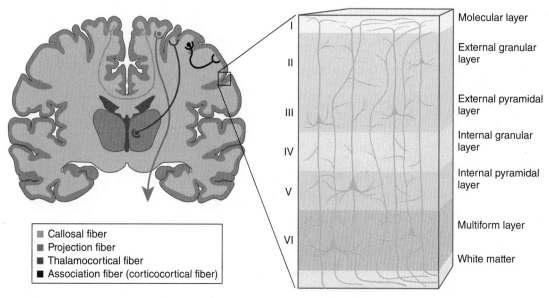

- Callosal fiber
- Projection fiber
- Thalamocortical fiber
- Association fiber (corticocortical fiber)

FIGURE 7-17 A coronal section of the brain showing the major types of fibers to and from the cerebral cortex (left) and the six layers of the cerebral cortex (right).

TABLE 7-2 The Lobes of the Brain and Their Major Functions	
Lobe	**Major Functions**
Frontal lobe	Cognitive functions (e.g., reasoning), speech, and expressive language
Parietal lobe	Touch perception and interpretation
Temporal lobe	Receptive language and long-term memory
Occipital lobe	Visual perception and interpretation

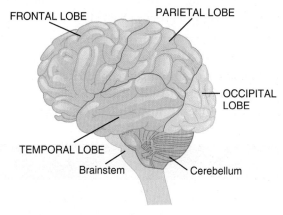

FIGURE 7-18 The lobes of the brain.

interpretation, and integration. Lying inferior to the parietal lobe is the **temporal lobe**, in which the processing of auditory information, including speech, takes place as well as some memory functions (e.g., long-term memory). Lastly, the **occipital lobe** lies posterior to the parietal and temporal lobes and makes up the very back part of the brain. Its main function is visual processing.

There is also what could be called a fifth lobe located underneath the four lobes just described, called the **limbic lobe**. It involves the cingulate gyrus and other brain structures (see Figure 7-13B).

▶ Hemispheric Specialization and Connections

Hemispheric Specialization

The two hemispheres of the brain do look like each other anatomically. The term **hemispheric specialization** captures the fact that, in terms of function, each hemisphere is not a mirror image of the other; rather, the two hemispheres function uniquely (**FIGURE 7-19**). The clearest example of hemispheric specialization is language. Ninety-six percent of right-handed people have their language functions lateralized to the left hemisphere, and we would say that these people are left brain dominant for both motor and language functions. In ambidextrous

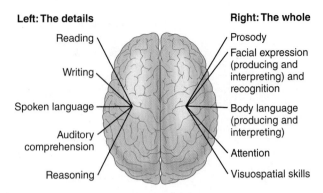

FIGURE 7-19 The function of the left hemisphere compared to the function of the right hemisphere.

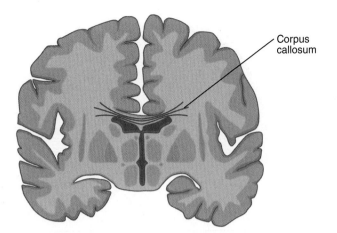

FIGURE 7-20 Coronal section of brain showing the corpus callosum.

people, that figure drops to 85%, and the percentage drops further in left-handed people to 73%. Reading this the opposite way, about 4% of right-handed, 15% of ambidextrous, and 27% of left-handed people have their language functions localized bilaterally or just in the right hemisphere (Knecht et al., 2000). Extra-linguistic features, such as intonation and stress, are lateralized to the right hemisphere rather than the left hemisphere (George et al., 1996; Ross & Monnot, 2008).

Inter- and Intrahemispheric Connections

Interhemispheric Connections

Although the cerebral hemispheres have specialized functions, they do communicate with each other. The **corpus callosum** is a band of axonal callosal fibers that connects the two cerebral hemispheres (Figure 7-13B and **FIGURE 7-20**). It has three major parts. The anterior part is called the genu, the middle part is the isthmus, and the posterior section is the splenium.

Functionally, the corpus callosum allows the cerebral hemispheres to communicate with one another. For example, a printed word presented in the left visual field passes to the right hemisphere and then to the left hemisphere via the corpus callosum for written language to be decoded by the language-dominant left hemisphere.

In patients who have undergone a surgical procedure called a **commissurotomy** to cut the corpus callosum (i.e., split-brain patients; see **BOX 7-2**), reading a word flashed in the left visual field is not possible, because the information cannot travel from the right hemisphere to the language-dominant left hemisphere (**FIGURE 7-21**).

The corpus callosum can be absent at birth (agenesis), thin and underdeveloped (hypoplasia), partially formed (hypogenesis), or malformed (dysgenesis). Kim Peek (1951–2009), a savant who was the inspiration for Raymond Babbitt in the movie *Rain Main*, had agenesis of the corpus callosum. Some believe that this abnormality, which leads to unique intrahemispheric connections, was involved in Peek's incredible memory skills. In an examination of Albert Einstein's brain, examiners found that he had more interhemispheric connections through a thicker corpus callosum than did people in control groups (Men et al., 2014).

Intrahemispheric Connections

Large bundles of neurons make connections within the cerebral hemispheres (**FIGURE 7-22**). One large notable bundle is the superior longitudinal fasciculus (SLF),

---

BOX 7-2 Split-Brain Research

Some people suffer from severe epilepsy, a condition in which uncontrollable, violent electrical storms arise in one hemisphere and migrate to the opposite hemisphere. Often, these storms can be managed with medications, but when this treatment option fails, patients may benefit from a commissurotomy. In this procedure, the corpus callosum is surgically severed, leaving the two hemispheres to work independently. In other words, the hemispheres no longer communicate with each other (and the epileptic electrical storms no longer pass from one hemisphere to the other, giving patients relief). In essence, it is like the patient now has two brains. It was through research on these patients in the 1950s and 1960s by Roger Sperry and Michael Gazzaniga that the idea of hemispheric specialization was explored. After the surgical procedure, patients had intact consciousness, intelligence, and emotions as well as the same personalities as before the surgery. However, testing showed that each hemisphere indeed had its own abilities (see Figure 7-19).

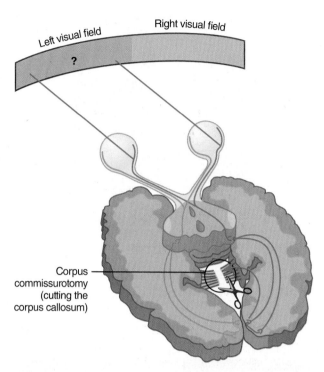

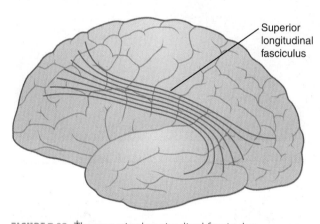

FIGURE 7-21 An illustration of a commissurotomy, a procedure that affects communication between the left and right hemispheres.

FIGURE 7-22 The superior longitudinal fasciculus.

an association fiber tract. This bundle is bidirectional and connects the back and front of the cerebrum and the four brain lobes so all can communicate with one another. The SLF is made up of four parts: SLF I, SLF II, SLF III, and the arcuate fasciculus (AF). The AF (**FIGURE 7-23**) has received much attention because it connects two important speech and language areas—Broca's area in the inferior frontal gyrus with Wernicke's area in the superior temporal gyrus. Damage to the AF can sometimes result in a condition called conduction aphasia, in which patients have difficulty repeating words said to them but have preserved speech fluency and auditory comprehension (Catani & Jones, 2005).

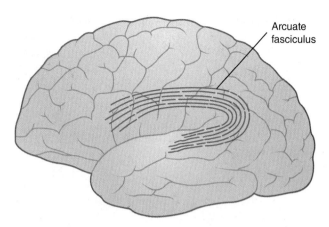

FIGURE 7-23 The arcuate fasciculus.

▶ Cerebral Disorders

There are various neurological conditions involving damage to the cerebral hemispheres. Those conditions that speech-language pathologists (SLPs) and audiologists are most likely to encounter are discussed here.

Cerebral Vascular Accident

A **cerebral vascular accident (CVA)**, commonly known as a stroke, is the fifth leading cause of death in the United States. The CDC estimates that about 795,000 Americans suffer a stroke each year, about one person every 40 seconds. Of these people, 610,000 are experiencing a stroke for the first time, and the remaining 185,000 have had a previous stroke. Many people think that strokes happen only to older adults, but about 34% of stroke victims are younger than 65 years of age. Strokes cost the United States approximately $34 billion each year (CDC, 2017).

CVAs involve some kind of interruption to the brain's blood supply. There are two types of CVA, ischemic CVA and hemorrhagic CVA (**FIGURE 7-24**). An **ischemic CVA** involves loss of blood flow to the brain, usually due to a blockage. The blockage originates in either the blood vessel itself (a **thrombus**) or somewhere else and lodges in a blood vessel (an **embolus**). A third type of ischemic event is a **transient ischemic attack (TIA)**. In a TIA, there is a loss of blood flow to the brain, but the loss is temporary and CVA symptoms resolve in a matter of minutes or within 24 hours. An ischemic event that lasts longer than 24 hours but less than 72 hours is called a reversible ischemic neurological deficit (Easton et al., 2009; Ferro et al., 1996).

Ischemic stroke damage is focal in nature. The area deprived of oxygen dies in about 1 hour or less (a process known as tissue necrosis); this dead tissue is called an **infarct** or an ischemic core (**FIGURE 7-25**). Surrounding the infarct is the ischemic penumbra

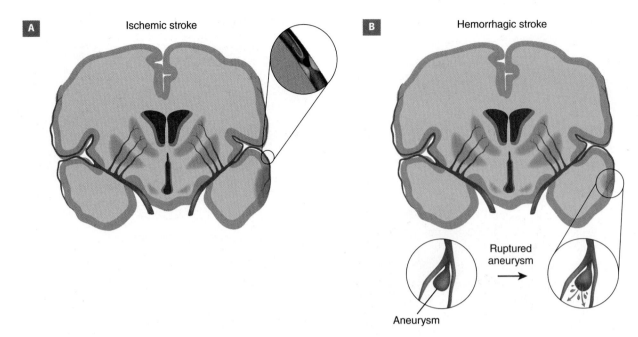

FIGURE 7-24 **A.** Ischemic cerebral vascular accident (CVA). **B.** Hemorrhagic CVA.

Modified from © Alila Medical Media/ShutterStock.

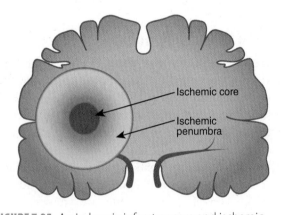

FIGURE 7-25 An ischemic infarct or core and ischemic penumbra.

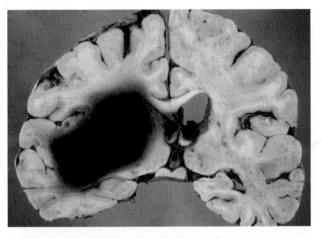

FIGURE 7-26 A large intracerebral hemorrhage.

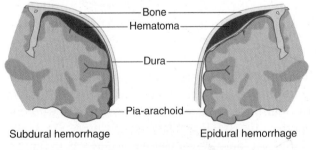

FIGURE 7-27 Comparison between subdural and epidural hematomas.

(Latin for "almost shadow"), an area of traumatized brain tissue that has lost some level of blood flow but has retained enough to stay alive. Though the infarct is lost through necrosis, there is hope the penumbra can be saved within 2 to 4 hours with appropriate medical treatment.

A **hemorrhagic CVA** is a bleeding type of CVA and is divided into two types, **intra-axial hemorrhage** and **extra-axial hemorrhage**. The term *axial* refers to what is central in the human body; thus anything inside the brain is intra-axial, and anything outside the brain is extra-axial. An intra-axial hemorrhage involves blood from a ruptured blood vessel inside the brain (an intraventricular hemorrhage would be in the brain ventricles), whereas an extra-axial hemorrhage involves blood in or around the meninges. Intra-axial hemorrhages are also known as intracerebral hemorrhages (**FIGURE 7-26**). In an extra-axial hemorrhage, the blood is inside the skull but outside the brain. Both intra- and extra-axial hemorrhages result in a hematoma, a collection of blood in a tissue or space. Extra-axial hemorrhages can result in three different kinds of hematomas (**FIGURE 7-27**).

First, **epidural hematomas** occur between the skull and the outer layer of the meninges (dura mater). Second, **subdural hematomas** occur between the dura mater and the middle layer of the meninges (arachnoid mater). Third, **subarachnoid hematomas** occur in the **arachnoid space**, the space below the arachnoid mater.

One mechanism of hemorrhagic CVA is an **aneurysm**, an abnormal ballooning of an artery's wall (Figure 7-24B and **FIGURE 7-28**). There are several different types, but the most common type is a saccular aneurysm, which is also known as a "berry" aneurysm. This type accounts for 80% to 90% of most aneurysms. Aneurysms are ticking time bombs; some people can live for years and never have issues with them, while others can experience a rupture of the aneurysm. Smoking and high blood pressure can further weaken the aneurysm's wall, leading to a rupture and a rapid flow of blood into the brain (**FIGURE 7-29**). When this happens, the victim will experience a severe headache, nausea and vomiting, a loss of consciousness, and possibly death if treatment is not immediate.

Because most strokes are ischemic in nature and this damage is typically focal, various communication disorders may or may not be present. If there is left hemisphere damage, many patients will experience receptive and/or expressive aphasia, apraxia of speech, dysarthria, alexia, dysgraphia, and/or acalculia. In right hemisphere damage, patients will exhibit signs

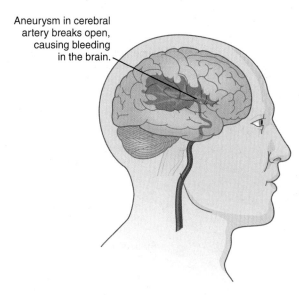

FIGURE 7-29 A ruptured aneurysm leading to severe bleeding in the brain.

of right hemisphere syndrome, including neuromuscular, perceptional, and/or cognitive-communicative issues. They may also experience dysarthria just as patients with left hemisphere damage sometimes do.

Stroke is diagnosed through a combination of clinical presentation and neuroimaging data via computed tomography (CT) or magnetic resonance imaging (MRI). In the case of hemorrhagic stroke, emergency surgery may be needed. A medication known as tissue plasminogen activator (tPA) has been shown to be effective in reducing disability in case of ischemic stroke if given within 4 hours of onset. This medication involves a protein enzyme that catalyzes the transformation of plasminogen to plasmin. Plasmin is the major enzyme for clot breakdowns in the human body.

After patients stabilize, recovery can involve months of hard work. This is accomplished through a rehabilitation team made up of occupational, physical, and speech therapists.

The American Heart Association, National Stroke Association, and CDC have all created campaigns to raise public awareness of strokes as well as awareness of the risk factors for the disease. In fact, the month of May is National Stroke Awareness Month. During this month, there is a push to raise awareness of the signs and symptoms of stroke. One specific educational campaign is Act FAST. This acronym highlights some of the key considerations in recognizing and responding to a stroke: F = face, A = arms, S = speech, and T = time (**FIGURE 7-30**). The hope of this campaign and others like it is for people to recognize when someone is having a stroke and to get the person to the hospital as soon as possible so he or she may benefit from newer treatments, such as tPA.

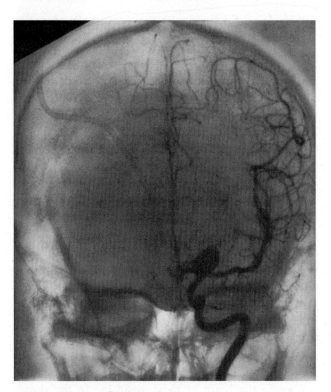

FIGURE 7-28 An angiogram showing a saccular aneurysm of the middle cerebral artery.

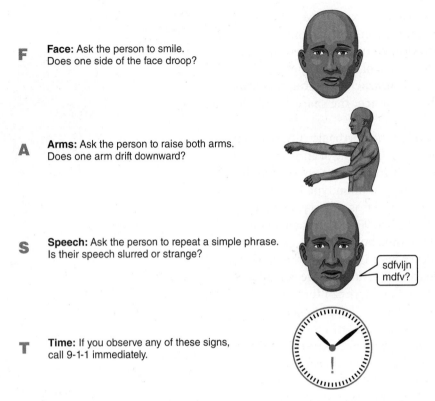

F **Face:** Ask the person to smile. Does one side of the face droop?

A **Arms:** Ask the person to raise both arms. Does one arm drift downward?

S **Speech:** Ask the person to repeat a simple phrase. Is their speech slurred or strange?

sdfvljn mdfv?

T **Time:** If you observe any of these signs, call 9-1-1 immediately.

FIGURE 7-30 The Act FAST campaign.

Traumatic Brain Injury

Traumatic brain injury (TBI) is defined as some type of traumatic blow to the brain that impairs the functioning of the brain. It can occur in one of two forms, open head injury and closed head injury. In **open head injury**, some object (e.g., bullet, shell fragment, rock) penetrates the skull and causes damage to the brain. In contrast, **closed head injury** involves forces that cause damage to the brain, but without penetrating the skull. There are two subtypes of closed head injury. Acceleration–deceleration closed head injury involves the body (and thus the brain) traveling at a high rate of speed and then suddenly coming to a stop (e.g., a car accident). The second type of closed head injury is impact based. In this situation, the body (and the brain) is stationary, but a moving object impacts the head (**FIGURE 7-31**). For example, this author once had a patient who had gotten into a verbal altercation in a bar. This patient decided to deescalate the situation and leave the bar but was followed out by the men and was hit in the head with a baseball bat, resulting in a severe impact-based closed head injury.

The CDC reports that around 1.7 million people sustain a TBI each year. In addition, TBI is a contributing factor in 30.5% of all injury-related deaths in the United States. Most TBI cases (75%) are in the form of a concussion or mild TBI. As a result, there are many "*walking wounded*" in our midst, people we would not immediately identify as having a TBI. Those most

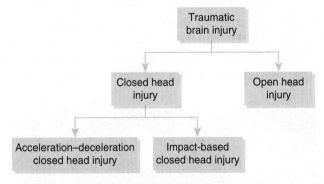

FIGURE 7-31 Types and subtypes of traumatic brain injury.

susceptible to sustaining a TBI include children, older adolescents, and adults older than 65 years (CDC, 2017; Faul, Xu, Wald, & Coronado, 2010).

Brain damage due to CVAs tends to be focused to a particular area of the brain (i.e., **focal damage**). The one exception is in the case of large intra-axial hemorrhages. In contrast, brain damage because of TBI tends to be widespread in nature (i.e., **diffuse damage**), especially in closed injury. This is because the forces applied to the brain in TBI can lead not only to the brain banging up against the inside of the skull (**coup damage**) and rebounding to the opposite site of the skull (**contrecoup damage**) but also to damage from rotational forces (**FIGURE 7-32**). These rotational forces can cause the brain to twist, resulting in the shearing and tearing of axonal fibers as well as metabolic changes (Garnett, Blamire, Rajagopalan, Styles, &

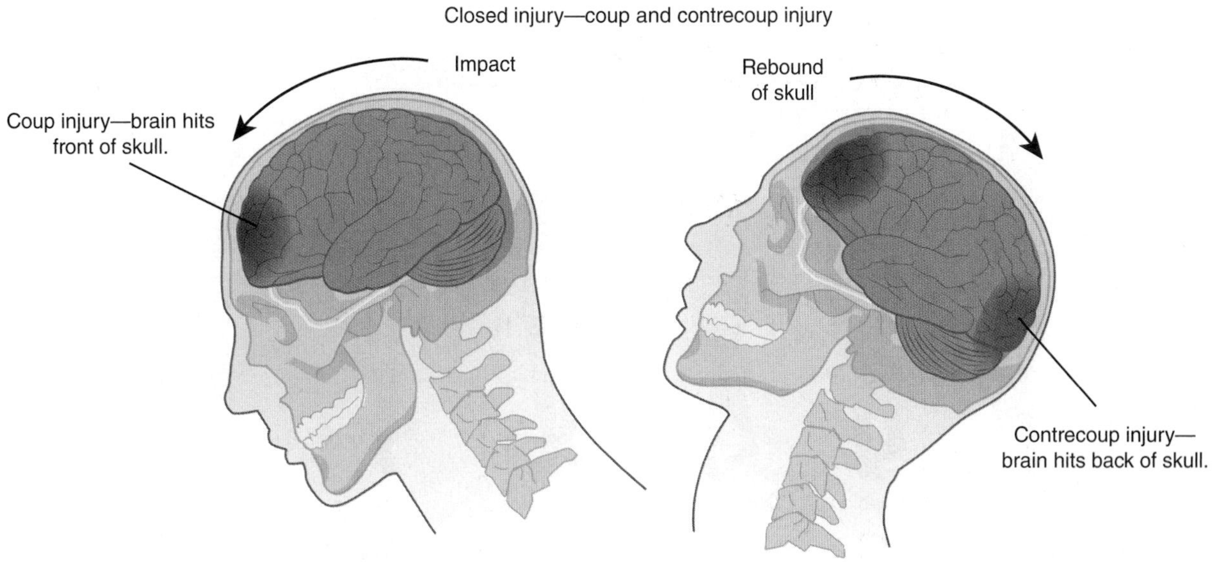

Closed injury—coup and contrecoup injury

Impact

Coup injury—brain hits
front of skull.

Rebound
of skull

Contrecoup injury—
brain hits back of skull.

FIGURE 7-32 Coup and contrecoup impact.

Cadoux-Hudson, 2000; Gennarelli, Thibault, & Graham, 1998). This type of damage typically does not show up on conventional imaging studies, though the results can be devastating to the patient. In terms of communication disorders, aphasia, right hemisphere syndrome, dysarthria, apraxia of speech, and/or dysphagia may be present due to the diffuse nature of damage associated with TBI.

The diagnosis of TBI is made through knowledge of the injury mechanism (e.g., motor vehicle accident), clinical presentation, and neuroimaging. Recovery may involve various medications and possibly surgery in some cases. The rehabilitation team will be crucial in a patient's recovery process.

Cerebral Palsy

Cerebral palsy (CP) is a nonprogressive brain disorder that affects movement, posture, and balance (**FIGURE 7-33**). It can also affect speech and swallowing in some cases. *Cerebral* refers to the brain and *palsy* refers to paralysis or uncontrolled movements. CP develops before birth (prenatal), during birth (perinatal), or shortly after birth (postnatal) and can be caused by a lack of oxygen, premature birth, infections, brain hemorrhages, jaundice, and head injury (CDC, 2018b). It is the most common childhood motor problem (CDC, 2018a).

There are four types of CP based on movement problems (**FIGURE 7-34**). *Spastic CP* is the most common form, occurring in 80% of cases; it involves damage to the cerebral hemispheres. It is characterized by muscle stiffness and rigidity. These issues can occur on one side of the body (hemiplegia), just in the legs (diplegia), or in all four limbs (quadriplegia). *Dyskinetic CP*

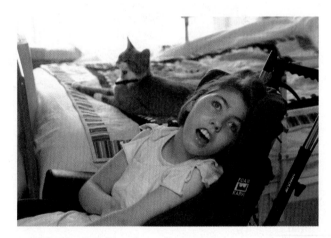

FIGURE 7-33 A child with cerebral palsy.

involves problems with muscle tone that affect the whole body because of damage to the basal ganglia system. Muscle tone can change from hour to hour or day to day. For example, a child may wake up with stiff, rigid muscle tone, which may normalize later in the day but then decrease at night. *Ataxic CP* involves discoordination between muscle groups because of cerebellar damage; it results in clumsy movement and difficulty walking. This type of CP is caused by damage to the cerebellum. Finally, *mixed CP* involves more than one type of motor issue (Pellegrino, 2002). CP can also be described by the body parts involved in the condition. Hemiplegic CP involves the arm and leg on one side of the body. When just the legs are involved, this is called diplegic CP. Quadriplegic CP involves all four extremities.

CP is initially diagnosed at birth through clinical presentation and reevaluated when a child is 18 to 24 months old. Neuroimaging is employed if the etiology of the child's CP is unknown. Occupational, physical,

Types of Cerebral Palsy and Areas of Brain Damage Involved

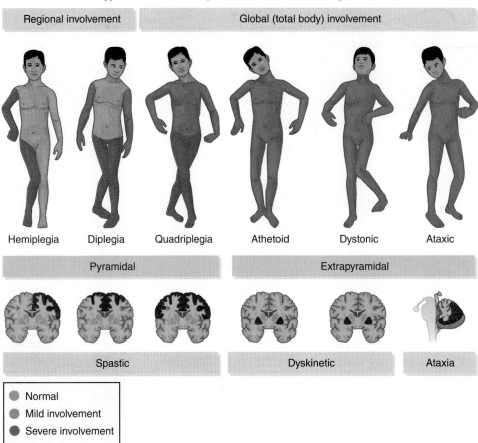

FIGURE 7-34 Types of cerebral palsy.

and speech therapy will be performed to reduce disability and get the child to his or her maximal functional capacity.

Stuttering

Stuttering (or *stammering*) may seem like an odd addition to this list of cerebral disorders, but there are probable neurophysiological differences in the brains of those who stutter versus those who do not stutter. **Fluency** refers to the smoothness with which sound, words, and sentences flow during oral language; **disfluency** is any interruption in this smoothness. All people are disfluent at one time or another, but stuttering is different from normal disfluency. Normal disfluency involves problems with whole words or between words. For example, an interjection ("um") is a disfluency that occurs between words. In stuttering, the disfluency often occurs within words (though there may be whole-word or between-word disfluencies also). For example, people who stutter will repeat or prolong sounds, or a sound will be blocked.

There is no one cause for stuttering. Genetics are involved in many cases, but the environment also seems to play a role in the condition. Whatever

the causes, there may be brain differences between those who stutter and those who do not. For example, the right nonlanguage hemisphere is overactive and the left language hemisphere is underactive in some people who stutter. More specifically, the right frontal operculum, which is in about the same place as Broca's area in the left hemisphere, is sometimes overactive. Another overactive area in some people who stutter is the right insula, an area of the cerebral cortex folded deep within the lateral fissure (Brown, Ingham, Ingham, Laird, & Fox, 2005; Fox, 2003). In contrast, speech motor areas and auditory areas in the left hemisphere are underactive in some people (Guitar, 2013).

Stuttering is diagnosed by an SLP through clinical presentation. The SLP will then use one of two (or both in some cases) therapy approaches, **stuttering modification** or **fluency shaping**. Stuttering modification focuses on the moment of stuttering and training patients to stutter more easily and with less tension. Fluency shaping does not focus on moments of stuttering, but rather on fluency itself and strategies that promote better fluent speech. There is evidence that the brain is changed through these therapies and that the right hemisphere quiets down while the left hemisphere ramps up its activity to more typical levels (Guitar, 2013). This evidence shows the principle of brain plasticity, which will be discussed next.

▶ Brain Plasticity

Brain plasticity or **neuroplasticity** refers to the adaptive capacity of the human brain. The brain is always changing, rewiring itself in response to internal and external influences. You are experiencing neuroplasticity right now as you read and study this text. Your brain is changing by the text (external influence) and by your own previous knowledge and experiences with neuroscience and neurological disorders (internal influence). How do our patients recover from some of the devastating conditions outlined in this chapter? The answer is through neuroplasticity.

Use It or Lose It and Use It and Improve It

There are many principles of neuroplasticity (TABLE 7-3). The first principle is "use it or lose it," which explains that failure to drive certain brain functions leads to loss. For example, a lack of cognitive activity in older adults can contribute to the loss of some cognitive skills (Burda, 2011). Another example is patients on prolonged mechanical ventilation who lose their swallowing ability, in part because of a lack of exercise of the swallowing muscles (Tolep, Getch, & Criner, 1996).

The second principle is the corollary to the first—"use it and improve it." This principle states that training of a specific brain function leads to improvement (Kleim & Jones, 2008). For example, continued cognitive activity into older adulthood reduces the risk of dementia (Gates & Valenzuela, 2010).

As discussed earlier, some stroke patients experience hemiparesis or hemiplegia. Physical therapists have taken advantage of the "use it or lose it" and "use it and improve it" principles of neuroplasticity through constraint-induced movement therapy (CIMT). In this therapy the patient's good arm is restrained, forcing the patient to use only the impaired hand in therapy. CIMT has resulted in some substantial functional improvements in many patients, but also imaging data showing increased cerebral metabolism. This same approach has been adapted in speech-language pathology, resulting in a therapy known as constraint-induced language therapy (CILT). In CILT, patients are forced to use verbal language only. In other words,

TABLE 7-3 Principles of Neuroplasticity	
Principle	**Description**
Use it or lose it	Failure to drive certain functions can lead to loss.
Use it and improve it	Training of certain brain functions can lead to improvement.
Specificity	The nature of the training experience dictates the nature of plasticity.
Repetition matters	Induction of plasticity requires sufficient repetition.
Intensity matters	Induction of plasticity requires sufficient training intensity.
Time matters	Different forms of plasticity occur at different times of training.
Salience matters	The training experience must be important to induce plasticity.
Age matters	Training-induced plasticity occurs more readily in younger people.
Transference	Plasticity in response to one training experience can enhance the acquisition of similar behaviors.
Interference	Plasticity in response to one experience can interfere with the acquisition of other behaviors.

Data from Kleim, J. A., & Jones, T. A. (2008). Principles of experience-dependent neural plasticity: Implications for rehabilitation after brain damage. *Journal of Speech, Language, and Hearing Research, 51,* S225–S239.

they cannot use another communication modality or compensatory strategy. Through two additional principles of neuroplasticity (intensity and shaping), patients play games like Go Fish while depending on their verbal skills only. Many patients have experienced gains in their verbal language because of this approach, which taps into the brain's natural ability to adapt (Pulvermüller et al., 2001).

Specificity Matters

Specificity means that the nature of training experience dictates nature of plasticity. In other words, specific, functional tasks can change the brain more than unspecific, general tasks can. Semantic feature analysis, a word-recall treatment, is an example of a specific treatment targeting a specific skill. In this treatment approach, clinicians help their patients to recall the semantic features of a noun (e.g., *lion*—fur, king, roars), with the intent of reestablishing semantic connections and improving naming. Identifying the semantic features of target words is a very specific therapy and is more likely to induce changes in the brain than is a less specific treatment.

Repetition and Intensity Matter

Repetition is defined as ongoing practice over time. It is sometimes referred to as dose frequency. For example, a patient's dose frequency might be 60-minute treatment sessions, three times per week for 12 weeks. This dose frequency would be a lot of repetition of therapy over this period (i.e., 36 total hours of therapy). While *repetition* refers to the treatment experience more broadly, *intensity* is focused on the dosage of treatment within individual therapy sessions. In other words, to how many teaching trials or episodes is a patient exposed in a treatment session? Some therapists practice high-intensity dosing, which is also known as massed practice. This practice is focused on teaching a patient a new skill. Other clinicians might choose a low-intensity dose (also called distributed practice) that is more focused on the maintenance of a learned skill. CILT often uses massed practice in the form of 20 to 25 teaching trials in a 1-hour session.

Time Matters

After injury, the brain is more plastic at some times and less plastic at other times. For example, in the acute phase of stroke recovery, the brain is in a state of shock for the first 3 to 4 days and is not very plastic. After 4 days to around 4 months, the brain is more plastic as it recovers. During the chronic phase of recovery (4 months and after), the brain is finding a new normal and is still plastic, but less so than in the post-stroke period (day 4 to 4 months).

Salience Matters

Salience refers to something that is important or meaningful. The principle of salience matters means that the training experience must be important to the patient in order to induce plasticity. A rewarding, functional, motivating therapy task is more likely to induce brain plasticity than is a nonrewarding, nonfunctional, boring task. For example, if a patient is a foodie, then therapy tasks that focus on menu reading and recipe following might be more beneficial than tasks focused on automobile maintenance, an area of noninterest for the patient.

Age Matters

This principle states that training-induced plasticity occurs more readily in younger people than in older people. *Younger* is defined as 50 years of age or younger. This distinction does not mean that plasticity is absent in people older than 50 years, but that it is less dramatic. This principle probably does not shock most readers, as we all remember being children and bouncing back from illness or accidents more quickly than we do now as adults.

Transference Matters

Transference (or generalization) means that plasticity in response to one training experience can enhance the acquisition of similar behaviors. For example, word-retrieval activities for atypical words (e.g., artichoke) may more readily generalize to untrained but related typical words (e.g., carrot). Or, a writing therapy that focuses on correct spelling of words might transfer to better reading ability.

Interference Matters

We are all familiar with bad habits and understand how they can interfere with learning. For example, many students complain that social media can distract them from studying. Interference, as its name suggests, means that as one experience changes the brain, it can interfere with gaining a new and possibly better behavior. Pain, seizures, psychological conditions, and substance abuse are all conditions or behaviors that can change the brain to the detriment of acquiring other behaviors, such as the knowledge and skills for a career in speech-language pathology or audiology.

▶ Conclusion

This look at the cerebrum surveyed structures that protect and support it, such as the meninges and vascular system. Macroscopic features, like sulci and gyri, were explored next. We discovered that the cerebral hemispheres are not mirror images of each other functionally; each has specialized functions.

Of great importance to those studying communication disorders is the left hemisphere, which is the language-dominant hemisphere for most people. Significant damage can occur to the speech, language, and swallowing systems due to CVAs and TBIs, but some of the effects of this damage can be overcome by applying the principles of neuroplasticity in therapy.

SUMMARY OF LEARNING OBJECTIVES

The following were the main learning objectives of this chapter. The information that should have been learned is below each learning objective.

1. The learner will list four structures/systems that nourish and protect the brain.
    *   *Protection:* the meninges and the blood–brain barrier
    *   *Nourishment:* the cerebral arteries
    *   *Waste removal:* the venous system
2. The learner will identify important features of the cerebral hemispheres, including the lobes of the brain.
    *   *Fissures:* deep grooves in the brain
    *   *Sulci:* shallower grooves in the brain
    *   *Gyri:* hills in the brain
    *   *Longitudinal fissure:* Separates the right and left hemispheres.
    *   *Central fissure:* Separates the frontal lobe from the parietal lobe.
    *   *Lateral fissure:* Separates the frontal and parietal lobes from the temporal lobe.
    *   *Frontal lobe:* Main functions include reasoning, planning, and voluntary motor movement.
    *   *Parietal lobe:* Functions in sensory perception and interpretation.
    *   *Temporal lobe:* Perception and comprehension of speech takes place as well as some memory functions.
    *   *Occipital lobe:* Main function is visual processing.
3. The learner will describe the phenomenon of hemispheric specialization, especially how it relates to language.
    *   In terms of function, each hemisphere is not a mirror image of the other; rather, the two hemispheres function uniquely. The clearest example of hemispheric specialization is language. Ninety-six percent of right-handed people have their language functions lateralized to the left hemisphere.
4. The learner will list and briefly describe causes of damage to the cerebral hemispheres.
    *   *Cerebral vascular accident (CVA):* Also known as stroke. A condition caused by an interruption to the brain's blood supply through either a blockage (ischemia) or bleeding (hemorrhage).
    *   *Traumatic brain injury (TBI):* a traumatic blow to the brain that impairs the functioning of the brain. There are two kinds, open and closed head injury. In open, the skull is penetrated by an object; in closed, the skull is not.
    *   *Cerebral palsy (CP):* a nonprogressive brain disorder acquired before, during, or shortly after birth that affects movement, posture, and balance.
    *   *Stuttering:* a condition characterized by in-word interruptions to the free flow of speech.
5. The learner will describe the phenomenon of brain plasticity and its principles.
    *   Brain plasticity refers to the adaptive capacity of the human brain. The brain is always changing, rewiring itself, in response to internal and external influences. The following are specific principles of neuroplasticity:
        *   *Use it or lose it:* Failure to drive certain functions can lead to loss.
        *   *Use it and improve it:* Training of certain brain functions can lead to improvement.
        *   *Specificity matters:* The nature of the training experience dictates the nature of plasticity.
        *   *Repetition matters:* Induction of plasticity requires sufficient repetition.
        *   *Intensity matters:* Induction of plasticity requires sufficient training intensity.
        *   *Time matters:* Different forms of plasticity occur at different times of training.

☐ *Salience matters:* The training experience must be important to induce plasticity.

☐ *Age matters:* Training-induced plasticity occurs more readily in younger people.

☐ *Transference:* Plasticity in response to one training experience can enhance the acquisition of similar behaviors.

☐ *Interference:* Plasticity in response to one experience can interfere with the acquisition of other behaviors.

KEY TERMS

Agyria
Aneurysm
Arachnoid mater
Arachnoid space
Blood–brain barrier (BBB)
Carotid artery
Central fissure
Cerebral palsy (CP)
Cerebral vascular accident (CVA)
Circle of Willis
Circumventricular organs (CVOs)
Closed head injury
Commissurotomy
Contrecoup damage
Corpus callosum
Coup damage
Deep cerebral veins
Diffuse damage
Disfluency

Dura mater
Embolus
Epidural hematomas
Epidural space
Extra-axial hemorrhage
Fissures
Fluency
Fluency shaping
Focal damage
Frontal lobe
Gyri (gyrus)
Hematoma
Hemispheric specialization
Hemorrhagic CVA
Infarct
Intra-axial hemorrhage
Ischemic CVA
Lateral fissure
Limbic lobe
Lissencephaly
Longitudinal fissure

Neuroplasticity
Occipital lobe
Open head injury
Parietal lobe
Pia mater
Stuttering
Stuttering modification
Subarachnoid hematomas
Subarachnoid space
Subdural hematomas
Subdural space
Sulci (sulcus)
Superficial cerebral veins
Temporal lobe
Thrombus
Transient ischemic attack (TIA)
Traumatic brain injury (TBI)
Venous system
Vertebral artery

DRAW IT TO KNOW IT

1. Sketch of the meninges, including the brain and skull. Label the following: dura mater, arachnoid mater, subarachnoid space, and pia mater.

2. Sketch of the left hemisphere (see Figures 7-13 and 7-14) and label all the major gyri and sulci as well as the lobes of the brain (see Figure 7-18).

QUESTIONS FOR DEEPER REFLECTION

1. List the four lobes of the brain and one function associated with each.
2. Describe the concept of hemispheric specialization as it relates to language.

3. Describe components of neuroplasticity that might be important to rehabilitation.

CASE STUDY

Ben is a 75-year-old male who suffered a sudden onset of right-sided weakness and aphasia. Upon admission to the hospital a CT scan was completed, which did not show any abnormalities. An MRI was completed later, which reveal a small infarct in the left frontal hemisphere near the lateral fissure. Ben was administered tPA and both his weakness and language abilities improved.

1. Explain what type of stroke Ben suffered.
2. Why do you think it is this type of stroke?
3. In thinking about the location of the stroke, why were motor and language functions affected?

SUGGESTED PROJECTS

1. Read the article by Kleim and Jones (2008) and give a presentation to the class on how neuroplasticity is important in speech-language therapy.

2. Find two or three sources on split-brain research and write a two- to three-page paper discussing how hemispheric specialization was discovered.

3. Read *My Stroke of Insight* by Jill Bolte Taylor and write a two- to three-page reflection paper. Half of the paper should be a summary of the book, and the other half should contain your reflections/reactions to the book.

4. Create a stroke prevention campaign that includes a poster, brochure, and public service announcement.

REFERENCES

Bhatnagar, S. C. (2008). *Neuroscience for the study of communicative disorders* (3rd ed.). Philadelphia, PA: Lippincott Williams & Wilkins.

Brown, S., Ingham, R. J., Ingham, J. C., Laird, A. R., & Fox, P. T. (2005). Stuttered and fluent speech production: An ALE meta-analysis of functional neuroimaging studies. *Human Brain Mapping, 25*(1), 105–117.

Burda, A. N. (2011). *Communication and swallowing changes in healthy aging adults.* Sudbury, MA: Jones & Bartlett Learning.

Catani, M., & Jones, D. K. (2005). Perisylvian language networks of the human brain. *Annals of Neurology, 57*(1), 8–16.

Centers for Disease Control and Prevention. (2017). *Stroke fact sheet.* Retrieved from https://www.cdc.gov/dhdsp/data _statistics/fact_sheets/fs_stroke.htm.

Centers for Disease Control and Prevention. (2018a). *Data and statistics for cerebral palsy.* Retrieved from https://www.cdc .gov/ncbddd/cp/data.html

Centers for Disease Control and Prevention. (2018b). *Basics about cerebral palsy.* Retrieved from http://www.cdc.gov/NCBDDD /cp/facts.html

Clarren, S. K., Alvord, E. C., Sumi, S. M., Streissguth, A. P., & Smith, D. W. (1978). Brain malformations related to prenatal exposure to ethanol. *The Journal of Pediatrics, 92*(1), 64–67.

Easton, J. D., Saver, J. L., Albers, G. W., Alberts, M. J., Chaturvedi, S., & Feldmann, E., . . . Sacco, R. L. (2009). Definition and evaluation of transient ischemic attack: A scientific statement for healthcare professionals. *Stroke, 40*(6), 2276–2293.

Faul, M., Xu, L., Wald, M. M., & Coronado, V. G. (2010). *Traumatic brain injury in the United States: Emergency department visits, hospitalizations, and deaths.* Atlanta, GA: Centers for Disease Control and Prevention, National Center for Injury Prevention and Control.

Ferro, J. M., Falcao, I., Rodrigues, G., Canhao, P., Melo, T. P., & Oliveira, V., . . . Salgado, A. V. (1996). Diagnosis of transient ischemic attack by the nonneurologist: A validation study. *Stroke, 27*(12), 2225–2229.

Fox, P. T. (2003). Brain imaging in stuttering: Where next? *Journal of Fluency Disorders, 28*(4), 265–272.

Garnett, M. R., Blamire, A. M., Rajagopalan, B., Styles, P., & Cadoux-Hudson, T. A. (2000). Evidence for cellular damage in normal-appearing white matter correlates with injury severity in patients following traumatic brain injury: A magnetic resonance spectroscopy study. *Brain, 123*(7), 1403–1409.

Gates, N., & Valenzuela, M. (2010). Cognitive exercise and its role in cognitive function in older adults. *Current Psychiatry Reports, 12*(1), 20–27.

Gennarelli, T. A., Thibault, L. E., & Graham, D. I. (1998). Diffuse axonal injury: An important form of traumatic brain damage. *The Neuroscientist, 4*(3), 202–215.

George, M. S., Parekh, P. I., Rosinsky, N., Ketter, T. A., Kimbrell, T. A., & Heilman, K. M., . . . Post, R. M. (1996). Understanding emotional prosody activates right hemisphere regions. *Archives of Neurology, 53*(7), 665.

Guitar, B. (2013). *Stuttering: An integrated approach to its nature and treatment.* Philadelphia, PA: Lippincott Williams & Wilkins.

Herculano-Houzel, S. (2009). The human brain in numbers: A linearly scaled-up primate brain. *Frontiers in Human Neuroscience, 3*(31), 1–11.

Hooper, R. (2013). Is this the most extraordinary human brain ever seen? *New Scientist, 219*(3924), 24–25.

Jones, E. G., & Peters, A. (1984). *Cerebral cortex: Cellular components of the cerebral cortex.* New York, NY: Plenum Press.

Kleim, J. A., & Jones, T. A. (2008). Principles of experience-dependent neural plasticity: Implications for rehabilitation after brain damage. *Journal of Speech, Language, and Hearing Research, 51,* S225–S239.

Knecht, S., Dräger, B., Deppe, M., Bobe, L., Lohmann, H., & Flöel, A., . . . Henningsen, H. (2000). Handedness and hemispheric language dominance in healthy humans. *Brain, 123*(12), 2512–2518.

Men, W., Falk, D., Sun, T., Chen, W., Li, J., & Yin, D., . . . Fan, M. (2014). The corpus callosum of Albert Einstein's brain: Another clue to his high intelligence? *Brain, 137*(4), e268–e268. doi:10.1093/brain/awt252

National Institute of Neurological Disorders and Stroke (NINDS). (2018). *Lissencephaly information page.* Retrieved from https:// www.ninds.nih.gov/Disorders/All-Disorders/Lissencephaly -Information-Page

Pellegrino, L. (2002). Cerebral palsy. In M. L. Batshaw (Ed.), *Children with disabilities* (pp. 443–466). Baltimore, MD: Paul H. Brookes Publishing.

Pulvermüller, F., Neininger, B., Elbert, T., Mohr, B., Rockstroh, B., Koebbel, P., & Taub, E. (2001). Constraint-induced therapy of chronic aphasia after stroke. *Stroke, 32*(7), 1621–1626.

Ross, E. D., & Monnot, M. (2008). Neurology of affective prosody and its functional–anatomic organization in right hemisphere. *Brain and Language, 104*(1), 51–74.

Tolep, K., Getch, C. L., & Criner, G. J. (1996). Swallowing dysfunction in patients receiving prolonged mechanical ventilation. *Chest, 109*(1), 167–172.

Toro, R., Perron, M., Pike, B., Richer, L., Veillette, S., Pausova, Z., & Paus, T. (2008). Brain size and folding of the human cerebral cortex. *Cerebral Cortex, 18*(10), 2352–2357.

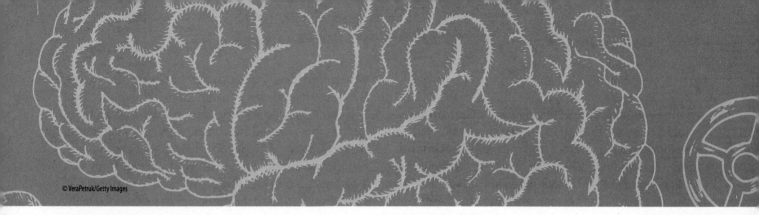

© VeraPetruk/Getty Images

CHAPTER 8

The Cerebrum: Cerebral Function

CHAPTER PREVIEW

Now it is time to explore the anatomy and functions of various cortical areas in more detail. We will begin at the front of the brain and make our way to the back of the brain using a special numbering system developed for this kind of journey.

IN THIS CHAPTER

In this chapter, we will . . .
- Describe the origins and use of the Brodmann map
- Survey the cerebral areas and functions using the Brodmann map, especially those functions related to communication and communication disorders

LEARNING OBJECTIVES

- The learner will state the main limitation of the Brodmann map.
- The learner will list the important areas in each lobe of the brain and ascribe at least one function to each area.

▶ Introduction

At the beginning of the 20th century, a German neurologist named Korbinian Brodmann (1868–1918) developed what is known today as the **Brodmann map** (FIGURE 8-1). With this map, he divided the human brain into 52 areas based on differences in gross anatomy and cytoarchitecture (i.e., cellular structure) and postulated that each of these areas, either individually or in connection with other areas, is responsible for certain functions. Today this map is a useful way to navigate around the human brain and discuss cerebral functions, with special attention to areas involved in speech, language, hearing, cognition, and swallowing. Instead of moving from area 1 to area 52 numerically, we will move anatomically from frontal to parietal to occipital lobe and, finally, to the temporal lobe.

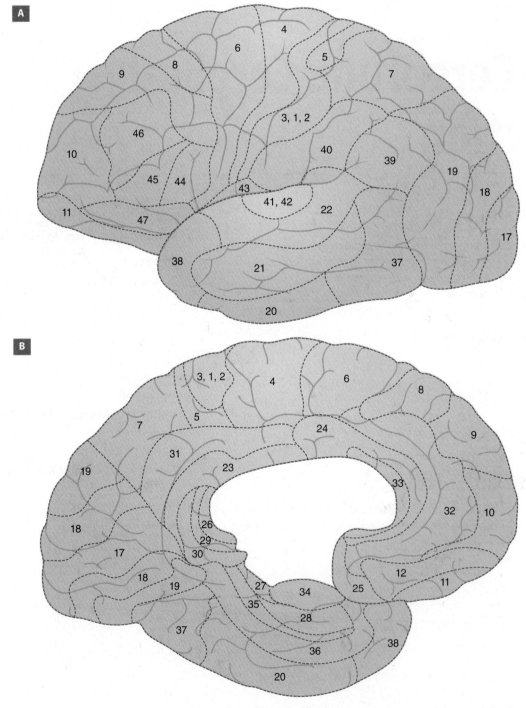

FIGURE 8-1 **A.** A lateral view of the left hemisphere with Brodmann numbers indicating cytoarchitecturally distinct areas. **B.** A medial view of the left hemisphere with Brodmann numbers. The blank white area in the middle would contain the corpus callosum, fornix, thalamus, and other structures.

There is one danger that needs to be mentioned before proceeding. Examining the cerebral cortex in this way could lead one to think that each area is responsible for a certain function and, correspondingly, that this particular function is managed by only that area. For example, is the Wernicke area (Brodmann area [BA] 22) in the superior temporal lobe the only area involved in the comprehension of human speech? The human brain is far more complex than this, with multiple areas in the cortex being involved in various functions, like auditory comprehension, as well as structures in the white matter under the cortex. The Brodmann map is meant to be a simple navigation tool that helps to survey the many complexities of the cerebral hemispheres.

▶ The Cerebral Cortex

Frontal Lobe

Prefrontal Cortex (Brodmann Areas 9, 10, 11, 12, 46, and 47)

The prefrontal cortex lies in the rostral end of the frontal lobe, with its caudal end being the premotor areas (e.g., BA 6). It is usually defined as areas 8, 44, and 45 in addition to 9, 10, 11, 12, 46, and 47, but for our purposes, we will leave these three areas (BAs 8, 44, 45) for a later discussion (**FIGURE 8-2**). Overall, the prefrontal cortex is associated with cognition, personality, decision making, and social behavior.

Much is known about the prefrontal cortex through cases of brain damage, the most famous case being that of **Phineas Gage** from the 19th century. Gage was a 25-year-old man who worked in railroad track installation, clearing rocks from the railroad path. To do this, a hole was drilled in a rock, which was then filled halfway with explosives. Sand was then added on top of the explosive powder to direct the explosion downward, which would split the rock into pieces. A long metal rod, known as a tamping iron, was used to ignite the powder and cause the explosion. On September 13, 1848, Gage became distracted and failed to realize his coworker had not added sand to the hole. When Gage tamped, the powder exploded, sending the metal rod up through Gage's head, with the entry wound being just under his cheek and the exit wound being at the top of his head where the frontal lobe lies (**FIGURE 8-3**). The rod fell some 100 yards away, showing the tremendous force of the explosion. Miraculously, Gage survived the tragic accident, but Gage was no longer Gage. Before his accident, Gage was known to be diligent, dependable, and likeable, but after his accident he was bad-tempered, foulmouthed, and antisocial. His injury, though tragic and sad, has taught neuroscientists much about the functioning of the prefrontal cortex.

Brodmann areas are anatomical in nature, being based on cytoarchitecture. These areas in the prefrontal cortex can be regrouped into at least three functional regions (**TABLE 8-1**).

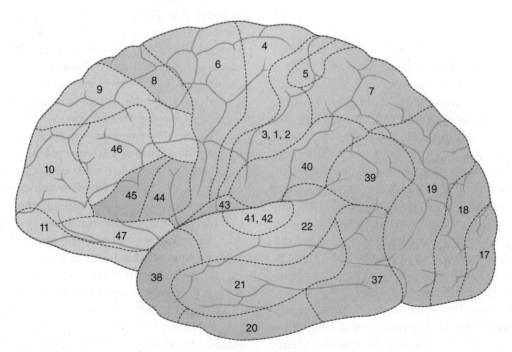

FIGURE 8-2 The prefrontal cortex occupies Brodmann areas 9, 10, 11, 12, 46, and 47. It sometimes includes areas 8, 44, and 45, which are not shaded but will be discussed later.

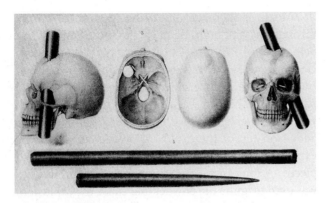

FIGURE 8-3 Phineas Gage and his injury.
Courtesy of the National Library of Medicine.

TABLE 8-1 Functional Regions of the Prefrontal Cortex

Functional Regions	Brodmann Area
Dorsolateral prefrontal cortex (DLPFC)	9, 10, 46
Ventrolateral prefrontal cortex (VLPFC)	45, 47
Orbitofrontal prefrontal cortex (OFC)	11, 12
Medial Prefrontal Cortex (MPFC)	24, 25, 32

Data from: Bateman, J. R. & Kaufer, D. I. (2018). The dorsolateral and cingulate cortex. In B. L. Miller & J. L. Cummings (Eds.), *The human frontal lobes: Functions and disorders* (3rd ed., pp. 29–41). New York, NY: Guilford Press.

The dorsolateral prefrontal cortex (DLPFC) region includes BAs 9, 10, and 46. The dorsal DLPFC is involved in working memory, a type of short-term memory used for temporarily holding information needed for different types of cognitive and linguistic processing. The ventral DLPFC is thought to be important for retrieving previously stored information needed to make judgments and decisions. For example, if someone challenged one of your deeply held political views with contradictory evidence, you would search through your stored information on the view and make a decision to either reject or accept the new evidence. You might even change your political view, though deeply held beliefs are difficult to overturn (Kaplan, Gimbel, & Harris, 2016).

The ventrolateral prefrontal cortex (VLPFC) region is BA 47 as well as BA 45. It appears to also be important in working memory as well as episodic memory. Episodic memory is our memory for space–time events, and the VLPFC plays a role in encoding these

memories and retrieving relevant memories for goal-directed tasks. A third type of memory that the VLPFC is involved in is autobiographical memory, a personal episodic memory. For example, you have the ability to recall your trip to France, but you also have the ability to insert your personal involvement in the trip into the retelling of those memories (Diamond & Levine, 2018). One additional function of the VLPFC is motor inhibition. For example, if you are walking and suddenly stop because a child ran in front of you, the VLPFC would be inhibiting the motor signals of walking (Aron, Robbins, & Poldrack, 2004). This motor stopping mechanism can be activated by an external signal (e.g., the child suddenly running in front of you) or an internal signal (e.g., you deciding to stop walking because you are tired) (Aron, Robbins, & Poldrack, 2014).

The orbitofrontal cortex (OFC) region, which includes BAs 11 and 12, is involved in learning and decision making. In particular, when you are about to perform an action, the OFC appears to evaluate the possible rewards or punishments associated with that action. In other words, it helps to guess the risks and rewards of certain behaviors. After the behavior is completed, the brain associates the behavior with the resulting reward or punishment, thus learning from the experience (Schoenbaum, Takahashi, Liu, & McDannald, 2011). This process is a type of learning called adaptive learning. Patients with damage to the OFC are often apathetic and irresponsible and demonstrate a lack of facial expression (i.e., flat affect) (Kim, Ogar, & Gorno-Tempini, 2018).

The medial prefrontal cortex (MPFC) region includes BAs 24, 25, and 32. This region is part of the cingulate cortex, which will be discussed later. Functionally, it is involved in working memory, but working memory that is spatial in nature. There are connections to the emotional parts of the brain (e.g., amygdala); thus, the MPFC is involved in emotional memory. Like the VLPFC, the MPFC is involved in autobiographical memory, specifically in one's ability to integrate a sense of self into episodic memories.

Overall, the prefrontal cortex is responsible for executive control, which involves goal-directed behavior. In other words, humans have the ability to order their cognitive functions to achieve goals, and the prefrontal cortex is the seat of this executive control. Important aspects of this executive control include restraint, initiative, and order (Fuster, 2008). Restraint involves the inhibition of inappropriate behaviors (e.g., sexual urges) due to having foresight (i.e., the ability to predict being rewarded versus being punished), whereas initiative has to do with the pursuit of productive activities (e.g., motivation, creativity). Order is the capacity to sequence information and events logically, and this task involves specific functions like reasoning, working memory, planning, insight, and organization.

Two distinct profiles can emerge after prefrontal cortex damage (TABLE 8-2). A depressive profile emerges with damage to the lateral prefrontal cortex regions, whereas a manic profile materializes with damage to the more anterior and medial regions (Fuster, 2008; Gazzaley & D'Esposito, 2007; Keeley, 2003). A person who fits the depressive profile will be apathetic and indifferent to people and situations, seemingly with a lack of will (abulia) to accomplish goals in life. The result is a lack of movement (akinesia) or talking (mutism), a virtual couch potato. When there is interest in something, it is a perseverative interest (i.e., getting stuck on one an idea). The person may be depressed and have little interest in sex, which can create tension in marital situations. In contrast, people who fit the manic profile will be explosively emotional, with seemingly small incidents triggering major explosions of anger. They will be distractible and unable to maintain motor acts (i.e., impersistence). Because of their distractedness and impersistence, they will appear frenzied (i.e., manic), moving from one task to another without completing the tasks. They will also confabulate or make up memories, often to compensate for memory gaps. Unlike people in the depressive profile, people with a manic profile often are obsessed with the topic of sex, which can create awkward social situations for those who interact with them. Having reviewed these two profiles, which one do you think better describes Phineas Gage after his injury?

TABLE 8-2 The Two Profiles Resulting From Prefrontal Cortex Damage	
Profile 1: Depressive	**Profile 2: Manic**
Apathetic, indifferent	Explosive emotional lability
Abulia	Environmental dependency
Akinesia	Distractibility
Perseveration	Impersistence
Mutism	Confabulation
Depression	Mania
Hyposexuality	Hypersexuality

Data from: Blumenfeld, H. (2010). *Neuroanatomy through clinical cases*. Sunderland, MA: Sinauer Associates.

Frontal Lobe: Frontal Eye Fields (Brodmann Area 8)

Area 8, known as the frontal eye fields, is an area located just anterior to the premotor cortex (BA 6) that controls left, right, up, and down eye movements (FIGURE 8-4). Typically, when damaged, a patient's eyes will deviate or look toward the side of injury. This area is more than a motor area for the eyes, though,

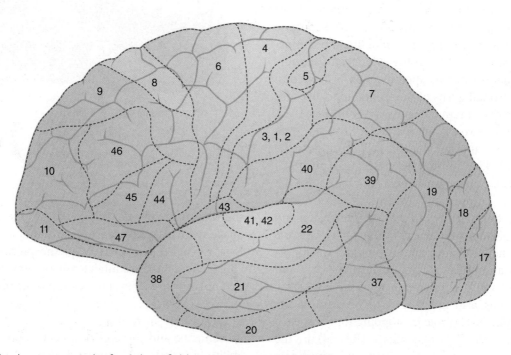

FIGURE 8-4 Brodmann area 8, the frontal eye fields.

as it appears to play a role in the management of uncertainty. Volz, Schubotz, and von Cramon (2005) demonstrated that when test subjects experienced increasing uncertainty, there was increased activation in this area. This area may also be involved in the experience of hope, the feeling that events will turn out for the best (Chew & Ho, 1994).

As can be seen by looking at the Brodmann map in Figure 8-4, area 8 is adjacent to the prefrontal cortex and, as mentioned earlier, is sometimes included as part of the prefrontal cortex. This makes sense given this area's role in uncertainty and hope, which could be thought of as part of the goal-directed behavior associated with executive control. In other words, as we plan a motor behavior, there is a certain amount of hope that the behavior will be successful, but also an uncertainty of its success.

Frontal Lobe: Broca's Area (Brodmann Areas 44 and 45)

The **Broca's area** is located in the inferior frontal gyrus of the frontal lobe and is sandwiched between the premotor cortex (BA 6) and the prefrontal cortex. It is involved in language processing and speech production. This area is named after the French physician Paul Broca (**FIGURE 8-5**), who first described it in 1861. Broca had a mysterious speech-impaired patient known only by his last name (Leborgne) and his nickname "Tan." He received this nickname because "tan" was the only word he could say. Tan suffered from language loss without loss of intellect. Tan's identity has only recently been discovered as Louis Victor Leborgne, an artisan in the shoe trade who suffered from epilepsy since his youth (Domanski, 2013). Leborgne died under Broca's care; after conducting a postmortem examination, Broca had the evidence to support his theory that the human speech center is located in the inferior frontal gyrus of the frontal lobe, because this is where Tan's brain damage was (**FIGURE 8-6**).

There are two main parts of Broca's area (**FIGURE 8-7**), an anterior portion called the *pars triangularis* (BA 45; Latin for the "triangular portion") and a posterior portion called *pars opercularis* (BA 44; Latin for the "lid portion"). As a whole, Broca's area has an important role in both the comprehension and production of language. For example, pars triangularis (BA 45) in the left hemisphere is thought to support the interpretation of language, especially syntax and the planning and programming of verbal responses. Since BA 45 is also considered to be part of the VLPFC, it may have a role in stopping motor speech processes as well. Pars opercularis (BA 44) in the left hemisphere is thought to initiate and coordinate

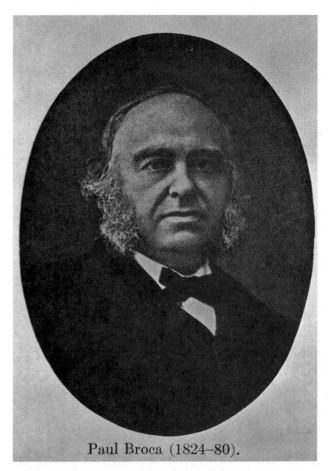

Paul Broca (1824–80).

FIGURE 8-5 Paul Broca.
Courtesy of the National Library of Medicine.

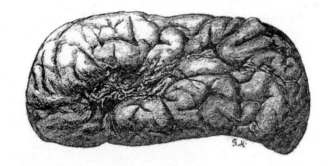

FIGURE 8-6 The brain of Mr. Leborgne (Tan).
Reproduced from Marie, P. (1906). Essai de critique historique sur la genèse de la doctrine de Broca. Semaine *Médicale, 26,* 565–571.

the speech organs for the actual production of language, which makes sense given its close proximity to a motor-related area called the premotor cortex (BA 6). Area 44 also contains mirror neurons, neurons that not only fire when a subject acts, but also when the subject observes someone else acting. Mirror neurons in area 44 fire in response to others' hand or mouth movements, and these cells appear important in our ability to imitate the hand and mouth movements of

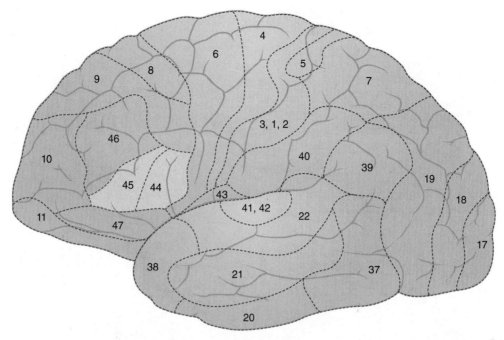

FIGURE 8-7 Brodmann areas 44 and 45, collectively known as the Broca's area.

others (Rajmohan & Mohandas, 2007; Rizzolatti & Craighero, 2004). Damage to these neurons can impair a person's ability to read lips and imitate mouth movements, two strategies often employed in both speech-language pathology and audiology. More generally, the left hemisphere's Broca area appears to be involved in the ability to retrieve and say verbs and the ability to spell words correctly in writing. Nouns appear to be activated in more posterior brain areas (González-Fernández & Hillis, 2018).

Broca's area is thought to be part of a larger dorsal stream of language that is strongly left hemisphere dominant. This is compared to a bilateral ventral stream of language that makes meaning out of heard sound. In short, the ventral stream maps meaning to sound while the dorsal stream maps sound to action (i.e., articulatory action). As already mentioned, the dorsal stream of language is more than Broca's area; it is theorized to also include the premotor cortex, the anterior insula, and the supramarginal gyrus in the parietal lobe, which acts as an interface between motor and sensory information (Hickok & Poeppel, 2007).

Broca's area in the right hemisphere is complementary to Broca's area in the left hemisphere and appears involved in the expression of emotional intonation (or prosody) in our expressive speech as well as the interpretation of intonation, especially the emotional content of others' prosody (Wildgruber, Ackermann, Kreifelts, & Ethofer, 2006). In addition, both right and left Broca areas seem to play some role in the phonological processing of heard speech (Hartwigsen et al., 2010).

Damage to Broca's area can cause what is called **Broca aphasia**, a condition in which people have limited verbal output that is agrammatic in nature. Agrammatism is a symptom of some aphasia types in which patients are not completely grammatical in their speaking. For example, a person with this symptom might say, "Dog . . . walk . . . park" instead of "I walked the dog to the park." The substantial words (nouns, verbs) are present, but the function words ("to" and "the") are absent. Patients can also have a cooccurring motor speech disorder called **apraxia of speech (AOS)**, which is difficulty planning or programming the articulators for speech. Patients with this condition experience great effort in speaking but have intact language functions (in pure forms of AOS). AOS leads to searching and groping for articulatory placement as well as random sound substitutions.

FIGURE 8-8 compares the language disorder aphasia to some other communication impairments. This figure divides communication into three processes: input of information (sensation and recognition), central processing of that information (language), and output of a response (planning and execution). Various dysfunctions or breakdowns in these processes are also listed. For example, if there were a breakdown in central processing, the person would then have aphasia. In comparison, if there is a breakdown in planning, a person would have apraxia of speech. This illustration is a helpful tool in summarizing neurogenic communication disorders and seeing the basic differences between them.

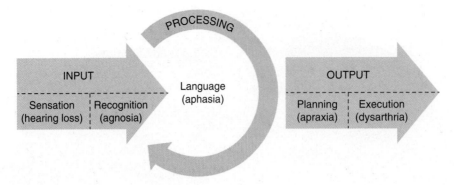

FIGURE 8-8 Comparison of different communication impairments.

Data from Davis, G. A. (2000). *Aphasiology: Disorders and clinical practice.* Needham Heights, MA: Allyn & Bacon.

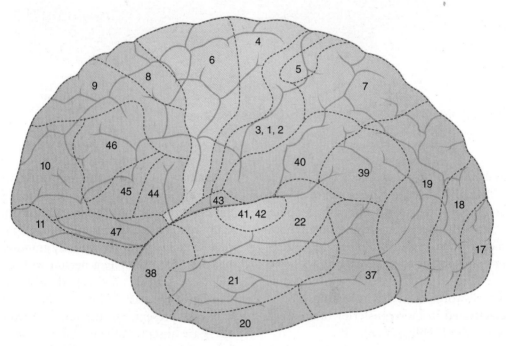

FIGURE 8-9 Brodmann area 6, the premotor cortex.

Frontal Lobe: Premotor Cortex (Brodmann Area 6)

The premotor cortex is anterior to the primary motor cortex (BA 4) and runs down the length of the frontal lobe to the lateral fissure (**FIGURE 8-9**). It is involved in selecting, planning, and sequencing of complex voluntary motor movements of the opposite side of the body in the absence of muscular weakness. When it comes to speech, it would appear that this area and area 44 (*pars opercularis*) have some relationship, because both are involved in motor movement planning and both contain mirror neurons. Damage to the premotor cortex can cause various forms of apraxia (**TABLE 8-3**). In other words, patients will have difficulty completing motor commands and tasks because they cannot pull up the appropriate motor plan to execute the request. For example, an examiner might ask

a patient to show him or her how to salute. The patient would comprehend the command, but then might move his or her hand in strange ways, trying to figure out the motor plan for saluting. This type of apraxia is known as limb-kinetic apraxia.

At the top of area 6 is another area without its own Brodmann number called the supplementary motor area (SMA). This area is thought to be involved with the sequencing of motor movements (Lee & Quessy, 2003), maintaining one's posture while walking (Penfield & Welch, 1951), initiating internally driven movement (Halsband, Matsuzaka, & Tanji, 1994), and using both hands to complete a task (i.e., bimanual coordination), such as tying a shoe (Serrien, Strens, Oliviero, & Brown, 2002). The SMA is thought to extend from BA 6 into the frontal eye fields (BA 8) (Schlag & Schlag-Rey, 1987).

TABLE 8-3 Different Types of Apraxia

Types of Apraxia	Description
Ideational apraxia	Loss of the idea of how to interact with an object because the knowledge and purpose of the object have been lost. Difficulty seen in sequencing multistep tasks due to this loss.
Ideomotor apraxia	Loss of ability to voluntarily carry out a motor action though the knowledge and purpose of the object have been retained.
Limb-kinetic apraxia	Loss of ability to voluntarily move the limbs (e.g., wave "hello").
Constructional apraxia	Loss of ability to voluntarily use the dominant hand in drawing figures (e.g., drawing a square).
Gait apraxia	Loss of ability to voluntarily move and coordinate the lower limbs in a walking motion.
Dressing apraxia	Loss of ability to voluntarily coordinate the limbs in the movements necessary to dress (e.g., button a shirt).
Oculomotor apraxia	Loss of ability to voluntarily move the eyes.
Oral (or buccofacial) apraxia	Loss of ability to voluntarily move the oral structures in nonspeech movements (e.g., sticking the tongue out).
Apraxia of speech	Loss of ability to voluntarily execute the movements of speech.

Data from: Wertz, R. T., LaPointe, L. L., & Rosenbek, J. C. (1991). *Apraxia of speech in adults: The disorder and its management.* San Diego, CA: Singular Publishing.

Frontal Lobe: Primary Motor Cortex (Brodmann Area 4)

The primary motor cortex is located on the precentral gyrus just anterior to the central fissure and posterior to the premotor cortex (**FIGURE 8-10**). In terms of function, it activates the motor plans from areas 44 and 6 by sending motor signals to muscles on the opposite side of the body to move. It has the form of a homunculus (Latin for "little man"), meaning certain areas of this cortex control the motor movements of certain body structures (Figure 8-11A in **FIGURE 8-11**). For example, the knee is controlled near the top of the primary motor cortex, while the tongue is near the bottom with other speech structures. The homunculus is exaggerated, though, with more motor fibers going to structures that are involved in fine motor movement, such as the tongue and the hands, and fewer fibers to gross motor structures, such as the knee (Figure 8-11B). Damage to the primary motor cortex can result in contralateral hemiplegia or hemiparesis. In terms of speech, damage to this region can result in dysarthria, a motor speech disorder where there is

significant weakness in the speech musculature and thus difficulty in executing the movements of speech.

Parietal Lobe

Primary Sensory Cortex (Brodmann Areas 1, 2, and 3)

The primary sensory cortex's anterior border is the central fissure, and its posterior border is made up of BAs 5, 7, and 40 (**FIGURE 8-12**). From anterior to posterior, the areas are organized 3, 1, and then 2.

Functionally, the primary sensory cortex is similar to the primary motor cortex in that a homunculus can be mapped on it, but instead of activating motor plans, it receives and perceives sensory information from the body (i.e., somatosensory information) (Figure 8-13A in **FIGURE 8-13**). Sensory fibers from the body project up through somatosensory tracts and are routed through the thalamus to the primary sensory cortex. The primary sensory cortex processes somatosensory information such as touch, temperature, vibration, proprioception (i.e., the body's eyes

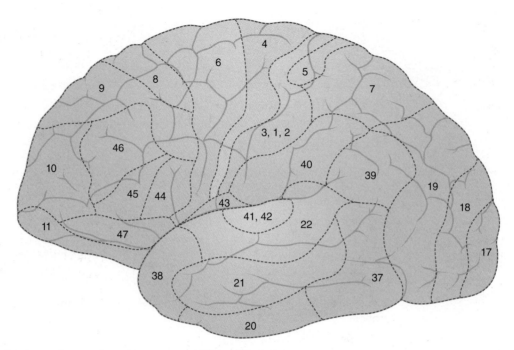

FIGURE 8-10 Brodmann area 4, the primary motor cortex.

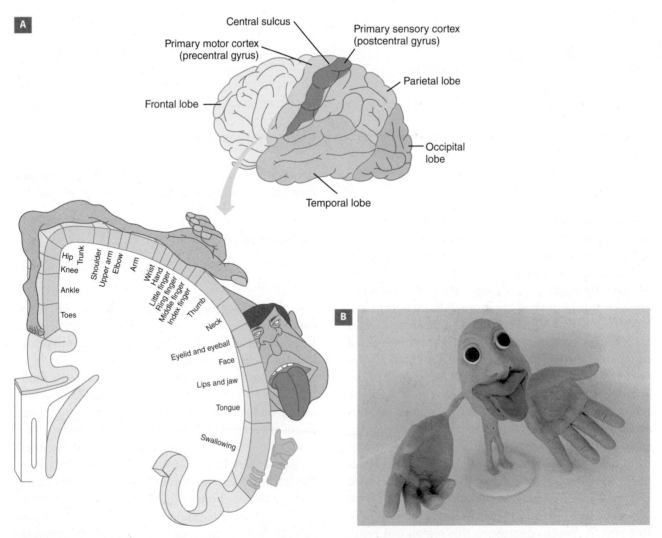

FIGURE 8-11 **A.** A coronal view of the left primary motor cortex with the homunculus mapped onto it.
B. A motor homunculus.

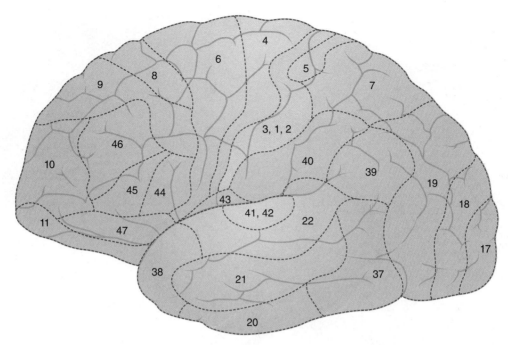

FIGURE 8-12 Brodmann areas 1, 2, and 3, the primary sensory cortex (or somatosensory cortex).

for itself), and stereognosia (i.e., tactile knowledge of three-dimensional forms). As mentioned earlier, the primary sensory cortex can be viewed as a homunculus that has exaggerated features corresponding to the amount of sensory fibers a structure requires (Figure 8-13B). For example, the lips of the homunculus are exaggerated because the lips are extremely sensitive structures as compared to the knee, which is less sensitive in comparison. The ears are exaggerated also because of their special sensory abilities.

Damage to the primary sensory cortex can result in decreased sensory abilities in touch (hemihypesthesia), temperature (thermoception), and pain (nociception), and in vibration on one side of the body. Damage can also result in an inability to discriminate the tactile characteristics of objects and an inability to identify objects via touch. Phantom limb syndrome, a condition in which amputees continue to sense their missing limb (e.g., feel pain in it), may be associated with this area (Ramachandran & Hirstein, 1998). Finally, the primary sensory cortex is remarkably plastic. For example, if a finger is amputated, the primary sensory cortex tissue assigned to that finger will be reassigned to other nearby body parts.

Somatosensory Association Cortex (Brodmann Areas 5 and 7)

BAs 5 and 7 are collectively known as the somatosensory association cortex. These areas lie on the dorsal part of the parietal lobe and are bordered by the primary sensory cortex anteriorly, the visual cortex posteriorly (BA 19), and the supramarginal gyrus (BA 40) ventrally (**FIGURE 8-14**).

Motor and sensory information are both important to speech. The motor system provides the basic movements needed, but the sensory system provides feedback to refine those movements. For example, if a person holds a paper cup of water, the sensory system influences the motor system so that the person does not hold the cup too loosely so as to drop it or too tightly so as to crush it. Speech is similarly controlled, and the somatosensory association cortex plays a role in influencing the fine movements needed for fluent speech (Dhanjal, Handunnetthi, Patel, & Wise, 2008; Premji, Rai, & Nelson, 2011). In addition, a writing circuit has been identified in the somatosensory association cortex through functional magnetic resonance imaging (Harrington, Farias, Davis, & Buonocore, 2007). **Astereognosis**, the inability to recognize three-dimensional forms via touch, is associated with damage to area 5 (Endo, Miyasaka, Makishita, & Yanagisawa, 1992; Nakamura, Endo, Sumida, & Hasegawa, 1998).

Angular Gyrus (Brodmann Area 39)

The angular gyrus lies in the parietal lobe, situated between BAs 19, 40, 22, and 37 (**FIGURE 8-15**). It wraps around the posterior end of the middle temporal gyrus.

The angular gyrus is another important language area in the left hemisphere and is associated with reading and math abilities. In terms of reading, it is involved with visual word form processing along with the middle temporal gyrus and ventral occipito-temporal cortex (Ischebeck et al., 2004; Price, 2012).

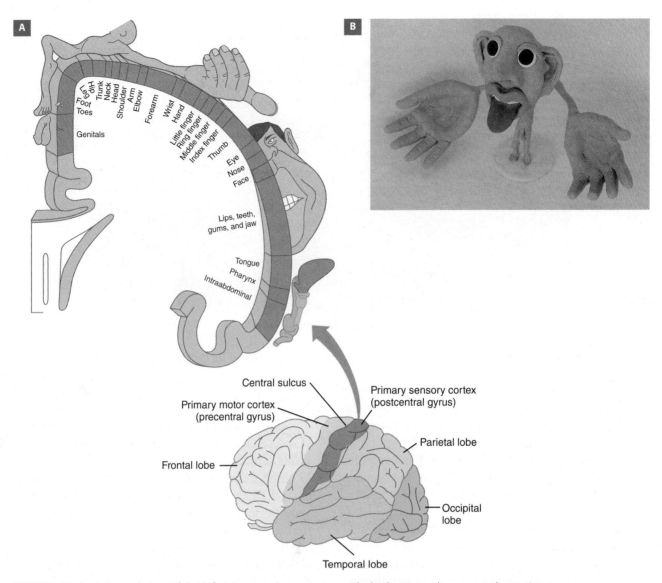

FIGURE 8-13 **A.** A coronal view of the left primary sensory cortex with the homunculus mapped onto it. **B.** A sensory homunculus.

Damage to the angular gyrus can result in alexia (i.e., difficulty reading) and acalculia (i.e., difficulty with math skills). Writing and disorders of writing have traditionally been associated with the angular gyrus, but Katanoda, Yoshikawa, and Sugishita (2001) found no evidence of angular gyrus activation during writing tasks. Hubbard and Ramachandran (2003) have theorized that the angular gyrus is a player in understanding metaphors. Out-of-body experiences, or the experience of floating outside one's body, have also been induced through stimulation of the angular gyrus (Blanke, Ortigue, Landis, & Seeck, 2002). Lastly, Gerstmann syndrome is associated with damage to this area. The symptoms of Gerstmann syndrome include agraphia, alexia, finger agnosia (i.e., difficulty identifying fingers), and right–left disorientation (Vallar, 2007).

The right hemisphere's angular gyrus is important for visuospatial processing, and damage to it can result

in a condition called hemispatial neglect (Mort et al., 2003). In this condition, a person technically "sees" information from both left and right visual fields, but neglects or ignores visual information from one of the visual fields. Sacks (1999) tells the story of a woman with this kind of deficit who, when she ate her meal, would eat only food on the right side of the plate. She would also put makeup on only one side of her face, ignoring the opposite side.

Supramarginal Gyrus (Brodmann Area 40)

The supramarginal gyrus (SMG) is just anterior to the angular gyrus in the parietal lobe and wraps around the posterior end of the lateral fissure (**FIGURE 8-16**). It is surrounded by the primary sensory cortex (anteriorly), the somatosensory association cortex (superiorly), the angular gyrus (posteriorly), and the temporal lobe (inferiorly). The SMG appears to have a

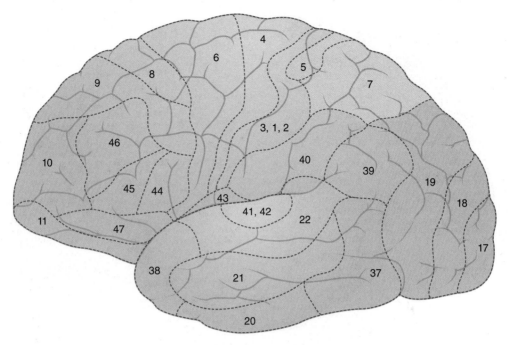

FIGURE 8-14 Brodmann areas 5 and 7, the somatosensory association cortex.

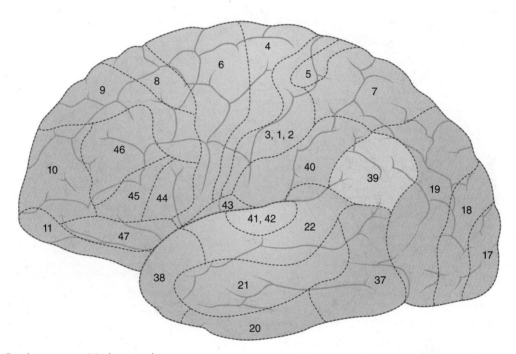

FIGURE 8-15 Brodmann area 39, the angular gyrus.

close connection to the angular gyrus. These two areas together are known as the inferior parietal lobe.

Functionally, the SMG appears to be involved with our phonological system, specifically in storing auditory representations of phonemes and phoneme combinations. Because of this role, it is thought to be a part of the dorsal stream of language mentioned earlier. It appears that when we see a written word, the SMG helps us form an auditory image (as opposed to a visual image) of the word, which would also be important in speaking. In other words, when we see a printed word, our SMG helps form the "sound of the word." **Phonological dyslexia** is a type of central dyslexia, which is a relatively mild form of dyslexia. It usually does not affect the reading of real words. The real difficulty comes in reading/sounding out new words or nonwords (i.e., pseudowords). For example, a nonword such as *phope* might be read as *phone*. Unfamiliar or new words can often be misperceived as being other known words (Stoeckel, Gough, Watkins, & Devlin, 2009). The SMG is also involved in our ability to write single letters (Rektor, Rektorová, Mikl, Brázdil, & Krupa, 2006).

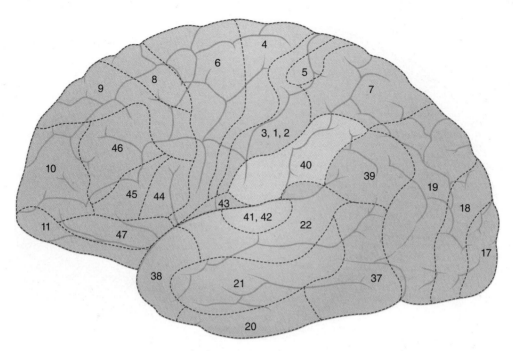

FIGURE 8-16 Brodmann area 40, the supramarginal gyrus.

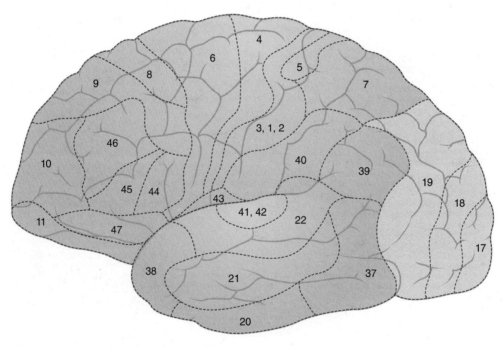

FIGURE 8-17 Brodmann areas 17, 18, and 19, the visual cortices.

Occipital Lobe: The Visual Cortex
(Brodmann Areas 17, 18, and 19)

BA 17 is the primary visual cortex, and BAs 18 and 19 make up the associative visual cortex. These three areas occupy the entire occipital lobe, the most posterior part of the brain (**FIGURE 8-17**).

The primary visual cortex (BA 17) is where visual information from the eyes is received via the optic tracts and processed. This cortex area is found in both hemispheres, with information from the left visual field traveling to the right visual cortex and information

from the right visual field going to the left visual cortex. Damage to this area from a stroke, brain injury, or other mechanism can result in **Anton syndrome** (also called cortical blindness), a rare condition in which patients have visual loss along with **visual anosognosia** (i.e., denial of visual deficits). With the lack of sight, patients with this condition often confabulate about things they are "seeing" (McDaniel & McDaniel, 1991).

Taking into consideration the associative visual cortex (BAs 18, 19) along with primary visual cortex (BA 17), it has been hypothesized that there are two streams of visual function (**FIGURE 8-18**) (Goodale &

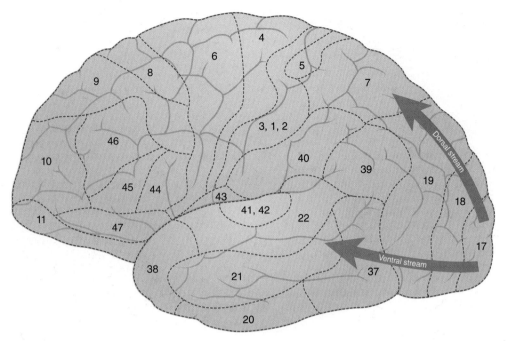

FIGURE 8-18 The two streams of vision. The dorsal stream is responsible for the *where of vision* while the ventral stream is responsible for the *what of vision*.

Milner, 1992). First, there is a dorsal stream beginning in BA 17 and extending into BAs 18, 19, 7, and perhaps 39. This dorsal stream is responsible for the *where of vision*. In other words, this stream analyzes motion and the spatial relationships between objects. Second, there is the ventral stream of vision, which also begins in BA 17 and involves BAs 18 and 19 along with BA 37. This is the *what of vision*, meaning this area analyzes forms, colors, faces, and other details, helping us identify objects and people visually.

Damage to the dorsal stream can result in **simultanagnosia**, a condition in which a patient cannot put the parts of a visual scene together into a comprehensive whole; **optic ataxia**, which is difficulty visually guiding the hand to touch an object; and **ocular apraxia**, which is difficulty voluntarily directing one's gaze to a certain object. Damage to the ventral stream can lead to **prosopagnosia** (inability to recognize familiar faces), color blindness, **micropsia** (where things look abnormally small), **macropsia** (where things look abnormally large), **palinopsia** (a reoccurring ghost image), and diplopia (double vision). It is obvious that damage to the visual cortices will significantly impair reading and writing.

Temporal Lobe

Inferior Temporal Area (Brodmann Areas 20 and 21)

The inferior temporal area takes up a majority of the inferior middle gyrus and middle temporal gyrus (**FIGURE 8-19**). It is involved in the processing of auditory information and language and may be best grouped as part of the Wernicke area (BA 22) due to this functioning. McGuire, Murray, and Shah (1993) have theorized that auditory hallucinations may be associated with dysfunction in this area. It may also play a role in reading facial emotions in conjunction with other areas (Sprengelmeyer et al., 1998).

Parahippocampal Gyrus (Brodmann Areas 27, 28, 34, 35, and 36)

The parahippocampal gyrus is located on the medial surface of the temporal lobe (**FIGURE 8-20**). There are eight components of this region:

- Piriform cortex (BA 27)
- Periamygdaloid cortex
- Presubicular cortex
- Parasubicular cortex
- Entorhinal cortex (BAs 28, 34)
- Prorhinal cortex
- Perirhinal cortex (BA 35)
- Parahippocampal cortex (BA 36)

Superior and medial to the parahippocampal cortex is the hippocampal formation (**FIGURE 8-21**). It is made up of the following three structures:

- Dentate gyrus
- Hippocampus
- Subiculum (BA 48)

The term **hippocampus** means "seahorse," and it was named this because of its compact *S* shape, like a seahorse's body. The hippocampus is a key structure

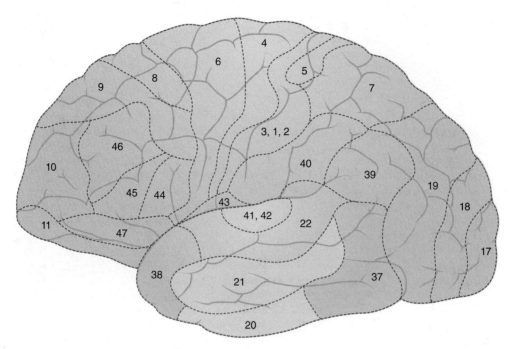

FIGURE 8-19 Brodmann areas 20 and 21, the inferior temporal area.

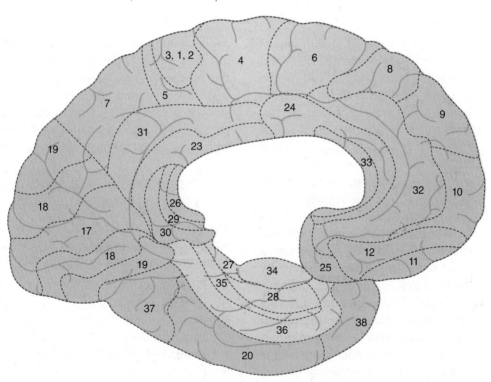

FIGURE 8-20 The parahippocampal gyrus.

for a type of long-term memory called **declarative memory**, which is our memory for facts (semantic memory) and space–time events (episodic memory) in our lives. The actual storage of memories is thought to take place not in the medial temporal lobe but in the whole of the cerebral cortex itself. The hippocampus is key to storing these memories as well as triggering their release when needed. One of the most important areas for memory in the parahippocampal cortex is the **entorhinal cortex** (BAs 28, 34), which is

a major input/output relay between the cerebral cortex and the hippocampus (Bear, Connors, & Paradiso, 2007; Blumenfeld, 2010).

Fusiform Gyrus (Brodmann Area 37)

The fusiform gyrus (FG) is also known as the occipito-temporal gyrus. It is part of the temporal and occipital lobes (**FIGURE 8-22**). This area is important for naming objects as well as recognizing and remembering

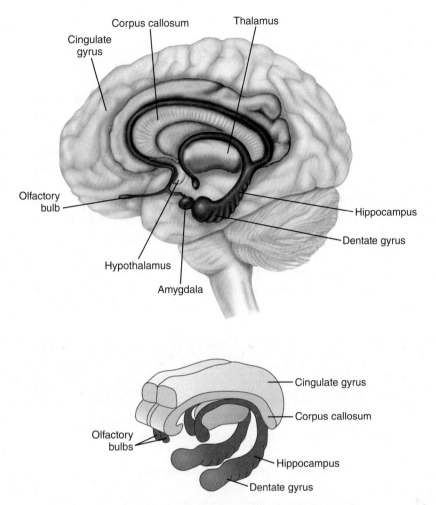

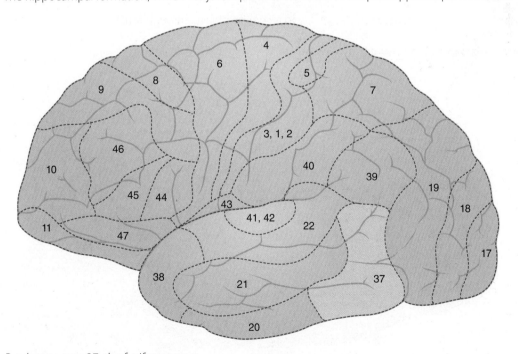

FIGURE 8-21 The hippocampal formation, which lies just superior and medial to the parahippocampal formation.

FIGURE 8-22 Brodmann area 37, the fusiform gyrus.

visual objects that have been seen (Tanaka, 1997). In other words, the FG functions as a lexicon; studies have shown that lesions can cause anomia and lexical

agraphia (Foundas, Daniels, & Vasterling, 1998; Rapcsak, Rubens, & Laguna, 1990; Raymer et al., 1997; Sakurai et al., 2000; Soma, Sugishita, Kitmura, Maruyama, &

Imanaga, 1989). Neurofibrillary tangles in the FG may be responsible for naming and object recognition problems (i.e., visual agnosia) that patients with Alzheimer disease face (Thangavel, Sahu, Van Hoesen, & Zaheer, 2008). The FG is also important for facial recognition (Blonder et al., 2004). It has the ability to draw the distinct features of a face into a specific identity. Difficulty recognizing faces is called prosopagnosia, or face blindness (TABLE 8-4). This condition can be developmental or acquired. Sacks (1999) named his book *The Man Who Mistook His Wife for a Hat* after a case of a music professor who developed prosopagnosia and could not recognize his own wife's face (and mistook it for a hat). People with this condition usually compensate by using people's distinct voices to identify them or by using a distinctive physical characteristic, like a scar or a tattoo.

The Temporal Pole (Brodmann Area 38)

The temporal pole is located on the anterior end of the temporal lobe (FIGURE 8-23). Its functions are many and complex, but only a few will be surveyed here. The left temporal pole is highly involved in language, including semantic processing, speech comprehension, and the comprehension of narratives (Collins et al., 2017; Giraud et al., 2004; Maguire, Frith, & Morris, 1999; Vandenberghe, Nobre, & Price, 2002). The right temporal pole plays a role in identifying familiar voices as well as integrating emotional content of language into narratives (Dupont, 2002; Nakamura et al. 2001). Both temporal poles appear involved in theory of mind (ToM) and empathy (Völlm et al., 2006). ToM is the ability to know you have a mind, that others have a mind, and that their perspectives are different than your own. Empathy, which is related to ToM,

TABLE 8-4 Select Types of Agnosia	
Category	**Examples**
Visual agnosia	Prosopagnosia—inability to recognize previously known faces Simultanagnosia—inability to synthesize all elements of a scene
Auditory agnosia	Pure word deafness—inability to recognize speech Auditory sound agnosia—inability to recognize environmental sounds Phonagnosia—inability to recognize familiar voices
Tactile agnosia	Astereognosis—inability to recognize objects through touch

Note: Agnosia of taste (gustatory agnosia) and of smell (olfactory agnosia) are also possible.

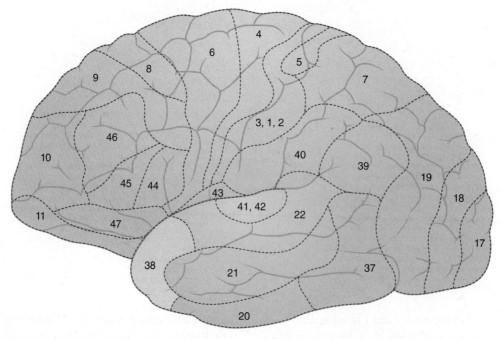

FIGURE 8-23 Brodmann area 38, the temporal pole.

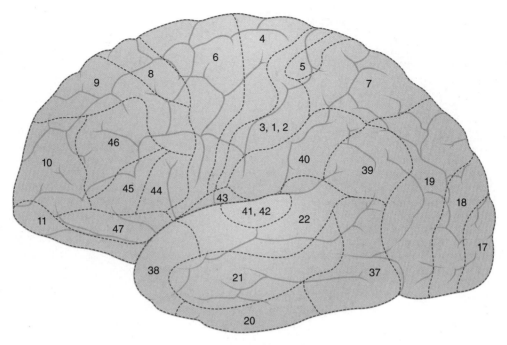

FIGURE 8-24 Brodmann areas 41 and 42, the primary and secondary auditory cortices.

describes a person's attempts to identify with another person's mental state.

Auditory Cortex (Brodmann Areas 41 and 42)

Situated on the ceiling of the superior temporal gyrus in roughly BA 41 and 42, the auditory cortex is crucial to the special sense of hearing (**FIGURE 8-24**). The auditory cortex is the initial cortical region that receives auditory information from the auditory pathway. It processes both sound intensity and frequency. In terms of frequency, this auditory cortex is tonotopically organized (**FIGURE 8-25**), meaning that neurons at one end of the cortex (the base) are sensitive to higher frequencies and neurons at the other end (the apex) are sensitive to lower frequencies.

One condition that can result from damage to the auditory cortex is **pure word deafness** (or auditory verbal agnosia), a rare type of auditory agnosia. Sufferers of pure word deafness have a pure deficit whereby they cannot understand speech; however, they do not have difficulties with speaking, reading, or writing. Patients report that they can hear the person talking but cannot understand what is being said. They do not have difficulty with nonspeech sounds, though, such as the ringing of a doorbell or the sound of a dog barking. Pure word deafness is produced by bilateral damage to the primary auditory cortex or by left hemisphere damage that destroys the connection of both auditory cortices to Wernicke's area (Papathanasiou, Coppens, & Potagas, 2013; Wolberg, Temlett, & Fritz, 1990).

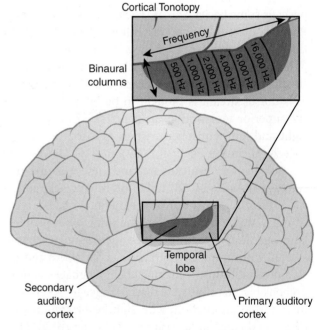

FIGURE 8-25 The tonotopic organization of Heschl's gyrus.

Wernicke's Area (Brodmann Area 22)

Named after the 19th-century German neurologist Karl Wernicke, **Wernicke's area** is traditionally thought to occupy BA 22 (**FIGURE 8-26**). It is involved in attaching meaning to auditory information, especially speech and language. In other words, it helps us understand what people say to us. Researchers using neuroimaging data suggest that the processing and understanding of speech is a much wider process that involves, in addition to Wernicke's area, Broca's area and other temporal areas, like BAs 20, 21, and 38, and

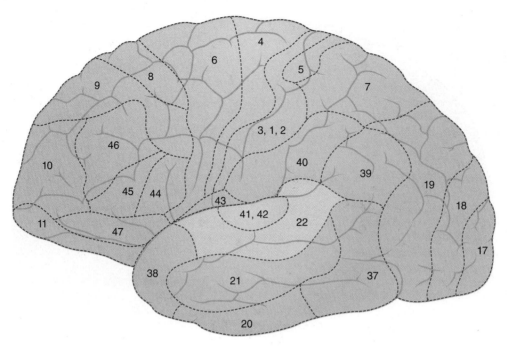

FIGURE 8-26 Brodmann area 22, Wernicke's area.

perhaps some parietal areas (Hickok & Poeppel, 2007; Poeppel, Idsardi, & Van Wassenhove, 2008). Based on this, some researchers have theorized a ventral stream of language that processes speech for comprehension. In short, this stream maps heard sound to meaning. This dorsal stream is thought to be bilateral because the superior temporal gyrus is activated in both the right and left hemispheres when exposed to human speech (Hickok & Poeppel, 2007).

Damage to Wernicke's area and these related cortical areas (BAs 20, 21, 38) can result in Wernicke aphasia, a form of fluent aphasia. Patients with this type of aphasia have trouble comprehending other people's language. They verbally produce fluent language, but it is filled with jargon and paraphasias (i.e., word and/or sound substitutions), making their language incomprehensible to others. Written language resembles their verbal production, with significant amounts of jargon and paraphasias (Halpern & Goldfarb, 2013).

Cingulate Cortex

(Brodmann Areas 23, 24, 25, 26, 29, 30, 31, 32, and 33)

The **cingulate** (Latin for "band that encircles") **cortex** is located in the medial surface of the brain between the corpus callosum and the cingulate sulcus (**FIGURE 8-27**). Above the cingulate sulcus are the frontal and parietal lobes. The cingulate cortex is a part of the limbic system, our emotional processing center. It receives inputs from the anterior thalamic nuclei and projects to the hippocampus via the parahippocampal

gyrus; thus it appears to play a role in memory. It also has many back-and-forth connections with the frontal, temporal, and occipital lobes. Overall, it is a very well-connected area of brain tissue.

Based on cell structure, Vogt (2005) divided the cingulate cortex into four areas, each with a main function:

- *Anterior cingulate cortex (ACC):* emotional and cognitive processing
- *Midcingulate cortex (MCC):* response selection
- *Posterior cingulate cortex (PCC):* personal orientation (autobiographical memory)
- *Retrosplenial cortex (RSC):* memory formation and access

Other researchers, such as Kozlovskiy, Vartanov, Nikonova, Pyasik, and Velichkovsky (2012), combine the ACC and MCC, resulting in a three-division model. There is disagreement in the literature about how to organize the cingulate cortex and what functions go where (Shackman et al., 2011). Because of this disagreement, the cingulate cortex will be discussed as a functional whole in the following discussion.

Functionally, the cingulate cortex is involved in cognitive control, which given its proximity to the prefrontal cortex is logical. For example, it appears that more anterior areas help in detecting errors when solving problems and the related function of detecting conflicts in information (e.g., uppercase vs. LOWERCASE). The cingulate is also involved in the perception of pain and the negative emotions associated with pain (e.g., fear) (Shackman et al., 2011).

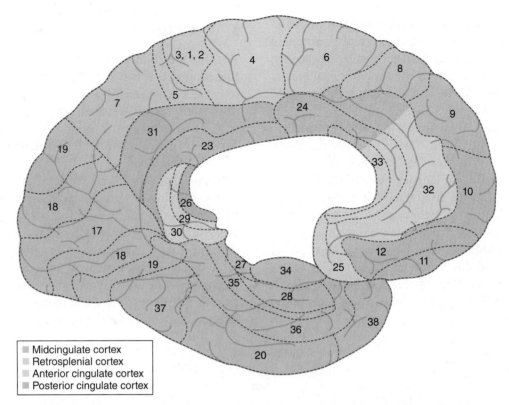

FIGURE 8-27 Brodmann areas 23, 24, 25, 26, 29, 30, 31, 32, and 33, the cingulate cortex divided into four regions.

Posterior areas appear involved in autobiographical memory, which is memory about ourselves and the events we have experienced. These areas may also play a role in managing risky behaviors. For example, if I decide to go skydiving, posterior areas might activate and convince me otherwise. Damage to the RSC has been associated with severe retrograde amnesia. Amnesia is a common word to most, meaning memory loss. Retrograde amnesia is a loss of memory before an event occurs, usually memory closer to the traumatic event. For example, many patients with traumatic brain injury after a motor vehicle accident do not remember the events leading up to the accident. The RSC also appears to be involved in emotional processing and in navigating in familiar places. The whole cingulate cortex appears involved in memory, with the ACC working to filter out irrelevant information and the PCC detecting useful information. If true, this filter and focus process would be an important component in our ability to remember things, like all the new terms in this text (Kozlovskiy et al., 2012).

Insular Cortex

Folded up and located deep within the lateral fissure is the **insular cortex** (FIGURE 8-28). It is sometimes referred to as just the *insula* (insula = "island"). Functionally, it can be divided into two parts, a posterior-dorsal portion involved in sensorimotor functions

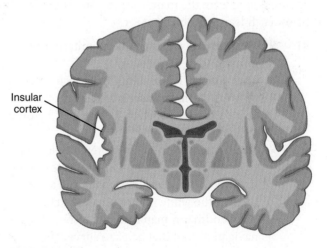

FIGURE 8-28 The insular cortex.

and an anterior part specializing in orofacial programs and emotions. The dorsal–caudal portion is highly connected to the parietal lobe's somatosensory areas (BAs 5, 7), and its function is similar to these areas' functions. The anterior part is a way station between the cerebral cortex and the main structures involved in emotions, including the hypothalamus, amygdala, and other subcortical gray areas. It also consists of motor programs for the mouth and face associated with emotion, such as ingestive behaviors (i.e., eating and drinking behaviors), negative food responses (e.g., the look of disgust), and behaviors related to vomiting (Jezzini, Caruana, Stoianov, Gallese, &

Rizzolatti, 2012). There is also evidence that this anterior area plays a role in awareness, a state important in consciousness and emotional processing. Awareness includes awareness of body movement, visual images of self, emotions, visual and auditory sensations, and time perception (Craig, 2009).

Clinical data suggest that in addition to these functions, the anterior insula has language functions. Ojemann and Whitaker (1978) concluded that the insula is an additional language area to the language centers located in the frontal lobe. It perhaps plays a role in our ability to pick the appropriate word, a process known as lexical decision making or semantic judgment. In addition, there have been cases of global aphasia reported due to lesions in the insular cortex (Shuren, 1993; Vignolo, Boccardi, & Caverni, 1986), suggesting that the insula does indeed play some important role in our language abilities.

▶ Conclusion

Korbinian Brodmann contributed his mapping of the cerebral cortex to neuroscience, and this system has been a useful tool in navigating it. Several important language areas have been highlighted (e.g., 44, 45) that cluster around the lateral or Sylvian fissure in an area of the left hemisphere known as the perisylvian region.

A word of warning is in order regarding the Brodmann mapping system, however. There is individual variation in the borders of these areas, meaning that every brain has a level of uniqueness. This mapping system is useful to researchers as a kind of shorthand to guide colleagues to general areas of the brain. For example, if one says, "Brodmann areas 44 and 45," another researcher's mind will immediately look at the inferior frontal lobe for the Broca area.

SUMMARY OF LEARNING OBJECTIVES

The following were the main learning objectives of this chapter. The information that should have been learned is below each learning objective.

1. The learner will state the main limitation of the Brodmann map.
   - The danger is thinking that each area is responsible for a certain function and that this particular function is managed by only that area.
   - The human brain is far more complex than this, with multiple areas in the cortex being involved in various functions as well as structures in the white matter under the cortex.
   - The Brodmann map is meant to be a simple navigation tool that helps to survey the cerebral cortex.
2. The learner will list the important areas in each lobe of the brain and ascribe at least one function to each area.
   - Frontal lobe areas
     - *Prefrontal cortex:* Associated with cognition, personality, decision making, and social behavior
     - *Frontal eye fields:* control of eye movements
     - *Broca area:* Involved in language processing and speech production
     - *Premotor cortex:* Involved in selecting and planning complex voluntary motor movements of the body

   - *Primary motor cortex:* Activates the motor plans from areas 44 and 6 by sending motor signals to muscles to move.
   - Parietal lobe areas
     - *Primary sensory cortex:* Perceives sensory information from the body.
     - *Somatosensory association cortex:* Plays a role in influencing the fine movements needed for fluent speech.
     - *Angular gyrus:* Associated with reading and math abilities.
     - *Supramarginal gyrus:* Involved with our phonological system, specifically in storing auditory representations of phonemes and phoneme combinations.
   - Occipital lobe
     - *Primary (BA 17) and associative visual cortex (BAs 18, 19):* visual processing
   - Temporal lobe
     - *Inferior temporal area:* Involved in the processing of auditory and language information.
     - *Parahippocampal gyrus:* a key structure for a type of long-term memory called declarative memory, which is our memory for facts (semantic memory) and

space–time events (episodic memory) in our lives.

☐ *Fusiform gyrus:* Important for naming objects as well as recognizing and remembering visual objects that have been seen.

☐ *Temporal pole:* Involved in semantic processing, speech comprehension, and the comprehension of narratives.

☐ *Auditory cortex:* Processes both sound intensity and frequency.

☐ *Wernicke area:* Involved in attaching meaning to auditory information, especially speech and language.

☐ *Cingulate cortex:* Involved in cognitive control, perception of pain and negative emotions associated with pain, autobiographical memory, and emotional processing.

☐ *Insular cortex:* Involved in sensorimotor functions and orofacial programs and emotions.

KEY TERMS

Anton syndrome

Apraxia of speech (AOS)

Astereognosis

Broca aphasia

Broca area

Brodmann map

Cingulate cortex

Declarative memory

Entorhinal cortex

Hippocampus

Insular cortex

Macropsia

Micropsia

Ocular apraxia

Optic ataxia

Palinopsia

Phineas Gage

Phonological dyslexia

Prosopagnosia

Pure word deafness

Simultanagnosia

Visual anosognosia

Wernicke area

DRAW IT TO KNOW IT

1. Sketch the left hemisphere and label all the important language and speech-related areas with their appropriate Brodmann number.

2. Recreate from memory Figure 8-8.

QUESTIONS FOR DEEPER REFLECTION

1. Given the blank diagram of the left cerebral hemisphere, locate and label all areas possible that were discussed in this chapter.

2. List the important language areas and describe what they contribute to language.

3. Discuss how the functions of the prefrontal cortex are relevant to a student.

CASE STUDY

Megan, a 32-year-old mother of two young children, reported a sudden loss in the ability to understand speech. Her motor functions were intact as well as her ability to speak, write, and read. She is able to correctly identify environmental sounds (e.g., a dog barking, a door bell ringing, etc.), but could not follow directions given to her auditorily or comprehend conversation. Megan reports that people's speech sounds like "gibberish".

1. What condition do you think Megan suffers from?

2. What brain lobe or lobes have been affected?

3. Can you identify a specific Brodmann area that is likely involved in her case?

SUGGESTED PROJECTS

1. Research the life of Phineas Gage and write a two- to three-page paper about his life and what his story contributes to our knowledge of the brain.

2. Take one of the specific Brodmann areas discussed in this chapter and perform a Google Scholar search for the most recent information about this area. What are the experts saying?

REFERENCES

Aron, A. R., Robbins, T. W., & Poldrack, R. A. (2004). Inhibition and the right inferior frontal cortex. *Trends in Cognitive Sciences, 8*(4), 170–177.

Aron, A. R., Robbins, T. W., & Poldrack, R. A. (2014). Inhibition and the right inferior frontal cortex: One decade on. *Trends in Cognitive Sciences, 18*(4), 177–185.

Bear, M. F., Connors, B. W., & Paradiso, M. A. (2007). *Neuroscience: Exploring the brain.* Baltimore, MD: Lippincott Williams & Wilkins.

Blanke, O., Ortigue, S., Landis, T., & Seeck, M. (2002). Stimulating illusory own-body perceptions. *Nature, 419*(6904), 269–270.

Blonder, L. X., Smith, C. D., Davis, C. E., Kesler, M. L., Garrity, T. F., Avison, M. J., & Andersen, A. H. (2004). Regional brain response to faces of humans and dogs. *Cognitive Brain Research, 20*(3), 384–394.

Blumenfeld, H. (2010). *Neuroanatomy through clinical cases.* Sunderland, MA: Sinauer Associates.

Chew, S. H., & Ho, J. L. (1994). Hope: An empirical study of attitude toward the timing of uncertainty resolution. *Journal of Risk and Uncertainty, 8*(3), 267–288.

Collins, J., Montal, V., Hochberg, D., Quimby, M., Mandelli, M. L., & Makris, N., . . . Dickerson, B. C. (2017). Focal temporal pole atrophy and network degeneration in semantic variant primary progressive aphasia. *Brain, 140*(2), 457–471.

Craig, A. D. (2009). How do you feel—now? The anterior insula and human awareness. *Nature Reviews Neuroscience, 10,* 59–70.

Dhanjal, N. S., Handunnetthi, L., Patel, M. C., & Wise, R. J. (2008). Perceptual systems controlling speech production. *Journal of Neuroscience, 28*(40), 9969–9975.

Diamond, N. B., & Levine, B. (2018). The prefrontal cortex and human memory. In B. L. Miller & J. L. Cummings (Eds.), *The human frontal lobes: Functions and disorders* (3rd ed., pp. 137–157). New York, NY: Guilford Press.

Domanski, C. W. (2013). Mysterious "Monsieur Leborgne": The mystery of the famous patient in the history of neuropsychology is explained. *Journal of the History of the Neurosciences, 22*(1), 47–52.

Dupont, S. (2002). Investigating temporal pole function by functional imaging. *Epileptic Disorders, 4*(1), 17–22.

Endo, K., Miyasaka, M., Makishita, H., & Yanagisawa, N. (1992). Tactile agnosia and tactile aphasia: Symptomatological and anatomical differences. *Cortex, 28*(3), 445–469.

Foundas, A. L., Daniels, S. K., & Vasterling, J. J. (1998). Anomia: Case studies with lesion localization. *Neurocase, 4*(1), 35–43.

Fuster, J. (2008). *The prefrontal cortex* (4th ed.). Waltham, MA: Academic Press.

Gazzaley, A., & D'Esposito, M. (2007). Unifying prefrontal cortex function: Executive control, neural networks, and top-down modulation. In B. L. Miller & J. L. Cummings (Eds.), *The human frontal lobes: Functions and disorders* (2nd ed., pp. 187–206). New York, NY: Guilford Press.

Giraud, A. L., Kell, C., Thierfelder, C., Sterzer, P., Russ, M. O., Preibisch, C., & Kleinschmidt, A. (2004). Contributions of sensory input, auditory search and verbal comprehension to cortical activity during speech processing. *Cerebral Cortex, 14*(3), 247–255.

González-Fernández, M., & Hillis, A. E. (2018). Language and the frontal cortex. In B. L. Miller & J. L. Cummings (Eds.), *The human frontal lobes: Functions and disorders* (3rd ed., pp. 158–170). New York, NY: Guilford Press.

Goodale, M. A., & Milner, A. D. (1992). Separate visual pathways for perception and action. *Trends in Neurosciences, 15*(1), 20–25.

Halpern, H., & Goldfarb, R. (2013). *Language and motor speech disorders in adults.* Burlington, MA: Jones & Bartlett Learning.

Halsband, U., Matsuzaka, Y., & Tanji, J. (1994). Neuronal activity in the primate supplementary, pre-supplementary and premotor cortex during externally and internally instructed sequential movements. *Neuroscience Research, 20*(2), 149–155.

Harrington, G. S., Farias, D., Davis, C. H., & Buonocore, M. H. (2007). Comparison of the neural basis for imagined writing and drawing. *Human Brain Mapping, 28*(5), 450–459.

Hartwigsen, G., Price, C. J., Baumgaertner, A., Geiss, G., Koehnke, M., Ulmer, S., & Siebner, H. R. (2010). The right posterior inferior frontal gyrus contributes to phonological word decisions in the healthy brain: Evidence from dual-site TMS. *Neuropsychologia, 48*(10), 3155–3163.

Hickok, G., & Poeppel, D. (2007). The cortical organization of speech processing. *Nature Reviews Neuroscience, 8*(5), 393–402.

Hubbard, E., & Ramachandran, V. S. (2003). The phenomenology of synaesthesia. *Journal of Consciousness Studies, 10*(8), 49–57.

Ischebeck, A., Indefrey, P., Usui, N., Nose, I., Hellwig, F., & Taira, M. (2004). Reading in a regular orthography: An fMRI study investigating the role of visual familiarity. *Journal of Cognitive Neuroscience, 16*(5), 727–741.

Jezzini, A., Caruana, F., Stoianov, I., Gallese, V., & Rizzolatti, G. (2012). Functional organization of the insula and inner perisylvian regions. *Proceedings of the National Academy of Sciences, 109*(25), 10077–10082.

Kaplan, J. T., Gimbel, S. I., & Harris, S. (2016). Neural correlates of maintaining one's political beliefs in the face of counterevidence. *Scientific Reports, 6,* 1–11.

Katanoda, K., Yoshikawa, K., & Sugishita, M. (2001). A functional MRI study on the neural substrates for writing. *Human Brain Mapping, 13*(1), 34–42.

Keeley, S. P. (2003). *The source for executive function disorders.* East Moline, IL: LinguiSystems.

Kim, E. J., Ogar, J., & Gorno-Tempini, M. L. (2018). The orbitofrontal cortex and the insula. In B. L. Miller & J. L. Cummings (Eds.), *The human frontal lobes: Functions and disorders* (3rd ed., pp. 42–54). New York, NY: Guilford Press.

Kozlovskiy, S. A., Vartanov, A. V., Nikonova, E. Y., Pyasik, M. M., & Velichkovsky, B. M. (2012). The cingulate cortex and human memory processes. *Psychology in Russia, 5*, 231–243.

Lee, D., & Quessy, S. (2003). Activity in the supplementary motor area related to learning and performance during a sequential visuomotor task. *Journal of Neurophysiology, 89*(2), 1039–1056.

Maguire, E. A., Frith, C. D., & Morris, R. G. M. (1999). The functional neuroanatomy of comprehension and memory: The importance of prior knowledge. *Brain, 122*(10), 1839–1850.

McDaniel, K. D., & McDaniel, L. D. (1991). Anton's syndrome in a patient with posttraumatic optic neuropathy and bifrontal contusions. *Archives of Neurology, 48*(1), 101.

McGuire, P. K., Murray, R. M., & Shah, G. M. S. (1993). Increased blood flow in Broca's area during auditory hallucinations in schizophrenia. *The Lancet, 342*(8873), 703–706.

Mort, D. J., Malhotra, P., Mannan, S. K., Rorden, C., Pambakian, A., Kennard, C., & Husain, M. (2003). The anatomy of visual neglect. *Brain, 126*(9), 1986–1997.

Nakamura, J., Endo, K., Sumida, T., & Hasegawa, T. (1998). Bilateral tactile agnosia: A case report. *Cortex, 34*(3), 375–388.

Nakamura, K., Kawashima, R., Sugiura, M., Kato, T., Nakamura, A., & Hatano, K., . . . Kojima, S. (2001). Neural substrates for recognition of familiar voices: A PET study. *Neuropsychologia, 39*(10), 1047–1054.

Ojemann, G. A., & Whitaker, H. A. (1978). Language localization and variability. *Brain and Language, 6*(2), 239–260.

Papathanasiou, I., Coppens, P., & Potagas, C. (2013). *Aphasia and related neurogenic communication disorders*. Burlington, MA: Jones & Bartlett Learning.

Penfield, W., & Welch, K. (1951). The supplementary motor area of the cerebral cortex: A clinical and experimental study. *Archives of Neurology and Psychiatry, 66*(3), 289.

Poeppel, D., Idsardi, W. J., & Van Wassenhove, V. (2008). Speech perception at the interface of neurobiology and linguistics. *Philosophical Transactions of the Royal Society B: Biological Sciences, 363*(1493), 1071–1086.

Premji, A., Rai, N., & Nelson, A. (2011). Area 5 influences excitability within the primary motor cortex in humans. *PLOS ONE, 6*(5), e20023. doi:10.1371/journal.pone.0020023

Price, C. J. (2012). A review and synthesis of the first 20 years of PET and fMRI studies of heard speech, spoken language and reading. *Neuroimage, 62*(2), 816–847.

Rajmohan, V., & Mohandas, E. (2007). Mirror neuron system. *Indian Journal of Psychiatry, 49*(1), 66.

Ramachandran, V. S., & Hirstein, W. (1998). The perception of phantom limbs. The DO Hebb lecture. *Brain, 121*(9), 1603–1630.

Rapcsak, S. Z., Rubens, A. B., & Laguna, J. F. (1990). From letters to words: Procedures for word recognition in letter-by-letter reading. *Brain and Language, 38*, 504–514.

Raymer, A. M., Foundas, A. L., Maher, L. M., Greenwald, M. L., Morris, M., Rothi, L. J. G., & Heilman, K. M. (1997). Cognitive neuropsychological analysis and neuroanatomic correlates in a case of acute anomia. *Brain and Language, 58*(1), 137–156.

Rektor, I., Rektorová, I., Mikl, M., Brázdil, M., & Krupa, P. (2006). An event-related fMRI study of self-paced alphabetically ordered writing of single letters. *Experimental Brain Research, 173*(1), 79–85.

Rizzolatti, G., & Craighero, L. (2004). The mirror-neuron system. *Annual Review of Neuroscience, 27*, 169–192.

Sacks, O. (1999). *The man who mistook his wife for a hat*. New York, NY: HarperCollins.

Sakurai, Y., Takeuchi, S., Takada, T., Horiuchi, E., Nakase, H., & Sakuta, M. (2000). Alexia caused by a fusiform or posterior inferior temporal lesion. *Journal of the Neurological Sciences, 178*(1), 42–51.

Schlag, J., & Schlag-Rey, M. (1987). Evidence for a supplementary eye field. *Journal of Neurophysiology, 57*(1), 179–200.

Schoenbaum, G., Takahashi, Y., Liu, T. L., & McDannald, M. A. (2011). Does the orbitofrontal cortex signal value? *Annals of the New York Academy of Sciences, 1239*(1), 87–99.

Serrien, D. J., Strens, L. H., Oliviero, A., & Brown, P. (2002). Repetitive transcranial magnetic stimulation of the supplementary motor area (SMA) degrades bimanual movement control in humans. *Neuroscience Letters, 328*(2), 89–92.

Shackman, A. J., Salomons, T. V., Slagter, H. A., Fox, A. S., Winter, J. J., & Davidson, R. J. (2011). The integration of negative affect, pain and cognitive control in the cingulate cortex. *Nature Reviews Neuroscience, 12*(3), 154–167.

Shuren, J. (1993). Insula and aphasia. *Journal of Neurology, 240*(4), 216–218.

Soma, Y., Sugishita, M., Kitmura, K., Maruyama, S., & Imanaga, H. (1989). Lexical agraphia in the Japanese language: Pure agraphia for Kanji due to left posteroinferior temporal lesions. *Brain, 112*(6), 1549–1561.

Sprengelmeyer, R., Rausch, M., Eysel, U. T., Przuntek, H., Sprengelmeyer, R., & Rausch, M., . . . Przuntek, H. (1998). Neural structures associated with recognition of facial expressions of basic emotions. *Proceedings of the Royal Society of London. Series B: Biological Sciences, 265*(1409), 1927–1931.

Stoeckel, C., Gough, P. M., Watkins, K. E., & Devlin, J. T. (2009). Supramarginal gyrus involvement in visual word recognition. *Cortex, 45*(9), 1091.

Tanaka, K. (1997). Mechanisms of visual object recognition: Monkey and human studies. *Current Opinion in Neurobiology, 7*(4), 523–529.

Thangavel, R., Sahu, S. K., Van Hoesen, G. W., & Zaheer, A. (2008). Modular and laminar pathology of Brodmann's area 37 in Alzheimer's disease. *Neuroscience, 152*(1), 5055.

Vallar, G. (2007). Spatial neglect, Balint-Homes' and Gerstmann's syndrome, and other spatial disorders. *CNS Spectrums, 12*(7), 527.

Vandenberghe, R., Nobre, A. C., & Price, C. J. (2002). The response of left temporal cortex to sentences. *Journal of Cognitive Neuroscience, 14*(4), 550–560.

Vignolo, L. A., Boccardi, E., & Caverni, L. (1986). Unexpected CT-scan findings in global aphasia. *Cortex, 22*(1), 55–69.

Vogt, B. A. (2005). Pain and emotion interactions in subregions of the cingulate gyrus. *Nature Reviews Neuroscience, 6*(7), 533–544.

Völlm, B. A., Taylor, A. N., Richardson, P., Corcoran, R., Stirling, J., & McKie, S., . . . Elliott, R. (2006). Neuronal correlates of theory of mind and empathy: A functional magnetic resonance imaging study in a nonverbal task. *Neuroimage, 29*(1), 90–98.

Volz, K. G., Schubotz, R. I., & von Cramon, D. (2005). Variants of uncertainty in decision-making and their neural correlates. *Brain Research Bulletin, 67*(5), 403–412.

Wildgruber, D., Ackermann, H., Kreifelts, B., & Ethofer, T. (2006). Cerebral processing of linguistic and emotional prosody: fMRI studies. *Progress in Brain Research, 156*, 249–268.

Wolberg, S. C., Temlett, J. A., & Fritz, V. U. (1990). Pure word deafness. *South African Medical Journal, 78*, 668–670.

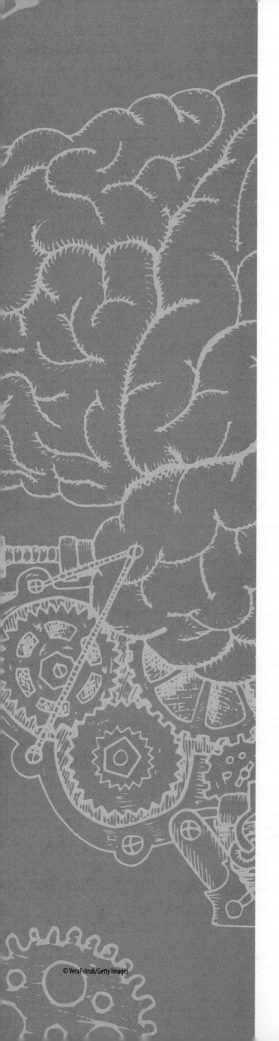

PART III

Neuroanatomy Applied to Communication and Communication Disorders

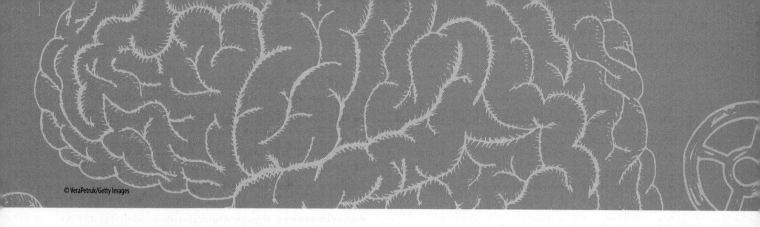

© VeraPetruk/Getty Images

CHAPTER 9

Consciousness and Disorders of Consciousness

CHAPTER PREVIEW

In this chapter we turn our attention to a specific neurological function: consciousness. This is an important topic in light of speech and language being conscious processes.

IN THIS CHAPTER

In this chapter, we will . . .
- Define the term *consciousness*
- Explore the neural basis of consciousness
- Describe how consciousness is assessed in a medical setting
- Describe different disorders of consciousness
- Explore the speech-language pathologist's role when helping patients with disorders of consciousness

LEARNING OBJECTIVES

1. The learner will define *consciousness, core consciousness*, and *extended consciousness*.
2. The learner will list and describe the primary neurological structures thought to be involved in consciousness.
3. The learner will list and briefly describe at least five specific disorders of consciousness.
4. The learner will list and describe the various mind–brain theories.
5. The learner will articulate the two main views of personhood.

▶ Introduction

Speech-language pathologists (SLPs) typically describe speech as being a *conscious voluntary motor activity*. To understand speech in this way, it is important to understand each of these terms. In this chapter, we will begin with the term *consciousness* and then consider different disorders of consciousness.

▶ What Is Consciousness?

The cognitive neuroscientist Daniel Dennett has called consciousness the last surviving mystery of our world (Dennett, 1992). What is consciousness? Neuroscientists think of **consciousness** as "the ability to be aware of self and surroundings" (Damasio & Meyer, 2009, pp. 4–5). This would mean that, as humans, we have internal, first-person, subjective, mental experiences that only we can be aware of and know. Examples of these experiences include our awareness and sense of ourselves, as well as our sensory, memory (creating and recalling), and decision-making experiences. Other people do not have access to these experiences (i.e., they are private to us), but others do have external, third-person, objective, and behavioral experiences of us. Examples include others seeing that we are awake, viewing emotional leakage (e.g., crying), watching us attending to an object or person (e.g., playing on our cell phone), and observing our behaviors (e.g., walking and talking) (Damasio & Meyer, 2009). Though others do not have access to our internal, first-person experiences, we can let others into these experiences through honest and transparent communication. This is what psychologists specialize in—accessing our first-person, private experiences in order to help us understand these experiences better, identifying unhealthy mental experiences (e.g., suicidal thoughts), and shaping these into healthier experiences.

There are two basic varieties of consciousness: core consciousness and extended consciousness. **Core consciousness** is the simpler of the two and involves our sense of ourselves in the here and now (i.e., at this very moment), objects in the world, and our relationship to those objects. For example, right now I have a sense of myself sitting at the computer typing on a keyboard. This is considered the "core self," and it is dependent on being awake (i.e., wakefulness). **Extended consciousness** is more complex and involves our sense of self in the flow of time. We think of ourselves in the past and anticipate ourselves living in a future. This form of consciousness is known as the "autobiographical self," and it depends on longer-term memory, whereas core consciousness does not. Extended consciousness obviously depends on intact core consciousness.

Philosophers use slightly different terms and speak of creature consciousness versus mental-state consciousness. **Creature consciousness** refers to the consciousness of whole organisms, whereas **mental-state consciousness** means consciousness as it relates to particular mental states and processes. Features of creature consciousness might include sentience (i.e., sensing the world around you), wakefulness, self-consciousness (i.e., being aware that you are aware), subjective experience (i.e., what is it like to be me?), and transitive consciousness (i.e., being conscious of various things) (Van Gulick, 2011). Mental-state consciousness would involve having a desire for something, like cake, and being able to step above the desire and reflect, "I am having a desire for cake right now." Creature consciousness combines wakefulness and core consciousness, and mental-state consciousness is akin to extended consciousness. For our purposes, we will focus on the terms *wakefulness*, *core consciousness*, and *extended consciousness* and ask, when is an organism considered conscious?

▶ The Neurology of Consciousness

Neural Mechanisms of Wakefulness

Perhaps a place to begin discussing the neurology of consciousness is with the question: What neural structures are involved in being awake and aware? Within the center of the brainstem's midbrain lies the **reticular** ("like a web") **formation** (FIGURE 9-1). The reticular formation is a series of nuclei, each of which serves specific function(s). These nuclei can be divided into four groups. First are classical reticular nuclei that contain glutaminergic (glutamate) projections. Second are monoaminergic nuclei specializing in adrenaline, serotonin, and dopamine. Third are cholinergic (acetylcholine) nuclei. Lastly, the reticular formation contains what are called autonomic nuclei that innervate the viscera (Damasio & Meyer, 2009; Parvizi & Damasio, 2001). Two of these nuclei, the classical reticular nuclei and the cholinergic nuclei, appear important in wakefulness. Glutaminergic projections from the classical reticular nuclei travel to the intralaminar nuclei of the thalamus, which the thalamus then projects to much of the cerebral cortex. Glutamate is excitatory, so it helps to stimulate cortical wakefulness. At the

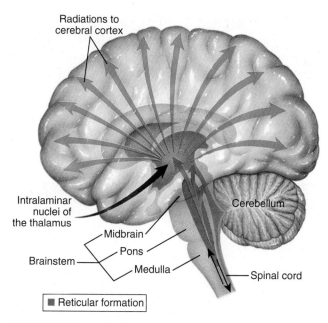

Radiations to
cerebral cortex

Intralaminar
nuclei of
the thalamus

Cerebellum

Brainstem

Midbrain

Pons

Medulla

Spinal cord

■ Reticular formation

FIGURE 9-1 The reticular activating system.

same time, cholinergic projections to the reticular thalamic nuclei hinder sleep.

Overall, the more anterior parts of the reticular formation modulate cerebral arousal and activity by controlling the responsiveness of cortical neurons, while the more posterior parts are involved in premotor functions, such as reflexes like sneezing and hiccupping (Purves et al., 2004). Damage to the reticular formation can lead to coma and other disorders of consciousness, which strongly suggests that it plays a role in consciousness through what is called the ascending **reticular activating system**. Putting the pieces together from the previous paragraph, this system begins in the midbrain's reticular formation and radiates out to the cerebral cortex through the thalamus, specifically through the intralaminar nuclei of the thalamus, in order to activate and coordinate the cerebral cortex for conscious experience. In reality, this system is still not well understood, being much more complicated than outlined here, probably involving other nuclei and nonthalamic pathways (Parvizi & Damasio, 2001). One can conclude that, though not well understood, the reticular formation does play an important role in consciousness (Blumenfeld, 2009). Massimini, Ferrarelli, Huber, Esser, Singh, and Tononi (2005) suggested that cortical connectivity is also crucial to consciousness. They examined the interconnectivity of cortical function in patients in deep sleep, a non–rapid eye movement sleep state in which a person is unconscious, and found that cortical interconnectivity is severely limited during deep sleep as compared to wakefulness.

Neural Mechanisms of Core Consciousness and Extended Consciousness

Damasio (1999) suggested that large portions of the cingulate cortex and its projections to almost all cortical regions are the crucial neural mechanism behind core consciousness's generation of our sense of self. Extended consciousness depends on those neural mechanisms responsible for working memory and explicit memory (e.g., semantic and episodic memory) (Damasio & Meyer, 2009). These mechanisms would include *at least* the prefrontal cortex, the anterior cingulate cortex, the parahippocampal region, and the hippocampal formation.

▶ Assessing Consciousness

As we have already discussed, there is a subjective, internal, first-person, mental perspective in being conscious and also an objective, external, third-person, behavioral perspective when it comes to consciousness. Professionals in communication sciences and disorders do not have access to other people's first-person perspectives other than through their reporting, but we can take the third-person perspective and observe behaviors in our patients that would lead us to determine whether they are conscious or not. The challenge was to develop a standard measure that would help in establishing a consciousness baseline. This tool would allow patient-to-patient comparison in addition to tracking progress in brain-injured patients.

The Glasgow Coma Scale

In 1974, neurosurgeons Teasdale and Jennett developed the **Glasgow Coma Scale (GCS)**, which is a 15-point scale that attempts to measure a patient's level of consciousness. It was developed to provide clear communication regarding a patient between hospitals and to track a patient's status upon admission with his or her ultimate outcome. The GCS was intended to supplement, rather than replace, other neurological assessments. The scale measures patient behavioral responses in three areas: eyes, motor, and verbal (**TABLE 9-1**).

This scale is administered by emergency medical services professionals in the field and by doctors and nurses in hospitals. The highest score a patient can receive is a 15, and the lowest score is a 3. A score more than 13 indicates possible minor brain injury; a score of 9 through 12 indicates moderate brain injury.

TABLE 9-1 The Glasgow Coma Scale

Eye Opening [E]

Spontaneous (open before a stimulus is given)	E4
To sound (open after spoken or shouted request)	E3
To pressure (open after squeezing fingertip stimulus)	E2
None (no opening at any time; no interfering factor [IF]*)	E1
Not testable (cannot test due to IF)	NT

Verbal Response [V]

Oriented (correctly gives name, place, and date)	V5
Confused (not oriented but communication coherent)	V4
Words (intelligible single words)	V3
Sounds (only moans or grunts)	V2
None (no audible response; no IF)	V1
Not testable (cannot test due to IF)	NT

Motor Response [M]

Obeys commands (obeys two-step commands)	M6
Localizing (brings hand above clavicle to stimulus)	M5
Normal flexion (bends arm at elbow rapidly, normal)	M4
Abnormal flexion (bends arm at elbow abnormally)	M3
Extension (extends arms at elbow)	M2
None (no movement in arms; no IF)	M1
Not testable (cannot test due to IF)	NT

*Interfering factors (IF) include drugs, cranial nerve injuries, intoxication, hearing impairment, intubation, tracheostomy, limb or spinal cord injuries, aphasia, dementia, psychiatric conditions, ocular trauma, orbital swelling, and language and culture differences.
Data from: Teasdale, G. (2014). *The Glasgow Coma Scale aid*. Retrieved from http://www.glasgowcomascale.org/download-aid/

Scores of 3 to 8 indicate severe head injury accompanied by significant changes in consciousness (e.g., a score of 3 indicates a deep coma or brain death). The majority of patients fall within the mild brain injury category (TABLE 9-2).

Although SLPs and audiologists do not administer this scale, they do consider GCS scores in their assessments of patients. A trauma center that treats people with traumatic brain injury might have the SLP assess every patient who has sustained a traumatic blow to the head. In the course of this assessment, the SLP might look at a patient's GCS score in the field and then upon admission to the hospital. The GCS might be a part of the screening where patients with a score of 14 or 15 pass, but all patients scoring below 13 fail and are followed for a time by the SLP. Of course, there are other factors to be considered before passing or failing a patient during a screening, but the GCS may play an important role.

TABLE 9-2 The Predictive Value of the Glasgow Coma Scale (Based on 34,977 Patients From 2003 to 2013)

GCS Score	Brain Injury Severity	% of Patients (% who died)
13–15	Mild brain injury	71% (8%)
9–12	Moderate brain injury	12% (20%)
3–8	Severe brain injury	22% (46%)

Data from: Teasdale, G., Maas, A., Lecky, F., Manley, G., Stocchetti, N., & Murray, G. (2014). The Glasgow Coma Scale at 40 years: Standing the test of time. *The Lancet Neurology, 13*(8), 844–854.

TABLE 9-3 Relationship of the Glasgow Coma Scale to Other Brain Injury Indicators

Brain Injury Level	GCS Score	Loss of Consciousness	Alteration of Consciousness	Post-traumatic Amnesia	Structural Brain Injury
Mild	13–15	0–30 minutes	<24 hours	<24 hours	Normal
Moderate	9–12	30 minutes to 24 hours	>24 hours	24 hours to 7 days	Abnormal
Severe	3–8	>24 hours	>24 hours	>7 days	Abnormal

Data from: Kimbarow, M.L. (2016). *Cognitive-communicative disorders* (2nd ed.). San Diego, CA: Plural Publishing.; Teasdale, G., Maas, A., Lecky, F., Manley, G., Stocchetti, N., & Murray, G. (2014). The Glasgow Coma Scale at 40 years: Standing the test of time. *The Lancet Neurology, 13*(8), 844–854.

Another situation could be if an SLP were asked to do a bedside swallowing evaluation on a patient and, upon evaluation, finds the patient has a GCS score less than 9 and an altered state of consciousness. Such a patient would most likely not be a good candidate for a swallowing examination, especially one that involves other personnel like for a videofluoroscopic exam.

In addition to the GCS, there are other predictors of brain injury and the resulting disorders of consciousness. Some of these include loss of consciousness, alterations in consciousness, post-traumatic amnesia, and the presence or absences of structural brain injury (**TABLE 9-3**). Imaging technology is used to assess structural brain injury. Electroencephalography (EEG), positron emission tomography (PET), and functional magnetic resonance imaging (fMRI) can all be used to assess brain function in patients suffering from disorders of consciousness. Special attention in this section will be paid to those structures known to play a role in consciousness, such as the midbrain and its reticular formation.

The Rancho Levels of Cognitive Functioning

In terms of tracking a person's emergence from coma, the **Rancho Levels of Cognitive Functioning (RLCF)** scale is a helpful tool to describe the process of recovery by tracking the behaviors the patient is and is not evidencing. There are eight cognitive levels, the lowest being one and the highest being eight (**TABLE 9-4**).

Cognitive Level I—No Response

At this level of the RLCF scale, patients are comatose. They are unresponsive to visual, auditory, and tactile stimuli. They also do not respond when their own limbs are moved (e.g., when the physical therapist does passive range-of-motion exercises).

Cognitive Level II—Generalized Response

This level describes beginning emergence from coma, when patients begin to respond to stimuli, but responses are slow, delayed, and often inconsistent. Their responses are also very general and not specific to the stimuli. For example, if a physical therapist begins to move the arm, the patient might start chewing, a response hardly connected with the stimulus. Patients at this level do not respond to verbal commands.

Cognitive Level III—Localized Response

When responses to stimuli become more specific, patients have entered the third level of the RLCF scale. These patients will not have a normal sleep–wake cycle but rather will sleep on and off throughout the day. When awake, their reactions to stimuli are more appropriate. For example, if their loved one talks to them, they might turn their head toward the side where the loved one is standing. Patients also begin to recognize their loved ones and will inconsistently follow simple commands, like "squeeze my hand." Verbal responses will begin to emerge, usually limited to saying "yes" and "no" in response to yes/no questions, though these responses may not be very accurate.

Cognitive Level IV—Confused, Agitated

This level is probably the most disconcerting level for family members to watch. Patients are disoriented and fearful and do not understand that people are trying to help them. They are highly focused on basic needs, like eating or going to the bathroom. They will overreact to stimuli, sometimes by thrashing around and hitting or through verbal abuse. Again, this is a very troubling stage for loved ones to experience, but it is important to counsel them that it actually marks progress in coma emergence.

TABLE 9-4 The Rancho Levels of Cognitive Functioning

Rancho Level	Level Title	Description
Cognitive Level I	No response	Unresponsive to visual, auditory, and tactile stimuli
Cognitive Level II	Generalized response	General responses not specific to the stimuli
Cognitive Level III	Localized response	Responses more specific to the stimuli
Cognitive Level IV	Confused, agitated	Disoriented, fearful, and easily agitated
Cognitive Level V	Confused, inappropriate, nonagitated	Disoriented with poor memory skills, but not agitated; confabulates
Cognitive Level VI	Confused, appropriate	Some level of disorientation; completes some activities of daily living with assistance; impulsive; cannot predict potential results of an action
Cognitive Level VII	Automatic, appropriate	Oriented; behaves appropriately in familiar settings; judgment impaired (e.g., unrealistic about the future)
Cognitive Level VIII	Purposeful, appropriate	Oriented; appropriate in social situations; has insight into impairments; abstract reasoning and judgment may still be impaired in new, unfamiliar situations

Data from Hagen, C., Malkmus, D., & Durham, P. (1979). *Levels of cognitive functioning, rehabilitation of the head injured adult: Comprehensive physical management.* Downey, CA: Professional Staff Association of Rancho Los Amigos National Rehabilitation Center.

Cognitive Level V—Confused, Inappropriate, Nonagitated

The second half of the scale is typically much more encouraging to family members because they begin to see the person they have known before the injury. At the fifth level, patients are still disoriented, but they are no longer agitated. They easily become overstimulated and require frequent rest breaks in therapy. These patients have poor memory skills and will sometimes confabulate to fill in their memory gaps, which is obviously inappropriate in normal daily life. They begin to complete tasks of daily living, like brushing their teeth, but often need step-by-step help to do so.

Cognitive Level VI—Confused, Appropriate

The next level describes patients who are still disoriented, but less so than at the previous levels. They will typically know the year and month but might be confused as to the day of the week or time. Patients will know they are in a hospital because of a brain injury, but their focus is more on physical problems than on issues in communication and cognition.

Memory issues will make it difficult to remember details from conversations or reading materials. They can complete activities of daily living with minimal assistance, but they remain impulsive, often acting without thinking about the consequences of actions.

Cognitive Level VII—Automatic, Appropriate

Patients at this level of the RLCF scale can follow a schedule and complete activities of daily living independently but have difficulty creating, completing, and assessing goals. They may also be unrealistic about future plans and activities, given their deficits. Cognitive processing speed is still slow, and stressful or unfamiliar situations may be frustrating.

Cognitive Level VIII—Purposeful, Appropriate

The final level involves patients who not only realize they have cognitive issues but also are beginning to compensate for those difficulties. For example, they may begin to use writing notes as a way to compensate for memory loss. At this point, they might be ready to take a driving examination or vocational evaluation. These patients' thinking will still be slower than normal, and they may need guidance in making decisions, especially in new situations. Level VIII patients are not normal. They still have cognitive deficits, but their thinking has improved to such a degree that new friends and acquaintances may not notice their cognitive deficits.

▶ Disorders of Consciousness

An Overview of Disorders of Consciousness

Patients who suffer brain injury and end up in a comatose state will either die or emerge from that state into another state within about 3 weeks postinjury.

Unlike Hollywood movies in which characters wake up from a coma like someone waking up from a nap, emergence from coma is a slow and difficult process, as described by the RLCF scale. Patients will transition from a comatose state into one of four states: chronic coma (rare), persistent vegetative state, minimally conscious state, or locked-in syndrome (**FIGURE 9-2**) (Blumenfeld, 2009).

Each of these conditions can be compared and contrasted through considering how responsive patients are to stimuli (e.g., "open your eyes"), whether brainstem reflexes are present (e.g., pupillary light reflex), whether there is some assemblage of a sleep–wake cycle, and the quality of the patient's EEG patterns (**TABLE 9-5**). A patient is considered to have experienced **brain death** when there are

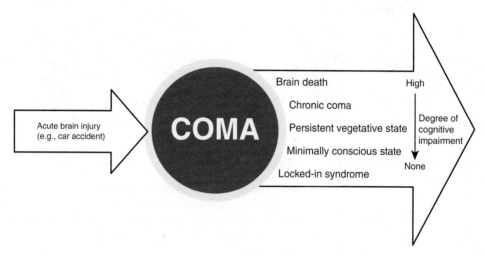

FIGURE 9-2 Disorders of consciousness.

Modified from Naci, L., Monti, M. M., Cruse, D., Kübler, A., Sorger, B., & Goebel, R., . . . Owen, A. M. (2012). Brain–computer interfaces for communication with nonresponsive patients. *Annals of Neurology, 72,* 312–323.

TABLE 9-5 Comparison of Different Disorders of Consciousness to Sleep

	Purposeful Response to Stimuli	Brainstem Reflexes	Sleep–Wake Cycle	EEG Patterns
Brain death	No	No	No	Flat
Coma	No	Yes	No	Severely depressed
PVS	No	Yes	Yes	Severely depressed
MCS	Yes, at times	Yes	Yes	Variable
LIS	Yes (eyes)	Yes	Yes	Normal
Sleep	Yes, at times	Yes	Yes	Normal sleep patterns

Abbreviations: EEG, electroencephalographic; LIS, locked-in syndrome; MCS, minimally conscious state; PVS, persistent vegetative state.
Data from: Blumenfeld, H. (2009). *Neuroanatomy through clinical cases.* Sunderland, MA: Sinauer Associates.

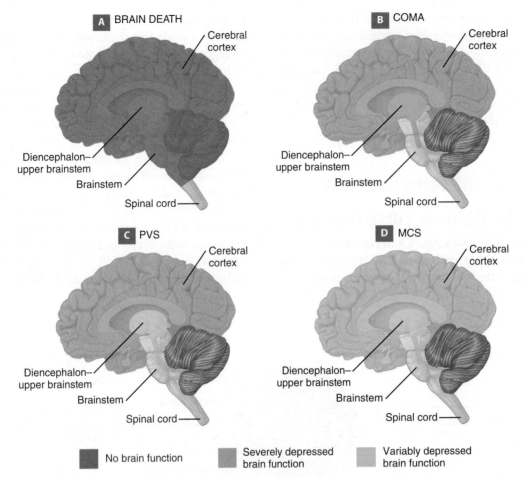

FIGURE 9-3 Levels of brain function in different disorders of consciousness. **A.** Brain death results in no brain function in the cortex, subcortex, or brainstem. **B.** Coma results in severely depressed function in the cortex, subcortex, and reticular activating system of the brainstem. **C.** Persistent vegetative state results in severely depressed cortical function, but variably depressed function in the subcortex and reticular activating system. **D.** Minimally conscious state results in variably depressed function in the cortex, subcortex, and reticular activating system.

no purposeful responses to stimuli, no brainstem reflexes, no sleep–wake cycle, and there are flat EEG patterns. Patients in a **coma** do not respond purposefully to stimuli but demonstrate brainstem reflexes (e.g., pupil constricts with introduction of a light source). Comatose patients do not have a sleep–wake cycle and demonstrate EEG patterns, though they are severely depressed. **Persistent vegetative state (PVS)** patients resemble comatose patients with one difference—they demonstrate a sleep–wake cycle. **Minimally conscious state (MCS)** patients can be thought of as being somewhere between PVS and fully conscious in that they transition between these two states. They at times respond purposefully to stimuli, but inconsistently. They also demonstrate brainstem reflexes and a sleep–wake cycle. Like their inconsistent responses to stimuli, their EEG patterns are variable depending on what state (PVS versus conscious) they are tending toward. Patients with locked-in syndrome (LIS) may be the most tragic

in that they are fully aware, conscious people locked inside bodies that do not work (Blumenfeld, 2009).

In addition to Table 9-5, **FIGURE 9-3** compares brain death, coma, PVS, and MCS in terms of overall brain function. Brain death results in absent function in the cerebral cortex, diencephalon, brainstem, or cerebellum. Coma results in severely depressed function in the cerebral cortex, diencephalon, and reticular formation. PVS results in severely depressed function in the cerebral cortex, but variable function in the diencephalon and the reticular formation. MCS involves variable depressed function in the cerebral cortex, diencephalon, and reticular formation.

Earlier, three aspects of consciousness were introduced: wakefulness, core consciousness, and extended consciousness. Using this grid, one can organize the various disorders of consciousness just surveyed. Conditions characterized by impaired wakefulness and core consciousness include general anesthesia, coma, and slow-wave sleep (or deep sleep). Conditions in which there is persistent wakefulness, but impaired core consciousness, include PVS, akinetic mutism, and some forms of epilepsy. Finally, patients with persistent wakefulness and core consciousness, but impaired extended consciousness, would be those with global amnesia and Alzheimer disease (Damasio & Meyer, 2009).

Specific Disorders of Consciousness

Now that an overview of some disorders of consciousness has been completed, it is time to survey these conditions more comprehensively. In addition to coma, brain death, PVS, MCS, and LIS, we will look at other conditions in which consciousness may be an issue, including dementia, aphasia, and epilepsy. In addition, two strange experiences (out of body and near death) will be touched on, because these also have implications for consciousness. Because some patients may report these odd experiences, it is good for SLPs and audiologists to be aware of them so they are not surprised and can help patients process these experiences.

Coma

Coma is a state in which a person is unarousable and does not make meaningful responses to stimuli in the environment. The person does not have any of the following: wakefulness, core consciousness, or extended consciousness. The GCS score would be a E2-V4-M2 or less (Pryse-Phillips, 2009). Neurologically, coma is due to either a damaged reticular activating system or global depression of cortical activity or both. Conditions that can produce this type of neurological damage include stroke, tumors, metabolic and nutritional disorders, toxins, central nervous system infections, seizures, trauma, and temperature-related conditions (hyperthermia or hypothermia). LIS mimics coma to the untrained eye, but patients with it are wakeful and have both core and extended consciousness. LIS looks like coma because people with it cannot interact with their environment due to full-body paralysis (Young, 2009).

Diagnosis of coma begins with an in-depth history taken from the family as well as a thorough neurological exam, including blood work, neuroimaging, lumbar puncture, and EEG. Comatose patients display brain wave patterns on EEG, but they are depressed. Supportive care in the form of ventilation and nutrition/hydration are key in keeping patients relatively healthy while in a coma. With 3 days of initial observation, a patient's outcome can be predicted. Poor outcomes are associated in part with absent ocular reflexes. For example, an absent pupillary light reflex and absent corneal reflex are associated with a poor outcome.

The pupillary light reflex is assessed by flashing light into the eyes and looking for constriction of the pupils. The corneal reflex is tested by lightly touching the cornea with a wisp of cotton, which produces a defensive blinking response. In addition to these ocular reflexes, an absent response to noxious stimuli and suppressed EEG patterns are consistent with poor outcomes (Bass & Gettleman, 2009). Comatose patients will typically emerge from their coma within 3 weeks or transition into one of the other disorders mentioned in this chapter (i.e., brain death, MCS, or PVS) (Young, 2009).

Brain Death

Brain death (also known as *cerebral death*) is the *irreversible* cessation of clinical function of the brain, involving the cerebral cortex and the brainstem (Pryse-Phillips, 2009). The clinical functions intended in this definition include respiration, circulation, and neuroendocrine control, as well as awareness. Not every neuron needs to be dead, but these major, life-sustaining systems have ceased functioning and the person is dead (Bernat, 2009). Like coma, wakefulness is absent, as are core and extended consciousness. Unlike coma, brain waves are flat on EEG, meaning there is no cortical or subcortical activity. GCS scores are E1-V1-M1. The criteria for the clinical determination of brain death are presented in **TABLE 9-6**, as is the process of declaring someone brain dead.

Persistent Vegetative State

PVS is defined as wakeful unawareness. Though wakefulness is present, there is no core or extended consciousness. The eyes may be open and even appear to briefly track, but there are no higher cortical functions like cognition or language. GCS score would be approximately E4-V4-M1. The diagnostic criteria for PVS are as follows (Pryse-Phillips, 2009):

- There is no evidence of awareness of self or surroundings.
- Reflexive or spontaneous eye opening may be present.
- There is no comprehensible speech or mouthing of words.
- There may be smiling, frowning, and even crying, but unconnected to a stimulus.
- Sleep–wake cycle is present.
- Brainstem and spinal cord reflexes are variable.
- There is no purposeful motor activity, though patient may withdraw from unpleasant stimuli.
- Cardiorespiratory functions are usually intact, but the patient is incontinent.

PVS is often challenging to diagnose. First, how long does a person need to demonstrate PVS symptoms before PVS is officially declared? One month? One year? Second, PVS is often confused with MCS or LIS because patients are noncommunicative in all three conditions. For example, a Belgian man was misdiagnosed as being in a PVS for 23 years. After neuroimaging was completed two decades after his injury, doctors found him to be fully aware and conscious (Hall, 2009). Monti et al. (2010) report that one in five patients diagnosed as in a PVS may actually be fully aware, like this Belgian man. Others may actually be in an MCS.

Minimally Conscious State

Patients with MCS have severely altered consciousness but do demonstrate minimal behavioral evidence that they are aware of self and their environment. In other words, they have periods of not only wakefulness but also core consciousness. The extent of their extended consciousness is unknown. Their GCS score would be about a E4-V6-M2 or E4-V6-M3. Patients have been said to emerge from MCS when they regain the ability to communicate functionally with others.

The patient in an MCS must show at least one of the following actions (Pryse-Phillips, 2009):

- Follow simple commands, though they may be inconsistent.
- Respond with gestures or yes/no answers, though they may be inaccurate.
- Speak intelligibly at times.
- Demonstrate purposeful behavior (e.g., crying) that is congruent with environmental stimuli.
- Perform sustained eye tracking of environmental stimuli (e.g., loved one's face).

MCS is an important diagnostic category because it distinguishes these patients from those with PVS or coma. **TABLE 9-7** summarizes some of the key differences among MCS, PVS, and coma.

TABLE 9-6 The Clinical Determination of Brain Death

Preconditions	Examination Elements	Process
■ Diffuse brain damage with coma and apnea ■ Structural brain lesion ■ No reversible metabolic or toxic conditions ■ Physicians treating have appropriate training	■ Coma with no responsiveness ■ Absent brainstem reflexes (e.g., pupillary light reflex) ■ Breathing suspension (apnea) in presence of elevated carbon dioxide levels (hypercapnea)	■ Findings confirmed by two separate exams ■ Second exam omitted if confirmatory test (e.g., EEG) performed ■ Patient declared dead after second exam or confirmatory test ■ Family offered opportunity for organ donation ■ Medical record reflects test results and declaration of death

Data from: Bernat, J. L. (2009). Brain death. In S. Laureys & G. Tononi (Eds.), *The neurology of consciousness*. London, UK: Elsevier.

TABLE 9-7 Comparison of Minimally Conscious State (MCS), Persistent Vegetative State (PVS), and Coma

Behavior	MCS	PVS	Coma
Eye opening	Spontaneous	Spontaneous	None
Spontaneous movement	Automatic/object manipulation	Reflexive/patterned	None
Response to pain	Localization	Posturing/withdrawal	Posturing/none
Visual response	Object recognition/pursuit	Startle/pursuit (rare)	None
Affective response	Contingent	Random	None
Commands	Inconsistent	None	None
Verbalization	Intelligible words	Random vocalization	None

Data from: Giacino, J. T., & Schiff, N. D. (2009). The minimally conscious state: Clinical features, pathophysiology, and therapeutic implications. In S. Laureys & G. Tononi (Eds.), *The neurology of consciousness*. London, UK: Elsevier.

Locked-in Syndrome

LIS was a relatively unknown condition until Jean-Dominique Bauby published his memoir *The Diving Bell and the Butterfly* in 1997. A film version of the same title was released in 2007. Bauby suffered a stroke in the ventral pons region of his brainstem and acquired LIS, which is characterized by total immobility but preserved wakefulness, core consciousness, and extended consciousness. A patient's GCS score would appear to be E4-V2-M1, but because of the whole-body paralysis, motor and verbal responses may be challenging to assess. In reality, these patients have a GCS score of E4-V6-M5 if they can obey commands with their eyes and communicate with others through a compensatory device like an alphabet board, as Bauby did.

Most LIS patients demonstrate sustained opening and movement of the eyes, quadriplegia or quadriparesis, anarthria (inability to produce known words), and aphonia (inability to speak) or hypophonia (inability to speak at normal volume). Their cognitive skills are intact. There are different forms of LIS. *Classical LIS* involves total body immobility but with preserved eye movements or blinking. Bauby acquired this form. *Incomplete LIS* is characterized by some very limited voluntary movement. *Total LIS* is the most devastating, with complete immobility of the body and the eyes. Any of these forms may be confused with PVS, MCS, or coma.

Dementia

Dementia refers to an acquired, usually progressive cognitive deterioration. Alzheimer disease (AD) is the most common form of dementia, affecting 5% of patients 65 years and older and almost 50% of people 85 years or older (Pietrini, Salmon, & Nichelli, 2009). The disease is caused by microscopic changes to cortical cells in the form of plaques, vacuoles, and neurofibrillary tangles (Pryse-Phillips, 2009).

People with AD progress through three stages of the disease: early, middle, and late. In the early stage of AD, patients have normal motor abilities but begin to have memory problems. In the middle stage, they have increasing problems with memory and other cognitive functions, including language. The late stage of the disease is characterized by severe cognitive deficits and deteriorating motor ability (Manasco, 2014). In terms of consciousness, wakefulness is preserved in the early through middle stages of the disease and will be affected in the later stages of AD. Core consciousness will follow the same pattern. It is extended consciousness that begins to be assaulted in the early stage of the disease as the autobiographical self begins to deteriorate under the weight of the disease.

Aphasia

Earlier in this chapter, we said that extended consciousness "depends on memory" and that our ability to share our memories depends on language. We have already seen that in AD, extended consciousness slowly declines as the disease progresses and impairs memory and language. AD patients lose the autobiographical self because they can no longer remember themselves in the past nor picture their future.

Aphasia is a multimodality acquired language disorder. People with this condition have impaired receptive and/or expressive language. The question is, when language is impaired, is extended consciousness impaired? Is a person with aphasia wakeful? Does he or she have core consciousness? Just spend 5 minutes with someone with aphasia and you will see that he or she is indeed awake and has a sense of his or her self in relationship to objects in the world.

Extended consciousness and the autobiographical self do appear to be preserved in aphasia. People who have experienced temporary aphasia due to transient ischemic attacks or hematomas have been able to report on their experiences with great detail and clarity. They note that thinking and recall were intact during the aphasic period. Some also report thinking about their future and what it would mean if the aphasic condition became a permanent part of life (Lazar, Marshall, Prell, & Pile-Spellman, 2000; Taylor, 2009).

Epilepsy

Epilepsy involves recurrent electrical storms in the brain that are involuntary and episodic in nature. They suddenly impair consciousness for short periods of time. Sufferers are awake during these events, but core and extended consciousness can both be impaired, depending on the type and severity of the seizure.

Out-of-Body Experiences

Out-of-body experiences (OBEs) are the experience of wakeful disembodiment. People feel as if they have left their physical body and even report seeing their body, sometimes with physicians trying to revive them. The following is a report from someone who experienced an OBE:

> I was in bed and about to fall asleep when I had the distinct impression that "I" was at the ceiling looking down at my body in the bed. I was very startled and frightened; immediately I felt that I was consciously back in the bed again. (Irwin, 1985)

OBEs are estimated to occur in approximately 5% to 10% of the population, and the precipitating factors range from neurological disorders to drugs (Blanke & Dieguez, 2009). They occur most frequently in people with epilepsy and migraine. They have been artificially created as well. Blanke, Ortigue, Landis, and Seeck (2002) were able to stimulate OBEs in normal subjects by applying electrical current to the right temporoparietal juncture, suggesting this may be an important area for our sense of embodiment.

Near-Death Experiences

OBEs are considered a key characteristic of a more elaborate phenomenon called near-death experience (NDE). Greyson (2005) defines NDEs as "profound subjective experiences with transcendental or mystical elements, in which persons close to death may believe they have left their physical bodies and transcended the boundaries of the ego and the confines of space and time." The incidence of NDEs is thought to be 6% to 12% in cardiac arrest patients but is unknown in other patient populations (Blanke & Dieguez, 2009).

Greyson (1983) constructed a scale to measure NDEs, which gives 16 experiential elements and their intensity (0–2) organized in four categories: cognitive, affective, paranormal, and transcendental (**TABLE 9-8**). The maximum score is 32, but a score of only 7 would qualify the experience as a true NDE because two of the four categories would be used to describe the experience. Using two or more categories indicates that the experience was complex, intense, and something out of the ordinary. **BOXES 9-1** and **9-2** offer further exploration of the mysterious nature of NDEs as well as the related topic of the mind–brain debate.

▶ Treatment of People With Disorders of Consciousness

There are several avenues of treatment available for people with disorders of consciousness; however,

---

BOX 9-1 Two Strange Cases of Near-Death Experience

Eben Alexander (2012), a Harvard neurosurgeon, contracted meningitis and fell into a coma in 2008. He asserts that his higher cortical functions ceased and that during this time he had an elaborate NDE that would score very high on the Greyson scale. Though many have criticized his account and have provided alternative, naturalistic explanations for his experience, Alexander continues to ask how a severely impaired brain such as his own could generate such an elaborate experience with vivid, detailed memories. It is a question worthy of further investigation.

This author once had a 24-year-old female patient, M. P. She was driving with a friend on a military base road when a drunken soldier struck her vehicle head on with his vehicle. M. P. suffered severe head trauma and was in a coma for approximately 3 weeks. The speech-language pathology team completed coma stimulation with her over the course of the 3 weeks and then began assessing her cognitive-communicative abilities as she began to emerge. After many weeks of recovery, M. P. regained the ability to converse with others and described a vivid experience, which would easily qualify as a genuine NDE using the Greyson scale. The story contained all the Greyson scale affective components and some paranormal and transcendental qualities. She also had a second experience while in the intensive care unit in a coma, but this one was an OBE only. She reported that she left her body, looked down, and saw a nurse with big blonde hair, red lips, and bright red fingernails. The therapists replied, "That sounds like Flo!"

Are stories like Alexander's and M. P.'s genuine disembodied NDEs or the product of oxygen deprivation or synaptic misfiring? Is there an immaterial mind as well as a material brain? If so, can the mind be separated from the body and exist independently from it? Further research should be conducted to find out. In the meantime, those SLPs and audiologists working in hospital settings should be prepared to hear about OBEs and NDEs from their patients.

TABLE 9-8 The Greyson Near-Death Experience Scale

Cognitive	Affective	Paranormal	Transcendental
Time distortion	Peace	Vivid sensory event	Sense of otherworld environment
Thought acceleration	Joy	Apparent extrasensory	Sense of mystical unity
Life review	Cosmic unity	perception	Sense of deceased/religious spirits
Revelation	Encounter with light	Precognitive visions	Sense of border/point of no return
		Out-of-body experience	

Data from Greyson, B. (1983). The near-death experience scale: Construction, reliability, and validity. *Journal of Nervous and Mental Disease, 185*, 327–334.

BOX 9-2 The Mind–Brain Debate

Strange phenomena like OBEs and NDEs and topics like consciousness make us think more about ourselves. Are we material only, meaning that all of our thinking and experiences are reducible to neurons and synapses? Alternatively, are we some mix of material and immaterial? In other words, do we have a soul and a body, and even more important to this text, do we have an immaterial mind and material brain? We will survey some of the different views on this topic (TABLE 9-9). We will begin with monistic (i.e., involving only one) views first and then proceed to dualistic (i.e., involving two) views.

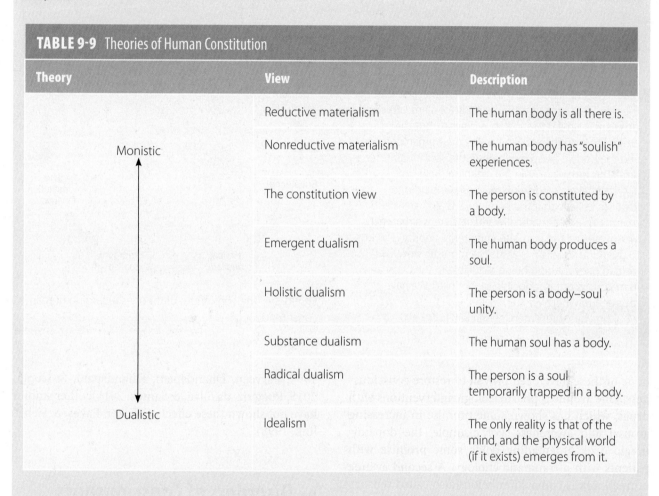

TABLE 9-9 Theories of Human Constitution

Theory	View	Description
Monistic ↕ Dualistic	Reductive materialism	The human body is all there is.
	Nonreductive materialism	The human body has "soulish" experiences.
	The constitution view	The person is constituted by a body.
	Emergent dualism	The human body produces a soul.
	Holistic dualism	The person is a body–soul unity.
	Substance dualism	The human soul has a body.
	Radical dualism	The person is a soul temporarily trapped in a body.
	Idealism	The only reality is that of the mind, and the physical world (if it exists) emerges from it.

There are three true monistic, materialistic views of human persons—reductive materialism, nonreductive materialism, and the constitution view. In **reductive materialism**, all of life is reduced to the material and to naturalistic explanations. As for mind, it is reduced to neurons and synaptic connections. OBEs, NDEs, and "miraculous" healings are all explained through neurophysiological processes. Most neuroscientists would probably affirm this position. **Nonreductive materialism** is also a materialistic view but says there is something more going on than neurons and synapses. Experiences of awe or beauty (or NDEs) do have neurological processes behind them, but these experiences cannot be reduced to mere neurological processes; rather, other processes (psychological, philosophical, and theological) are needed to explain these complex, nonreducible experiences. The **constitution view** is a materialistic view as well. It purports that humans are material only but are different from animals because we have a first-person perspective (i.e., extended consciousness). This first-person perspective is what makes us a person and not an animal.

Emergent dualism and holistic dualism attempt to bridge the divide between monists and dualists. **Emergent dualism** is the belief that the human mind emerges or arises from a combination of many brain activities. This view attempts to mediate between monism and dualism. It agrees with materialism that the mind is produced by the brain, but it also agrees with dualism that the mind is a separate entity, not completely explainable, reducible, or identifiable with specific brain functions. **Holistic dualism** involves the idea that human persons are integrated wholes. In other words, bodily existence is what it is to be human. There is no separation between material and immaterial because they

(continues)

BOX 9-2 The Mind–Brain Debate *(continued)*

are intertwined with each other. If there is an afterlife, it is somehow an embodied afterlife. Although both emergent and holistic dualism have the word *dualism* in their title, they are both essentially monistic views, but with dualistic elements.

True dualistic views include substance dualism and radical dualism. **Substance dualism** holds that humans are both material and immaterial and that the immaterial can exist apart from the material for a time. It is like holistic dualism in that it holds that to be human is to be embodied, but material and immaterial are not as tightly integrated. Proponents of this view would believe that OBEs and NDEs are evidence that the immaterial part can separate from the physical. In terms of brain–mind, supporters of substance dualism would believe that the brain is material and the mind is immaterial and that the mind can exist outside the body for a time. **Radical dualism** is similar to substance dualism, but the emphasis is on the soul; the soul *is* the human person and the body is just a mechanism the soul inhabits for a time. This is the "ghost in the machine" view.

The final view is **idealism**. Those who hold to idealism believe that the immaterial is all there is and that things in the material world (if there is a material world) are created from the immaterial. Priority is given to the mind. Idealism is actually a monistic view, but instead of everything being reducible to the body as in materialism, it is reducible to the mind. We have returned to where we started, because these views would be best presented in a circle (**FIGURE 9-4**).

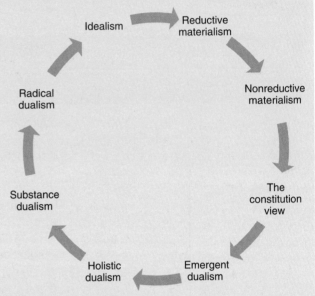

FIGURE 9-4 The continuum of theories regarding human constitution.

---

none of these have been proven to restore consciousness. One avenue is pharmacologic interventions with drugs, which has shown some promise in increasing arousal and awareness. For example, the dopaminergic drug amantadine holds some promise with patients with a traumatic etiology. A second avenue of treatment is coma stimulation (also called sensory stimulation), which can be unimodal (i.e., one sensory route) or multimodal. This approach attempts to increase arousal and awareness through systemically stimulating one or more of the five senses, thus stimulating the nervous system (Bass & Gettleman, 2009). For example, the sense of smell can be stimulated through presentation of both good (e.g., vanilla) and noxious (e.g., smelling salts) stimuli. Vision can be stimulated by showing photographs of loved ones and encouraging eye tracking. It is important to note that there is little evidence to support the efficacy of coma stimulation, though some studies have shown some increase in body movements, facial expressions, pulse rate, and respiration rate in response to auditory stimulation with audio recordings of family and friend voices (Jones, Hux, Morton-Anderson, & Knepper,

1994; Parveen, Dhandapani, Dhandapani, & Gupta, 2015; Puggina, da Silva, & Santos, 2011); other studies have not shown these effects (Walker, Eakes, & Siebelink, 1998).

▶ Disorders of Consciousness and Personhood

As we have been exploring this mysterious thing we call consciousness and disorders of consciousness, the discussions raise other questions. If the definition of being brain dead presented in this chapter is followed, then we can conclude that being brain dead means that the human person is dead as well. There is only a body left. However, what about people in other not-so-clear states? Are people who are comatose or in a PVS or MCS state, or who have dementia, still people? Has the spark of humanness left them? These questions raise one of the most significant questions in life: What makes a person a person? We will use a story to help us frame this question.

Terry was only 19 years old at the time of his accident. He was married and had a baby girl named Amber. One night, while out with a friend, he lost control of his pickup truck and ran into a guardrail that hugged a curve in the road. His truck was launched straight up and came down on its tailgate. Terry's friend walked away from the accident unharmed; however, Terry immediately fell into a coma. He did not have a scratch on his body except for a small cut on his forehead, but he was unable to take care of himself or communicate with his family. One day, after 19 years in this coma, he mysteriously woke up and began to talk to his family. His memory was impaired for recalling recent events, but it was sharp for everything that occurred before the accident. Terry was both a medical miracle and a mystery.

Why start a discussion on human personhood with this story? The answer is that this story can help us ask important questions about personhood. Is a person defined by what external behaviors he or she can or cannot do? Is a person simply a machine who is the sum of his or her parts, and when a part does not work, is he or she not a person anymore? Alternatively, is a person defined by something else, perhaps an internal essence that orders and unifies the parts a person possesses?

Two Broad Views of Personhood

There is an ongoing debate regarding human personhood, and this debate narrows down to how you define a human person. There are two basic views that revolve around this question.

The first view is to define a person as being physical only (i.e., physicalism). He or she is a body only and there is no real difference between humans and animals. Thus, a person's abilities or disabilities become paramount in defining whether he or she is truly a person. In this view, a person is merely the sum of his or her parts, essentially a machine like a computer (Rae & Cox, 1999). Does the person have all the typical capacities, functions, and parts (e.g., consciousness, memory, the ability to communicate) we think of when we think of a human person? If the answer to this question is "yes," then a proponent of this view might say that the person is truly a person. If someone has never attained some or all of these capacities, or if a person has lost these abilities, as in the case of Terry, is he or she still a human person?

Proponents of this view might say "no" and a practice like euthanasia becomes not only possible but in some cases necessary to increase what Princeton philosopher Peter Singer calls the total amount of happiness in the world (Will, 1999).

The second way to define a person is to say that his or her substance is a body and a soul, material and immaterial, and that something mysterious (e.g., the human spirit or essence?) orders and unifies the parts of this substance. This could be called an internal essence view. For example, a dog has dog essence, which orders and unifies its parts. It is defined by its essence, not its parts or capacities. If a dog loses the capacity to bark, is it still a dog (Beckwith, 2000)? Most reasonable people would answer in the affirmative. In addition, if a human person loses certain capacities and functions (e.g., the capacity to walk, remember things, speak), is he or she still a human person? Proponents of this view would argue that Terry, though he has severe disabilities, is still a human person.

However, what makes humans different from dogs? Singer would say "nothing" and that anyone who argues for humanity being of a different and better essence is committing *speciesism*, the intentional act of promoting one species over another (Will, 1999). Yet others would argue that there is something unique about humans, something that separates man and woman from beast. What do you think? Does monistic physicalism make more sense to you? Or does some kind of soul–body, mind–brain dualism make more sense? These are important and interesting questions because they do affect life decisions, like living wills and end-of-life decisions. They also may affect the way we see and work with our patients.

▶ Speech-Language Pathology, Audiology, and Disorders of Consciousness

SLPs may be involved with patients who have disorders of consciousness. This may take the form of completing coma stimulation with patients; assessing speech/language function in a patient suspected of being PVS, MCS, or LIS; or assessing swallowing function. Coma stimulation is a systematic application of stimulation to a patient's five senses with the purpose of increasing the patient's responsiveness to stimuli. Vision can be stimulated through blinking lights, gustatory through applying different tastes, auditory through music or family voices, olfaction through applying different smells, and touch through applying different textures or temperatures to the skin. Some coma stimulation programs also add kinesthetic stimulation in the form of posture changes and/or range-of-movement exercises. Studies have been completed examining the effectiveness of this therapy approach; the results of these studies are mixed. Some studies have shown improvement in cognitive status and responsiveness and a decrease in mean length of time in a coma (Karma & Rawat, 2006; Kater, 1989; Mitchell, Bradley, Welch, & Britton, 1990; Wilson, Powell, Elliott, & Thwaites, 1991). Other studies have shown that coma stimulation does not appear to make a difference in these patients (Pierce et al., 1990; Rader, Alston, & Ellis, 1989). Audiologists may work with these populations in conducting nonbehavioral hearing assessment measures, such as auditory brainstem response.

▶ Conclusion

Thomas Nagel wrote an article in 1974 titled "What Is It Like to Be a Bat?" He challenged the reductionist tendencies of many neuroscientists with the fact that both humans and animals (like the bat) have conscious, personal, first-person experiences that are unique, rich, and private to us and difficult to reduce to neurons, synapses, and action potentials. Only I know what it is truly like to be Matt. You, the reader, do not know and cannot know anything of my private experience as I write this book unless I decide to reveal something to you. Even then, you will never have a true or complete first-person perspective of my first-person experience. Consciousness is certainly an interesting, complex, and mysterious topic of study.

SUMMARY OF LEARNING OBJECTIVES

The following were the main learning objectives of this chapter. The information that should have been learned is below each learning objective.

1. The learner will define *consciousness, core consciousness*, and *extended consciousness*.
   - *Consciousness:* the ability to be aware of self and surroundings
   - *Core consciousness:* our sense of ourselves in the here and now (i.e., at this very moment), objects in the world, and our relationship to those objects
   - *Extended consciousness:* our sense of self in the flow of time as we think of ourselves in the past and anticipate ourselves living in a future

2. The learner will list and describe the primary neurological structures thought to be involved in consciousness.
   - *Reticular formation:* Two nuclei, the classical reticular nuclei and the cholinergic nuclei, appear important in wakefulness. Glutaminergic projections from the classical reticular nuclei travel to the intralaminar nuclei of the thalamus, which the thalamus then projects to much of the cerebral cortex. Because glutamate is excitatory, it helps to stimulate cortical wakefulness. At the same time, cholinergic projections to the reticular thalamic nuclei hinder sleep.
   - *Ascending reticular activating system:* This system begins in the midbrain's reticular formation and radiates out to the cerebral cortex through the thalamus, specifically through the intralaminar nuclei of the thalamus, in order to activate and coordinate the cerebral cortex for conscious experience.

3. The learner will list and briefly describe at least five specific disorders of consciousness.
   - *Coma:* a condition in which the person does not respond purposefully to stimuli but does demonstrate brainstem reflexes. Comatose patients do not have a sleep–wake cycle and demonstrate EEG patterns, although they are severely depressed.
   - *Brain death:* a condition in which the person has no purposeful responses to stimuli, no brainstem reflexes, no sleep–wake cycle, and flat EEG patterns.
   - *Persistent vegetative state (PVS):* a condition in which the person does not respond purposefully to stimuli but does demonstrate brainstem reflexes. PVS patients have a sleep–wake cycle and demonstrate EEG patterns, although they are severely depressed.
   - *Minimally conscious state (MCS):* a condition in which the person responds purposefully to stimuli, but inconsistently. MCS patients also demonstrate brainstem reflexes and a

sleep–wake cycle. Like their inconsistent responses to stimuli, their EEG patterns are variable depending on what state (PVS vs. conscious) they are tending toward.

- *Locked-in syndrome (LIS):* a condition in which the person is fully aware and conscious but locked inside a body that does not work.
- *Dementia:* a condition in which the person is wakeful in the early through middle stages of the disease and will begin to be affected in the later stages of Alzheimer disease. Core consciousness will follow the same pattern. It is extended consciousness that begins to be assaulted in the early stage of the disease as the autobiographical self begins to deteriorate under the weight of the disease.
- *Aphasia:* a condition in which the person has an acquired language disorder but intact consciousness.
- *Epilepsy:* a condition in which the person has recurrent electrical storms in the brain that are involuntary and episodic in nature that suddenly impair consciousness for short periods of time.
- *Out-of-body experience (OBE):* the experience of wakeful disembodiment.
- *Near-death experience (NDE):* a profound subjective experience with transcendental or mystical elements, in which persons close to death may believe they have left their physical bodies and transcended the boundaries of the ego and the confines of space and time.

4. The learner will list and describe the various mind–brain theories.
- *Reductive materialism:* belief that all of life is reduced to the material and to naturalistic explanations

- *Nonreductive materialism:* belief that experiences (e.g., beauty) cannot be reduced to mere neurological processes, but rather, other processes (psychological, philosophical, and theological) are needed to explain these complex, nonreducible experiences
- *Constitution view:* belief that humans are material only, but are different from animals because we have a first-person perspective (i.e., extended consciousness)
- *Emergent dualism:* belief that the human mind emerges or arises from a combination of many brain activities
- *Holistic dualism:* belief that human persons are integrated wholes
- *Substance dualism:* belief that humans are both material and immaterial and that the immaterial can exist apart from the material for a time
- *Radical dualism:* belief that the soul *is* the human person and the body is just a mechanism the soul inhabits for a time
- *Idealism:* belief that all there is, is the immaterial and that things in the material world (if there is a material world) are created from the immaterial

5. The learner will articulate the two main views of personhood.
- *Physicalism:* belief that a person is a body only and there is no real difference between humans and animals. Thus, a person's abilities or disabilities become paramount in defining whether he or she is truly a person.
- *Internal essence view:* belief that a person is both a body and a soul, material and immaterial, and that something mysterious (e.g., the human spirit or essence?) orders and unifies the parts of this substance.

KEY TERMS

Brain death
Coma
Consciousness
Constitution view
Core consciousness
Creature consciousness
Emergent dualism
Extended consciousness
Glasgow Coma Scale (GCS)

Holistic dualism
Idealism
Mental-state consciousness
Minimally conscious state (MCS)
Nonreductive materialism
Persistent vegetative state (PVS)
Radical dualism

Rancho Levels of Cognitive Functioning (RLCF)
Reductive materialism
Reticular activating system
Reticular formation
Substance dualism

DRAW IT TO KNOW IT

1. Draw four coronal sections of the brain and shade in impaired areas in the following conditions: brain death, coma, PVS, and MCS (see Figure 9-3).

QUESTIONS FOR DEEPER REFLECTION

1. Pick a view of human constitution and write one paragraph supporting this view.
2. Why should a communication disorders professional be aware of consciousness?
3. Describe the neural basis for consciousness.

CASE STUDY

Teresa is a 21-year-old female who was involved in a motor vehicle accident. She was ejected from her truck upon impact with another vehicle and suffered a significant brain injury. Her GCS in the field was E4-V6-M2 that improved to E4-V6-M3 upon admission to the emergency room. Currently, Teresa demonstrates appropriate behavior in response to environmental stimuli (e.g., will move head toward a source of sound), but arousal is inconsistent. She also attempts to utter sounds during her periods of arousal though her speech is unintelligible. She can move all four extremities, but is inconsistent upon command.

1. Which of the following states is Teresa most likely to be in?
   a. Coma
   b. Minimally conscious state
   c. Persistent vegetative state
   d. Locked-in syndrome
2. Explain why you picked the answer you did.
3. Do you think Teresa is aware of herself and her surroundings?

SUGGESTED PROJECTS

1. Research the reticular activating system and write a short paper outlining its structure and function.
2. Obtain and read Thomas Nagel's 1974 article "What Is It Like to Be a Bat?" (A Google search will turn up free copies.) Write a two-page reflection paper on it. Include a brief summary of the article, and state whether you agree or disagree with Nagle and why.
3. Write a two- to three-page paper on one of the disorders of consciousness presented in this chapter.
4. Explore the literature on coma/sensory stimulation and present the evidence for and against this approach.
5. Write a two- to three-page paper on how you define personhood.

REFERENCES

Alexander, E. (2012). *Proof of heaven: A neurosurgeon's journey into the afterlife.* New York, NY: Simon & Schuster.

Bass, H., & Gettleman, M. (2009, November). *Is anyone in there? Treatment of the minimally conscious patient.* Seminar presented at the American Speech-Language-Hearing Association's Annual Convention, New Orleans, LA.

Beckwith, F. J. (2000). Abortion, bioethics, and personhood: A philosophical reflection. *Southern Baptist Journal of Theology, 4,* 20.

Bernat, J. L. (2009). Brain death. In S. Laureys & G. Tononi (Eds.), *The neurology of consciousness: Cognitive neuroscience and neuropathology* (pp. 151–162). London, UK: Academic Press.

Blanke, O., & Dieguez, S. (2009). Leaving body and life behind: Out-of-body and near-death experience. In S. Laureys & G. Tononi (Eds.), *The neurology of consciousness: Cognitive neuroscience and neuropathology* (pp. 303–325). London, UK: Academic Press.

Blanke, O., Ortigue, S., Landis, T., & Seeck, M. (2002). Neuropsychology: Stimulating illusory own-body perceptions. *Nature, 419*(6904), 269–270.

Blumenfeld, H. (2009). The neurological examination of consciousness. In S. Laureys, & G. Tononi (Eds.), *The neurology of consciousness: Cognitive neuroscience and neuropathology* (pp. 15–30). London, UK: Academic Press.

Damasio, A. (1999). *The feeling of what happens.* Orlando, FL: Houghton Mifflin Harcourt.

Damasio, A., & Meyer, K. (2009). Consciousness: An overview of the phenomenon and of its possible neural basis. In S. Laureys &

G. Tononi (Eds.), *The neurology of consciousness: Cognitive neuroscience and neuropathology* (pp. 3–14). London, UK: Academic Press.

Dennett, D. (1992). *Consciousness explained.* New York, NY: Back Bay Books.

Greyson, B. (1983). The near-death experience scale: Construction, reliability, and validity. *Journal of Nervous and Mental Disease, 185,* 327–334.

Greyson, B. (2005). "False positive" claims of near-death experiences and "false negative" denials of near-death experiences. *Death Studies, 29*(2), 145–155.

Hall, A. (2009, November 23). Conscious man "in coma" for 23 years. *The Telegraph.* Retrieved from http://www.telegraph .co.uk/news/worldnews/europe/belgium/6632518/Conscious -man-in-coma-for-23-years.html

Irwin, H. J. (1985). *Flight of mind: A psychological study of the out-of-body experience.* Metuchen, NJ: The Scarecrow Press.

Jones, R., Hux, K., Morton-Anderson, K. A., & Knepper, L. (1994). Auditory stimulation effect on a comatose survivor of traumatic brain injury. *Archives of Physical Medicine and Rehabilitation, 75*(2), 164–171.

Karma, D., & Rawat, A. K. (2006). Effect of stimulation in coma. *Indian Pediatrics, 43,* 856–860.

Kater, K. M. (1989). Response of head-injured patients to sensory stimulation. *Western Journal of Nursing Research, 11*(1), 20–33.

Lazar, R. M., Marshall, R. S., Prell, G. D., & Pile-Spellman, J. (2000). The experience of Wernicke's aphasia. *Neurology, 55*(8), 1222–1224.

Manasco, M. H. (2014). *Introduction to neurogenic communication disorders.* Burlington, MA: Jones & Bartlett Learning.

Massimini, M., Ferrarelli, F., Huber, R., Esser, S., Singh, H., & Tononi, G. (2005). Breakdown of cortical effective connectivity during sleep. *Science, 309,* 2228–2232.

Mitchell, S., Bradley, V. A., Welch, J. L., & Britton, P. G. (1990). Coma arousal procedure: A therapeutic intervention in the treatment of head injury. *Brain Injury, 4*(3), 273–279.

Monti, M. M., Vanhaudenhuyse, A., Coleman, M. R., Boly, M., Pickard, J. D., & Tshibanda, L., . . . Laureys, S. (2010). Willful modulation of brain activity in disorders of consciousness. *New England Journal of Medicine, 362*(7), 579–589.

Nagel, T. (1974). What is it like to be a bat? *Philosophical Review, 83*(4), 435–450.

Parveen, Y., Dhandapani, M., Dhandapani, S., & Gupta, S. K. (2015). A randomized controlled trial to assess the efficacy of auditory stimulation on selected parameters of comatose patients with traumatic brain injury. *Indian Journal of Neurotrauma, 12*(02), 128–134.

Parvizi, J., & Damasio, A. (2001). Consciousness and the brainstem. *Cognition, 79,* 135–159.

Pierce, J. P., Lyle, D. M., Quine, S., Evans, N. J., Morris, J., & Fearnside, M. R. (1990). The effectiveness of coma arousal intervention. *Brain Injury, 4*(2), 191–197.

Pietrini, P., Salmon, E., & Nichelli, P. (2009). Consciousness and dementia: How the brain loses its self. In S. Laureys & G. Tononi (Eds.), *The neurology of consciousness: Cognitive neuroscience and neuropathology* (pp. 204–216). London, UK: Elsevier.

Pryse-Phillips, W. (2009). *Companion to clinical neurology.* Cary, NC: Oxford University Press.

Puggina, A. C. G., da Silva, M. J. P., & Santos, J. L. F. (2011). Use of music and voice stimulus on patients with disorders of consciousness. *Journal of Neuroscience Nursing, 43*(1), E8–E16. doi:10.1097/JNN.0b013e3182029778.

Purves, D., Augustine, G. J., Fitzpatrick, D., Hall, W. C., LaMantia, A. S., McNamara, J. O., & Williams, S. M. (2004). *Neuroscience* (3rd ed.). Sunderland, MA: Sinauer Associates.

Rader, M. A., Alston, J. B., & Ellis, D. W. (1989). Sensory stimulation of severely brain-injured patients. *Brain Injury, 3*(2), 141–147.

Rae, S. B., & Cox, P. M. (1999). *Bioethics: A Christian approach in a pluralistic age.* Grand Rapids, MI: William B. Eerdmans.

Taylor, J. B. (2009). *My stroke of insight: A brain scientist's personal journey.* New York, NY: Viking Penguin.

Teasdale, G., & Jennett, B. (1974). Assessment of coma and impaired consciousness: A practical scale. *The Lancet, 2*(7872), 81–84.

Van Gulick, R. (2011). Consciousness. In N. Zalta (Ed.), *Stanford encyclopedia of philosophy (Summer 2011 ed.).* Wellesley, MA: Babson Press. Retrieved from https://plato.stanford.edu/entries/consciousness/

Walker, J. S., Eakes, G. G., & Siebelink, E. (1998). The effects of familial voice interventions on comatose head-injured patients. *Journal of Trauma Nursing, 5*(2), 41.

Will, G. F. (1999, September 13). Life and death at Princeton. *Newsweek,* 80–81.

Wilson, S. L., Powell, G. E., Elliott, K., & Thwaites, H. (1991). Sensory stimulation in prolonged coma: Four single case studies. *Brain Injury, 5*(4), 393–400.

Young, G. B. (2009). Coma. In S. Laureys & G. Tononi (Eds.), *The neurology of consciousness: Cognitive neuroscience and neuropathology* (pp. 137–150). London, UK: Academic Press.

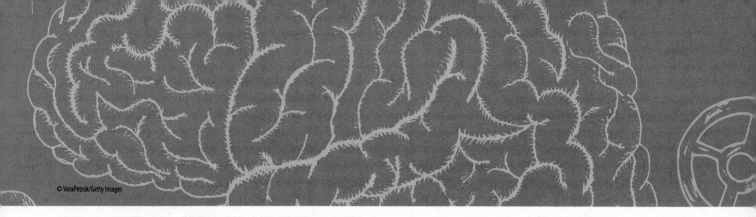

CHAPTER 10

The Neurology of Hearing and Balance

CHAPTER PREVIEW

It is time to apply neuroscience to communication and communication disorders. This chapter will discuss the neurology of both hearing and balance as well as survey select disorders that affect these systems.

IN THIS CHAPTER

In this chapter, we will . . .

- Survey the anatomy and physiology of the peripheral hearing system
- Explore the anatomy and physiology of the central auditory system
- Examine disorders of the auditory system
- Survey the anatomy and physiology of the peripheral vestibular system
- Explore the anatomy and physiology of the central vestibular system
- Examine disorders of the vestibular system

LEARNING OBJECTIVES

1. The learner will list and briefly describe the peripheral auditory system.
2. The learner will list and briefly describe the central auditory system.
3. The learner will list and describe the function of the main central auditory structures.
4. The learner will define the following auditory disorders: *sensorineural hearing loss, auditory processing disorder, pure word deafness,* and *other disorders that may affect auditory comprehension.*
5. The learner will briefly describe the peripheral and central vestibular systems.
6. The learner will define the following vestibular disorders: *vestibular schwannoma* and *labyrinthitis.*

▶ Introduction

Hearing, also known as **audition**, is a process whereby acoustic or sound energy waves are changed into neural impulses. This is why the ear is known as a **transducer** or energy changer. Anatomically, the ear can be divided into the peripheral auditory system and the central auditory system (**FIGURE 10-1**). The **peripheral auditory system** includes the outer ear, middle ear, inner ear, and cranial nerve VIII, while the **central auditory system** involves several structures in the brainstem, thalamus, and cerebral cortex. The purpose of this chapter is to survey these two systems, perform an in-depth exploration of the central auditory system, and examine select neurological disorders of hearing.

▶ The Neurology of Hearing

The Peripheral Auditory System

The outer ear includes the pinna (or auricle) and the external auditory meatus. In the **outer ear**, hearing involves the pinna locating, collecting, and funneling acoustic energy (i.e., sound) to the middle ear via the external auditory canal or meatus (**FIGURE 10-2**). In the **middle ear**, acoustic energy is changed, or transduced, into mechanical energy as the tympanic membrane begins to vibrate due to sound waves hitting it. This mechanical energy is then transmitted through the ossicular chain, which is composed of three small bones—the malleus, incus, and stapes (**FIGURE 10-3**). This causes the footplate of the stapes to rock in and out of the vestibule's oval window. At this point, the **inner ear** has been reached and several other energy changes will occur. The cochlea is filled with two fluids, perilymph and endolymph. Perilymph occupies the scala vestibuli and scala tympani, and endolymph is found in the scala media. As the footplate of the stapes rocks in and out of the cochlea, mechanical energy from the middle ear is changed into hydraulic energy through the creation of waves in these cochlear fluids. Hydraulic energy is the power of moving fluids. As these waves travel through the cochlea, hair cells in the organ of Corti are displaced, causing two more energy changes at these hair cells. First, there is a hydraulic to mechanical energy change at the hair cell cilia as they bend. Second, there is a mechanical to electrochemical energy change at the synapse of the hair cell to the afferent auditory neuron at the base of the hair cell.

Resting hair cells in the organ of Corti are in a highly polarized state, just like neurons. The environment outside an individual hair cell is positively charged, whereas the environment in the hair cell is negatively charged. The movement of the stapes

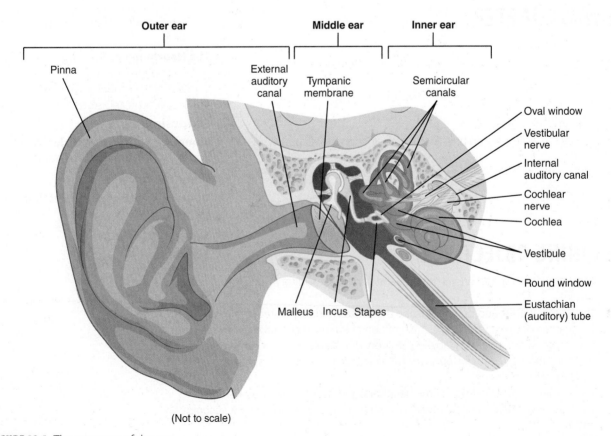

(Not to scale)

FIGURE 10-1 The anatomy of the ear.

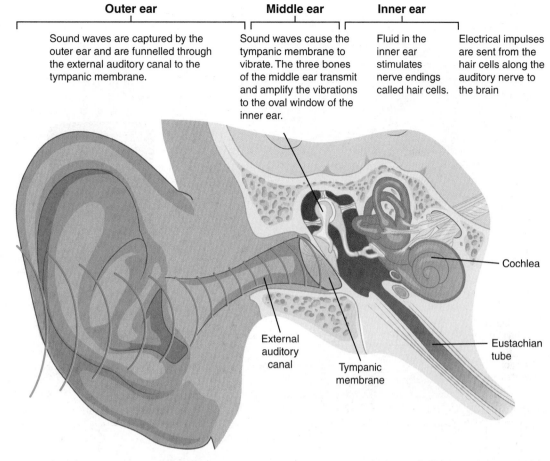

| Outer ear | Middle ear | Inner ear |

Sound waves are captured by the outer ear and are funnelled through the external auditory canal to the tympanic membrane.

Sound waves cause the tympanic membrane to vibrate. The three bones of the middle ear transmit and amplify the vibrations to the oval window of the inner ear.

Fluid in the inner ear stimulates nerve endings called hair cells.

Electrical impulses are sent from the hair cells along the auditory nerve to the brain

Cochlea

External auditory canal

Tympanic membrane

Eustachian tube

FIGURE 10-2 The process of hearing in the peripheral auditory system. Movements of fluid in the inner ear stimulate the hairs of the auditory hair cells, which result in stimulation of auditory nerve endings.

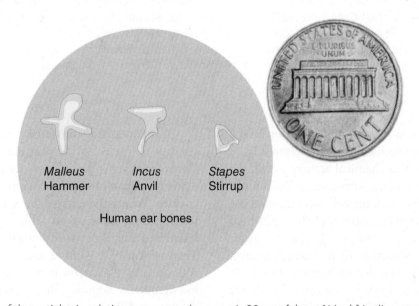

Malleus Hammer

Incus Anvil

Stapes Stirrup

Human ear bones

FIGURE 10-3 The size of the ossicles in relation to a penny (a penny is 20 mm [about ¾ inch] in diameter).

causes perilymph displacement that leads to disruption of the basilar membrane. This disruption causes stereocilia at the very end of the hair cells to bend, leading to potassium channels opening at the ends of the stereocilia. Potassium ions (K^+) enter the hair cell from the endolymph through the cilia and change the hair cell's inner environment from negative to positive (**FIGURE 10-4**). This is the process of depolarization. The hair cell will repolarize later through active transport facilitated by the sodium–potassium pump. Hair cell

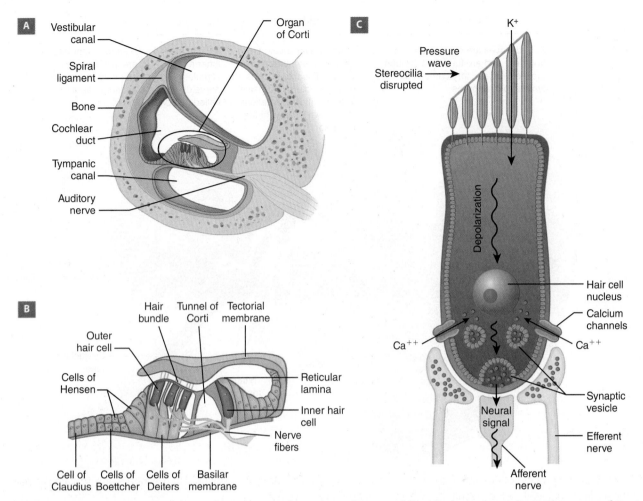

FIGURE 10-4 A. A cross-section of the cochlea showing the scalas and organ of Corti in the scala media. **B.** The organ of Corti and the inner and outer hair cells. **C.** An individual hair cell undergoing depolarization. A pressure wave bends the hair cell's cilia, causing potassium channels to open and allow potassium to enter the hair cell. As a result, the hair cell depolarizes. Depolarization causes calcium channels at the bottom of the hair cell to open and allow calcium to enter the hair cell. This activity triggers the synaptic vesicles to fuse with the cell membrane and release glutamate across the synaptic cleft to the afferent neuron.

© Sakurra/Shutterstock.

depolarization causes calcium channels to open on the bottom sides of the hair cells, allowing calcium (Ca^{++}) to enter the hair cell. This chemical activity within the hair cell triggers the opening of vesicles at the bottom of the hair cells to fuse with the cell membrane; these vesicles release the neurotransmitter glutamate, which travels across the synaptic cleft and excites the auditory nerve branch's dendrites. At this point, neuron function takes over and an electrochemical impulse is sent from the organ of Corti to the central auditory system via cranial nerve VIII. Approximately 30,000 cochlear nerve fibers pass from the cochlea through the internal auditory canal (or meatus) to cranial nerve VIII (Martin & Clark, 2000). In addition to these fibers, vestibular nerve fibers course through the internal auditory canal to the brainstem. Cranial nerve VII fibers and the internal auditory artery also pass through the internal auditory canal.

As mentioned previously, hydraulic energy is changed into electrochemical energy in the organ of Corti. These energy changes occur at specific places along the organ of Corti, which runs the length of the cochlea. Where the energy change occurs is related to the frequency of the sound. Different sensitivities to different frequencies occur all along the basilar membrane. The cochlear base is more sensitive to high-frequency sounds, and the cochlear apex is more sensitive to low-frequency sounds. The basilar membrane's sensitivity to different sound frequencies is known as **tonotopic organization** (**FIGURE 10-5**). Nerve fibers leave their corresponding hair cells along the basilar membrane; each is responsible for communicating different frequencies and intensities to the brain, which we will see is tonotopically arranged also. In conclusion, the cochlea is a finely tuned instrument, able to decipher different sound intensities and frequencies.

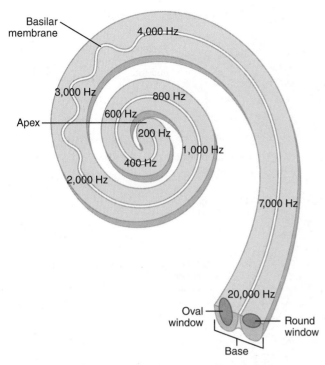

FIGURE 10-5 The tonotopic organization of the cochlea.

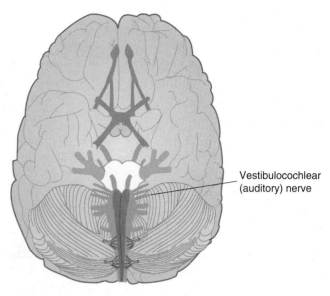

FIGURE 10-6 Inferior view of the brain showing where cranial nerve VIII inputs into the brainstem.
Modified from: © illustrator/Shutterstock.

The Central Auditory System

Brainstem Organization

Cochlear Nucleus

Cranial nerve VIII carries the neural impulse approximately 17 to 18 mm (about 0.7 in) from the internal auditory meatus to the brainstem (Martin & Clark, 2000). It inputs near where the pons and cerebellum meet to form the cerebellopontine angle (**FIGURE 10-6**). It is here that the vestibular and cochlear portions of cranial nerve VIII diverge and go their separate ways. All cochlear fibers synapse at the **cochlear nucleus (CN)**. A nucleus is a collection of neuron cell bodies that function to relay and integrate neural signals as well as play an important role in the reflex arc.

The CN resembles a fish tail, as can be seen in **FIGURE 10-7**, and it has a few important divisions. The posterior CN (also called the dorsal CN) is an area made up of what are called pyramidal cells, so named because the cells look like little pyramids. Their function is a bit of a mystery because destroying them in animals does not seem to affect their hearing. The anterior CN (also called the ventral CN) is made up of three different nuclei. First, the most anterior nucleus is made up of spherical bushy cells. Second, the middle nucleus is made up of globular bushy cells, which are sensitive to very specific frequencies. The last nucleus is made up of octopus cells, so named because of their long, tentacle-like dendrites. These cells are sensitive to a wider range of frequencies. The rest of the CN is made up of various multipolar neurons, sensitive to the beginning, ending, or change of a sound in terms of frequency and/or intensity.

As one can see, the anterior CN preserves the tonotopic arrangement of the basilar membrane. It is represented not just once but several times throughout the nervous system, which is key to our ability to hear complex sounds. As we will see shortly, this tonotopic organization is also preserved in the primary auditory cortex of the cerebral cortex.

Superior Olivary Complex

Vast arrays of neural connections are made throughout the central auditory nervous system projecting through the brainstem, diencephalon, and cerebrum, as can be seen in **FIGURE 10-8**. From the CN, fibers course to the trapezoid body where most (about two-thirds) of nerve fibers decussate from the CN to the superior olivary complex, giving binaural representation in the central auditory nervous system. The **superior olivary complex (SOC)** in the pons gets the name *olivary* because its shape resembles that of an olive. Overall, this complex is important in integrating auditory information together. It has two major components, the **medial superior olivary complex (MSOC)** and the **lateral superior olivary complex (LSOC)**. The MSOC (the center, or pit, of the olive) specializes in low-frequency hearing, specifically integrating low-frequency hearing from the right and left ears to create binaural hearing. **Binaural hearing** is hearing with two ears that provides us with several benefits—principally, our ability to determine the

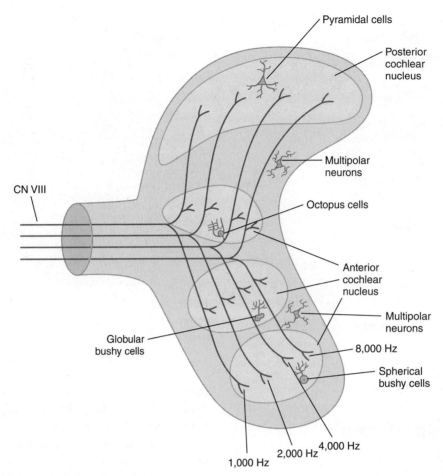

FIGURE 10-7 The cochlear nucleus.

location of a sound. Because of the decussation of nerve fibers at the trapezoid body, each superior olive in the complex receives information from both ears. The SOCs on both sides of the brainstem analyze the slight differences in time and intensity of sound coming from each ear to locate the sound. Our ears are quite tuned for localizing sound and can do it precisely. The MSOC is the first place in the central auditory system to do this type of integration of our two ears. The LSOC (the fleshy part of the olive) specializes in higher frequency hearing. Both the medial SOC and the lateral SOC play a role in sound localization.

In addition, the medial and lateral SOCs are responsible for the stapedius reflex, which is when the stapedius muscle contracts during loud sounds to stiffen the ossicular chain, thus preventing damage to the cochlea. When a sound is too loud, it does not need to travel all the way to the cerebral cortex. The SOC determines if it is too loud and, if so, sends a signal down the facial nerve (cranial nerve VII) to the stapedius muscle in both ears to contract. This action pulls the stapes out of the oval window, decreasing the intensity of the vibrations and protecting the delicate

hair cells in the cochlea. This reflex lasts 45 seconds, so it is protection only for transient loud sounds. Its presence is used routinely by audiologists as a valid diagnostic test to evaluate the outer ear to the SOC.

Lateral Lemniscus and Inferior Colliculus

There are two other important brainstem regions. The **lateral lemniscus** (Latin for "ribbon") is a tract of six pathways (or axons) that travel from the CN and SOC to the inferior colliculus in the midbrain. Two pathways travel directly from the CN to the inferior colliculus, and the remaining four travel to the inferior colliculus via the SOC. There are also nuclei scattered throughout the lateral lemniscus. The **inferior colliculus** (Latin for "lower mound" or "lower hill") is the auditory center of the midbrain. There are two inferior colliculi, one of the right and one of the left. They maintain the tonotopic organization we first discussed in the cochlea. They also regulate our acoustic startle reflex, which is when we suddenly move in response to an unanticipated sound. People with hyperacusis (hypersensitivity to sound) are easily startled (Davis, Gendelman, Tischler, & Gendelman, 1982).

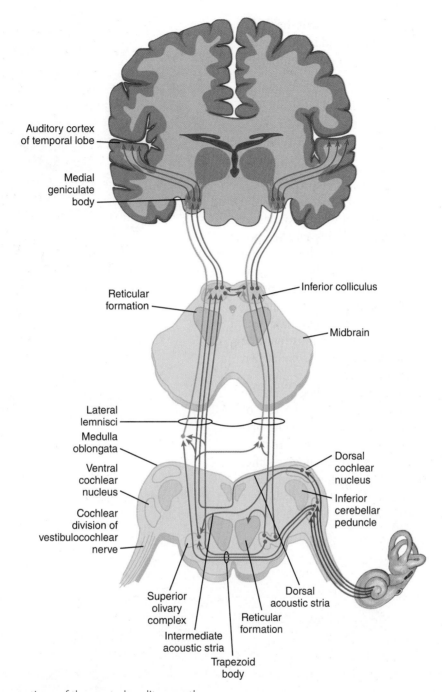

Auditory cortex of temporal lobe

Medial geniculate body

Reticular formation

Inferior colliculus

Midbrain

Lateral lemnisci

Medulla oblongata

Ventral cochlear nucleus

Cochlear division of vestibulocochlear nerve

Dorsal cochlear nucleus

Inferior cerebellar peduncle

Superior olivary complex

Intermediate acoustic stria

Dorsal acoustic stria

Reticular formation

Trapezoid body

FIGURE 10-8 The connections of the central auditory pathway.

Diencephalon Organization

The thalamus's auditory center is the medial geniculate body (Latin for "knee" or "bent abruptly") as compared to the lateral geniculate body, which is the thalamic visual center. Overall, the medial geniculate body acts as a relay station, directing auditory tracts from the inferior colliculus to the auditory cortex of the cerebrum's temporal lobe. It has three parts: the ventral, medial, and dorsal divisions. Most auditory tracts input into the ventral division, which maintains the tonotopic organization previously discussed.

Specifically, the ventral division receives the following auditory information: sound source, sound location, sound onset and offset, frequency, intensity, and binaural information. Axons leave the ventral division and pass into the internal capsule, ascending to the primary auditory cortex.

The dorsal division is thought to play a role in establishing and maintaining our attention to a sound source (i.e., auditory attention). Similar to the reticular formation, the medial division may play a role in our arousal system (i.e., telling the brain to pay attention to something). These two divisions also exit the thalamus, pass into the internal capsule, and input into the cerebral cortex. All these connections are summarized in **FIGURE 10-9**.

Cerebral Cortex Organization

The Primary Auditory Cortex

The central auditory pathway ends at the primary auditory cortex (Brodmann areas [BAs] 41 and 42), which sits on the superior part of the temporal lobe on the superior temporal gyrus and what is known as the gyri of Heschl (also called the transverse temporal gyri) (**FIGURE 10-10**). As can be seen by the name *gyri* (as opposed to *gyrus*) of Heschl, there are typically multiple gyri (one to three) that make up this area. The number of gyri also differs between the left and right temporal lobe (e.g., the left might have two, but the right might have three). This fact illustrates the variability between human brains. There is no known functional reason for this difference.

The tonotopic organization that began in the cochlea and that is maintained through the rest of the central auditory system is preserved in the primary auditory cortex. In other words, there are neurons in this area that are sound frequency specific. Neurons at one end respond best to low frequencies, and neurons on the other end react best to higher frequencies. Functionally, BAs 41 and 42 locate,

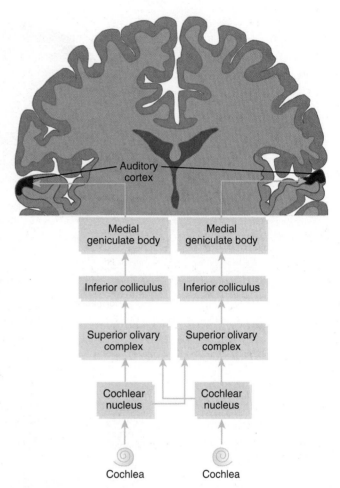

FIGURE 10-9 A simplified diagram of the central auditory pathways.

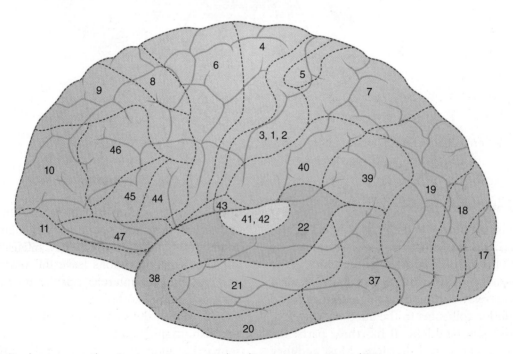

FIGURE 10-10 Brodmann map showing important cortical auditory areas 41, 42, and 22.

perceive (i.e., recognize it is there), and discriminate (i.e., identify auditory segments in terms of frequency and intensity) sound; damage to these areas can result in a loss of awareness of sound, but with preserved auditory reflexes due to anatomical integrity at the level of the SOC.

Wernicke's Area

The auditory information processed in the primary auditory cortex is then sent to BA 22 in the dominant cerebral hemisphere (Figure 10-10). This area consists of the posterior two-thirds of the superior temporal gyrus and a structure called the **planum temporale** (Latin for "temporal plain"). BA 22 is known as Wernicke area (named after the German neurologist Karl Wernicke's) or the **auditory association cortex.** The planum temporale is in the shape of a flat triangle and is larger in the dominant cerebral hemisphere, which in most people is the left hemisphere. For those who are not left hemisphere dominant for language, this structure will be of equal size in both hemispheres or larger in the right hemisphere than in the left hemisphere.

The function of Wernicke's area is not well understood, but those with damage to this area have what is called Wernicke aphasia. One of the hallmark characteristics of this aphasia type is severely impaired auditory comprehension. Because of this observation, neuroscientists believe Wernicke's area in the dominant hemisphere is important in attaching meaning to others' speech. Specifically, they believe that it processes dominant word meanings of ambiguous words (e.g., if I say "bank," you associate the word "teller").

The area corresponding to Wernicke's area in the nondominant hemisphere may play a role in nondominant word meanings of ambiguous words (e.g., if I say "bank," you associate "river") (Harpaz, Levkovitz, & Lavidor, 2009).

Broca's Area

Wernicke's area (BA 22) connects to Broca's area (BAs 44, 45) via the arcuate fasciculus (Latin for "curved bundle"), an axonal tract that leaves BA 22 and inputs into BAs 44 and 45 and the prefrontal cortex as well as the angular gyrus (BA 39) and supramarginal gyrus (BA 40). Because those with Broca aphasia have difficulty understanding complex grammatical constructions, Broca's area appears to be recruited into the task of understanding these constructions.

Select Disorders of the Auditory System

Sensorineural Hearing Loss

A **sensorineural hearing loss** is a hearing loss caused by problems with either the inner ear or the vestibulocochlear nerve (cranial nerve VIII). When the loss is located in the inner ear, it is usually due to damage in the hair cells located in the organ of Corti. This damage can be induced by loud noise (**noise-induced hearing loss**) or by other conditions, such as **Meniere disease**, which is caused by a buildup of endolymph in the inner ear. Most cases of sensorineural hearing loss are due to inner ear issues involving the hair cells (**BOX 10-1**).

BOX 10-1   Sensorineural Hearing Loss and Cochlear Implants

Cochlear implants (**FIGURE 10-11**) are a treatment option for people with severe to profound cochlear hearing losses. When inner ear hair cells are damaged, the sound processing flow is broken in the inner ear and does not reach the brain. Cochlear implants are designed to fill in for this broken inner ear link. There are four parts to a cochlear implant, three of which are external and one that is internal. The one internal part is the intracochlear electrode array, which is tonotopically arranged. It is surgically implanted in the cochlea and takes advantage of the inner ear's tonotopic organization by stimulating the nerve directly. The inner ear's hair cells are essentially bypassed by this electrode, which directly stimulates the auditory branch of the vestibulocochlear nerve. The nerve then takes the auditory signal to the brain through the central auditory pathway, where it is processed. This signal is not perceived as in normal hearing, so it requires time and training to learn to interpret the signals. The external parts of the cochlear implant are the microphone, the processor, and the transmitter. The microphone picks up auditory signals from the environment and sends this signal to the processor, which turns it into an electrical signal. The processor then turns over this electrical signal to the transmitter (or coil), which sends it to the internal electrode array. This last external piece is held in place by a magnet implant just under the skin near the mastoid bone (**FIGURE 10-12**).

(continues)

BOX 10-1 Sensorineural Hearing Loss and Cochlear Implants *(continued)*

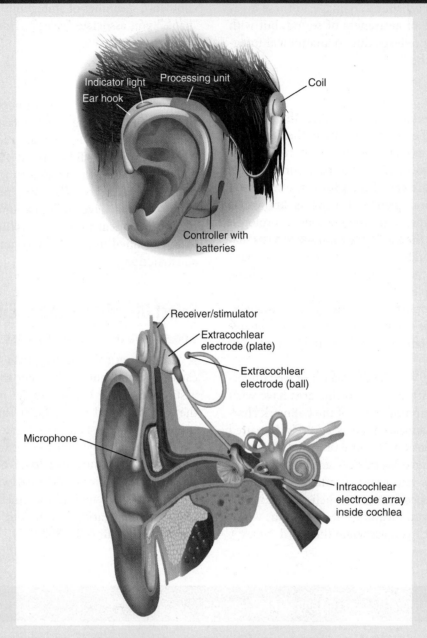

FIGURE 10-11 The external and internal components of a cochlear implant.

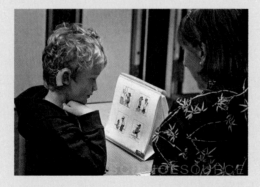

FIGURE 10-12 A 7-year-old boy who has been fitted with a cochlear implant.

Auditory Processing Disorder

Auditory processing is "what we do with what we hear" (Katz, 1992). An **auditory processing disorder (APD)** can be thought of as *dyslexia of the ears* in that there is difficulty processing and interpreting auditory symbols similar to how people with dyslexia have difficulty interpreting written symbols. The peripheral auditory system is intact in those who suffer from APD, but their brain struggles to process auditory information. The condition can be congenital or acquired through brain injuries, strokes, or other mechanisms.

In terms of specific difficulties, the American Speech-Language-Hearing Association (2005) reports that APD can include problems with the following:

- Sound localization and lateralization
- Auditory discrimination
- Auditory pattern recognition
- Temporal aspects of audition, including temporal integration, temporal discrimination (e.g., temporal gap detection), temporal ordering, and temporal masking
- Auditory performance in competing acoustic signals (including dichotic listening)
- Auditory performance with degraded acoustic signals

These problems are not believed to be caused by general attention problems, language disorders, or cognitive impairments, but APD may have associations with these conditions. Hearing and intelligence are intact in children with APD.

The National Institute on Deafness and Other Communication Disorders (2004) has listed warning signs of APD, which include the following:

- Trouble paying attention to and remembering information presented orally
- Problems carrying out multistep directions
- Poor listening skills
- Increased time to process information
- Low academic performance
- Behavior problems
- Language difficulty (e.g., they confuse syllable sequences and have problems developing vocabulary and understanding language)
- Difficulty with reading, comprehension, spelling, and vocabulary

Auditory training is the main method of treating APD; however, auditory training methods lack evidence to support their efficacy. There is some evidence that treatment targeting phonological disorders improves not only phonology but also auditory processing (Leite, Wertzner, & Matas, 2010).

Pure Word Deafness

Pure word deafness or auditory verbal agnosia is caused by bilateral damage to the superior temporal lobes, resulting in the inability to distinguish phonemes and, thus, comprehend speech. Patients do retain the ability to hear and comprehend nonspeech sounds, like a doorbell ringing or a bird singing, as well as the abilities to speak, read, and write. Pure word deafness is one of the first symptoms of Landau-Kleffner syndrome (LKS), a rare epileptic syndrome that occurs in children between 3 and 7 years of age (Metz-Lutz, 2009). It can also be a symptom of Alzheimer disease (Kim et al., 2011).

Deficits in Auditory Comprehension

Though not technically a disorder of the central auditory system, aphasia is a multimodality language disorder that can affect mapping meaning to sounds. Most patients with aphasia suffer from at least some high-level difficulties in auditory comprehension. When thinking about the classical aphasias, three stand out in terms of significant deficits in auditory comprehension: global, Wernicke, and transcortical sensory aphasia. What these three types of aphasia have in common is damage to the temporal lobe where the primary auditory cortex and Wernicke's area are located.

The name **global aphasia** sounds bad, and the name is fitting because this is the most severe form of aphasia. Severe deficits are found in all the modalities of language, including verbal formulation, auditory comprehension, reading, and writing. Verbally, patients are nonfluent and are either mute or produce just a few sounds or words. Repeating words is often very difficult. In terms of auditory comprehension, patients struggle to follow even one-step commands and to complete simple tasks like pointing to a picture in a field of two pictures after being given the name of one picture. Reading is equally compromised, with patients unable to match a single written picture to a picture in a field of two pictures. Often patients with global aphasia cannot write their name or other identifying information.

Wernicke aphasia causes severe deficits in auditory comprehension; however, unlike with global aphasia, these patients have fluent verbal output (100–200 words per minute), though it is filled with paraphasias (sound or word substitutions). They are described as having word salad in their verbal output, meaning it seems someone placed their words in a bowl, stirred them up, and then what was dumped out was their verbal output. Repeating is severely impaired, as is writing and reading.

Patients with **transcortical sensory aphasia (TSA)** are fluent like patients with Wernicke aphasia but have paraphasias in their speech. They also demonstrate echolalia, which is repeating what other people say. Unlike people with Wernicke aphasia, patients with TSA can repeat words said to them. Auditory comprehension is poor, as is reading and writing.

▶ The Neurology of Balance

Human beings are sensory creatures. We have five senses through which we experience the world: vision, hearing, smell, taste, and touch. Right now, if you are reading the print version of this text, the most prominent sense you are using is vision. Touch is also used as you touch and turn the pages, as is perhaps smell if the book still has that "new book" smell. However, there is a sixth sense working in the background of which you are probably not aware. It keeps you sitting upright as you read this text and coordinates your head and eye movements. The only time you may have been aware of the stealthy system behind this sense is when you had an inner ear infection and experienced vertigo or when you were on a boat in choppy waters and felt seasick. The sense is your sense of balance, and the main system behind it is called the vestibular system.

The vestibular system contributes to spatial orientation by constantly sending information about your head's position in space to your brain. When there is a change in head position, information concerning the direction and speed is relayed to the brain. This system does not work alone to maintain spatial orientation but rather works with your sense of vision and proprioception. (Proprioception is your body's eyes for itself.) This redundancy illustrates how important this sense is to living in and navigating our environment. The vestibular system will be examined in this chapter.

The Peripheral Vestibular System

The vestibular system is located in the same place as the cochlea—the inner ear. In fact, these two structures are connected to each other (**FIGURE 10-13**). Just as the cochlea contains the main organ of the hearing system, so the semicircular canals and the vestibule's utricle and saccule contain the main organs of the vestibular system.

Three semicircular canals are interconnected with each other. All three branch from the labyrinth and are filled with endolymph. Because we live in a three-dimensional world, each canal senses head movement in a particular dimension. The canals sit at right angles to each other to accomplish this (**FIGURE 10-14**). To imagine this arrangement, look over to a corner of the

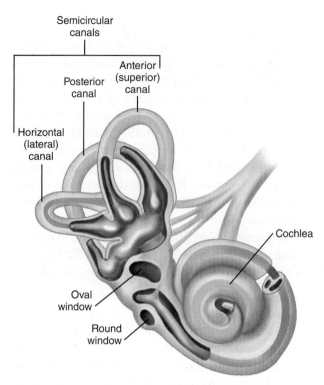

FIGURE 10-13 The semicircular canals.

room you are sitting in. Look at where the floor and two walls meet. The floor is the horizontal semicircular canal, which is sometimes referred to as the lateral canal; it senses head movement in the transverse or horizontal plane. For example, you use this canal when crossing the street, looking left and then right to make sure your path is free of cars. Continuing the analogy, one of the walls is the anterior semicircular canal, also known as the superior canal, which senses movement in the coronal plane. For example, if you touch your ear to your shoulder, you are activating this canal. The final wall is the posterior semicircular canal. It senses movement in the sagittal plane. This canal is activated when you nod your head yes. You can see that all planes of head movement are covered by these canals: horizontal, coronal, and sagittal. Movement can be a combination of multiple planes (e.g., left upward movement); when this is the case, multiple canals are involved. How this movement is specifically sensed is our next topic.

Each semicircular canal has an enlargement called an ampulla, and each ampulla contains a sensory epithelium called a crista (**FIGURE 10-15**). Each of these cristae contains a ridge of epithelium, the ampullary crest, which contains sensory hair cells similar to the organ of Corti in the cochlea. Each hair cell has stereocilia that protrude into a gelatinous structure called the cupula. These stereocilia are sensitive to rotary movements of the head (i.e., head turning left and right in relation to the body) in the horizontal plane.

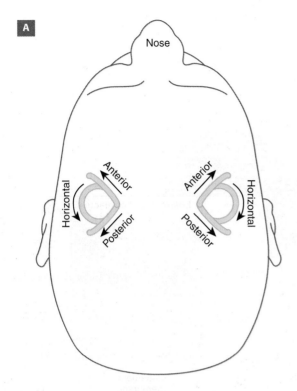

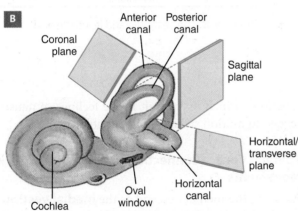

FIGURE 10-14 A. The arrangement of the semicircular canals. **B.** The semicircular canals and their planes. Notice the enlargement of each semicircular canal as it attaches at the vestibule. This enlargement is the ampulla.

When these movements occur, waves are produced in the endolymph that cause the stereocilia to move, triggering depolarization of the hair cell.

In the vestibule, there are two important structures, the utricle and the saccule. Each of these structures contains a sensory epithelium, called the macula, that is similar to the crista. One macula is called the macula utriculus (located in the utricle), and the other is the macula sacculus (located in the saccule). In both the utricle and saccule, the macula is made up of support cells layered with hair cells with stereocilia embedded in a gelatinous otolithic membrane with otoconia (calcium carbonite crystals) imbedded in it.

In the utricle, the macula is on the "floor" and the hair cells point up. These hair cells respond to linear acceleration on the horizontal plane (forward/backward) and right and left head tilt. The otolith membrane with the otoconia "leans" with the motion, causing depolarization of the hair cells. In contrast, in the saccule the macula is situated on the "back" and the hair cells point out. These hair cells respond to linear acceleration on the vertical plane, or moving up and down (as in an elevator). The depolarization of the hair cells with Ca^{++} and K^+ entering the cell occurs as in the cochlea, but now it happens with movement.

Like in the cochlea, the hair cells are transducers of hydraulic energy into nerve impulses. At the end of the hair cells are two kinds of cilia, stereocilia and kinocilia. There are approximately 100 stereocilia on each hair cell, but only 1 kinocilium per hair cell. When the stereocilia bend toward the kinocilium, potassium and calcium channels open, allowing K^+ and Ca^{++} to flow from the endolymph into the hair cells. This action depolarizes the hair cell (i.e., neural firing), exciting it to release the neurotransmitter glutamate at its base into the synaptic cleft. The neural signal is then transferred to the Scarpa ganglion of the vestibular branch of cranial nerve VIII, which transmits the signal to the brain. If the stereocilia sway away from the kinocilium, then the signal produced is inhibitory in nature, meaning action potentials are not sent to the brain. This is quite useful information to the brain. When the sensory structures from one inner ear are sending action potentials to the brain because the stereocilia are moving toward the kinocilium, the other inner ear's structures are not if the stereocilia are moving away from the kinocilium (such as when turning the head to the right). This dynamic tells the brain which way the head is turning.

The Central Vestibular System

Brainstem Organization and Connections

Vestibular Nucleus

The vestibular portion of cranial nerve VIII leaves the semicircular canals and the utricle and saccule serving the left and right vestibules, joins the cochlear portion, and travels through the internal auditory canal before inputting into the brainstem at the cerebellopontine angle. Fibers from it input into the **vestibular nucleus (VN)**, a structure consisting of four nuclei on each side of the brainstem—the superior, inferior, medial, and lateral (Deiter) nuclei. Axons from these nuclei make connections with various nervous system structures that form the five functional systems that will be considered next.

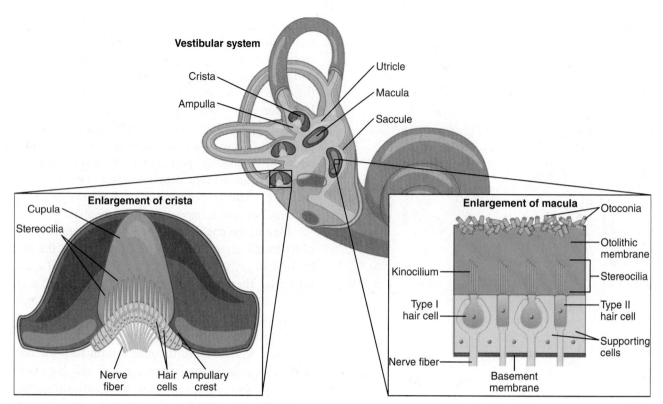

FIGURE 10-15 **A.** A semicircular canal's ampulla and an enlarged picture of its crista. **B.** The vestibule and its utricle and saccule with an enlarged picture of the saccule's macula.

Cerebellar Connections and Balance

Vestibular fibers project to the cerebellum and back from the cerebellum to the VN. The cerebellum coordinates motor movement, so these connections facilitate the coordinated movements necessary to preserve the body's balance.

Brainstem Nuclei Connections and Eye Movements

Fibers project from the VN to form the medial longitudinal fasciculus that inputs into various nuclei in the brainstem that control eye movements (**FIGURE 10-16**). These nuclei include the abducens nucleus in the pons, the trochlear nucleus in the midbrain, and the oculomotor nucleus in the midbrain. From these nuclei, cranial nerves III, IV, and VI project to the extrinsic eye muscles that move the eyeballs. These connections allow you to keep your eyes fixed on a target while moving your head (try it now). We do this without thinking about it, so this ability is called the **vestibulo-ocular reflex**.

Brainstem Connections and Nausea

The VN make connections to the reticular formation (RF). The RF coordinates visceral/autonomic functions, which may result in the feelings of nausea related to motion sickness and possible vomiting.

Spinal Cord Connections and Head/Neck Movements

Axons of the medial descend as the **medial vestibulospinal tracts** (**FIGURE 10-17**). These tracts input in the lower motor neuron portions of the cervical spinal cord. This results in our ability to rotate our head in one direction and our body in the other direction. This is a reflex called the **vestibulocollic reflex**.

Spinal Cord Connections and Arm/Leg Adjustments

Axons from the lateral VN descend to form the **lateral vestibulospinal tract** (Figure 10-17). This ipsilateral tract terminates in the thoracic and lumbar lower motor neurons of the spinal cord. The lower motor neuron's axons then pass to the extensor muscles of the arms and legs, resulting in the **vestibulospinal reflex**. You can test this reflex by bending over to pick something up. When you do, you will usually unconsciously extend one or more of your limbs to keep yourself balanced.

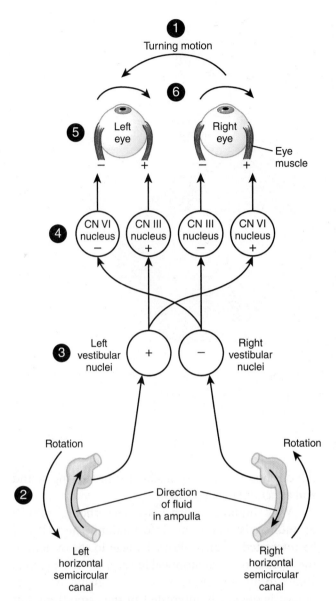

FIGURE 10-16 An example of vestibular neural organization using the horizontal semicircular canal as an example. 1. The turning motion of the head. 2. The effect of the head's motion on the horizontal canals and their fluid. 3. The left and right vestibular nuclei. 4. Important cranial nerve nuclei and their connections to eye muscles. 5. The effect on particular eye muscles and the turning of the eyes in the opposite direction of the head movement.

The vestibular system works in the background, hardly being noticed. This is because there are few connections between this system and the cerebral cortex. An indirect pathway does exist between the VN and the thalamus. The thalamus then projects to a small part of the postcentral gyrus (sensory cortex) and the middle temporal gyrus. It would appear that the cortex activates our conscious awareness of our vestibular system when there is something wrong with

it (e.g., vertigo), such as in the case of the following select examples of vestibular disorders.

Select Vestibular Disorders

Vestibular Schwannoma

Schwann cells are the myelin producers of the peripheral nervous system. A schwannoma is a slow-growing, unilateral, benign tumor that occurs in the peripheral nervous system, most commonly on cranial nerves. When a schwannoma occurs on cranial nerve VIII, it typically arises on one of the two vestibular branches of the nerve and therefore is properly called a vestibular schwannoma. The first symptoms patients typically report are hearing loss in one ear and tinnitus (i.e., a sensation of a sound, typically, a high-pitched ringing) in the same ear. Other symptoms include headache, balance issues, vertigo, and nausea. Schwannomas are diagnosed through neuroimaging techniques, like magnetic resonance imaging. Once diagnosed, treatment is usually surgery to remove the tumor (Victor & Ropper, 2001). All cranial nerve VIII schwannomas begin in the internal auditory canal; and as they grow, they expand out this canal; into the base of the skull. Preservation of hearing in surgical cases is dependent on time of detection and location in the internal auditory canal. Schwannomas that are completely within the internal auditory canal ("intracanalicular") have a better chance of hearing preservation postoperatively. With larger tumors expanding into the skull base, most likely hearing will be lost postoperatively, and as well, there is an attendant risk of damage to the facial nerve (cranial nerve VII) because it is in this same region. Compression of cranial nerve VII can cause facial paresis or paralysis. Schwannomas are generally unilateral (95% of the time) but can be bilateral and develop at a younger age in people with a genetic problem called neurofibromatosis-2.

Labyrinthitis

Labyrinthitis is an infection of the inner ear that affects the vestibular nerve. It is usually caused by a virus but can also be bacterial in origin. Onset is usually rapid, with patients reporting vertigo, nausea, and vomiting. People suffering from this condition report that they need to remain in bed to lessen the symptoms. Interestingly enough, patients do not usually report tinnitus or hearing loss, illustrating that the condition is affecting only the vestibular portions of the inner ear. Virally caused labyrinthitis usually will go away on its own in a matter of a few days to a week without

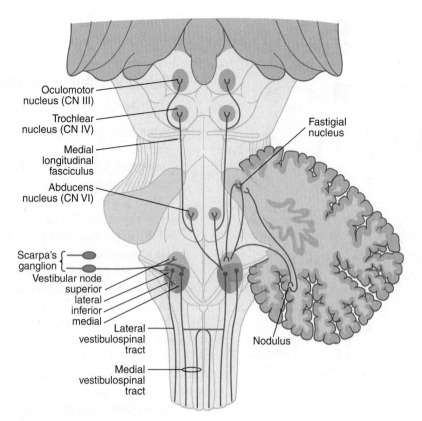

FIGURE 10-17 Dorsal view of the brainstem illustrating the central vestibular pathway.

treatment. Bacterial labyrinthitis may require antibiotics (Victor & Ropper, 2001).

▶ Conclusion

In this chapter, the route of the central auditory pathway has been traced from the cochlea to the CN through various brainstem structures and finally to the cerebral cortex via the thalamus. The route of the central vestibular pathway was also traced. An important observation was made in this chapter about hearing: Tonotopic organization, which begins in the cochlea, is maintained through the whole pathway and even in

the cerebral tissues responsible for processing sound and attaching meaning to it.

Why should a speech-language pathologist (SLP) or audiologist know this information? The SLP will be interested to know how damage to the system at the various neuroanatomical levels impairs a person's ability to understand speech and language. An audiologist is obviously interested in the same thing but also in how tests, like auditory brainstem response, examine this pathway and assess where damage is in the system (**BOX 10-2**). Knowing this information leads to appropriate treatment for the patient, especially babies and others incapable of behavioral audiological measures.

BOX 10-2 Auditory Brainstem Response

Auditory brainstem response (ABR) is a test that evaluates the integrity of cranial nerve VIII and the central auditory pathway. It is also sometimes known as an auditory evoked potential. ABR is used on people who cannot respond to typical hearing examinations. For example, pure tone hearing tests require the listener to raise a hand on the side on which he or she hears a short beep. Some people, such as babies or people with disorders of consciousness, cannot respond to these types of tests, so ABR is an appropriate substitute. To perform the test, electrodes are placed on the subject's skin and then hooked to a computer (**FIGURE 10-18**). Sounds are then played through earphones, and the

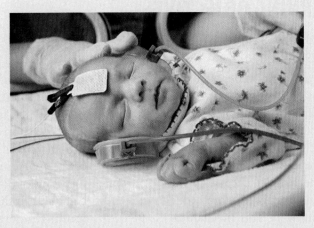

FIGURE 10-18 A child undergoing an auditory brainstem response screening.

Courtesy of Natus Neurology Incorporated (Grass Brand), 3150 Pleasant View Road, Middleton, WI.

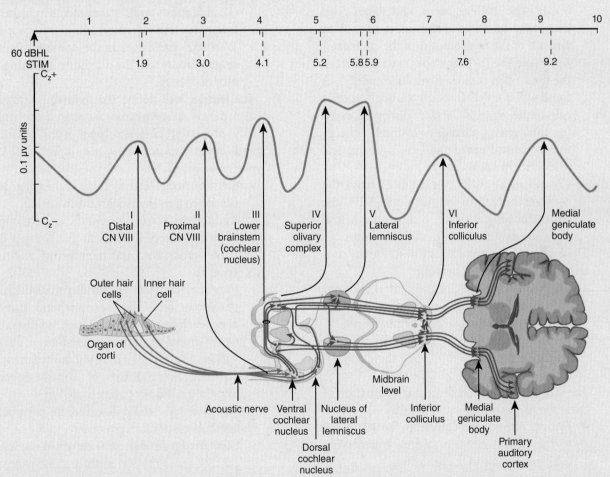

FIGURE 10-19 Auditory brainstem response (ABR). ABR involves waves I through V.

Courtesy of Natus Neurology Incorporated (Grass Brand), 3150 Pleasant View Road, Middleton, WI.

equipment records the evoked potentials generated (**FIGURE 10-19**). ABR and otoacoustic emissions (OAE), a test that tests up to the outer hair cells in the cochlea, are the instruments of choice for screening the hearing of newborn infants. If the baby fails the screening, further audiological examination is warranted. Screening infants is part of the Early Hearing Detection and Intervention (EHDI) program in which every newborn infant receives a hearing screening using ABR and/or OAE. All 50 states have EHDI programs in place (American Speech Language Hearing Association, 2018).

SUMMARY OF LEARNING OBJECTIVES

The following were the main learning objectives of this chapter. The information that should have been learned is below each learning objective.

1. The learner will list and briefly describe the peripheral auditory system.
   - *Outer ear:* Involves the location, collection, and funneling of acoustic energy to the middle ear via the external auditory meatus.
   - *Middle ear:* Involves acoustic energy being transduced into mechanical energy as the tympanic membrane begins to vibrate due to sound waves hitting it. This mechanical energy is then transmitted through the ossicular chain, which is composed of three small bones—the malleus, incus, and stapes. This causes the footplate of the stapes to rock in and out of the oval window of the cochlea.
   - *Inner ear:* The rocking stapes causes waves in the fluid-filled cochlea (hydraulic energy); as these waves travel through the cochlea, hair cells in the organ of Corti are disrupted, causing final energy changes—hydraulic energy to mechanical energy and then mechanical to electrochemical energy.
   - *Cranial nerve VIII:* Nerve fibers from the cochlear branch of cranial nerve VIII, the vestibulocochlear nerve, pick up the neural impulses and transmit them to the brain.

2. The learner will list and briefly describe the central auditory system of hearing.
   - *The brainstem:* It begins the central auditory system by receiving and routing auditory information to the cerebral hemispheres.
   - *The cerebral hemispheres:* Auditory areas of the brain decode and identify the electrical impulses.

3. The learner will list and describe the function of the main central auditory structures.
   - *Cranial nerve VIII:* Connects the inner ear to the central nervous system, transferring cochlear signals to the brainstem.
   - *Cochlear nucleus (CN):* several groups of nuclei that receive auditory signals from cranial nerve VIII.
   - *Superior olivary complex (SOC):* Integrates auditory information and specializes in low-frequency hearing, specifically integrating low-frequency hearing from the right and left ears into what is called binaural hearing.
   - *Lateral lemniscus:* a tract of six pathways/axons that travels from the CN and SOC to the inferior colliculus in the midbrain.
   - *Inferior colliculus:* the auditory center of the midbrain that regulates our acoustic startle reflex, which is when we suddenly move in response to an unanticipated sound.
   - *Medial geniculate body:* the auditory center of the thalamus that acts as a relay station, directing auditory tracts from the inferior colliculus to the auditory cortex of the cerebrum's temporal lobe.
   - *Primary auditory cortex:* Locates, perceives (i.e., recognizes it is there), and discriminates (i.e., identifies auditory segments in terms of frequency and intensity) sound information.
   - *Wernicke's area:* area in the dominant hemisphere important in attaching meaning to others' speech.

4. The learner will define the following auditory disorders: *sensorineural hearing loss, auditory processing disorder, pure word deafness,* and *other disorders that may affect auditory comprehension.*
   - *Sensorineural hearing loss:* a hearing loss caused by problems with the inner ear.
   - *Auditory processing disorder:* Can be thought of as dyslexia of the ears in that there is difficulty processing and interpreting auditory symbols.
   - *Pure word deafness:* an inability to distinguish phonemes and, thus, comprehend speech; nonspeech sound interpretation is preserved.
   - *Other disorders that affect auditory comprehension.* Aphasia is a multimodality language disorder. Some forms of aphasia involve impaired auditory comprehension.

5. The learner will briefly describe the peripheral and central vestibular systems.
   - *Semicircular canals:* three canals in the inner ear that sense motion in three dimensions
   - *Utricle and saccule:* structures in the vestibule of the inner ears that sense linear acceleration in the horizontal and vertical planes
   - *Vestibular nucleus:* a group of nuclei that contain axons that make connections with various nervous system structures that form the five functional systems: balance, eye movements, nausea, head/neck movements, and arm/leg adjustments

6. The learner will define the following vestibular disorders: *vestibular schwannoma* and *labyrinthitis.*

- *Vestibular schwannoma:* a slow-growing, benign peripheral nervous system tumor of cranial nerve VIII

- *Labyrinthitis:* an infection of the inner ear that can affect the vestibular branch of cranial nerve VIII

KEY TERMS

Audition

Auditory association cortex

Auditory brainstem response (ABR)

Auditory processing disorder (APD)

Binaural hearing

Central auditory system

Cochlear nucleus (CN)

Global aphasia

Inferior colliculus

Inner ear

Lateral lemniscus

Lateral superior olivary complex (LSOC)

Lateral vestibulospinal tract

Medial superior olivary complex (MSOC)

Medial vestibulospinal tracts

Meniere disease

Middle ear

Noise-induced hearing loss

Outer ear

Peripheral auditory system

Planum temporale

Sensorineural hearing loss

Superior olivary complex (SOC)

Tonotopic organization

Transcortical sensory aphasia (TSA)

Transducer

Vestibular nucleus (VN)

Vestibulocollic reflex

Vestibulo-ocular reflex

Vestibulospinal reflex

Wernicke aphasia

DRAW IT TO KNOW IT

1. Draw a cross-section of the cochlea (see Figure 10-4) and label the following: scala vestibuli, scala media, scala tympani, organ of Corti, inner hair cells, and outer hair cells.

2. Draw and label the central auditory pathway (see Figure 10-9).

QUESTIONS FOR DEEPER REFLECTION

1. In essay form, describe the process of hearing from when a sound is heard through when the brain processes the signal.

2. In essay form, describe how the vestibular system works.

3. List and define the central auditory disorders discussed in this chapter.

CASE STUDY

Julie is a 46-year-old college professor who has experienced tinnitus and a slow loss of her hearing in her left ear over the past year and a half. Her neurologist ordered an MRI, which revealed a mass on the vestibular branch of her left cranial nerve VIII. Julie's neurologist counseled her that it would be best to monitor the growth of the tumor, but that a day might come when she might need to have it surgically removed.

1. What condition to you think Julie has? Why do you think this?

2. What could happen to Julie is the mass continues to grow?

SUGGESTED PROJECTS

1. Borrow a portable audiometer from your clinic and test the hearing of five people. Did you detect any hearing losses? Is so, what kind?

2. Choose one of the disorders discussed in this chapter and write a two- to three-page paper with the following sections: cause, signs and symptoms, diagnosis, and treatment.

3. Read Chapter 3 of Oliver Sack's *The Man Who Mistook His Wife for a Hat*. Write one or two pages about how this clinical tale relates to the vestibular system.

REFERENCES

American Speech-Language-Hearing Association (ASHA). (2005). *ASHA practice policy*. Retrieved from http://www.asha.org/policy

American Speech-Language-Hearing Association. (2018). *Early hearing detection and intervention (EHDI)*. https://www.asha.org/Advocacy/federal/Early-Hearing-Detection-and-Intervention/

Davis, M., Gendelman, D. S., Tischler, M. D., & Gendelman, P. M. (1982). A primary acoustic startle circuit: Lesion and stimulation studies. *Journal of Neuroscience*, *2*(6), 791–805.

Harpaz, Y., Levkovitz, Y., & Lavidor, M. (2009). Lexical ambiguity resolution in Wernicke's area and its right homologue. *Cortex*, *45*(9), 1097–1103.

Katz, J. (1992). Classification of auditory processing disorders. In J. Katz, N. A. Stecker, & D. Henderson (Eds.), *Central auditory processing: A transdisciplinary view* (pp. 81–92). St. Louis, MO: Mosby Year Book.

Kim, S. H., Suh, M. K., Seo, S. W., Chin, J., Han, S. H., & Na, D. L. (2011). Pure word deafness in a patient with early-onset Alzheimer's disease: An unusual presentation. *Journal of Clinical Neurology*, *7*(4), 227–230.

Leite, R. A., Wertzner, H. F., & Matas, C. G. (2010). Long latency auditory evoked potentials in children with phonological disorder. *Pró-Fono Revista de Atualização Científica*, *22*(4), 561–566.

Martin, F. N., & Clark J. G. (2000). *Introduction to audiology* (7th ed). Needham Heights, MA: Allyn & Bacon.

Metz-Lutz, M. N. (2009). The assessment of auditory function in CSWS: Lessons from long-term outcome. *Epilepsia*, *50*(s7), 73–76.

National Institute on Deafness and Other Communication Disorders. (2004). *Auditory processing disorders in children* (NIH Pub. No. 01-4949). Retrieved from http://www.ldonline.org/article/8056

Victor, M., & Ropper, A. H. (2001). *Principles of neurology*. New York, NY: McGraw-Hill Medical.

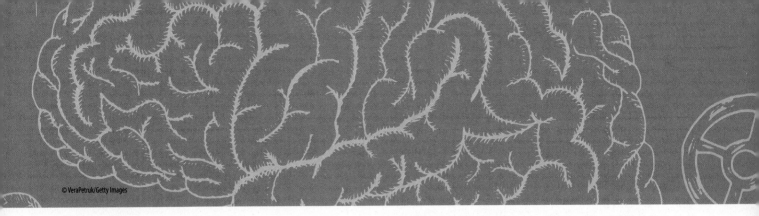

© VeraPetruk/Getty Images

CHAPTER 11

The Neurology of Speech

CHAPTER PREVIEW

We now turn to the neurology of speech. Speech is a complex motor act involving many muscles and nerves. The nervous system acts as a conductor coordinating a great orchestra of instruments that together produce human speech.

IN THIS CHAPTER

In this chapter, we will . . .

- Survey the motor speech system
- Examine different forms of dysarthria and apraxia of speech as they relate to motor pathways
- Review important sensory pathways for speech

LEARNING OBJECTIVES

1. The learner will outline the major components of the motor speech system.
2. The learner will connect different places of damage in the motor speech system to different forms of dysarthria.
3. The learner will identify places of damage associated with apraxia of speech.
4. The learner will describe the importance of the sensory system to speech.
5. The learner will describe the human response space and the communication disorders professional's role in expanding it.

▶ Introduction

The motor system is a complex system involving a number of pathways and structures that make movement of both voluntary and involuntary muscles possible. The motor speech system is a subunit of the motor system, and an understanding of the motor system gives the student an understanding of the motor speech system as well as motor speech disorders.

The motor speech system is one possible language route. Humans can also express language through writing or through gestures, such as those used in American Sign Language (ASL). Speech is a dynamic motor process involving the coordination of respiration, phonation, resonance, and articulation in order to produce strings of speech sounds grouped together in words. The purpose of this chapter is to survey the neurology of the motor speech system and to discuss motor speech disorders.

▶ The Motor Speech System

A multilevel division of control is helpful in grasping the complexity of the motor speech system (**FIGURE 11-1**). These levels are as follows:

- The conceptual level
- The linguistic planning level
- The motor planning and programming levels
- The motor control circuits
- The direct motor pathway
- The indirect motor pathway
- The final common pathway
- The sensory system

The Conceptual Level

We all have ideas, thoughts, and feelings swimming around in our heads. This is our first-person perspective. These ideas, thoughts, and feelings are known only to us (i.e., they are private to us), unless of course we decide we would like to let someone into our first-person perspective through communication. When we make this decision to communicate, we then decide how to communicate. If we choose the route of producing language orally through speech, we then form an intention to express our ideas, thoughts, and feelings (**BOX 11-1**). Where do these thoughts swim and intentions reside? It is best thought of as being a whole-brain activity, involving the entire cerebral cortex, with the prefrontal

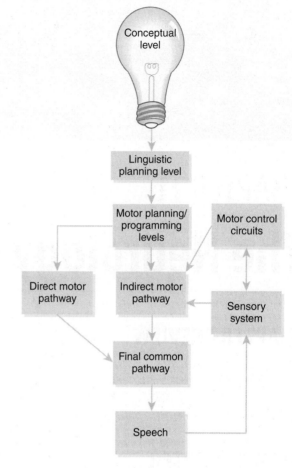

FIGURE 11-1 The motor speech system.

cortex and limbic system taking primary roles in the process.

The Linguistic Planning Level

There are two parts of the planning level, linguistic planning and motor planning. Linguistic information, which includes content, form, and use, makes up the substance of our speech. Content or semantics is the meaning of our language. Form is the structure or grammar of language and includes phonology (sound system structure), morphology (word structure), and syntax (sentence structure). Lastly, language use involves all the pragmatic rules we use as we express language through speech.

Linguistic planning is nonmotor in nature. It involves taking one of our ideas, thoughts, or feelings and *dressing it* in language, what is called encoding. This planning engages the dominant language hemisphere, which is the left hemisphere in most people. Specifically, the dominant dorsal perisylvian region (i.e., the region around the lateral fissure) is highly engaged in linguistic planning.

BOX 11-1 Speech and Free Will

It has always been assumed that speech is a voluntary act of our free will. In other words, the typical order of events is that I create an intention to speak of my own volition, which then sets off a series of neural impulses to accomplish the very thing I intended to do.

In the 1980s, a researcher named Benjamin Libet produced a series of experiments that challenged this notion (Libet, Gleason, Wright, & Pearl, 1983; Libet, 1993). His research question was: What happens in the brain just before we make a voluntary, free-will action like speaking? Libet hooked his test subjects up to electroencephalography (EEG) equipment to detect the brain's electrical activity and to an electromyogram (EMG) on their finger (**FIGURE 11-2**). This way, he could measure the time it took from the generation of a neural impulse to when a subject actually moved his or her finger. In addition, a specialized clock was placed in front of the subjects so they could report the exact time they first had an intention to move their finger. In summary, Libet was attempting to measure three things:

1. The time at which a person formed an intention to move his or her finger
2. The time at which a neural impulse to move the finger was initiated
3. The time at which the finger actually moved

One would expect that the order of events would occur as follows: 1, 2, 3. Instead, Libet found the order was 2, 1, 3. In other words, the neural impulse came first, then the intention, and finally the action. It would appear that a so-called voluntary free act is not so free if neural impulses precede the conscious intention to act. If this is true, what do we do with the concept of free will? The brain seems to be doing all the choosing before I am consciously aware of it. Can I truly claim ownership of my acts, including my speech acts? There has been much criticism of Libet and his experiments in this arena (see Seifert, 2011). For example, some have criticized him for not considering other brain states that may be occurring before the intention was formed (a kind of deliberating stage).

Historically, there have been two views of free will, libertarianism and compatibilism. Libertarians define free will as a person's capacity for choosing otherwise, whereas compatibilists define it as acting without coercion. A libertarian would believe that free will and determinism are incompatible, whereas a compatibilist would believe that they are compatible. Typically, the discussion is centered around whether we have free will or not (i.e., a binary property), but

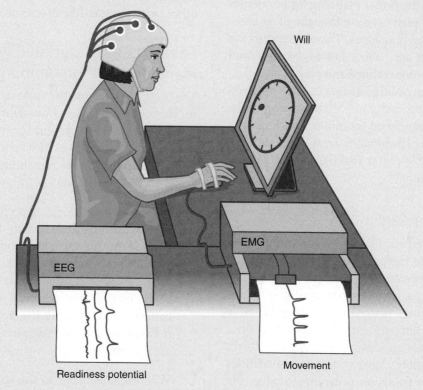

FIGURE 11-2 The Libet experiments attempted to demonstrate that the brain decides to initiate motor functions before a person consciously chooses to make any movements.

(continues)

BOX 11-1 Speech and Free Will   *(continued)*

perhaps it is better defined as a scalable property. In other words, free will is something of which we have more or less, depending on the constraints on us. Spence (2009) calls this the *human response space*. This is the space within a person can act, a space with constraints or walls around it. Some people have more space to act; others have less. What are some of these constraints? One example might be an anatomical restraint. A person who has a stroke might experience paralysis and thus might not be able to speak in the way that he or she wants. His or her response space has been narrowed by the stroke. Another example of a restraint is society. We might refrain from a certain action (e.g., eating one's grandmother) because society frowns on such an act. Other restraint categories include the physical environment, brain anatomy, neurochemistry, physiology, psychology, phenomenology (e.g., lack of "feeling emotion"), and genetics. Spence notes, "It is not the instant of the act but its context that seems to matter" (p. 395).

Perhaps it is time to reconsider what we mean by free will and move our attention away from the instant of action to the context of that action. Our patients with motor speech disorders (MSDs), like dysarthria and apraxia of speech (AOS), experience the restraint of their impaired neuroanatomy, which limits their ability to act as they desire. This is where speech-language pathologists (SLPs) and audiologists come in. Our job is to work hard in therapy with our patients and try to increase their human response space for communication.

The Motor Planning and Programming Levels

Motor Planning

The second part of planning is motor planning. Once phonological assembly (i.e., assigning correct phonemes in correct order) has taken place in the linguistic planning phase, the motor planning for phonemes takes place. Motor plans can be thought of as blueprints for actualizing phonemes. These blueprints are unrefined when we are babies, but as we grow and learn, they become more refined and precise and need only to be recalled in order to be executed (as opposed to being created anew each time). Neuroanatomically, the frontal lobe is important for motor planning, specifically Broca's area (Brodmann areas [BAs] 44, 45), parts of the premotor cortex (BA 6), and the supplementary motor area.

Motor Programming

Motor plans are prerequisites for a motor program to be executed; without them, motor programs would be aimless. Programs have to do with the execution of phonemes in time and space. It takes many motor programs to accomplish a motor plan. An illustrative example is the Ford Motor Company. Ford has a planning division that designs cars, producing blueprints for them. Ford also has assembly plants with robotic machines that actually follow computer programs to make the car plans come into existence. Many different computer programs have to be executed to fulfill a car plan. It is similar with motor plans. Motor plans contain the specific, individual movements of the speech organs to produce speech sounds (i.e., motor programs).

Proper speech sound production requires that the speech organs move accurately and precisely in terms of articulatory target, timing, muscle tone, and force. Sensory information is also incorporated into the process to give feedback, allowing for midcourse corrections of the articulators. The neurological structures involved in programming include the cerebellum, basal ganglia, and supplementary motor area as well as other cortical areas, like Broca's area.

Speech Issues Associated With the Motor Planning and Programming Levels

The umbrella term **motor speech disorders (MSDs)** includes two disorders, dysarthria and apraxia of speech (AOS). The different forms of dysarthria collectively make up 92% of MSD cases, while apraxia of speech accounts for the remaining 8% (Duffy, 2005). Duffy (2005) defines AOS as follows:

> AOS is a neurologic speech disorder that reflects an impaired capacity to plan or program sensorimotor commands necessary for directing movements that result in phonetically and prosodically normal speech. It can occur in the absence of physiologic disturbances associated with the dysarthrias and in the absence of disturbance in any components of language. (p. 307)

When lesions occur to the structures vital to the motor planning and programming levels, AOS may result.

Duffy (2005) combines the motor planning and programming levels into what he calls the motor speech programmer (MSP), which anatomically is spread throughout the left hemisphere, particularly in the left perisylvian region. It is influenced by numerous other structures, such as the motor control circuits as well as the limbic system and the right hemisphere. The MSP relies heavily on the frontal lobe, particularly Broca's area, and the supplementary motor area. Lesions in these areas can lead to AOS, but lesions to the insula or the basal ganglia can also lead to it.

The hallmark characteristic of AOS is searching and groping for articulatory placement when attempting to speak in the absence of any musculature abnormality. These patients know what they want to say, but they cannot "pull up" the appropriate motor plans and programs to execute saying the word. They are like a professional tennis player who suddenly "forgets" how to hit a forehand or backhand but retains his or her muscle strength and range of motion. The motor plans and programs, developed over years of practice, are absent or impaired even though the player's muscles are intact.

In addition to searching and groping behavior, patients make more substitution errors than omissions, distortions, or additions. Errors also occur more in place rather than manner or voice. Consonants are more difficult to produce than vowels, and consonant clusters are more difficult than single consonants. These patients are more successful in producing sounds in the front of the mouth as compared to back sounds, probably because frontal sounds are highly visible and easier to mimic. Overall, people with AOS make inconsistent errors in articulation, differing from children with phonological disorders, who have discernable error patterns called phonological processes. One of the most amazing phenomena is the occasional periods of error-free speech. After struggling for many minutes, a patient might suddenly exclaim, "Oh damn it" as clear as a bell.

The Motor Control Circuits

There are two control circuits important to speech, the basal ganglia and the cerebellum. These circuits are important in motor programming of speech by coordinating, integrating, and refining the movements of the direct and indirect pathways, which will be discussed in a moment. These circuits can be thought of as fine tuners, just as tuning up a car makes it run smoother and more efficiently. Both these circuits could be discussed under the indirect motor pathway, but we will discuss them separately so they receive their due attention.

The Basal Ganglia Circuit

The basal ganglia are a collection of nuclei including the caudate nucleus, putamen, globus pallidus, substantia nigra, and subthalamic nucleus. This system is central to the indirect motor system, also known as the extrapyramidal system. The basal ganglia nuclei form various afferent and efferent loops connecting the cerebral cortex, premotor cortex, supplementary motor area, thalamus, and substantia nigra (**FIGURE 11-3**). In addition to these connections, the basal ganglia use several neurotransmitters to regulate motor functioning, including acetylcholine (ACh), dopamine, and gamma-aminobutyric acid (GABA). The purpose of these loops and neurotransmitters is specifically to regulate muscle tone and posture and to smooth or refine muscle contraction. They also seem to have a dampening effect on the motor signals sent from the cerebral cortex. Damage to the basal ganglia system results in dyskinesias and conditions like Parkinson disease and Huntington disease. In these conditions, we can witness the loss of this dampening effect as we observe tremors and other dyskinesias.

The Cerebellar Circuit

The **cerebellar circuit** could also be subsumed under the indirect motor pathway (i.e., extrapyramidal system), but it will be discussed separately to highlight the cerebellum's contribution to speech production. As discussed previously, the cerebellum rests posterior to the pons and inferior to the temporal lobe. The cerebellum can be divided into two hemispheres, the right cerebellar hemisphere and the left cerebellar hemisphere. Each hemisphere has three lobes: the flocculonodular, anterior, and posterior. Of these three, the posterior lobe plays the most important role in speech production. Specifically, it automatically incorporates feedback "for coordinating skilled, sequential voluntary muscle activity" (Duffy, 2005, p. 54). This type of movement is obviously crucial in speech production. The cerebellum also has a number of afferent and efferent tracts that run to and from it (**FIGURE 11-4**). Afferent tracts greatly outnumber efferent ones, which demonstrates how important sensory feedback (e.g., proprioception of the speech muscles) is to coordinated motor function like speech.

Functionally, the cerebellum plays a role in a motor feedback loop between the cerebellum and the premotor cortex (BA 6) and the precentral gyrus (BA 4). When the primary motor strip (BA 4) sends a motor signal through the direct motor system, the signal is most likely unrefined and needs the refining effect of the cerebellum. A copy of this message travels

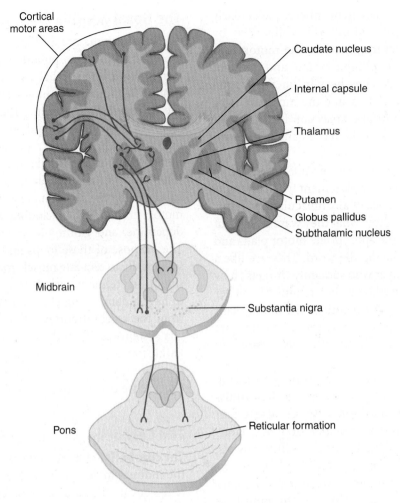

FIGURE 11-3 The basal ganglia control circuit.

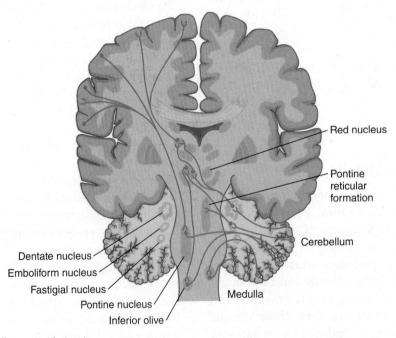

FIGURE 11-4 The cerebellar control circuit.

to the cerebellum via the corticopontine-cerebellar tract. The cerebellum then compares this information with the proprioception and kinesthetic information it receives from muscles and joints and coordinates muscle activity so that it is smooth and precise. Thus, the cerebellum makes an important contribution to the **diadochokinesia** (i.e., precise, rapid, alternating movements) necessary for speech. Disruptions in this ability lead to ataxia, a lack of order and coordination between muscles, and adiadochokinesia, an inability to perform rapid, alternating movements. Diadochokinesia can be tested in speech by having a patient say "pa-ta-ka" as rapidly and accurately as possible. Cerebellar damage can lead to a dysarthria called **ataxic dysarthria** that is characterized by harsh voice, monopitch, loud voice, imprecise consonants, and irregular breakdown in articulation. Often, patients with ataxic dysarthria sound drunk to the listener; as a result, listeners are not always empathetic regarding the patient's disorder and may even accuse him or her of being intoxicated.

The Direct Motor Pathway

The direct motor pathway is also known as the pyramidal system. This system is made up of two motor pathways, the lateral corticobulbar tract and the lateral corticospinal tract, and one medial motor pathway, the anterior corticospinal tract (TABLE 11-1). The lateral corticobulbar tract will be the focus in this section because it controls the movement of the speech muscles. The *cortico* portion of this name refers to the cerebral cortex, and the *bulbar* part refers to the brainstem because it is bulbous (i.e., "bulging"). This tract controls the muscles of the neck and face, including those important for speech and swallowing.

The pyramidal system receives its name from the primary type of cell in this system, **pyramidal neurons**. The neurons' cell bodies are in the shape of pyramids, hence their name (FIGURE 11-5). Betz cells, the largest type of pyramidal cell, are found only in the fifth layer of the cerebral cortex and the lateral corticospinal and lateral corticobulbar tracts of the pyramidal system; they occur nowhere else in the nervous

TABLE 11-1 The Motor Pathways

Pathway	Tract	Origin	Decussation	Ending	Function
Lateral motor pathways	Lateral corticobulbar	Primary motor cortex (BA 4)	Medulla/spinal cord juncture	Brainstem	Movement of contralateral head region
	Lateral corticospinal	Primary motor cortex (BA 4)	Medulla/spinal cord juncture	Spinal cord	Movement of contralateral limbs
	Rubrospinal	Midbrain	Midbrain	Cervical spinal cord	Flexor tone
Medial motor pathways	Anterior corticospinal	Primary (BA 4) and premotor (BA 6) cortex	None	Cervical and thoracic spinal cord	Movement of trunk muscles
	Vestibulospinal	Pons and medulla	None	Throughout whole spinal cord	Extensor tone and spinal reflexes
	Reticulospinal	Pons and medulla	None	Throughout whole spinal cord	Posture and gait
	Tectospinal	Midbrain	Midbrain	Cervical spinal cord	Coordination of head and eye movements

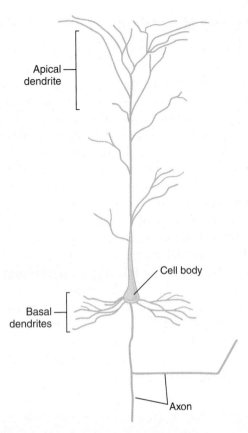

FIGURE 11-5 A pyramidal neuron.

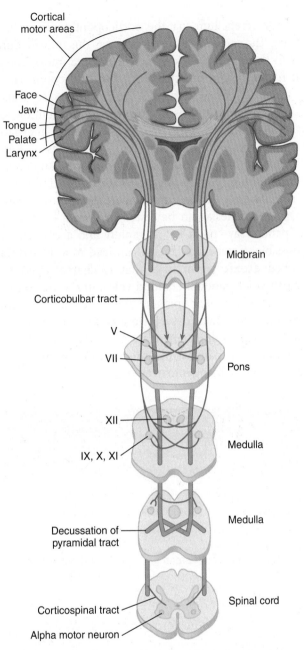

FIGURE 11-6 The direct motor system. Note the directness of this pathway and the decussation at the level of the medulla.

system. The Betz cell bodies are located in the cerebral cortex, and their axons course down through the lateral corticospinal tract and synapse directly to the ventral horn cells of the spinal cord, which then synapse directly with muscles. The lateral corticobulbar tract follows the same pattern as the lateral corticospinal tract, except it synapses with cranial nerve nuclei in the brainstem rather than the spinal cord. Overall, pyramidal cells are crucial for the modulation of the pyramidal system as well as the nervous system overall (Spruston, 2009).

The **pyramidal system** is a voluntary motor system that controls gross motor movement. In other words, it controls those actions we consciously make (e.g., I will now stick out my tongue), but in an unrefined way. The refinement comes through the basal ganglia and cerebellar control circuits. The tracts that make up this system are very direct, like an express train (**FIGURE 11-6**). They begin in the primary motor cortex (BA 4), which lies on the frontal lobe's postcentral gyrus, and in the premotor cortex (BA 6). When mapped out, a homunculus (Latin for "little person") can be generated from the primary motor cortex's motor areas. Exaggerated parts of the homunculus illustrate that more motor fibers are associated with that area than others are, primarily because that body

part (e.g., hand or mouth) performs fine motor activity and needs more motor fibers to make this type of activity happen. A similar homunculus can be created for the primary sensory cortex. Many of the same structures (e.g., hands and mouth) are enlarged, indicating a larger number of sensory fibers going to those structures. This illustrates the importance of sensory feedback to motor activities.

The pyramidal tracts then descend through the corona radiata and into the internal capsule. Because tracts like the corticobulbar and corticospinal run through the internal capsule, even small lesions from strokes can cause catastrophic motor problems. The pyramidal tracts travel to the brainstem where they decussate (i.e., cross over) to the other side at the medulla and spinal cord juncture. This decussation is responsible for what is called **contralateral innervation**, meaning that the right side of the brain controls the left side of the body, and the left side of the brain controls the right side of the body. In the case of the lateral corticobulbar tract, once it has decussated at the medulla, it leaves the brainstem as a cranial nerve that then innervates various muscles in the head and neck. The cranial nerves that are important to speech include V, VII, IX, X, and XII.

Upper Motor Neuron Damage Versus Lower Motor Neuron Damage

Neuroscientists have made a useful distinction in the pyramidal system (and the extrapyramidal system to be discussed next), calling the part that courses from the cortex to the brainstem the upper tract, or **upper motor neurons (UMNs)**, and calling the part that leaves the brainstem as a cranial nerve the lower tract, or **lower motor neurons (LMNs)**. UMNs are housed entirely within the central nervous system (CNS) and control LMNs. LMNs are housed in the peripheral nervous system (PNS). UMNs also include both the direct and indirect motor pathways (i.e., pyramidal and extrapyramidal). We will mainly discuss the UMNs here and provide a lengthier discussion on the LMNs under "The Final Common Pathway."

The distinction between UMNs and LMNs is helpful because UMN damage differs from LMN damage (TABLE 11-2). Damage to the UMNs results in spastic muscles due to overactive muscle tone (hypertonia) and reflexes (hyperreflexia), whereas damage to the LMNs results in the opposite—flaccid muscles due to

lack of muscle tone (hypotonia) and reflexes (hyporeflexia). **Clonus**, a jerky resistance when putting a limb into extension, is present in UMN damage, but not in LMN damage.

Clonus, which involves larger movements, can be contrasted to fasciculations, which are small spontaneous twitches. There are no fasciculations in UMN damage, but it is evidenced in LMN damage. A **Babinski sign** is elicited when scratching the bottom of the foot. A normal (negative) Babinski sign occurs when the toes curl and withdraw from the scratching. An abnormal (positive) Babinski sign occurs when the big toe moves back and the toes spread out, which is what occurs in UMN damage. In LMN damage, there is no Babinski sign at all (i.e., the toes do nothing when the bottom of the foot is scratched). Finally, atrophy refers to muscle shrinking and wasting; this is seen in LMN damage, but not in UMN damage.

Why does LMN damage differ symptomatically from UMN damage? Reflexes are mediated at the level of the brainstem or spinal cord, depending on which reflex is being discussed. In UMN damage, the reflex arc is left intact, but in LMN damage, this arc is interrupted. Remember that reflexes occur along the route of cranial and spinal nerves, the very structures that make up the LMNs. When the LMNs are damaged and the reflex arc is interrupted, reflexes will be absent (hyporeflexia, no Babinski sign) and muscles will shrink due to lack of tonal stimulation (hypotonia, marked atrophy). LMN fasciculations occur because of spontaneous depolarization of the LMNs, leading to contraction, not of the whole muscle, but of individual muscle fibers.

Speech Issues Associated With Pyramidal System Damage

Dysarthria is speech that is slurred and/or uncoordinated due to CNS or PNS problems that affect one or more of the following: respiration, phonation, resonance, and articulation. There are seven types of dysarthria; of these, three are associated with pyramidal system damage (TABLE 11-3). **Spastic dysarthria** is due to bilateral UMN damage and results in stiff, rigid muscles. Speech is characterized by a harsh/strained voice, monopitch intonation, hypernasality, slow speech rate, and imprecise consonants. When there is unilateral UMN damage, the condition is called **unilateral UMN dysarthria**, a milder form of dysarthria that affects only one side of the face and mouth. It usually has minimal impact on speech because the person still has one functional side of the face and mouth. The third type of dysarthria associated with pyramidal system damage is **flaccid dysarthria**. It is caused by

TABLE 11-2 Symptoms of Upper Versus Lower Motor Neuron Damage

Upper Motor Neuron Damage	Lower Motor Neuron Damage
Spastic muscles due to:	Flaccid muscles due to:
▪ Hypertonia	▪ Hypotonia
▪ Hyperreflexia	▪ Hyporeflexia
Clonus	No clonus
No fasciculations	Fasciculations
Positive Babinski sign	No Babinski sign
No atrophy	Marked atrophy

TABLE 11-3 Types of Dysarthria

Dysarthria Type	Place of Damage	Signs
Spastic	Bilateral upper motor neuron	Bilateral spasticity and weakness
Unilateral upper motor neuron	Unilateral upper motor neuron	Unilateral spasticity and weakness
Flaccid	Lower motor neuron	Hypotonia and weakness
Hyperkinetic	Basal ganglia and its connections	Extra and abnormal movements
Hypokinetic	Basal ganglia and its connections	Reduced movement and range of motion
Ataxic	Cerebellum and its connections	Incoordination of muscles
Mixed	Variable; any mix of the above places of damage	Variable; depends on what type of dysarthria mix

Adapted from: Manasco, M. H. (2017). *Introduction to neurogenic communication disorders*. Burlington, MA: Jones & Bartlett Learning.

LMN damage and results in speech that is breathy in voice, monopitch, and hypernasal and that uses short phrases and imprecise consonants.

The Indirect Motor System

The indirect motor system is also known as the extrapyramidal system. Whereas the pyramidal system controls voluntary motor movement, the **extrapyramidal system** controls involuntary movements involved in posture, muscle tone, and reflexes, as well as the coordination or modulation of movements.

There are several tracts involved in the extrapyramidal system (**FIGURE 11-7**). Two that originate in the cortex are the corticoreticular and corticorubral tracts. The corticoreticular tract begins at the premotor (BA 6), motor (BA 4), and sensory cortices (BAs 1, 2, 3) and inputs into the reticular formation of the brainstem, which projects to various other structures like the cerebellum and cranial nerve nuclei. The corticorubral tract also arises from the cortex but inputs into the midbrain's red nucleus.

The other four extrapyramidal tracts, which originate in the brainstem, are the rubrospinal, vestibulospinal, reticulospinal, and tectospinal tracts. The rubrospinal tract arises from the midbrain's red nucleus and inputs along the cervical spinal cord. It influences flexor tone in the limbs. Its involvement in speech is uncertain, but damage to it has led to cases of myoclonus in speech muscles. The vestibulospinal tract originates at the vestibular nucleus (where the medulla and pons meet) and inputs into motor neurons throughout the spinal cord. Functionally, it regulates muscle tone to maintain balance and posture. Like the rubrospinal tract, the vestibulospinal tract's function in relation to speech, if any, is unknown. The reticulospinal tract begins in the reticular formation and ends at motor neurons in the spinal cord. This tract has connections to cranial nerve nuclei and plays a role in certain reflexes, like swallowing. The tectospinal tract originates from the tectum ("roof") of the midbrain and ends in the cervical spinal cord. It functions to coordinate head posture with eye movements and does not appear to play any meaningful role in speech.

In addition to the functional difference with the pyramidal system, the extrapyramidal system is different anatomically in that it is made up of many short tracts that are very indirect, much like a commuter train that makes numerous stops along its route. These stops include the basal ganglia, cerebellum, and thalamus (pictured in Figures 11-3 and 11-4), as well as their final destination at either brainstem cranial nerve nuclei or the ventral horn cells of the spinal cord.

Damage to the extrapyramidal system causes a loss of coordination and modulation, leading to dyskinesias, or movement disorders. Some common dyskinesias include **tremors** (rhythmic shaking), **chorea** (quick movements of the hands and feet), **athetosis** (slow writhing movements of extremities), **dystonia** (distorted posture), and clonus (large muscle contractions). All of these conditions are involuntary in nature.

little; *kinesis* = movement) is typically due to problems in the substantia nigra, specifically with dopamine production. Dopamine is an important neurotransmitter for the smoothing and regulation of motor behavior. High levels of dopamine can lead to abnormally increased motor behaviors and impulsivity; low levels lead to stiff, rigid, and slow movements. Parkinson disease is characterized by low levels of dopamine. Patients with Parkinson disease suffer from hypokinetic dysarthria, which involves breathy voice, monopitch, reduced syllable stress, variable speech rate, and imprecise consonants.

The Final Common Pathway

Alpha and Gamma Motor Neurons

The final common pathway (FCP) was briefly introduced in the discussion of the LMN system. It is called the final common pathway because it is the last leg of the journey for all motor signals. Speech is a voluntary motor activity that occurs through the contraction of skeletal muscles. We will begin to discuss the FCP by examining its relationship to skeletal muscles.

Skeletal muscles are made up of many individual muscle fibers. Some of these fibers are extrafusal and others are intrafusal. Extrafusal fibers are innervated by alpha motor neurons that contract these fibers, facilitating muscle movement, whereas intrafusal fibers are innervated by gamma motor neurons and are involved in proprioception. The motor neuron and the fibers it innervates are known as **motor units**. Both alpha and gamma motor neurons are part of the LMN system. Alpha motor neurons are influenced more by the direct motor system, whereas the indirect motor system has more influence on gamma motor neurons. We will focus on alpha motor neurons and their involvement in speech muscle contraction.

The alpha motor neuron axon leaves the brainstem as part of a cranial nerve and courses to a muscle. The axon divides into many terminal branches. Because of this branching, an axon might innervate many muscle fibers. In addition, each muscle fiber may be innervated by multiple alpha motor neurons. This arrangement allows for greater control of contraction. Motor units vary in size depending on the number of fibers an axon innervates. Muscles involved in fine motor activity (e.g., speech) have fewer fibers per axon (e.g., 15:1), whereas gross motor movement involves larger ratios of fibers per axon (e.g., 500:1).

Alpha and gamma motor neurons have a relationship in maintaining muscle tone. Normal, healthy muscles are neither too tight nor too floppy. They constantly receive some level of neurological

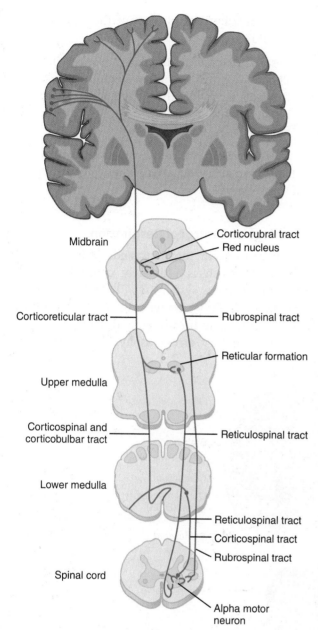

Midbrain

Corticorubral tract
Red nucleus

Corticoreticular tract

Rubrospinal tract

Reticular formation

Upper medulla

Corticospinal and
corticobulbar tract

Reticulospinal tract

Lower medulla

Reticulospinal tract
Corticospinal tract
Rubrospinal tract

Spinal cord

Alpha motor
neuron

FIGURE 11-7 The indirect motor system. Note the many stops this pathway makes, leading it to be called an indirect pathway.

In terms of speech problems, either hyperkinetic or hypokinetic dysarthria is possible in extrapyramidal system damage, depending on where in the system the damage takes place. **Hyperkinetic dysarthria** (*hyper* = too much; *kinesis* = movement) is usually due to damage in the basal ganglia and is associated with conditions like Huntington disease, a progressive, hereditary disorder. The speech of patients with this form of dysarthria is characterized by a harsh voice, monopitch, loud voice level, imprecise consonants, and distorted vowels. These symptoms are due to the constant involuntary motion from which these patients suffer. **Hypokinetic dysarthria** (*hypo* = too stimulation to keep them in a state of readiness; thus, muscles are never completely relaxed. The gamma motor system firing causes intrafusal fibers to contract, which is detected by sensors in these fibers. The intrafusal fibers send sensory signals back to the brainstem and to alpha motor neurons, which in turn send motor signals to extrafusal fibers to shorten and match the length of the intrafusal fibers. The result is that instead of being completely relaxed, the indirect motor system keeps muscles stimulated and prepared for voluntary movements, such as those that occur in speech.

The FCP and Speech

The FCP for speech includes the cranial and spinal nerves involved in phonation, resonance, and articulation as well as spinal nerves involved in respiration. Respiration, phonation, resonance, and articulation are the four main subsystems of speech,

and the contributions of each of these subsystems are as follows:

- Respiration provides the power for speech.
- Phonation provides the raw sound for speech.
- Resonance provides the tonal qualities for speech.
- Articulation provides the speech sounds for speech.

We will briefly look at the neurological control of each of these subsystems with their relevant cranial and spinal nerves.

Neurological Control of Respiration

Several neurons in the pons and medulla regulate respiration, which is ultimately controlled by the autonomic nervous system (**FIGURE 11-8**). The pontomedullary respiratory center is the CNS area responsible for automatic breathing, and damage to it can lead to respiratory arrest, asphyxiation, and death.

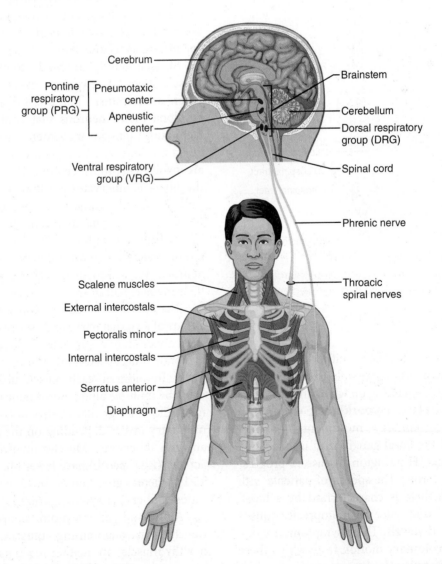

FIGURE 11-8 Neurological control of respiration.

This control center has three groups. The dorsal respiratory group (DRG) is found in the dorsomedial portion of the medulla and is responsible for respiratory rhythm and inspiration (i.e., breathing in). It is driven by the apneustic (Greek for "not breathing") center and inhibited by the pneumotaxic (Greek for "breathing arrangement") center, both of which are in the pons and are collectively called the pontine respiratory group (PRG). The ventral respiratory group (VRG) is located in the ventrolateral area of the medulla and is responsible for inspiration and expiration during forced breathing (e.g., breathing during exercise). Lesions in this system can produce irregular breathing patterns, sometimes found in dysarthric patients. For example, Cheyne-Stokes respiration is a common phenomenon in which breathing switches back and forth from hyperventilation to hypoventilation. Another example is ataxic breathing where respiration is irregular and uncoordinated with speech.

Some spinal nerves support speech by innervating muscles of respiration. LMNs that innervate respiration are found in the cervical and thoracic spinal cord. The diaphragm is the main muscle of inspiration, and it increases the vertical dimensions of the thoracic cavity when contracted. It is innervated by cervical nerves C3, C4, and C5, which combine to form the phrenic nerves. Each phrenic nerve innervates one-half of the diaphragm. The external intercostal muscles contract to pull the ribs up, thus increasing the horizontal dimensions of the thoracic cavity. The internal intercostal muscles assist the external intercostals, but also appear to be involved in expiration. These muscles are innervated by thoracic spinal nerves T2 through T11.

Neurological Control of Phonation

The vagus nerve (cranial nerve X) is a crucial nerve for proper phonatory function. Lateral corticobulbar fibers arise from the primary motor cortex (BA 4) and input into the nucleus ambiguous (NA) in the brainstem (**FIGURE 11-9**). The vagus nerve projects from the NA and splits into two branches, the superior laryngeal nerve (SLN) and the recurrent laryngeal nerve (RLN). The RLN innervates all the intrinsic laryngeal muscles with the exception of the cricothyroid muscle, which is innervated by the SLN.

Unilateral UMN damage to the vagus nerve has little effect on the voice other than possible vocal harshness. Bilateral UMN lesions can paralyze both vocal cords in a paramedian position due to spasticity and lead to a more significant strained-strangle phonation. LMN lesions of the vagus nerve cause paresis or paralysis of the larynx. For example, unilateral damage to the RLN leads to unilateral vocal fold

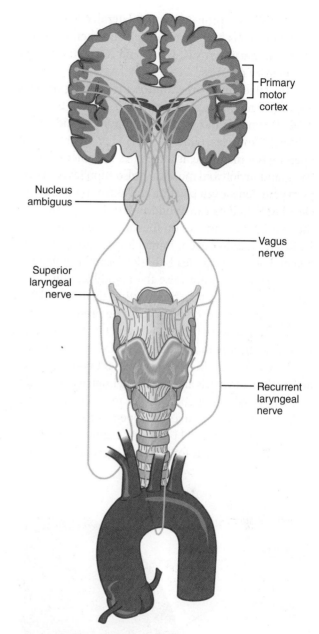

FIGURE 11-9 Neurological control of phonation.

paralysis and a breathy or hoarse voice. Bilateral LMN lesions cause severe deficits in phonation due to bilateral vocal fold paralysis. The voice will be very breathy. Damage to the SLN is less catastrophic than is damage to the RLN, causing damage to pitch control in light of the cricothyroid being an important muscle in raising and lowering vocal pitch.

Neurological Control of Resonance and Articulation

Neurological control of articulation and resonance is a complicated process controlled by at least five cranial nerves: the trigeminal (V), facial (VII), glossopharyngeal (IX), vagus (X), and hypoglossal (XII). The pathway for motor control arises in the primary motor cortex (BA 4), projects as the lateral corticobulbar tract to various brainstem nuclei, and then continues as cranial nerves V, VII, IX, X, and XII to the various articulatory muscles.

The trigeminal nerve controls the opening and closing of the mandible. In elevating or closing the mandible, it controls the masseter, temporalis, and medial pterygoid muscles (**FIGURE 11-10**). For depressing or opening the mandible, it innervates the anterior digastricus and mylohyoid muscles. It also supplies the lateral pterygoid, tensor veli palatini, and tensor tympani muscles. LMN lesions can produce paresis or paralysis of the mandibular muscles on the same side as the lesion. Unilateral lesions have minimal impact on speech, but bilateral lesions can lead to significant problems in which patients cannot raise the mandible, which prevents other articulators from hitting their articulatory targets. Vowel distortions may also be present. Because the trigeminal nerve receives bilateral UMN input, there is no real effect with unilateral UMN damage. Bilateral UMN damage can limit jaw movement and thus affect articulation of vowels and labial and lingual consonants.

The facial nerve controls the muscles of the face, including muscles that purse, open, raise, lower, and retract the lips (Figure 11-10). For example, orbicularis oris is a crucial muscle for lip rounding that is important

for the /w/ sound, a labial sound, among others. The facial nerve also innervates two mandibular openers, the posterior digastricus and the platysma. Unilateral UMN lesions lead to paresis or paralysis of the contralateral lower two-thirds of the face muscles, but have little effect on speech (**FIGURE 11-11**). Bilateral UMN lesions will have more serious consequences, affecting all the face muscles and labial and labiodental sounds. Unilateral LMN lesions result in ipsilateral paresis or paralysis of the upper and lower face muscles. Fasciculations and atrophy of the speech muscles are also present. Speech will be affected only mildly, if at all, as compared to bilateral LMN damage, which involves significant difficulty producing labial and labiodental sounds.

The stylopharyngeus muscle is innervated by the glossopharyngeal nerve. This muscle plays a role in elevating and opening the pharynx, so it may play some role in resonance but is more relevant for swallowing. It also mediates the gag reflex. LMN damage will not affect speech, but it may lead to a loss of pharyngeal sensation, diminished gag, and decreased pharyngeal elevation during swallowing.

The vagus nerve's role in phonation has already been discussed, but this nerve also innervates muscles of the soft palate (or velum) with the exception of the tensor veli palatini and the three pharyngeal constrictor

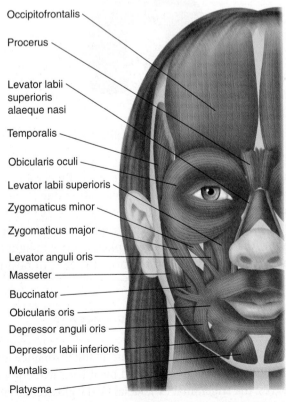

Occipitofrontalis

Procerus

Levator labii superioris alaeque nasi

Temporalis

Obicularis oculi

Levator labii superioris

Zygomaticus minor

Zygomaticus major

Levator anguli oris

Masseter

Buccinator

Obicularis oris

Depressor anguli oris

Depressor labii inferioris

Mentalis

Platysma

FIGURE 11-10 The muscles of the jaw and face. These muscles are innervated by the facial nerve (cranial nerve VII).

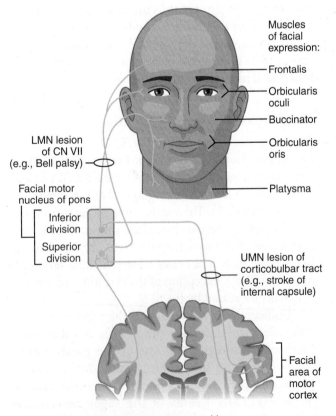

Muscles of facial expression:

Frontalis

Orbicularis oculi

Buccinator

Orbicularis oris

Platysma

LMN lesion of CN VII (e.g., Bell palsy)

Facial motor nucleus of pons

Inferior division

Superior division

UMN lesion of corticobulbar tract (e.g., stroke of internal capsule)

Facial area of motor cortex

FIGURE 11-11 Upper motor neuron and lower motor neuron damage involving the facial nerve (cranial nerve VII).

muscles. The vagus nerve functions with the assistance of the spinal accessory nerve (cranial nerve XI). Unilateral UMN damage has little effect on resonance because of the nerve's bilateral innervation, but bilateral UMN damage will lead to hypernasality due to a faulty, spastic velar mechanism. Like unilateral UMN damage, unilateral LMN damage has little effect on speech. Patients demonstrate a droopy palate ipsilateral to the lesion and a mild hypernasality. Bilateral UMN damage results in complete palatal drooping and severe hypernasality.

There are two sets of tongue muscles, the intrinsic tongue muscles that control fine motor movement and the extrinsic tongue muscles that control gross motor function (**FIGURE 11-12**). The hypoglossal nerve controls all of these muscles with the exception of one extrinsic tongue muscle, the palatoglossus muscle. Thus, this nerve and the muscles it supplies are crucial for speech. The brainstem nucleus of the hypoglossal nerves receives bilateral UMN innervation with the exception of the genioglossus muscle, which receives only contralateral UMN input. Patients with unilateral UMN damage to this nerve have some paresis on the contralateral side of the tongue. The tongue deviates on protrusion, but there is only a mild impact on articulation. Bilateral UMN damage results in bilateral tongue weakness and more significant articulatory problems. Unilateral LMN lesions result in weakness (with the tongue deviating toward the side of lesion), atrophy, and fasciculations ipsilateral to the lesion and mild articulatory problems. Bilateral LMN lesions do not result in tongue deviation due to bilateral weakness but are consistent with more significant speech issues.

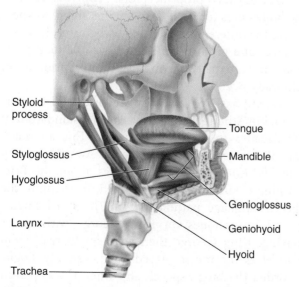

Styloid process

Styloglossus

Hyoglossus

Larynx

Trachea

Tongue

Mandible

Genioglossus

Geniohyoid

Hyoid

FIGURE 11-12 The extrinsic tongue muscles. The intrinsic tongue muscles make up the tongue itself and are not visible in this view.

▶ Multisystem Damage

As discussed in this section, damage to one system leads to one or two types of dysarthria, whereas damage to another system leads to one or two other types of dysarthria. What happens when multiple systems are damaged, such as in the case of amyotrophic lateral sclerosis (ALS)? People with conditions like ALS will have **mixed dysarthria**, which is a mixture of two or more of the pure dysarthrias discussed earlier. For example, both the UMN and LMN systems are damaged in ALS, causing patients to have characteristics of both spastic and flaccid dysarthria. This flaccid-spastic subtype accounts for about 42% of mixed dysarthria cases (Duffy, 2013). Sometimes one form of dysarthria will characterize the beginning of the disease process and then the other form will appear as the disease progresses. Other conditions, such as traumatic brain injury or multiple strokes, can lead to mixed dysarthria. Many patients with dysarthria have the mixed form, because neurological injury often involves more than one neurological system component. Duffy (2013) found that mixed dysarthria accounted for nearly one-third of all dysarthric conditions.

▶ Sensory Pathways Important for Speech

Ascending Sensory Pathways

Descending neural pathways are motor in nature, whereas ascending neural pathways are sensory. Three major ascending sensory pathways relay sensory information like touch, pressure, temperature, and proprioception to various brain structures (**TABLE 11-4**). The first and most important of these to speech is the **dorsal column medial lemniscal pathway**, which is made up of two bundles, the fasciculus gracilis (slender bundle) and the fasciculus cuneatus (wedge-shaped bundle) (**FIGURE 11-13**). Sense receptors in the skin and muscles send sensory signals to the dorsal root ganglion of the spinal nerve or the ganglia of sensory cranial nerves in the brainstem. Neurons in the spinal cord or brainstem then carry the signal through the thalamus to the postcentral gyrus of the parietal lobe. The sensory functions of this pathway include fine touch (as is found in the hands and mouth), vibratory sense, and proprioception. This sensory feedback is important to the speech process, and heightened awareness of it is often targeted in stuttering therapy.

The second tract is the spinothalamic tract, which follows the same course as the dorsal column but has final connections in the cingulate and insular cortices

TABLE 11-4 Ascending Sensory Tracts

Tract	Site of Origin	Site of Ending	Function(s)
Dorsal column	Spinal cord	Primary sensory cortex via thalamus	Fine touch, vibratory sense, proprioception
Spinothalamic	Spinal cord	Primary sensory cortex via thalamus	Crude touch, pain, pressure, temperature
Spinocerebellar	Spinal cord	Cerebellum	Proprioception

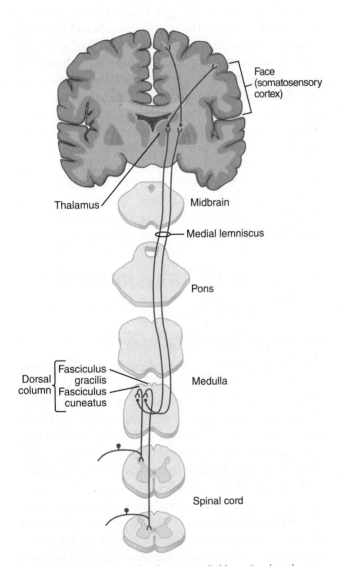

FIGURE 11-13 The dorsal column medial lemniscal pathway.

as well as the postcentral gyrus. The spinothalamic tract is the primary route for pain information as well as temperature, pressure, and crude touch.

The third tract is the spinocerebellar tract. This tract has the same origin as the previous two, but its final input is in the cerebellum. Its function is to relay proprioceptive information from the arms, legs, and trunk of the body to the cerebellum, where it is then processed. The cerebellum is an important neural structure for our balance, and it uses proprioceptive information from the body to help us maintain our balance.

Kinesthesia

It is a common assumption that the brain uses only our sense of hearing as a source of feedback for how our motor speech system is performing. For example, if we mispronounce a word (as we all tend to do at times), we hear the error and make the appropriate corrections in order to say the word correctly. Auditory feedback is not the only sensory system the brain uses to monitor speech, however; if it were, how would a person who is deaf ever learn to speak? Some people who are deaf have speech that is as good as any hearing person's. How is this possible? The answer is that the brain also uses somatosensory information to achieve the precision needed in speech (Nasir & Ostry, 2006). Specifically, the brain uses **kinesthesia**, which is the brain's awareness of the position and movement of the articulators through sense organs imbedded in muscles called proprioceptors. **Proprioception** is the body's eyes for itself or the brain's ability to know where the different parts of the body (arms, legs) are in space at a given time. Kinesthesia and joint position sense are the two components of proprioception (Konradsen, 2002).

Deemphasizing auditory feedback and emphasizing kinesthetic feedback has been a standard tool for decades in treating stuttering. This approach was illustrated in the Academy Award–winning film *The King's Speech*, which was about the British king George VI, who stuttered. In the film, the speech-language pathologist (SLP), Lionel Logue, placed headphones on King George with music playing. King George then went on to read from *Hamlet* as the music played in his ear. Mr. Logue recorded the king's speech and when it was played later in the film, the king was perfectly fluent. How did this happen? King George was deprived of auditory feedback, which is thought to be flawed in those who stutter, and relied solely on the kinesthetic feedback from his mouth. This proves to be a more reliable form of feedback for those who stutter, and SLPs have taken advantage of this insight in stuttering therapy. Often, delayed auditory feedback, rather than music, is used with people who stutter. In this therapeutic technique, the person who stutters wears headphones connected to a system (or a smartphone with an app) that sends auditory feedback back to him or her, but in a delayed fashion. Because it is delayed, it is of no use to the person because it does not match up with what is currently happening with the articulators. Delayed auditory feedback thus forces the person to depend on kinesthetic feedback rather than auditory feedback and helps to produce improved fluency.

▶ Conclusion

The motor and sensory systems important for speech have been surveyed, as have AOS and the types of dysarthria associated with damage to the motor systems. Spastic, unilateral UMN, and flaccid dysarthria result from pyramidal system damage, whereas hypokinetic dysarthria and hyperkinetic dysarthria are a consequence of extrapyramidal system damage. The sixth dysarthria type, ataxic, is due to impairment in the cerebellar system. A seventh type, mixed dysarthria, results from diffuse brain damage that impacts multiple speech systems. ALS is one example of a condition that leads to this type of dysarthria. As the disease progresses, the patient will eventually deteriorate to the point of having **anarthria**, which means no speech at all.

SUMMARY OF LEARNING OBJECTIVES

The following were the main learning objectives of this chapter. The information that should have been learned is below each learning objective.

1. The learner will outline the major components of the motor speech system.
   - *The conceptual level:* Includes the ideas, thoughts, and feelings in our minds.
   - *The motor planning level:* Involves phonological assembly and motor planning for phonemes.
   - *The motor programming level:* Involves the actual execution of phonemes in time and space.
   - *The motor control circuits:* Include the basal ganglia and cerebellar circuits, which are important in motor programming of speech by coordinating, integrating, and refining the movements of the direct and indirect pathways.
   - *The direct motor pathway:* A voluntary motor system that controls gross motor movement; also known as the pyramidal system.
   - *The indirect motor pathway:* Controls involuntary movements involved in posture, muscle tone, and reflexes, as well as the coordination or modulation of movements; also known as the extrapyramidal system.
   - *The final common pathway:* the last leg of the journey for all motor signals, which occurs through the lower motor neurons (LMNs).
2. The learner will connect different places of damage in the motor speech system to different forms of dysarthria.
   - *Spastic dysarthria:* bilateral upper motor neuron (UMN) damage

   - *Unilateral UMN dysarthria:* unilateral UMN damage
   - *Flaccid dysarthria:* LMN damage
   - *Hyperkinetic dysarthria:* basal ganglia, extrapyramidal system
   - *Hypokinetic dysarthria:* substantia nigra, extrapyramidal system
   - *Ataxic dysarthria:* cerebellar circuit
   - *Mixed dysarthria:* multisystem damage
3. The learner will identify places of damage associated with apraxia of speech.
   - *Apraxia of speech:* Can be caused by lesions to the perisylvian region, insula, or basal ganglia.
4. The learner will describe the importance of the sensory system to speech.
   - Both kinesthesia and proprioception are used in the speech system to provide the brain with information regarding where the articulators are and to make last-minute adjustments and corrections.
5. The learner will describe the human response space and the communication disorders professional's role in expanding it.
   - Speech is thought to be an act of our free will.
   - Free will may be better thought of as a scalable property—you have more or less of it.
   - Patients with motor speech disorders, like dysarthria and apraxia of speech, experience the restraint of their impaired neuroanatomy, which limits their ability to act as they desire.

KEY TERMS

Anarthria
Ataxic dysarthria
Athetosis
Babinski sign
Cerebellar circuit
Chorea
Clonus
Contralateral innervation
Diadochokinesia
Dorsal column medial
  lemniscal pathway

Dysarthria
Dystonia
Extrapyramidal system
Flaccid dysarthria
Hyperkinetic dysarthria
Hypokinetic dysarthria
Kinesthesia
Lower motor neurons (LMNs)
Mixed dysarthria
Motor speech disorders
  (MSDs)

Motor units
Proprioception
Pyramidal neurons
Pyramidal system
Spastic dysarthria
Tremors
Unilateral upper motor
  neuron dysarthria
Upper motor neurons
  (UMNs)

DRAW IT TO KNOW IT

1. Draw the flowchart of the motor speech system found in Figure 11-1 from memory.

2. Given the following figure (**FIGURE 11-14**), roughly draw the pyramidal and extrapyramidal pathways.

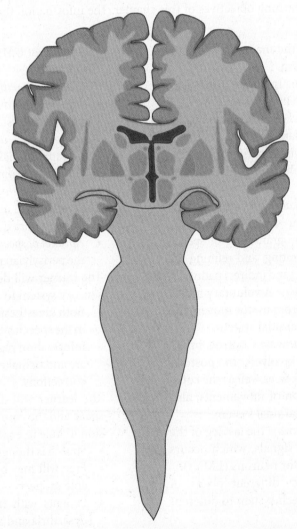

FIGURE 11-14 Unlabeled coronal section of the brain and brainstem.

QUESTIONS FOR DEEPER REFLECTION

1. List the basic levels of the motor speech system beginning with the conceptual level.
2. Compare and contrast UMN damage to LMN damage.
3. Write out the names of the seven types of dysarthria along with where damage occurs in the motor speech system to cause each. Use Table 11-3 as a guide.

CASE STUDY

William is a 70-year-old male with a 6-year history of stiffness and difficulty transferring from chairs and bed to standing. He reports "difficulty talking". The neurologist's report states that William demonstrates diminished arm swinging and shuffling steps while walking. He also demonstrates tremors in both hands with the tremors being more pronounced on the right.

Overall movements are slow (bradykinesia). His facial expression is masked.

1. What neurological condition do you think the neurologist diagnosed William as having? Why do you think this?
2. What kind of dysarthria does William most likely have?

SUGGESTED PROJECTS

1. Write a five- to six-page paper surveying the seven types of dysarthria.
2. Search the scholarly literature and locate two or three recent articles (i.e., from the last 3 years) regarding apraxia of speech. Share what you found with your class.
3. Read the Libet studies found in the References and summarize his experimental design. Do you see any flaws in it?
4. Write a three- to four-page paper on the concept of free will.

REFERENCES

Duffy, J. R. (2005). *Motor speech disorders: Substrates, differential diagnosis, and management* (2nd ed.). St. Louis, MO: Mosby.

Duffy, J. R. (2013). *Motor speech disorders: Substrates, differential diagnosis, and management* (3rd ed.). St. Louis, MO: Mosby.

Konradsen, L. (2002). Factors contributing to chronic ankle instability: Kinesthesia and joint position sense. *Journal of Athletic Training, 37*(4), 381–385.

Libet, B. (1993). Unconscious cerebral initiative and the role of conscious will in voluntary action. In B. W. Libet (Ed.), *Neurophysiology of consciousness* (pp. 269–306). Boston, MA: Birkhäuser.

Libet, B., Gleason, C. A., Wright, E. W., & Pearl, D. K. (1983). Time of conscious intention to act in relation to onset of cerebral activity (readiness-potential). The unconscious initiation of a freely voluntary act. *Brain, 106*(3), 623–642.

Nasir, S. M., & Ostry, D. J. (2006). Somatosensory precision in speech production. *Current Biology, 16*(19), 1918–1923.

Seifert, J. (2011). In defense of free will: A critique of Benjamin Libet. *The Review of Metaphysics, 65,* 377–407.

Spence, S. A. (2009). *The actor's brain: Exploring the cognitive neuroscience of free will.* New York, NY: Oxford University Press.

Spruston, N. (2009). Pyramidal neuron. *Scholarpedia, 4*(5), 6130. Retrieved from http://www.scholarpedia.org/article/Pyramidal_neuron

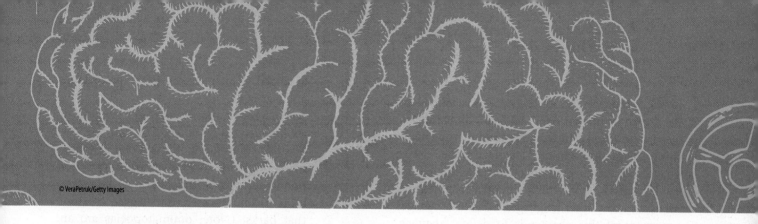

© VeraPetruk/Getty Images

CHAPTER 12

The Neurology of Language

CHAPTER PREVIEW

Language is a code we use to express ourselves through speech or writing. We not only express language but also receive it through listening/comprehending and reading. Language is complex, and many brain regions appear to be involved in our production and comprehension of it. We will survey the neural substrates of language in this chapter.

IN THIS CHAPTER

In this chapter, we will . . .
- Define language
- Discuss three components of language—content, form, and use
- Survey how language comprehension and production may be processed in the neurological system
- Survey several language disorders, including aphasia, alexia, and agraphia

LEARNING OBJECTIVES

1. The learner will define *language*.
2. The learner will list and define the components of language.
3. The learner will outline how language is thought to be neurologically processed in comprehending, reading, speaking, and writing.
4. The learner will describe the following disorders: aphasia, alexia, and agraphia.

▶ Introduction

There are an estimated 6,000 to 7,000 different languages in the world. Students spend numerous hours learning at least one additional language to their native language; thus, language is not only something we use every day but also something we intentionally think about as we learn other languages. What is language? The purpose of this chapter is to define language, sketch out its components, discuss the neurology of language, and survey several language disorders.

A Definition of Language

There are eight main characteristics of all languages to consider before defining what we mean by the term *language* (**FIGURE 12-1**).

1. *Language is a code*; it is a system of symbols used for transmitting messages.
2. *Language is used to represent ideas about the world.* If person A wanted to communicate with person B, A could bring all the objects necessary and point to them to convey a thought, but language makes this task much easier. We use words to represent these real objects; thus we do not need objects at hand to talk about them.
3. *Language is conventional, meaning that it is shared by a speaking community.* A nonconventional language is a dead language, such as Latin.
4. *Language is systematic.* Languages have rules and regulations for how the code is arranged, which makes them predictable and learnable.
5. *Languages use mostly arbitrary symbols to communicate with others.* For example, the word *dog* does not look like a dog or sound like a dog. This word is an arbitrary set of phonemes that is understood to represent a furry, domesticated, four-legged creature that barks. (Note: onomatopoeias are an exception to this [e.g., the word *buzz* represents the sound "buzz"].)
6. *Languages are generative in that speakers are continually creating novel utterances.* For example, when I teach my classes, what I say one semester is never exactly what I say the next semester; I am always creating new sentences even though the topics are the same semester after semester.
7. *Languages are dynamic in that they change over time.* Old English developed into Middle English, then went through the Great Vowel Shift, and emerged into Modern English.
8. *Languages have universal characteristics.* All languages have nouns, verbs, adjectives, and, most of all, rules.

Taking all these characteristics into consideration, a working definition of language can be developed before discussing the neural basis of language. The following is an adaptation of Bloom and Lahey's (1978) definition of language: **Language** is a generative and dynamic code containing universal characteristics whereby ideas about the world are expressed through a conventional system of arbitrary symbols for communication. Having defined language, it is now time to discuss the basic components of language before taking on the difficult task of outlining a neurology of language.

The Components of Language

Language consists of three basic components: content, form, and use (**FIGURE 12-2**). **Content** (i.e., semantics) refers to word meaning. For example, if one says the

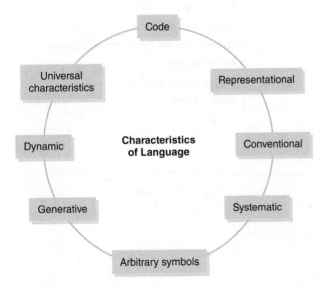

FIGURE 12-1 Characteristics of language.

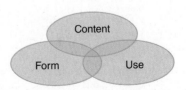

FIGURE 12-2 The three components of language.

word *dog*, there is meaning attached to this word (i.e., a furry, domesticated, four-legged creature that barks). Language **form** or grammar refers to the shape or structure of language. This involves the language's sound structure (**phonology**), word structure (**morphology**), and phrase/sentence structure (**syntax**). Lastly, language use is also known as **pragmatics**, which refers to how we practically use language with other human beings. The two primary ways are through monologues (e.g., telling a story) and through dialogues or conversation. Just from laying out these three components and some of their subcomponents, one can see the incredible complexity of language. It is simply amazing that humans can produce such a complex feat and often with little thought behind how to do it. We just open our mouths and it usually flows out (**BOX 12-1**).

▶ The Neural Basis of Language

How does the brain comprehend and produce language? The short answer is no one really understands all the inner workings of how the brain does this. The longer answer is that although a comprehensive understanding of the brain's language functioning still eludes neuroscientists, there is evidence of brain regions important to language skills.

If one were to peruse textbooks on neuroanatomy, one would find references to the **Wernicke-Geschwind model** of language processing, named after Karl Wernicke (1848–1905) and Norman Geschwind (1926–1984). This model uses a connectionist framework, connecting the following structures in language tasks: Broca's area, the arcuate fasciculus, Wernicke's area, the angular gyrus, and the supramarginal gyrus. It has to be said up front that this model is woefully inadequate in explaining the complex process of language comprehension and expression, as will be explained later. However, it, along with newer research on a ventral and dorsal stream of language, is useful in getting a general neurological flow of language during various language tasks.

Important language regions of the cortex have been known since the time of Wernicke. These include the inferior frontal gyrus (Brodmann areas [BAs] 44, 45), the superior temporal gyrus (BAs 41, 42, 22), some of the middle temporal gyrus (BAs 20, 21, 37, 38), and the inferior parietal lobe (BAs 39, 40). Together, these are known as the perisylvian region because they all border the sylvian fissure, also known as the lateral fissure (**FIGURE 12-4**). These areas, among

BOX 12-1 Is American Sign Language a Language?

For those who are deaf and for whom language does not always flow out of the mouth, manual sign language, like American Sign Language (ASL), is the preferred communication modality **FIGURE 12-3**. Is a manual communication system like ASL a true language? Does it have content, form, and use? The simple answer is "yes." It is obvious that ASL has content or meaning since each sign conveys meaning to those who observe the signs. It is also obvious that ASL has use or pragmatics since it is used in conversations and in telling stories. The hard question is: Does ASL have form that is similar to the form of spoken English? The answer is that "yes," it does.

For example, in English phonology, we talk about three major features of consonants—manner, place, and voice. ASL has something akin to these features: *configuration* of the hand, *movement* of the hands/arms in the signing space, and the *location* of the hands in the signing space. For the sign "mother," the fingers and thumb are flared out and the thumb taps the chin. The sign's configuration is the fingers and thumb spread out, its movement is the tapping, and the location is the chin. ASL also has both bound and free morphemes like in English. For example, extra gestures can be added to a sign to alter its meaning (e.g., negation through hand turning). Finally, ASL has syntax because it has rules for ordering signs. Specifically, it uses a subject-verb-object ordering similar to English. In conclusion, ASL has content, form, and use and is thus a language.

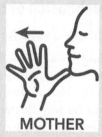

FIGURE 12-3 The ASL sign for "mother" or "mom."

others, will be discussed in the following sections. We will first focus on receptive language modalities by looking at auditory comprehension and reading. We will then shift our focus to language expression modalities and explore the oral production of language (i.e., verbal formulation) as well as its written expression (**TABLE 12-1**).

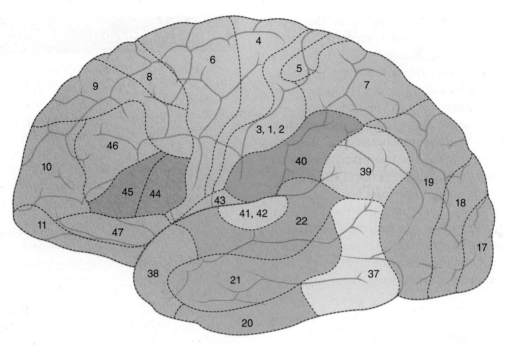

FIGURE 12-4 The perisylvian region. Notice how important language areas congregate around the lateral or Sylvian fissure.

TABLE 12-1 An Overview of Language Modalities

Input: Modalities of Language Reception	Output: Modalities of Language Expression
Auditory comprehension Reading comprehension	Verbal formulation Written expression

Auditory Comprehension of Language

Peripheral Auditory System

When someone asks us a question (e.g., "What is your name?"), how is this auditory information processed (**FIGURE 12-5**)? The auditory information in this question makes its way through the peripheral auditory system first. The auditory components of the question are located and collected by the pinna and then funneled to the tympanic membrane. The sound waves vibrate the tympanic membrane, changing this acoustic energy into mechanical energy. These mechanical vibrations are sent through the ossicles to the oval window of the cochlea. The footplate of the stapes rocks in and out of the window, causing waves in the cochlear perilymph fluid. A second energy change takes place where mechanical energy becomes hydraulic energy. The perilymphatic waves cause waves in the cochlea duct, which disrupt hair cells in its organ of Corti. As these hair cells are disrupted, they depolarize and generate a chemical-electrical signal. The change from hydraulic energy to chemical-electrical energy is the third and final energy change.

The cochlear branch of the cochleovestibular nerve (cranial nerve VIII) picks up the chemical-electrical signal produced in the organ of Corti and transmits it to the cochlear nucleus of the brainstem. The cochlear nucleus routes this information through various brainstem structures to the thalamus, which, in turn, routes the signal to the primary auditory cortex (PAC).

Temporal Lobe Processing

In regard to the cerebral cortex, primary analysis of the auditory information (i.e., phonological analysis) begins at the Heschl gyrus, where the PAC is located. This area shows activation by any type of sound (i.e., speech and nonspeech sounds). The PAC analyzes the

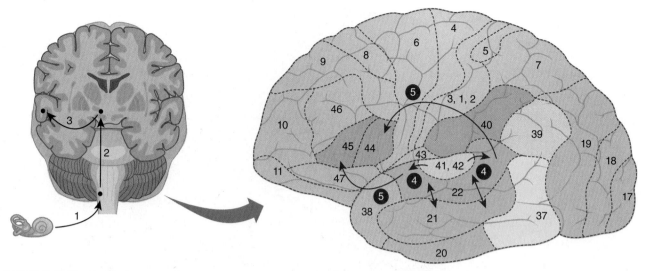

FIGURE 12-5 The auditory comprehension of language. 1. The ear converts acoustic energy into electrochemical energy and transmits it to the brainstem's cochlear nuclear complex (CNC) via cranial nerve VIII. 2. The CNC sends this information to the thalamus. 3. The thalamus relays the information to the primary auditory cortex (PAC) for signal processing. 4. The PAC routes to Wernicke's area and other temporal areas for meaning attachment. 5. Wernicke's area projects to Broca's area for higher-level syntactical processing.

primary auditory signal, with the left PAC sensitive to speech sound characteristics (i.e., distinctive features) and the right PAC sensitive to pitch. After this first processing step, the information is sent in two directions. First, it is sent to the planum temporale (PT) on the posterior superior temporal gyrus (i.e., Wernicke's area) via a short-range rostral fiber pathway. Wernicke's area was once thought to be where meaning was attached to speech, but it might act as more of a hub, drawing information from a surrounding network consisting of parietal (BAs 39, 40) and temporal regions (BAs 21, 37) in the meaning attachment process. Second, the auditory information is sent to the planum polare, which is situated anterior to the Heschl gyrus, via a short-range caudal fiber pathway. (Compare these short-range pathways to the long-range pathways discussed in the next section.) This region may be involved in acoustic analysis, but the planum polare's role is not understood at this time. Phonological processing and semantic processing have been mentioned so far, but what happens in syntactic processing?

Syntax has to do with the rules that guide phrase and sentence structure in a given native language. For example, the sentence "I kicked the red ball" is in correct syntactic order for English, but not Spanish. In Spanish, the sentence would be "I kicked the ball red" because adjectives come after the word they describe in Spanish, but before in English. Semantics has to do with the meaning of words. Neurologically, what part

or parts of the brain appear involved in syntactic and semantic processing? Researchers have performed studies looking at what part of the brain is activated during activities where subjects are exposed to grammatically correct and incorrect sentences. From these and other studies, a picture of syntactic processing begins to emerge.

First, the superior temporal gyrus appears to be involved in the processing of syntactic structure. Second, the posterior temporal lobe is thought to be activated in processing a verb and its arguments. An argument involves the syntactic and semantic relationship between a noun phrase and a verb. For example, syntactically intransitive verbs require a subject (e.g., Bill giggled), whereas transitive verbs require a subject and an object (e.g., Bill built a house). In terms of semantics, a subject is an agent (i.e., one who does an action), whereas an object is a patient (i.e., one who undergoes an action).

Connections Between the Frontal and Temporal Lobes

In terms of connectivity within the perisylvian region, there are two sets of pathways—two dorsal pathways and two ventral pathways (**FIGURE 12-6**). Dorsal pathway 1 connects Wernicke's area (BA 22) to the premotor cortex (BA 6) via two axonal tracts, the arcuate fasciculus and the superior longitudinal fasciculus.

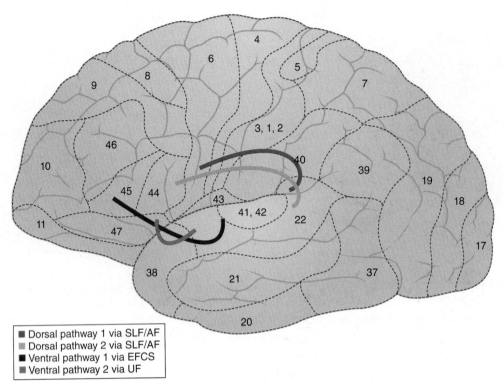

- ■ Dorsal pathway 1 via SLF/AF
- ■ Dorsal pathway 2 via SLF/AF
- ■ Ventral pathway 1 via EFCS
- ■ Ventral pathway 2 via UF

FIGURE 12-6 Fronto-temporal language regions and their connections via two dorsal and two ventral pathways. Dorsal pathway 1 (DP1) and 2 (DP2) both involve the arcuate fasciculus (AF) and the superior longitudinal fasciculus (SLF). DP1 connects Wernicke's area (BA 22) to the premotor cortex (BA 6) while DP2 connects Wernicke's area to Broca's area (BA 44). Ventral pathway 1 involves the extreme fiber capsule system (EFCS) and connects the superior temporal gyrus (BA 41, 42) to Broca's area (BA 45). Ventral pathway 2 uses the uncinate fasciculus (UF) to connect the anterior superior temporal gyrus to the frontal operculum.

Dorsal pathway 2 connects Wernicke's area to the pars opercularis of Broca's area (BA 44) via the same two tracts associated with dorsal pathway 1. Ventral pathway 1 connects the superior temporal gyrus (i.e., PAC, BA 41, BA 42) to the pars triangularis of Broca's area (BA 45) using an axonal tract called the extreme fiber capsule system. Finally, ventral pathway 2 connects the anterior superior temporal gyrus to the frontal operculum via the uncinate fasciculus. This dizzying array of connections illustrates one important point: The superior temporal gyrus is highly connected to the inferior frontal gyrus (Friederici & Gierhan, 2013).

The ventral pathways are thought to facilitate the attachment of meaning to sounds and sound combinations, whereas the dorsal pathways support auditory-motor integration. The dorsal and ventral pathways are considered "dual stream," meaning that information flows back and forth on them.

Frontal Lobe Processing

It appears that when syntax becomes complex, the inferior frontal gyrus is recruited to the comprehension task via the pathways mentioned previously. Broca's area (BAs 44, 45) shows activation during complex syntactic activities. This observation accords with clinical evidence of patients with Broca's aphasia who not only are expressively agrammatic but also struggle with higher-level comprehension tasks such as passive constructions (e.g., "The leopard was killed by the lion. Which animal died?"). It is possible that Broca's area also contributes working memory to the task of comprehension (Dapretto & Bookheimer, 1999). Working memory is a type of temporary, scratch pad–like holding space that we use to work out information (e.g., a math problem). Experientially, this would seem to be true for when someone says something to us that has a level of complexity to it; we need the mental space to work it out. Patients with Broca's aphasia would appear to lack this space for complex or odd grammatical constructions.

Visual Comprehension of Language

We can comprehend language through our auditory system, but we can also visually comprehend language through reading. We now turn to the topic of reading to explore how our eyes gather visual information and pass it through the visual pathways to cortical areas for processing and how the left hemisphere then decodes written language (**FIGURE 12-7**).

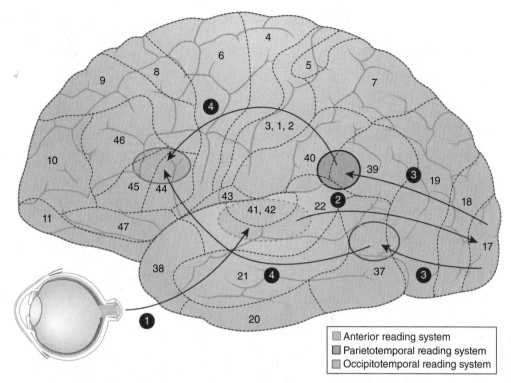

FIGURE 12-7 The visual comprehension of language. 1. Visual information is projected to the thalamus's lateral geniculate nucleus via the optic tracts. 2. The thalamus projects back to the occipital lobe's visual areas (BAs 17–19) for visual processing via the geniculocalcarine tract. 3. The visual areas project a dorsal stream of vision (i.e., the "where" of vision) to the parietotemporal reading system and a ventral stream of vision (i.e., the "what" of vision) to the occipitotemporal reading system. 4. An anterior reading system area is activated in silent reading and in decoding infrequently used words.

The Eyes

Our eyes are precious resources that we use to navigate the world around us. We also use them as a first step in the process of reading because they gather written visual information and then pass that information on to the visual pathways.

The eyes have three layers: the external, middle, and inner layers (**FIGURE 12-8**). The external layer contains a tough, white covering called the sclera and a thin mucous membrane with numerous sensory receptors called the cornea. The middle layer of the eye is continuous with the pia mater of the meninges. This layer contains the choroid, which contains blood vessels that nourish the retina. It also has what is called the ciliary body whose muscles shape the lens and control the optics of the eye. The iris is also a part of the middle layer. It is made of smooth muscle with an opening in the middle called the pupil through which light passes. The inner layer is the retina, which is continuous with the brain through the optic nerve. The retina contains three layers of cells: a photoreceptor layer, a bipolar cell layer, and a ganglion layer. Photoreceptors come in two varieties, rods and cones. Rods are sensitive to blue to green light (not red) and are most useful in low-light situations. Cones come in three varieties: red, green, and blue. Overall, cones

are sensitive to a wide spectrum of light wavelengths and thus are sensitive for colors and are most useful in bright-light situations.

The photoreceptors transduce light into neural impulses. When light strikes a photoreceptor, it excites a pigment in the photoreceptor. Each pigment is sensitive to a specific wavelength of light. The excitation of the pigment sets off a chemical chain reaction that leads to the creation of an electrical impulse from the photoreceptors to the bipolar cells to the ganglion cells, and eventually to the optic nerve.

The Visual Pathways

The optic nerves enter the eyes at the medial posterior side and branch to the lateral (temporal) and medial (nasal) sides of each eye (**FIGURE 12-9**). We have two visual fields, a left visual field and a right visual field. A common misunderstanding is that the left eye is responsible for the left visual field and the right eye is responsible for the right visual field. In actuality, both eyes participate in each visual field. The temporal retina of the left eye and the nasal retina of the right eye are responsible for the right visual field, and the right temporal retina and left nasal retina take care of the left visual field. Retinal ganglion cell axons project from the eyes to the optic chiasm.

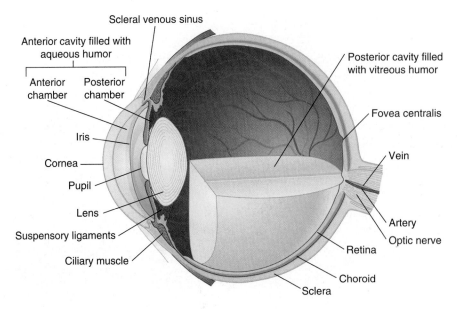

FIGURE 12-8 The structure of the eye.

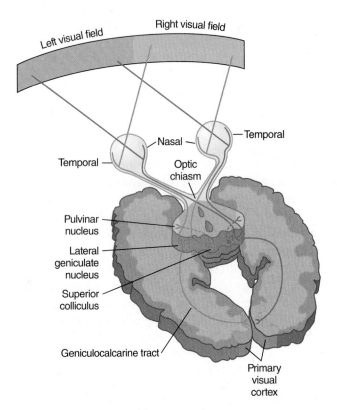

FIGURE 12-9 The visual pathway.

The **optic chiasm** ("crossing") is a structure between the optic nerves and the optic tracts. The optic nerve fibers from the nasal retinas cross at this point, whereas the temporal retinas do not cross. The optic tracts begin at the optic chiasm and conduct retinal ganglion cell axons to the lateral geniculate nucleus of the thalamus. Ninety percent of these axons terminate at the lateral geniculate nucleus; the remaining 10% project to the pretectal area and the superior colliculus. The pretectal area is a region of the midbrain composed

of seven nuclei that make up the subcortical vision system. It is here that the pupillary light reflex is mediated. The superior colliculus is also found in the midbrain; it is involved in the control of eye movements.

From the lateral geniculate nucleus, the **geniculocalcarine tract** projects to the medial part of the occipital lobe surrounding the calcarine sulcus (BA 17). The fibers from the left visual field are projected to the right part of BA 17, and the right visual field to the left. In other words, the visual fields are received by the cortex in a contralateral fashion.

Cortical Processing of Visual Information

Cortical processing involves handling color, location, motion, depth, and identifying features of objects. All this processing happens at the same time and is known as parallel processing. Visual information is sent from BA 17 to BAs 18 and 19. A dorsal stream of vision occurs as information is sent to the superior occipital lobe and inferior parietal lobe for further processing. This dorsal stream represents the "where" of vision (i.e., where an object is located in the visual field). A ventral stream of processing, involving the inferior occipital lobe and posterior and inferior temporal lobe, processes the "what" of vision, or the identity of an object. Lesions in the ventral stream sometimes result in agnosia, the inability to recognize the object.

Cortical Reading Areas

The posterior part of the brain is focused on recognizing patterns, whether they are auditory, visual, or olfactory patterns. We read a book and the words we read form a pattern. If we hear our friend speak, we recognize the pattern of his or her voice. If our neighbor grills a steak, we recognize the smell pattern and can identify what is cooking. Humans have not always read, but as we developed the ability to do so, we took advantage of the pattern-recognition system already built into our brains. Pattern recognition is crucial in reading. As we read, we recognize combinations of letters. For example, the d-o-g pattern is recognized as "dog."

Shaywitz and Shaywitz (2008) proposed that there are three reading systems in the left hemisphere, one in the anterior portion and two in the posterior portion. The term *systems* is used rather than *areas* because these systems encompass more than one Brodmann area.

The first posterior reading system is called the **parietotemporal reading system**. This system focuses on word analysis, meaning the decoding of words at the phonemic level (i.e., phonics). It is also involved in the comprehension of written and spoken language (Heim & Keil, 2004; Joseph, Nobel, & Eden, 2001). The angular gyrus (BA 39), the supramarginal gyrus (BA 40), and the posterior part of the superior temporal lobe are all part of this system. The other posterior reading system is the **occipitotemporal reading system**, which is also known as the visual word-form area. As the name implies, this system is concerned with visual word

form recognition (i.e., sight-reading) and rapid access to whole words. In addition, it integrates printed letters to their corresponding sounds (i.e., grapheme-to-phoneme conversion). Cortical areas involved with this system include the left inferior occipital area, left inferior-posterior temporal area, and fusiform gyrus.

In addition to the two posterior reading systems, there is the **anterior reading system**, which involves Broca's area as well as the ventral and dorsal premotor areas. This system has long been known to play an important role in word analysis in terms of spoken language syntax and articulation, but it may also play a role in silent reading (Shaywitz & Shaywitz, 2004, 2008) and in decoding infrequently encountered words (Cornelissen, Hansen, Kringelbach, & Pugh, 2010).

The Oral Production of Language

The Prefrontal Cortex

Our decision to speak to another human most likely originates in the prefrontal cortex (**FIGURE 12-10**). This structure lies in the frontal lobe anterior to the motor areas. It is highly connected to the parietal, temporal, and occipital lobes, and the rest of the frontal lobe by way of the dorsal pathways (i.e., the arcuate

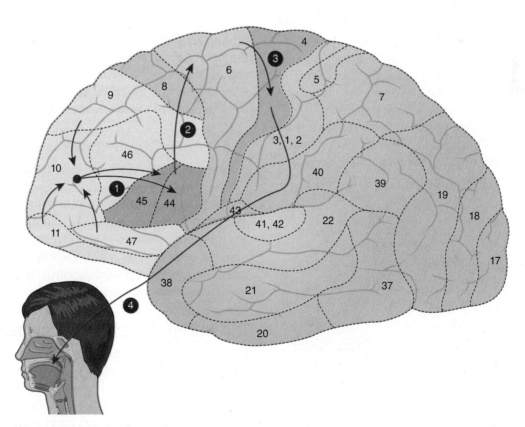

FIGURE 12-10 The oral production of language. 1. Desire and thoughts to communicate originate in the prefrontal cortex and are sent to Broca's area for language encoding and speech planning/programming. 2. Broca's area projects to the supplementary motor area (top of area 6), which activates speech plans. 3. Supplementary motor area relays now-active plans to the primary motor cortex. 4. Primary motor cortex sends plans to the speech muscles for execution.

fasciculus and the superior longitudinal fasciculus). In addition, the prefrontal cortex receives information from the limbic system, our emotional center, via the thalamus. Because of this substantial connectivity, the prefrontal cortex is wired for decision making. When a decision to talk is made, the thought is likely transferred to the left inferior frontal cortex for semantic and phonological assembly.

One of the reasons the prefrontal cortex is thought to help us make decisions, like when to talk, is due to the experience of those who have received **prefrontal lobotomies** (**FIGURE 12-11**). This surgical procedure, which was once done to help psychiatric patients, disconnects the prefrontal cortex from the rest of the brain. One of the characteristics of those who have undergone this procedure is that they lack rational decision-making abilities and act more on impulse.

The Left Inferior Frontal Cortex

Anatomically, the left inferior frontal cortex (LIFC) consists of Broca's area (BAs 44, 45) as well as the pars orbitalis. It is associated with syntactic comprehension, as mentioned earlier. It is also involved in language production, though probably in addition to other subregions (e.g., insular cortex, fusiform gyrus). In the LIFC, there appears to be language specialization with the anterior (i.e., pars orbitalis) and ventral parts (i.e., BA 45, pars triangularis) specializing in semantics (e.g., verb selection) and in the posterior regions (i.e., BA 44, pars opercularis) handling phonology. The posterior dorsal part of the LIFC could be thought of as an extension of the prefrontal motor cortex (BA 6) where motor plans for speech are stored. Damage to this area can result in apraxia of speech. In this condition, people cannot pull up the motor plans necessary for speech, though their language may be intact.

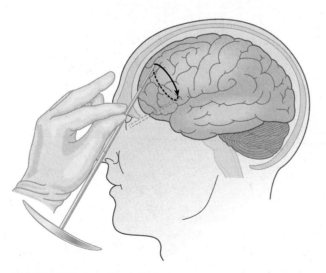

FIGURE 12-11 A prefrontal lobotomy.

From this discussion, Broca's area can be described as *necessary* for properly formed oral language, but not *sufficient*. It networks with other cortical and subcortical areas, such as the pars orbitalis, frontal operculum, insular cortex, and fusiform gyrus, to name just a few. The relationship among these areas can be seen in patients with transcortical motor aphasia who suffer lesions just anterior to Broca's area. They can understand others and repeat what is said to them, but they struggle in initiating speech. Again, Broca's area is necessary, but not sufficient, for expressive language. In fact, neuroimaging studies have provided evidence that regions anterior to Broca's area (e.g., BA 47) are involved in semantic tasks, such as semantic retrieval (Wagner, Koutstaal, Maril, Schacter, & Buckner, 2000; Wagner, Paré-Blagoev, Clark, & Poldrack, 2001), verb generation (Thompson-Schill, Aguirre, Desposito, & Farah, 1999), and judging whether semantic choices are acceptable (Dapretto & Bookheimer, 1999).

The Supplementary Motor Area

After semantic assembly has been performed in the anterior ventral LIFC, it is most likely passed on to the posterior dorsal LIFC for phonological planning and assembly. From here, the language product is most likely sent to the supplementary motor area (SMA), which has been implicated in internally initiated activity. The product may be sent directly to the SMA or first relayed through cerebral motor regions, such as the basal ganglia and thalamus, before arriving at the SMA. The SMA then initiates the motor plans, much like turning the key in a car turns the car on, making it ready to drive.

The Primary Motor Cortex

The SMA sends the motor information for the intended language production to the primary motor cortex (BA 4). If the SMA turns the car on, the primary motor cortex puts the car into drive by relaying the motor information to the speech muscles via the motor speech system, which includes the pyramidal and extrapyramidal systems, control circuits, and sensory feedback mechanisms.

The Written Expression of Language

Writing, like reading, is a uniquely human function that relies upon our language abilities. Writing is a powerful skill in conveying ideas not only to large groups of people but also to people living in different eras. Sitting on my shelves are many books written by people who have long been dead. These authors may be deceased, but their ideas live on and continue to influence people.

In thinking about writing, there appear to be three key processes involved in our ability to write. First, there is the language involved in our written communication. This means language processing and production are intimately linked with the skill of writing, with the LIFC probably involved in encoding. Second, there is the motor control necessary to manipulate pen in hand in relation to paper. This motor control involves not only the gross movements of the arm and hands but also the precise, fine motor movements of the fingers as they wield a writing instrument. Third, there is significant visuospatial involvement because writing involves the use of vision guiding motor movements in the three-dimensional writing space. Because we have already surveyed linguistic regions of the brain, next we will look at the visuospatial and motor control aspects of writing (**FIGURE 12-12**).

Visuospatial Elements: Left Superior Parietal Lobe

As mentioned, writing requires significant visuospatial skills because it involves visual guidance of the hand and fingers in forming graphemes. Graphemes are the written equivalent to phonemes and require the same precision to produce as phonemes. Neurologically, where does the control of writing reside?

Part of the writing circuit is the somatosensory association cortex (BAs 5, 7) that lies inferior to the primary sensory cortex (BAs 1, 2, 3) and superior to the angular gyrus (BA 39) and supramarginal gyrus (BA 40). It received its name because it coordinates motor and sensory information, including tactile and visual sensation. Several studies using functional magnetic resonance imaging (Harrington, Farias, Davis, & Buonocore, 2007; Katanoda, Yoshikawa, & Sugishita, 2001; Menon & Desmond, 2001) have found the left superior parietal lobe (SPL), part of the somatosensory association cortex, active during writing activities. The left SPL is thought to construct graphic images of letters. In other words, as we write, we imagine what letters look like just before and as we write them. The left SPL also is thought to direct the sequence of movements that occur during writing. Harrington et al. (2007) found that drawing activates the right and left SPLs.

Motoric Elements: Broca's Area and the Premotor Cortex

It has long been known from lesion studies that an area in the premotor cortex (BA 6) adjacent to Broca's area is important for the motor aspects of writing. This area is known as Exner's area, named after Sigmund Exner (1846–1926), an Austrian physiologist who first theorized that this region is important to writing.

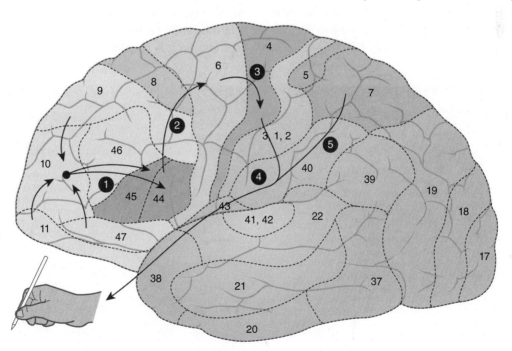

FIGURE 12-12 The written expression of language. 1. Desire and thoughts originate in the prefrontal cortex and are sent to Broca's area for language encoding. 2. Language-encoded thoughts are sent to the premotor cortex (BA 6; Exner's area) for handwriting motor planning. 3. Motor plans are sent to the primary motor cortex. 4. The primary motor cortex sends writing motor plans to the dominant hand. 5. The left superior parietal lobe coordinates the visuospatial elements of writing.

The main brain areas involved in the motoric aspects of writing appear to be Broca's area (BAs 44, 45), Exner's area in the premotor cortex (BA 6), and the precentral gyrus (BA 4). In fact, Exner's area is anterior to the hand area in the precentral gyrus. The graphemic images generated in the SPL are sent to Broca's area, which has extensive connections with Exner's area. Broca's area is thought to organize the impulses from the SPL and relay them to Exner's area for conversion into graphemic motor plans. These plans are then sequenced in the SMA and sent to the precentral gyrus, which activates muscle motor movements of the dominant writing hand (Joseph, 2000; Longcamp, Anton, Roth, & Velay, 2003; Roux et al., 2009).

▶ Language Disorders

Aphasia

Aphasia is an acquired multimodality language disorder. *Acquired* means that it is a condition caused by a stroke or some other form of brain injury; *multimodality* means that it affects all language modalities, such as auditory comprehension, verbal formulation, reading, and writing. Aphasia involves *language* in that people with it struggle with comprehending or using language symbols. Lastly, aphasia is a *disorder* in that a system, the language system, does not function as it should function, and this dysfunction may disable the person with aphasia. It should be said that aphasia

should not be confused with conditions like mental confusion, memory problems, or dementia. Aphasia is not an intellectual disorder, but rather an acquired disorder of language.

One basic way of describing aphasia is through the categories of fluent versus nonfluent aphasia. Typically, fluency is thought to be a category reserved for fluency disorders, like stuttering. In these cases, fluency is thought of as the smoothness with which sounds, words, and sentences are produced. In aphasia, fluency is thought of a bit differently. It is thought of as the effort that goes into speech and the quantity of words produced. The speech of people with fluent aphasia is effortless, and they produce a normal quantity of words, between 100 and 200 words per minute. Their speech is empty, though, because they produce more function words (prepositions, pronouns) than content words (nouns, verbs). People with nonfluent aphasia have the opposite features; speech is effortful and labored, and they produce fewer than 100 words per minute. Their language is rich in content words, but short on function words, which are critical for seeing the relationships between words. These criteria along with others can be explored further in **TABLE 12-2**.

In addition to fluency, aphasias can be distinguished from each other through other features. For example, a patient's auditory comprehension and ability to repeat words can be useful pieces of information in differentiating one form of aphasia from another. Naming ability is typically impaired across all forms of aphasia, so it is usually not a helpful indicator of type

TABLE 12-2 Fluent Versus Nonfluent Aphasia

Category or Feature	Nonfluent Aphasia	Fluent Aphasia
Articulation	Affected	Normal
Effort	Effortful, labored	Normal
Quantity of words	Sparse	Normal
Words per minute	<100	100–200
Phrase length	1–2 words	5–8 words
Prosody	Impaired	Normal
Content	Excessive content words, but few function words	Lacks content words, but lots of function words

Data from Davis, G. A. (2006). *Aphasiology: Disorders and clinical practice* (2nd ed.). Upper Saddle River, NJ: Pearson.

of aphasia. Impairment in naming is called **anomia**. Sometimes anomia can be due to motor issues, like those found in Broca's aphasia. Other times, anomia is due to word selection issues, which is considered true anomia and is the most common type of anomia in aphasia. Finally, in severe cases of aphasia, sometimes anomia is due to entire semantic fields being wiped out, as is the case with semantic anomia (TABLE 12-3).

In addition to these features, some types of aphasia have paraphasias. Paraphasias are either word and sound substitutions that can be lexical (real words) or nonlexical (nonwords) in nature. An example of a lexical paraphasia is a semantic paraphasia where a word is substituted for the target word and is related to it in meaning. For example, if the target word is *cat*, a semantic paraphasia might be *dog*. An example of a nonlexical paraphasia is a neologism (literally "new word"). If the target word is again *cat*, a neologistic error might be *repuco*, a production that is not a known word in English. These and other types of paraphasias are described in TABLE 12-4.

Of all the features mentioned earlier, the most useful to differentially diagnose aphasia are fluency, auditory comprehension, and word repetition. These three categories lead to eight types of "classical" aphasias, four that are fluent in nature and four that are nonfluent. These types of aphasia are useful for professional communication between speech-language

TABLE 12-3 Types of Anomia

Anomia Type	Does Patient Know Word?	Can Patient Produce Word in Another Modality (e.g., writing)?	Description of Patient Anomic Error
Word production anomia	Yes	Yes	Labored speech due to motor issues (Broca's aphasia, apraxia of speech)
Word selection anomia	Yes	No	Tip-of-the-tongue phenomenon ("Oh, it's . . . uh . . ."); true anomia
Semantic anomia	No	No	Semantic field lost; no response from the patient; usually accompanied by poor auditory comprehension

Data from Code, C. (1991). *The characteristics of aphasia*. London, UK: Lawrence Erlbaum Associates.

TABLE 12-4 Classification of Aphasic Paraphasias

Paraphasia Category	Paraphasia Types	Definitions	Examples	
			Target	*Error*
Lexical (real words)	Semantic	Word related to target in meaning	Cat	Dog
	Formal	Word related to target in sound	Cat	Mat
	Mixed	Word with sound and meaning relationship	Cat	Rat
	Unrelated	Word with no apparent relationship to target	Cat	Bucket
Nonlexical (nonwords)	Phonemic	Nonword obviously related in sound	Cat	Zat
	Neologistic	Nonword with no apparent relationship	Cat	Repuco

Data from Davis, G. A. (2007). *Aphasiology: Disorders and clinical practice* (2nd ed.). Upper Saddle River, NJ: Pearson.

pathologists (SLPs) as well as between SLPs and physicians. However, we should keep in mind that some people do not cleanly fit into these categories and that labels like these only tell so much about a patient. The goal of assessment is to describe the language strengths and weaknesses of the patient, as this information is what we use to plan therapy. These eight aphasias are compared and contrasted in TABLE 12-5. They are also graphically laid out in FIGURE 12-13.

Broca's Aphasia

Broca's aphasia is probably the most well-known form of aphasia thanks to Paul Broca's famous case involving his patient, Tan (discussed in Chapter 1). It occurs in about 27% of aphasic cases, making it the most common form of aphasia (Hoffmann & Chen, 2013). The exact site or sites of damage are debated, but the condition can be due to lesions in and axonal areas under deep to Broca's area (BAs 44,45) as well as frontal, parietal, and temporal areas surrounding Broca's area (FIGURE 12-14).

Looking at Table 12-5, Broca's aphasia is characterized as a nonfluent aphasia with relatively intact auditory comprehension, but impaired repetition. Struggles in auditory comprehension become apparent when the length and complexity of auditory information increase. Patients are agrammatic, meaning their

TABLE 12-5 Comparison of Classical Aphasias								
	Nonfluent Aphasias				**Fluent Aphasias**			
Category or Feature	**Broca's**	**Transcortical Motor**	**Mixed Transcortical**	**Global**	**Wernicke's**	**Transcortical Sensory**	**Conduction**	**Anomic**
Fluency	−	−	−	−	+	+	+	+
Auditory comprehension	+	+	−	−	−	−	+	+
Repetition	−	+	+	−	−	+	−	+

+, relatively intact; −, impaired.

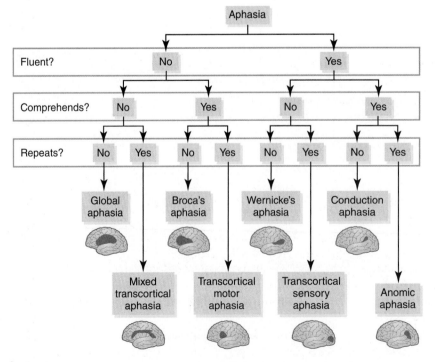

FIGURE 12-13 Types of aphasia.

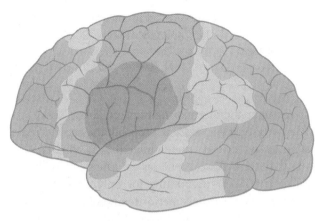

FIGURE 12-14 The neuropathology of Broca's aphasia. Darker areas mark primary lesion areas; lighter shading denotes other possible areas of involvement.

expressions lack grammatical completeness. For example, a patient might say, "I . . . walk . . . dog . . . park" in place of *I walked the dog in the park*. Paraphasias are not typically observed in this form of aphasia. Reading comprehension is functional for short, simple material, but will break down with longer and more complex reading passages. Writing is impaired and often follows the pattern of the patient's oral output.

Despite these challenges, patients with Broca's aphasia are generally good communicators because they can produce heavy content words (e.g., nouns). They also have good awareness, are cooperative, and have some ability to self-correct. Apraxia of speech and dysarthria may co-occur with Broca's aphasia (Davis, 2006; Hedge, 2018; LaPointe, 2005).

Transcortical Motor Aphasia

Hoffmann and Chen (2013) report that all of the transcortical aphasia types together account for 1.8% of all cases of aphasia, so transcortical motor aphasia is exceedingly rare. It is caused by lesions in the frontal lobes above or below Broca's area and in the supplementary motor area (**FIGURE 12-15**). Like Broca's aphasia, it is a nonfluent form of aphasia with relatively preserved auditory comprehension. Unlike Broca's aphasia, patients have intact repeating abilities. Patients are usually initially mute, but as this subsides, their speech will be echolalic with some paraphasias and agrammatism. Reading comprehension will be relatively intact except for syntactically complex material, but writing will have significant deficits that mirror oral communication deficits (Davis, 2006; Hedge, 2018; LaPointe, 2005).

Mixed Transcortical Aphasia

Another rare transcortical aphasia is mixed transcortical aphasia, which is a mixture of transcortical motor

and transcortical sensory aphasia. It is caused by damage to what is called the watershed area, a region that receives blood supply from the small branches at the end of the three cerebral arteries (**FIGURE 12-16**). Mixed transcortical aphasia is like global aphasia in that patients are severely nonfluent, with severely impaired auditory comprehension, reading, and writing, but with preserved repetition, which often manifests as echolalia (Davis, 2006; Hedge, 2018).

Global Aphasia

Global aphasia is the most devastating type of aphasia to the language system. It accounts for about 19% of aphasia cases (Hoffmann & Chen, 2013). It is caused by extension damage in the perisylvian language region that is supplied by the middle cerebral artery (Figure 12-4 and **FIGURE 12-17**). All language modalities are severely impaired. Co-occurring conditions include hemiparesis or hemiplegia, oral apraxia, apraxia of speech, and hemineglect. If there is a bright spot with this aphasia type it is that it can

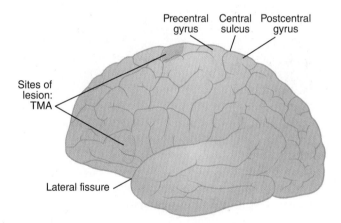

FIGURE 12-15 The neuropathology of transcortical motor aphasia (TMA).

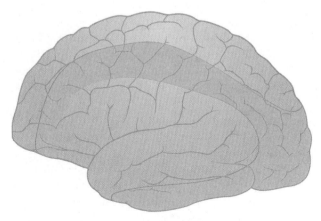

FIGURE 12-16 Mixed transcortical aphasia results from damage to the brain's watershed area (see gray shading).

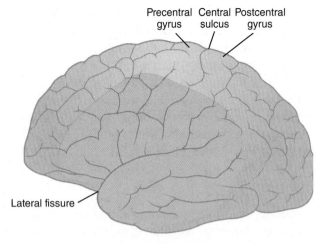

FIGURE 12-17 The neuropathology of global aphasia. The condition is due to extensive damage to the perisylvian language region.

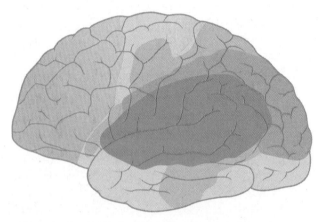

FIGURE 12-18 The neuropathology of Wernicke's aphasia. Darker areas mark primary lesion areas; lighter shading denotes other possible areas of involvement.

morph into a less severe form of aphasia, such as Broca's or Wernicke's aphasia (Davis, 2006; Hedge, 2018; LaPointe, 2005).

Wernicke's Aphasia

Named after the German neuropsychiatrist, Karl Wernicke, Wernicke's aphasia is probably the second most well-known form of aphasia after Broca's aphasia. It is rarer than transcortical aphasias according to Hoffmann and Chen (2013), accounting for only 1.6% of cases. Damage occurs in the superior temporal gyrus, supramarginal gyrus, or angular gyrus (**FIGURE 12-18**). It is a fluent aphasia where verbal output flows easily and effortlessly, so much so that patients are described as having logorrhea, a diarrhea of the mouth. This verbal output is full of semantic paraphasias and neologisms; as a result, the speech of patients with Wernicke's aphasia is said to be empty or devoid of meaning. Example, for the target sentence "The dog needs to go out, so I will take him for a walk," someone with Wernicke's aphasia might say, "You know that smoodle pinkered and that I want to get him round and take care of him like you want before" (The Internet Stroke Center, n.d.). In these patients, auditory comprehension is severely impaired, as is their repetition and writing. Reading comprehension is impaired also, but not as severely as the other modalities, being a relative strength compared to the other modalities (Davis, 2006; Hedge, 2018; LaPointe, 2005).

Transcortical Sensory Aphasia

The final form of transcortical aphasia is transcortical sensory aphasia. It is caused by lesions to the temporoparietal region, including the angular gyrus and the posterior temporal lobe (**FIGURE 12-19**). People

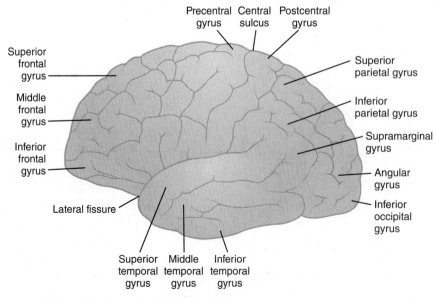

FIGURE 12-19 The neuropathology of transcortical sensory aphasia.

with transcortical sensory aphasia are fluent, but their verbal output is filled with paraphasias (semantic and neologistic paraphasias), echolalia, and empty speech. Auditory comprehension is impaired as well as reading and writing, but repetition abilities are preserved. It is interesting that repetition is intact and echolalic behavior is present in a condition with impaired auditory comprehension (Davis, 2006; Hedge, 2018; LaPointe, 2005).

Conduction Aphasia

Conduction aphasia is an extremely rare form of aphasia occurring only in about 1% of cases. Its neuropathology has been controversial, with the traditional site of damage being the arcuate fasciculus. However, damage anywhere between Broca's area and Wernicke's area can result in this classification (**FIGURE 12-20**). The condition itself is characterized by fluent verbal output with some paraphasias at times. Auditory and reading comprehension are also relatively intact, but its hallmark characteristic is impaired repetition. Writing is also impaired (Davis, 2006; Hedge, 2018; LaPointe, 2005).

Anomic Aphasia

Hoffmann and Chen (2013) report that anomic aphasia is the second most common type of aphasia, representing 26% of aphasia cases, after Broca's aphasia. Some lesion sites include the temporoparietal area, including the angular gyrus, middle temporal gyrus, supramarginal gyrus, and posterior inferior temporal gyrus (**FIGURE 12-21**). In many ways, anomic aphasia is the least severe form of aphasia because patients are fluent, with persevered auditory comprehension, repetition, reading, and writing. The hallmark characteristic

is word selection anomia with semantic paraphasias (Davis, 2006; Hedge, 2018; LaPointe, 2005).

Alexia

Alexia is a term that refers to an acquired disorder of reading. This condition is different from **dyslexia**, a term this text reserves for developmental problems in acquiring reading skills. Alexia is caused by a stroke, head injury, or some other mechanism. Premorbid reading abilities are normal but then suddenly change due to one of these neurological conditions.

A Dual-Route Reading Model

Riley, Brookshire, and Kendall (2017) have proposed a dual-route model for reading, developed by Coltheart, Rastle, Perry, and Langdon (2001), that is helpful for explaining different types of alexia (**FIGURE 12-22**). The two routes include a lexical reading route and a nonlexical reading route. The lexical route is our sight-reading route for already-known words, while the nonlexical route is our phonics, or "sounding things out," route, which is important as we encounter new words.

Figure 12-22 applies the written word example of *dog* to this model. When we see this written word, our brains first perform a visual analysis of each grapheme in the word. For example, an analysis of *d* would be that it has a straight vertical line with a curve on its lower left side. Next, our brains do a letter analysis and determine the letter-to-sound correspondences contained in the word. Dog has three letters and three sounds. Another word, *shoe*, has four letters but only three sounds. If the word is familiar to us and already a part of our lexicon, it moves through the

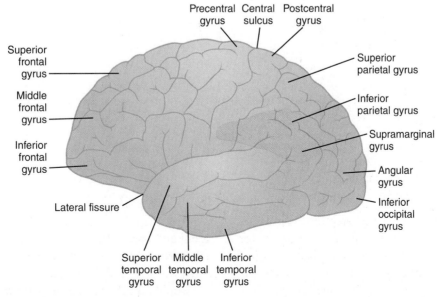

FIGURE 12-20 The neuropathology of conduction aphasia.

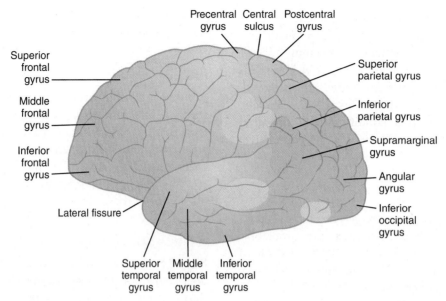

FIGURE 12-21 The neuropathology of anomic aphasia. Darker areas mark primary lesion areas; lighter shading denotes other possible areas of involvement.

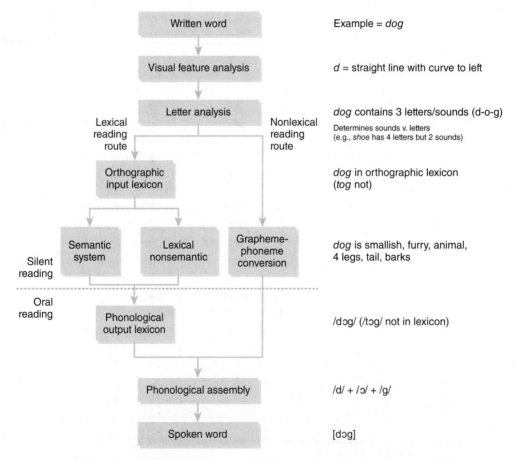

FIGURE 12-22 The dual-route reading model.

lexical reading route. As the first step of this process, our brains scan our orthographic input lexicon for a match for what word is being seen. Then the word moves into the semantic system for meaning attachment. In our example of *dog*, the meaning revolves around a smallish, furry, four-legged animal that has a tail and barks. This is the point at which we stop in silent reading because meaning has been attached to what we have read. If we wanted to read out loud, then we would take the further step of running *dog* through our phonological output lexicon. This is a dictionary of known words we can say. Phonemes are then assembled, and we speak the word out loud. Again, if the word we are trying to read is not in our sight-reading mechanism, then our reading switches to the nonlexical reading route, where graphemes are converted to phonemes and we sound the word out.

Types of Alexia

Alexia comes in two basic forms—peripheral alexia and central alexia. **Peripheral alexia** involves reading problems caused by visuospatial and attention problems. There is difficulty in matching the word seen with the word representation stored in the brain. It is nonlinguistic in nature and does not affect the underlying reading system. **Central alexia** is a linguistic problem that affects the underlying reading system. Examples from each form will be discussed in the following sections. Taking the dual-route model of reading into consideration, peripheral alexia occurs at the beginning of the model (i.e., visual feature analysis and letter analysis), while central alexia is due to a breakdown within the lexical reading route itself (e.g.,

the semantic system). With the dual-route model of reading and these two general categories of alexia in mind, we can now discuss the subtypes of central and peripheral alexia (TABLE 12-6).

Peripheral Alexias

There are four types of peripheral alexia: pure alexia, neglect alexia, attentional alexia, and visual alexia. **Pure alexia** is also known as alexia without agraphia, verbal alexia, or letter-by-letter reading. People who suffer from it have difficulty reading, but writing ability is left intact. In fact, they would not be able to read their own writing. In pure alexia there is a disconnection between the visual information taken in (i.e., visual feature analysis and letter analysis) and the left hemisphere's word recognition system, which lies in the occipitotemporal reading system. In other words, the sight-reading mechanism is damaged. These patients can read, but it has to be done with a letter-by-letter, sounding-out approach (i.e., phonic approach using the nonlexical reading route). This makes reading possible, but also slow and inefficient.

TABLE 12-6 Summary of Peripheral and Central Alexia Subtypes

Alexia Category	Alexia Subtype	Definition	Place of Breakdown in Dual-Route Model
Peripheral alexia	Pure	Sight-reading impaired	Visual feature analysis and letter analysis
	Neglect	Ignoring left or right visual field	Letter analysis
	Attentional	Poor visual attention	Letter analysis
	Visual	Letter or syllable substitutions, additions, or omissions	Letter analysis system and/or the orthographic input lexicon
Central alexia	Phonological	Trouble reading unfamiliar or nonwords	Nonlexical reading route
	Surface	Trouble reading words with irregular print-to-sound correspondences	Lexical reading route
	Deep	Misreading one word for another	Lexical and nonlexical reading routes
	Nonsemantic	Reading without meaning or comprehending	Semantic system in the lexical reading route

Data from Riley, E. A., Brookshire, C. E., & Kendall, D. L. (2017). The acquired disorders of reading. In I. Papathanasiou & P. Coppens (Eds.), *Aphasia and related neurogenic communication disorders* (pp. 195–218). Burlington, MA: Jones & Bartlett Learning.

Neglect alexia occurs usually because of damage to the right hemisphere. Sufferers will fail to identify the initial portions of a word or sentence as they try to read, which is a defect in letter analysis. In other words, they begin reading in the middle of words and/ or sentences (e.g., *tiger* might be read as *-ger*). People who have this form do better reading familiar words because they can predict the word.

The next form, **attentional alexia**, is usually caused by damage to the prefrontal cortex that helps mediate attention. People with this condition can read single words, but when there are multiple words on a page, they become distracted and unable to read. Like neglect alexia, this is a failure at the letter analysis level. This form of alexia is common in people with head injury.

Lastly, **visual alexia** is an impairment in the way that written words are perceived and analyzed during reading. It manifests as letter or syllable substitutions, additions, or omissions (e.g., *butter* instead of *better*; *prince* instead of *price*). This problem is caused by issues with the letter analysis system and/or the orthographic input lexicon.

Central Alexias

Central alexias affect the underlying linguistic reading system. There are four forms to mention: phonological alexia, surface alexia, deep alexia, and nonsemantic reading. **Phonological alexia** is a relatively mild form of dyslexia, which usually does not affect the reading of real words. If people with this condition do have trouble reading real words, it is usually in misperceiving visually similar words. Their real difficulty comes in reading/sounding out new or nonwords (i.e., pseudowords). For example, a nonword such as *phope* might be read as *phone*. Unfamiliar or new words can often be misperceived as being other known words. Phonological alexia is probably due to damage to the parietotemporal reading system, where word analysis occurs. In the dual-route reading model, it is a breakdown in the nonlexical reading route.

In comparison, patients with **surface alexia** have difficulty reading words with irregular print-to-sound correspondences. For example, they would have difficulty reading words like *colonel, yacht, island,* and *borough*. This deficit should be compared to those with phonological alexia, who usually do not have this difficulty. These patients read words with regular print-to-sound correspondences (e.g., *state, hand*) well. These issues are thought to be due to problems with the occipitotemporal reading system, which appears to be important in the lexical reading route.

Deep alexia, also known as semantic alexia, is a breakdown in both the lexical and nonlexical reading routes. In this condition, people recognize words as other words. For example, the word *castle* is perceived as *knight*. Another example might be the word *bird* being read as *canary*. They can also misperceive similar-looking words, like *scale* versus *skate*. Concrete words (e.g., *chair, table*) are read better than abstract words (e.g., *fate, destiny, wish*). Nonwords cannot be read either, which is a breakdown in the nonlexical reading route. Patients with deep alexia are usually not aware of their errors, and these errors are not circumlocutions due to word finding errors. Deep alexia occurs because of disruptions to the occipitotemporal reading system plus probably the perisylvian language area.

Nonsemantic reading is also called reading without meaning. People with this form of alexia can read real and nonwords, and regular and irregular words without difficulty; however, they do not comprehend what they are reading. In other words, they correctly pronounce but do not understand what they are pronouncing. In the dual-route model, it is a problem with the semantic system in the lexical reading route. Neuroanatomically, these issues are most likely due to lesions in and around Wernicke's area (BA 22) and perhaps the fusiform gyrus (BA 37) (Hillis, 2004). We joke in my neuroanatomy class that college students have this condition, which becomes evident as they wade through hundreds of pages of reading each semester.

Agraphia

Agraphia (or dysgraphia) is an acquired disorder of writing. Premorbid writing abilities were normal, but after a stroke or other neurological disorder, writing abilities are impaired. Because writing and spelling are crucial to skills of daily living (e.g., writing checks, making grocery lists), agraphia can be a devastating disorder, especially when it co-occurs with other neurogenic language disorders like aphasia and/or alexia.

A Dual-Route Writing Model

Just as there is a dual-route reading model, so there is a dual-route writing model with lexical and nonlexical writing routes (**FIGURE 12-23**). The lexical writing route is for spelling words we already know, while the nonlexical writing route is for spelling words that are unfamiliar to us. Imagine you are sitting across from a client and you ask him or her to write the word *dog*. If this person's writing were unimpaired, meaning would be attached to the heard word using

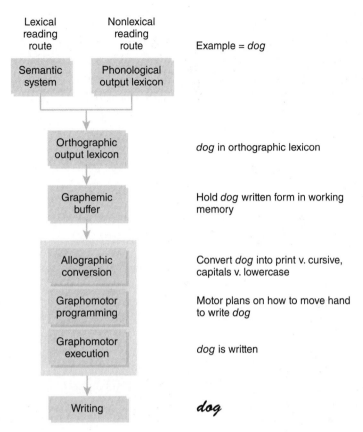

FIGURE 12-23 The dual-route writing model.

the semantic system. His or her brain would then search for a known written word in the orthographic output lexicon to match this auditory stimulus. Next this item would be sent to the graphemic buffer, a type of working memory meant to store this written word form long enough to write it. The process would then move into actual preparing to write stages. The first of these is the allographic conversion stage. Here the word *dog* would be converted into print or cursive and into uppercase and lowercase as appropriate. The next stage, graphomotor programming, involves motor planning for the hand to make the correct motions with a pen to write the word *dog*. Graphomotor execution is the final stage, in which the word *dog* is written. The nonlexical writing route accounts for writing words that are new to a person. This route is used heavily in childhood as we learn to write and spell. This model is used to explain the different types of agraphia in the next section (**TABLE 12-7**).

Types of Agraphia

There are two basic types of agraphia, peripheral and central agraphia. **Peripheral agraphia** includes writing problems due to visuospatial processing and attentional problems. They occur lower in the dual-route writing model, leaving the patient's underlying core

linguistic reading system intact. **Central agraphia** involves impairment in the underlying linguistic writing system and occurs higher in the dual-route model. Both of these categories of agraphia are discussed in the following sections along with their subtypes.

Peripheral Agraphias

Graphemic agraphia is a problem with graphomotor execution of writing and spelling due to attentional issues. Patients omit, substitute, add, or transpose letters. This form of agraphia is caused by lesions to the left prefrontal cortex and left parietal lobe. Patients with **spatial agraphia** have difficulty writing accurately on a horizontal line. They may also write on one side of the paper or the other or will make extra marks on a letter. This form sometimes accompanies visual neglect or hemianopsia. It is a deficit in graphomotor execution usually caused by damage to the right hemisphere. **Allographic agraphia** involves errors in allographic conversion of lowercase versus uppercase letters (e.g., mR. sMitH). It can also include confusion of print and cursive scripts. Left parieto-occipital lesions are associated with allographic agraphia. The final form of peripheral agraphia is **apraxic agraphia**, a disorder of graphomotor programming, in which people have impairments carrying out the motor plans

TABLE 12-7 Summary of Peripheral and Central Agraphia Subtypes

Agraphia Category	Agraphia Subtype	Definition	Place of Breakdown in Dual-Route Model
Peripheral agraphia	Graphemic	Letter or syllable substitutions, additions, or omissions	Graphomotor execution
	Spatial	Writing on a slant and/or including additional marks	Graphomotor execution
	Allographic	Errors in lowercase vs. uppercase and printing vs. cursive	Allographic conversion
	Apraxic	Motor plans for writing graphemes lost	Graphomotor programming
Central agraphia	Deep	Semantic paragraphias (e.g., substituting one word for another)	Semantic system and/or orthographic output lexicon
	Phonological	Trouble writing nonwords	Phonological output lexicon
	Surface	Inability to spell irregular words (e.g., island)	Orthographic output lexicon
	Semantic	Difficulty spelling homophones	Semantic system
	Graphemic buffer	Trouble holding word form in memory in order to write it	Graphemic buffer

Data from Papathanasiou, I., & Cséfalvay, Z. (2017). Written language and its impairments. In I. Papathanasiou & P. Coppens (Eds.), *Aphasia and related neurogenic communication disorders* (pp. 219–244). Burlington, MA: Jones & Bartlett Learning; McNeil, M. R., & Tseng, C. H. (2005). Acquired neurogenic agraphias: Writing problems. In L. L. LaPointe (Ed.), *Aphasia and related neurogenic language disorders*. New York, NY: Thieme.

for writing. They will struggle to hold a writing utensil correctly and will search and grope to write letters correctly. Apraxic agraphia is associated with the main components of the brain's writing centers, including SPL, premotor cortex, and SMA damage (Beeson & Rapcsak, 2004).

Central Agraphias

Central agraphias are linguistically based and occur higher in the dual-route writing model. For example, **deep agraphia** (or semantic agraphia) is characterized by semantic paraphasias (i.e., substituting one word for another) due to issues with the semantic system. In addition, patients have trouble with spelling, especially homophones (e.g., *night* versus *knight*). **Phonological agraphia** is a relatively mild form of agraphia caused by damage to the nonlexical route's phonological output lexicon. These patients can write regular and irregular words but have difficulty with nonwords or nonconcrete words (e.g., pride). Spelling

is affected in both deep and phonological agraphias. These two conditions typically occur due to damage to the language regions of the left hemisphere, including Broca's area, Wernicke's area, and supramarginal gyrus. **Surface agraphia** involves impairments in spelling irregular words (e.g., island), but spelling of regular words is preserved. This type of agraphia is due to problems with the orthographic output lexicon. Damage to the extrasylvian temporoparietal regions of the left hemisphere are usually associated with this form of agraphia (Beeson & Rapcsak, 2004). **Semantic agraphia** is difficulty spelling homophones and is a deficit in the lexical writing route's semantic system. Finally, **graphemic buffer agraphia** is a deficit in the dual-route model's graphemic buffer system. Patients with this type of agraphia cannot hold written forms in their linguistic working memory long enough to write the word. Shorter words are easier to write than longer words are because shorter words require less graphemic buffer space (Papathanasiou & Cséfalvay, 2017).

▶ Conclusion

There are many things we humans take for granted in our lives, and our ability to express ourselves through language may be one of those things. It is certainly extremely complicated neurologically, using a vast array of networked structures. Its complexity is very difficult to capture, as the Wernicke-Geschwind model illustrates. Imaging studies as well as case studies do lend support to some kind of altered form of this model. The major problem with the Wernicke-Geschwind model is that it is too simplistic. First, the size and location of language areas are different from patient to patient. Second, the model does not take into consideration subcortical regions that may be involved in language. Third, the reliance on case and imaging studies may be problematic, especially if these studies are not taking into consideration areas that are subtly involved.

SUMMARY OF LEARNING OBJECTIVES

The following were the main learning objectives of this chapter. The information that should have been learned is below each learning objective.

1. The learner will define *language*.
   - Language is a generative and dynamic code containing universal characteristics whereby ideas about the world are expressed through a conventional system of arbitrary symbols for communication.
2. The learner will list and define the components of language.
   - *Content (semantics):* the meaning of language
   - *Form (grammar):* the form of language
     - □ *Phonology:* the study of a language's sound structure
     - □ *Morphology:* the study of a language's word structure
     - □ *Syntax:* the study of a language's sentence structure
   - *Use (pragmatics):* how language is used practically (e.g., conversation)
3. The learner will outline how language is thought to be neurologically processed in comprehending, reading, speaking, and writing.
   - *Auditory comprehension:* The sounds of spoken language pass through the peripheral auditory system where their acoustic energy is changed into neural impulses. These impulses are conducted through cranial nerve VIII to the cochlear nuclear complex and through the brainstem to the medial geniculate of the thalamus. The thalamus routes the neural impulses to the temporal lobe's primary auditory cortex where the signal is analyzed. The signal then goes to the planum temporale (Wernicke's area), which acts as a hub, drawing help from surrounding areas in the meaning attachment process. Syntax appears to be processed by the superior and posterior temporal lobes. If syntax is complex, Broca's area is recruited into syntax processing.
   - *Reading:* The eyes receive visual information, and photoreceptors in the eyes transduce light into neural impulses. These impulses travel down the visual pathways to the lateral geniculate nucleus of the thalamus. The geniculocalcarine tract projects to the medial part of the occipital lobe surrounding the calcarine sulcus (BA 17). The visual areas of the occipital lobe (BAs 17–19) process the signal and send it to three reading centers for decoding: the parietotemporal system (analysis at the phonemic level), the occipitotemporal reading system (sight-reading), and the anterior reading system (analysis at the syntactic level and silent reading).
   - *Speaking:* The prefrontal cortex is important in the generation of our desire and intention to speak. Our idea is sent to the left inferior frontal cortex where semantic and phonological encoding occurs, probably with the help of surrounding areas (e.g., insular cortex). The plan to speak is sent to the supplementary motor area that initiates the motor plans. These plans are sent to the primary motor cortex, which activates speech muscles via the motor speech system.
   - *Writing:* The prefrontal cortex is important in the generation of our desire and intention to write. Writing occurs through the cooperation of the superior parietal lobe (imagining

graphemes and directing sequence of movements) and the following frontal lobe areas: Broca's area, Exner's area in the premotor cortex, and precentral gyrus. Motor signals are sent to the hand from the precentral gyrus.

4. The learner will describe the following disorders: aphasia, alexia, and agraphia.
   - *Aphasia:* an acquired multimodality language disorder in which patients are either fluent (produce 100–200 words/minute) or nonfluent (produce fewer than 100 words/minute).
   - *Alexia:* an acquired disorder of reading that can be peripheral or central in nature.

Peripheral alexia involves reading problems due to visuospatial and attention problems. It is nonlinguistic in nature and does not affect the underlying reading system. Central alexia is a linguistic problem that affects the underlying reading system.

   - *Agraphia:* an acquired disorder of writing that can be peripheral or central in nature. Peripheral agraphia includes writing problems due to visuospatial processing and attentional problems. The patient's underlying core linguistic reading system is left intact. Central agraphia involves impairment in the underlying linguistic reading system.

KEY TERMS

Agraphia
Alexia
Allographic agraphia
Anomia
Anterior reading system
Aphasia
Apraxic agraphia
Attentional alexia
Central agraphia
Central alexia
Conduction aphasia
Content
Deep agraphia
Deep alexia
Dyslexia

Form
Geniculocalcarine tract
Graphemic agraphia
Graphemic buffer agraphia
Language
Morphology
Neglect alexia
Nonsemantic reading
Occipitotemporal reading
    system
Optic chiasm
Parietotemporal reading
    system
Peripheral agraphia
Peripheral alexia

Phonological agraphia
Phonological alexia
Phonology
Pragmatics
Prefrontal lobotomies
Pure alexia
Semantic agraphia
Spatial agraphia
Surface agraphia
Surface alexia
Syntax
Visual alexia
Wernicke-Geschwind
    model

DRAW IT TO KNOW IT

1. Using the following Brodmann map, sketch a flow of neural information in the following tasks: auditory comprehension, visual comprehension, oral production, and written expression of language. You will have to sketch in the peripheral structures, like the ears, eyes, and so on.

2. Draw a diagram that displays the different classical aphasias, including their similarities and differences.

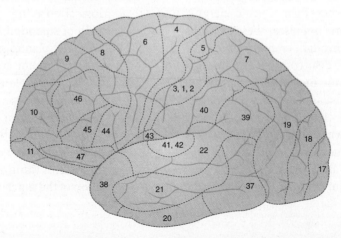

QUESTIONS FOR DEEPER REFLECTION

1. Define *language*.
2. List and define the components and subcomponents of language.
3. Compare and contrast fluent versus nonfluent aphasia.
4. Fill out the following chart using a positive sign (+) for relatively intact and negative sign (−) for impaired. See Table 12-5 as a reference.
5. Compare and contrast central alexia versus peripheral alexia. Give examples.
6. Compare and contrast central agraphia versus peripheral agraphia. Give examples.

Category or Feature	Nonfluent Aphasias				Fluent Aphasias			
	Broca's	Transcortical Motor	Mixed Transcortical	Global	Wernicke's	Transcortical Sensory	Conduction	Anomic
Fluency								
Auditory comprehension								
Repetition								

CASE STUDY

Megan is a 27-year-old television sports reporter who had a sudden onset of difficulty talking on the air. While trying to describe a basketball game that had just ended, she said the following: "well, a very, very heava-ah-heavy-de-bertation tonigh. We had a very deris-derison by let's go hit teris tazen go for the bit had the pit!" In addition to these speech problems, Megan had difficulty auditorily understanding her producer as he expressed concern for her behavior.

After about 30 minutes, Megan's speech returned to normal.

1. What communication disorder was Megan experiencing?
2. What specific subtype of this disorder is the most likely type in Megan's case?
3. What might have caused her to have this episode and then quickly recover?

SUGGESTED PROJECTS

1. Search the scholarly literature and find a case study involving aphasia, alexia, or agraphia. Prepare to present the case to your class.
2. Visit the National Aphasia Association's website, prepare a summary of the resources available, and share with your class.
3. Pretend you have been asked to write an encyclopedia entry on aphasia, alexia, or agraphia. The entry you write should be no more than 750 words long.

REFERENCES

Beeson, P. M., & Rapcsak, S. Z. (2004). Agraphia. In R. D. Kent (Ed.), *The MIT encyclopedia of communication disorders* (pp. 233–236). Cambridge, MA: MIT Press.

Bloom, L., & Lahey, M. (1978). *Language development and language disorders*. London, UK: Pearson.

Cornelissen, P., Hansen, P., Kringelbach, M., & Pugh, K. (2010). *The neural basis of reading*. Oxford, UK: Oxford University Press.

Dapretto, M., & Bookheimer, S. Y. (1999). Form and content: Dissociating syntax and semantics in sentence comprehension. *Neuron, 24*(2), 427–432.

Davis, G. A. (2006). *Aphasiology: Disorders and clinical practice* (2nd ed.). Upper Saddle River, NJ: Pearson.

Friederici, A. D., & Gierhan, S. M. (2013). The language network. *Current Opinion in Neurobiology, 23*(2), 250–254.

Harrington, G. S., Farias, D., Davis, C. H., & Buonocore, M. H. (2007). Comparison of the neural basis for imagined writing and drawing. *Human Brain Mapping, 28*(5), 450–459.

Hedge, M. N. (2018). *A coursebook on aphasia and other neurogenic language disorders* (4th ed.). San Diego, CA: Plural Publishing.

Heim, S., & Keil, A. (2004). Large-scale neural correlates of developmental dyslexia. *European Child and Adolescent Psychiatry, 13*, 125–140.

Hillis, A. E. (2004). Alexia. In R. D. Kent (Ed.), *The MIT encyclopedia of communication disorders* (pp. 236–240). Cambridge, MA: MIT Press.

Hoffmann, M., & Chen, R. (2013). The spectrum of aphasia subtypes and etiology in subacute stroke. *Journal of Stroke and Cerebrovascular Diseases, 22*(8), 1385–1392.

Joseph, J., Noble, K., & Eden, G. (2001). The neurobiological basis of reading. *Journal of Learning Disabilities, 34*, 566–579.

Joseph, R. (2000). *Neuroscience: Neuropsychology, neuropsychiatry, behavioral neurology, brain and mind.* New York, NY: Academic Press.

Katanoda, K., Yoshikawa, K., & Sugishita, M. (2001). A functional MRI study on the neural substrates for writing. *Human Brain Mapping, 13*(1), 34–42.

LaPointe, L. L. (2005). *Aphasia and related neurogenic language disorders.* New York, NY: Thieme.

Longcamp, M., Anton, J. L., Roth, M., & Velay, J. L. (2003). Visual presentation of single letters activates a premotor area involved in writing. *Neuroimage, 19*(4), 1492–1500.

Menon, V., & Desmond, J. E. (2001). Left superior parietal cortex involvement in writing: Integrating fMRI with lesion evidence. *Cognitive Brain Research, 12*(2), 337–340.

Papathanasiou, I., & Cséfalvay, Z. (2017). Written language and its impairments. In I. Papathanasiou & P. Coppens (Eds.), *Aphasia and related neurogenic communication disorders* (pp. 219–244). Burlington, MA: Jones & Bartlett Learning.

Riley, E. A., Brookshire, C. E., & Kendall, D. L. (2017). The acquired disorders of reading. In I. Papathanasiou & P. Coppens (Eds.), *Aphasia and related neurogenic communication disorders* (pp. 195–218). Burlington, MA: Jones & Bartlett Learning.

Roux, F. E., Dufor, O., Giussani, C., Wamain, Y., Draper, L., Longcamp, M., & Démonet, J. F. (2009). The graphemic/motor frontal area: Exner's area revisited. *Annals of Neurology, 66*(4), 537–545.

Shaywitz, S. E., & Shaywitz, B. A. (2004). Reading disability and the brain. *Educational Leadership, 61*(6), 7–11.

Shaywitz, S. E., & Shaywitz, B. A. (2008). Paying attention to reading: The neurobiology of reading and dyslexia. *Development and Psychopathology, 20*, 1329–1349.

The Internet Stroke Center. (n.d.). *What is aphasia?* Retrieved from http://www.strokecenter.org/patients/caregiver-and-patient-resources/aphasia-information/

Thompson-Schill, S. L., Aguirre, G. K., Desposito, M., & Farah, M. J. (1999). A neural basis for category and modality specificity of semantic knowledge. *Neuropsychologia, 37*(6), 671–676.

Wagner, A. D., Koutstaal, W., Maril, A., Schacter, D. L., & Buckner, R. L. (2000). Task-specific repetition priming in left inferior prefrontal cortex. *Cerebral Cortex, 10*(12), 1176–1184.

Wagner, A. D., Paré-Blagoev, E. J., Clark, J., & Poldrack, R. A. (2001). Recovering meaning: Left prefrontal cortex guides controlled semantic retrieval. *Neuron, 31*(2), 329–338.

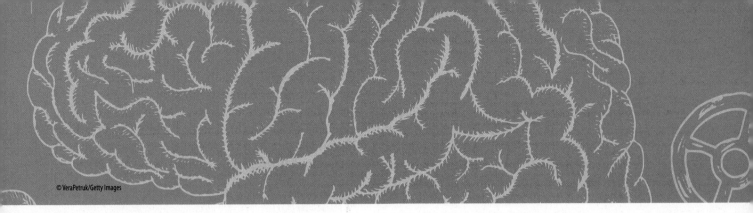

CHAPTER 13

The Neurology of Swallowing

CHAPTER PREVIEW

Swallowing has become a major component of many speech-language pathologists' (SLPs') caseloads, even though it has nothing to do with communication. It does take advantage of the same anatomy as speech, though, so SLPs are capable professionals in the assessment and treatment of swallowing disorders. Like speech, swallowing is a complex process involving a number of muscles, nerves, and even glands. We will be surveying central control of swallowing in this chapter.

IN THIS CHAPTER

In this chapter, we will . . .
- Review the steps and events in the normal swallow
- Analyze the central swallowing system
- Briefly discuss neurogenic swallowing disorders

LEARNING OBJECTIVES

1. The learner will briefly describe each stage of the normal swallow.
2. The learner will correctly identify the cranial nerves involved in each step of the normal swallow.
3. The learner will describe the main components of the central swallowing system.
4. The learner will list neurological disorders that cause dysphagia and note the specific nature of the swallowing problem for each disorder.

▶ Introduction

When not eating, the average person swallows approximately two times per minute while awake and once a minute when sleeping. This adds up to 2,400 swallows every day *not* associated with eating. If the number of swallows when eating were factored in, human beings swallow many thousands of times during an average day. It is a process that we take for granted until something happens to it. In this chapter, both the peripheral and central swallowing systems will be surveyed.

▶ The Normal Swallow

The normal swallow can be thought of as occurring in four dynamic stages: the oral preparatory, oral, pharyngeal, and esophageal stages (**FIGURE 13-1**). Each of these stages will be briefly discussed along with the type of neural control associated with each stage (voluntary versus involuntary), the time it takes to complete each stage, and the muscles involved (**TABLE 13-1**). Of the 12 pairs of cranial nerves, half of them are involved in normal swallowing: V, VII, IX, X, XI, and XII. (As in Chapter 5, cranial nerve numbers are noted in parentheses throughout this chapter.) These nerves and their relationship to swallowing are also surveyed in this section.

The Oral Preparatory Stage

The **oral preparatory stage** is voluntary and variable in length, depending on the substance being eaten. In this stage, food is placed in the mouth and is prepared for swallowing. Essentially, solid and semisolid foods are masticated and mixed with saliva, forming a puree consistency, which makes swallowing safer and more efficient. Oral breathing ceases and nasal breathing takes over due to a labial seal being established and maintained in order to keep food in the oral cavity.

Mastication

The trigeminal nerve's (V) mandibular branch innervates the muscles for mastication (chewing). The main chewing muscles include the following mandibular elevators: masseters, temporalis, and pterygoid muscles. The masseter closes the mandible, which facilitates cutting food using the central and lateral incisors. The temporalis and the medial and lateral pterygoids are the prime muscles for grinding food via the molars. The trigeminal nerve also innervates muscles that depress or open the mandible. These muscles include the mylohyoid and the anterior belly of the digastric muscle.

Gland Secretion

Saliva is an important component in the process of breaking foods down for swallowing. It consists mostly of water, with the remaining portion being enzymes that break down foods. Three major salivary glands secrete saliva and mix it into the **bolus** (i.e., a food or liquid ball) during chewing (**FIGURE 13-2**). The parotid gland is stimulated by the general visceral efferent fibers of the glossopharyngeal nerve (IX), and the submandibular and sublingual glands are innervated by the general visceral efferent fibers of the facial nerve (VII).

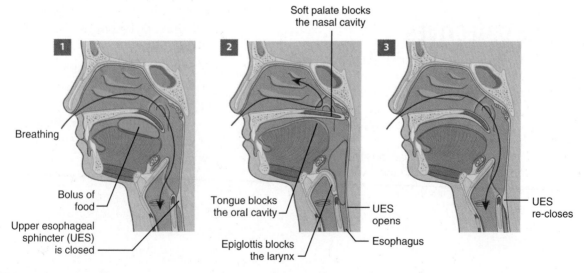

FIGURE 13-1 The stages of the normal swallow. (Note: The oral preparatory stage is not pictured.) **1.** The oral stage. **2.** The pharyngeal stage. **3.** The esophageal stage.

TABLE 13-1 Summary of the Normal Swallow Stages

Swallow Stage	Type of Neural Control	Timing (in secs)	Cranial Nerve Involvement	Muscle Involvement
Oral preparatory	Voluntary	Variable (depends on bolus type)	V—chewing IX—gland VII—gland	Mandibular elevators and depressors
Oral	Voluntary	1 second	VII—labial seal; taste XII—anterior-to-posterior bolus movement	Face muscles (e.g., orbicularis oris) Intrinsic and extrinsic tongue muscles
Pharyngeal	Involuntary*	1 second	V—soft palate closure; laryngeal elevation VII—laryngeal elevation X—laryngeal, velar closure; pharyngeal constriction XI—soft palate closure; pharyngeal constriction XII—laryngeal elevation	Soft palate elevators and depressors Intrinsic laryngeal muscles Supra- and infrahyoid muscles Pharyngeal constrictors
Esophageal	Involuntary	Variable (depends on bolus type)	X— upper esophageal sphincter control; esophageal peristalsis	Cricopharyngeus muscle Esophageal muscles

* It is possible to exercise voluntary control in the pharyngeal stage, but this is not typical behavior. However, the fact that you can exercise voluntary control is used in some swallowing therapy maneuvers.

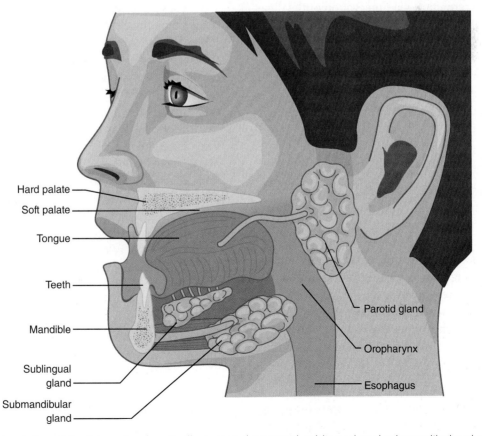

FIGURE 13-2 A lateral view of the internal oral cavity illustrating the parotid, sublingual, and submandibular glands.

The Oral Stage

The **oral stage** is also a voluntary stage lasting approximately 1 second. It begins once mastication ceases. A bolus is formed and placed on the tongue. The anterior tip of the tongue rises and its posterior portion drops, forming a ramp. The bolus is then squeezed posteriorly through the oral cavity by the tongue's rolling contact against the palate. During this activity, the labial seal is maintained and nasal breathing continues.

Labial Seal

The facial nerve (VII) controls motor and sensory function in swallowing. It innervates the muscles of the face via special visceral efferent fibers, especially the lip muscles (e.g., orbicularis oris, buccinator) responsible for compressing and sealing the lips to keep the bolus in the oral cavity. Its special visceral afferent fibers convey taste information to the brain from the anterior two-thirds of the tongue; its general visceral efferent fibers stimulate the production of saliva used to keep the mouth moist and to help in the breakdown of food during mastication.

Tongue Retraction

In addition to playing an important role in innervating the chewing muscles, the trigeminal nerve is responsible for tongue retraction via innervation of the digastric and mylohyoid muscles. This action is important in the oral stage of the swallow when the tongue forms a ramp to move the bolus from the anterior portion of the mouth to the posterior. The trigeminal's general somatic afferent fibers carry information regarding temperature, pressure, and touch from the oral cavity to the brain.

Anterior-to-Posterior Bolus Movement

The hypoglossal nerve (XII) is a motor nerve. It controls all the intrinsic and most of the extrinsic tongue muscles. The tongue is obviously crucial to the oral stage of the swallow in gathering up the bolus and moving it posteriorly to the pharynx. The intrinsic and extrinsic tongue muscles control the shape of the tongue and are responsible for not only forming the ramp the bolus will travel down but also squeezing the bolus through the oral cavity.

The Pharyngeal Stage

The **pharyngeal stage** is essentially involuntary, though one could exert conscious control over it. Like the oral stage, it lasts approximately 1 second. As the bolus contacts the faucial arches, the soft palate elevates, the vocal cords adduct, and respiration pauses. The larynx elevates and moves forward and the epiglottis lowers, directing the bolus toward the esophageal segment. Simultaneously, the **cricopharyngeus** muscle at the top of the esophagus relaxes, allowing the bolus to enter the esophagus.

Soft Palate Closure

Soft palate elevation is crucial in keeping liquids and solids out of the nasal cavity during swallowing. Five muscles control the soft palate during swallowing. The levator veli palatini and palatoglossal muscles, innervated by the vagus (X) and accessory (XI) nerves, raise the soft palate and seal off the nasal cavity. The tensor veli palatini muscle assists these muscles by tensing the soft palate. It is innervated by the trigeminal nerve (V). The musculus uvulae muscle, innervated by the vagus and accessory nerves, also assists these muscles by shortening and raising the uvula. The palatopharyngeus muscles pull the pharynx up and constrict it. They also help to open the soft palate once the bolus has passed. They are innervated by the vagus and accessory nerves.

Laryngeal Closure

During the pharyngeal stage of the swallow, the larynx closes three valves to prevent food and liquid from penetrating the airway, which could lead to aspiration. First, the cartilaginous epiglottis closes over the top of the larynx and, thus, guards the airway. The aryepiglottic and thyroepiglottic muscles, when contracted, lower the epiglottis. Both of these muscles are controlled by the recurrent laryngeal branch of the vagus nerve.

The second valve is the false vocal folds, or the ventricular folds. These thick folds of mucous membrane are brought toward midline as the true vocal folds contract. They do not contain muscle.

The third and final valve is the true vocal folds. There are a number of intrinsic laryngeal muscles that control the vocal folds. The intrinsic adductor muscles are the most relevant in swallowing because these adduct the vocal folds during swallowing. There are three adductor muscles, the lateral thyroarytenoid and the oblique arytenoids, which are paired, and the transverse arytenoid. All three of these muscles are innervated by the recurrent laryngeal nerve of the vagus.

Laryngeal Elevation

During the pharyngeal stage of swallowing, the larynx elevates under the epiglottis. This is achieved through several extrinsic suprahyoid muscles, which include the digastricus, stylohyoid, mylohyoid, geniohyoid, hyoglossus, and genioglossus. The digastricus muscle has an anterior belly innervated by the mandibular branch of the trigeminal nerve (V) and a posterior belly controlled by the facial nerve (VII). The mylohyoid also has its nerve supply from the mandibular branch of the trigeminal nerve. The stylohyoid receives stimulation from the facial nerve (VII). The hypoglossal nerve (XII) innervates the hyoglossus and genioglossus. The geniohyoid is controlled by cervical spinal nerve 1 through the hypoglossal nerve.

Pharyngeal Constriction

The vagus (X) and accessory (XI) nerves innervate the superior, middle, and inferior pharyngeal constrictor muscles. These muscles form a muscular tube that, when contracted, squeezes the bolus through the pharynx to the esophagus. This squeezing action is initiated when the bolus meets sensory receptors near the faucial pillars, tonsils, and soft palate. Sensation is then sent through cranial nerves VII, IX, and X to the medulla, which then sends motor commands through cranial nerves X and XI.

The Esophageal Stage

The **esophageal stage** is an involuntary stage; like the oral preparatory stage it is variable in length (8–20 seconds), depending on the substance eaten. After the bolus enters the esophagus, peristaltic waves (i.e., involuntary wavelike contractions) move the bolus to the stomach in conjunction with gravity. When not swallowing, the cricopharyngeus muscle contracts to prevent reflux, and respiration resumes.

Esophageal Opening

The esophagus lies posterior to the trachea. At its superior end is a muscular valve called the upper esophageal sphincter. The cricopharyngeus muscle, which powers this valve, is normally contracted but relaxes as the bolus reaches the posterior pharyngeal wall. This muscle is innervated by the pharyngeal branch of the vagus nerve.

Esophageal Constriction

The esophagus is an 18- to 25-centimeter (cm)-long tube that is collapsed when not containing food or liquids. It can be divided into three segments: the cervical, thoracic, and abdominal esophagus.

The cervical esophagus is approximately 4 to 5 cm long and is made up of striated muscle. The thoracic esophagus is approximately 18.5 to 20.5 cm long; the upper half consists of a mix of striated and smooth muscle, and the inferior portion is smooth muscle only. Striated muscle is voluntary in nature, whereas smooth muscle is involuntary. The abdominal esophagus is 0.5 to 2.5 cm long and made of smooth muscle. It meets the stomach at the lower esophageal sphincter (Corbin-Lewis, Liss, & Sciortino, 2005).

Sequential, wavelike muscle contractions, referred to as **peristalsis**, move food through the esophagus. These contractions are coordinated by the medulla, with the proximal end of the esophagus contracting while the distal end is relaxed. The striated muscle in the cervical segment is controlled by parasympathetic fibers of the vagus nerve, and the thoracic and abdominal portions are controlled by the enteric nervous system. The vagus nerve is the prime controller of esophageal peristalsis.

The process of swallowing is a complicated, dynamic process, and staging it is a helpful but artificial way of conceptualizing it. **FIGURE 13-3** illustrates these stages' interdependent and highly coordinated nature and summarizes the main events we have discussed so far.

▶ The Central Swallowing System

Brainstem Involvement

Like the cochlear nucleus in the central auditory system, the swallowing system has specialized nuclei in the brainstem as well (**FIGURE 13-4**). The first of these is the **nucleus tractus solitarius (NTS)**, which is Latin for "nucleus of the solitary tract." The NTS is located in the medulla. It acts as a swallowing sensory center by receiving afferent information, such as touch and taste, from cranial nerves V, VII, IX, and X, as well as sensory input from the respiratory and cardiovascular brainstem nuclei. This sensory information is then transferred to the second brainstem nucleus, the **nucleus ambiguus (NA)** or "ambiguous nucleus," also located in the medulla. The NA is the motor swallowing center that innervates the swallowing muscles via cranial nerves in the peripheral swallowing system. These cranial nerves include IX, X, and XII. Because of the tight functional integration between the NTS and NA, these are sometimes referred to as the swallowing center of the medulla.

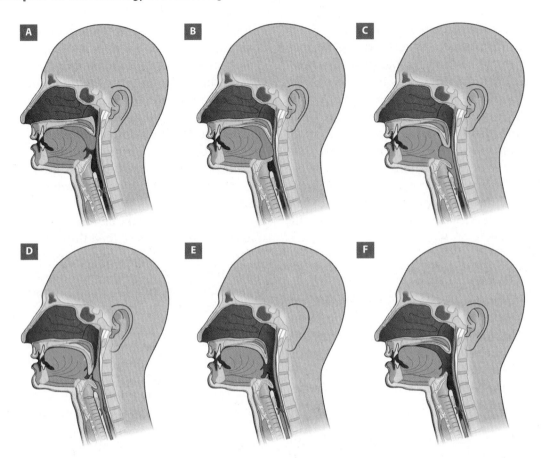

FIGURE 13-3 The normal swallow involves four separate stages that are interdependent and highly coordinated: the oral preparatory stage, the oral stage, the pharyngeal stage, and the esophageal stage. This series of illustrations demonstrates a lateral view of bolus propulsion during the swallow: **A.** The oral stage uses the tongue to voluntarily move the bolus toward the back of the mouth; the soft palate raises to prevent nasal regurgitation. **B.** The pharyngeal stage is initiated and the larynx raises, causing the epiglottis to drop down to cover the larynx and prevent penetration of food or liquid. Both the true and false vocal folds close to prevent material from falling into the trachea. **C.** The epiglottis descends completely and the bolus reaches the upper esophageal valve. **D.** The upper esophageal valve opens, allowing the bolus to enter the esophagus. **E.** The upper esophageal valve closes once the bolus has completely passed. **F.** The larynx descends, causing the epiglottis to rise to its normal position, and the true and false vocal folds open. The base of the tongue and soft palate move to their resting positions. Esophageal peristalsis helps propel the bolus to the lower esophageal valve, which opens and allows the bolus to enter the stomach.

Subcortical and Cortical Controls

The NTS ascends to the pons, hypothalamus, and thalamus and terminates in the primary sensory cortex (Brodmann areas [BAs] 1–3) of the parietal lobe (**FIGURE 13-5**). The hypothalamus regulates hunger and thirst, so it is connected to the eating and swallowing process. The thalamus relays the NTS's fibers to the primary sensory cortex for processing.

Motor fibers leading to the NA begin in the inferior primary motor cortex (IPMC) and descend to the substantia nigra and then to the reticular formation of the pons. The fibers then course down to the medulla where they terminate in the NA. In addition to these fibers, there are fibers from the hypothalamus and cerebellum that may influence swallowing.

Cortical control of swallowing most likely includes additional areas besides the IPMC because cortical and subcortical lesions outside this area lead to **dysphagia** (i.e., swallowing trouble). Zald and Pardo (1999) used positron emission tomography (PET) scans to measure cerebral blood flow in eight patients during swallowing. In addition to the activity in the inferior primary motor cortex, there was substantial activity in the **claustrum** (a sheetlike membrane of neurons under the cortex), cerebellum, basal ganglia, thalamus, and right temporal lobe. Hamdy et al. (1999) used functional magnetic resonance imaging and detected cortical activity during swallowing in the sensorimotor cortex, anterior insula, premotor cortex, frontal operculum, anterior cingulate and prefrontal cortex, anterolateral and posterior parietal cortex, precuneus, and superiomedial temporal cortex. Less consistent activations were also observed in the posterior cingulate cortex and the basal ganglia. Martin,

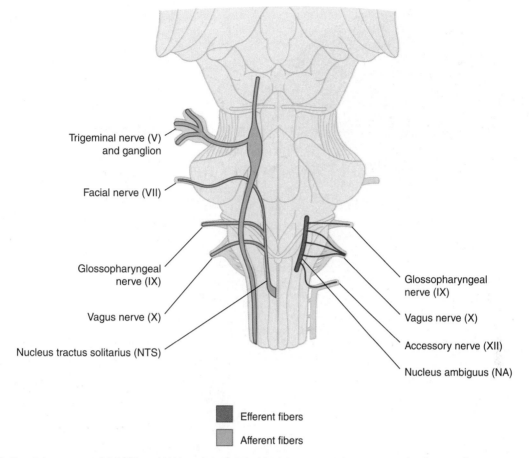

Trigeminal nerve (V)
and ganglion

Facial nerve (VII)

Glossopharyngeal
nerve (IX)

Vagus nerve (X)

Nucleus tractus solitarius (NTS)

Glossopharyngeal
nerve (IX)

Vagus nerve (X)

Accessory nerve (XII)

Nucleus ambiguus (NA)

Efferent fibers

Afferent fibers

FIGURE 13-4 Cranial nerve nuclei (NTS and NA) and their relationship to cranial nerves involved in swallowing.

Goodyear, Gati, and Menon (2001) observed activation within the lateral precentral gyrus, lateral postcentral gyrus, right insula, superior temporal gyrus, middle and inferior frontal gyri, and frontal operculum. Daniels and Foundas (1997) also found activation in the anterior insula. Cola et al. (2010) reported that subcortical stroke in the left periventricular white matter caused dysphagia involving oral control and transfer. These studies suggest that there is a large cortical and subcortical network responsible for swallowing in addition to the IPMC and the swallowing center (NTS + NA) in the medulla. How do these cortical and subcortical structures function in swallowing?

The primary motor cortex (BA 4) is probably the easiest to explain given that it activates muscles via the pyramidal system. Thus, the primary motor cortex activates the oral, pharyngeal, and cervical esophageal muscles for swallowing. Across the central fissure, the primary sensory cortex (BAs 1–3) likely processes sensation from the oral cavity as a person manipulates food in the oral preparatory and oral stages of the swallow. The insula is thought to mediate motor and sensory information in the oral and pharyngeal cavities as well as the esophagus. It may also play some role in the control of the swallow. The frontal operculum (BA 44) may play a role in some

of the motor and sensory functions in the oral cavity. The anterior cingulate cortex may provide the attention necessary for swallowing. The premotor cortex (BA 6) plays a role in motor planning, so it would be logical to assume it plays a role in swallowing motor planning. Activations in the posterior part of the brain (parietal and temporal lobes) most likely relate to sensorimotor integration. The thalamus and basal ganglia may incorporate sensory information from food and liquid as the bolus passes through the swallowing structures into the actual movements of swallowing (Daniels, Brailey, & Foundas, 1999; Daniels & Foundas, 1997, 1999; Kern, Jaradeh, Arndorfer, & Shaker, 2001; Malandraki, Perlman, Karampinos, & Sutton, 2011; Martin et al., 2001; Mosier & Bereznaya, 2001).

Neurology of the Cough Response

Coughing is an important defensive reflex in swallowing. It clears not only secretions from the airway but also any food or drink that has penetrated the laryngeal defenses and made it to the vocal folds.

There are three main components in the cough reflex arc (**FIGURE 13-6**). First, the afferent fibers from the vagus nerve convey signals from cough receptors

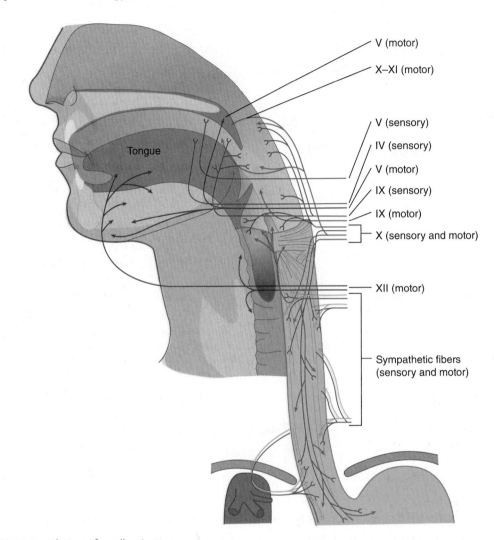

- V (motor)
- X–XI (motor)
- V (sensory)
- IV (sensory)
- V (motor)
- IX (sensory)
- IX (motor)
- X (sensory and motor)
- XII (motor)
- Sympathetic fibers (sensory and motor)

Tongue

FIGURE 13-5 Neuroregulation of swallowing.

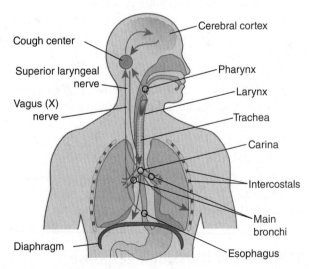

- Cough center
- Superior laryngeal nerve
- Vagus (X) nerve
- Diaphragm
- Cerebral cortex
- Pharynx
- Larynx
- Trachea
- Carina
- Intercostals
- Main bronchi
- Esophagus

FIGURE 13-6 Neural pathways for the cough. Cough receptors are shown in red.

located in the pharynx, larynx, and trachea. These cough receptors are sensitive to chemical stimulation. Second, these signals go to a cough center located in the upper brainstem and the pons. Third, efferent signals are sent from the cough center via the vagus, phrenic, and spinal nerves to the respiratory muscles and via the vagus nerve to the larynx. Inhalation of air occurs that is needed to generate the cough's power, and the larynx closes. Pressure is thus built up. The glottis suddenly opens and releases the built-up air, which results in the coughing behavior (Polverino et al., 2012).

Neurology of Silent Aspiration

Aspiration occurs when food or liquid penetrates below the vocal cords and then has a clear path to the lungs. Typically, the cough reflex arc is stimulated when material penetrates the larynx; however, neurological damage can suppress this reflex arc, and patients can experience silent aspiration, which is aspiration without any apparent signs of it (i.e., no cough or throat clearing). Silent aspiration is estimated to occur in one-third of dysphagic patients (Corbin-Lewis, Liss, & Sciortino, 2005). Daniels, Ballo, Mahoney, and Foundas (2000) attempted to compile a list of clinical indicators of aspiration broader than just cough.

In addition to watching for cough after swallow, they suggested looking for dysphonia, dysarthria, abnormal gag reflex, abnormal volitional cough, and any voice changes after swallow (TABLE 13-2). A patient demonstrating two or more of these indicators should be labeled an aspiration risk and have further evaluation with a videofluoroscopic swallow study or a fiberoptic endoscopic evaluation of swallowing (**BOX 13-1**).

TABLE 13-2 Six Clinical Indicators of Aspiration Risk

Indicator	Description
Dysphonia	A voice disturbance in the parameters of vocal quality, pitch, or intensity
Dysarthria	A speech disorder resulting from disturbances in muscular control affecting the areas of respiration, articulation, phonation, resonance, or prosody
Abnormal gag reflex	Either absent or weakened velar or pharyngeal wall contraction, unilaterally or bilaterally, in response to tactile stimulation of the posterior pharyngeal wall
Abnormal volitional cough	A weak response, verbalized response, or no response when given the command to cough
Cough after swallow	Cough immediate or within 1 minute of ingestion of calibrated volumes of water (5, 10, and 20 mL presented in duplicate)
Voice change after swallow	Alteration in vocal quality following ingestion of calibrated volumes of water

Data from Daniels, S. K., Ballo, L. A., Mahoney, M. C., & Foundas, A. L. (2000). Clinical predictors of dysphagia and aspiration risk: Outcome measures in acute stroke patients. *Archives of Physical Medicine and Rehabilitation, 81*(8), 1030–1033.

BOX 13-1 Evaluation for Dysphagia

SLPs are the main health care professionals for assessing swallowing mechanism, diagnosing dysphagia, and providing treatment. The evaluation process begins at the bedside with what is called the bedside swallowing evaluation. An SLP performs an oral motor examination and small trials of swallowing water or ice chips, watching for the clinical indicators listed in Table 13-2. If the patient is identified as an aspiration risk, further evaluation takes place with either a videofluoroscopic swallow study (VSS; also known as a modified barium swallow study [MBSS], FIGURE 13-7) in the radiology department or a fiberoptic endoscopic evaluation of swallowing (FEES) at the bedside. There are benefits and drawbacks to each procedure. For example, FEES does not expose patients to radiation and can be done at the bedside without the use of barium (i.e., a radiopaque substance used in MBSS that patients do not enjoy swallowing); however, FEES cannot be used to assess the oral preparatory, oral, or esophageal stages of the swallow. It is focused on what happens just before and after the pharyngeal stage. The clinician can observe all stages of the swallow with VSS. The FEES procedure is more sensitive to detecting aspiration, while the VSS procedure is better at seeing the whole of the swallowing process (Gerek, Atalay, Çekin, Ciyiltepe, & Ozkaptan, 2005).

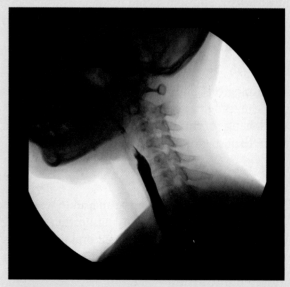

FIGURE 13-7 A videofluoroscopic swallow study. Note: the dark substance in the pharynx and esophagus is the bolus mixed with barium.

▶ Neurological Swallowing Disorders

Deglutition (Latin for "to swallow down") is the medical term for the process of swallowing, and dysphagia is the formal term for a swallowing disorder. *Dysphagia* literally means "impaired eating." It can be caused by a variety of conditions, so it is a common occurrence in the medical field. Prior to the 1970s, there were few articles published on dysphagia, and, thus, little medical expertise was available in assessment or treatment (Massey & Shaker, 2003). Patients with swallowing trouble typically receive a gastric tube and may never eat by mouth again. With the explosion of imaging technology in the 1970s and 1980s, research attention shifted to swallowing and swallowing disorders. In fact, in 1986 the journal *Dysphagia* was established, which greatly advanced knowledge in this important area.

Causes

There are numerous neurological disorders in which dysphagia is a symptom. Cerebrovascular accident is one of the most common reasons people experience dysphagia. Swallowing problems will vary in these patients, depending on the location and site of lesion. Traumatic brain injury, which causes diffuse brain injury, can also lead to disorders of swallowing. Other neurological conditions include neoplasms (cancerous or benign tumors), infections (e.g., meningitis, encephalitis), toxin exposure (**BOX 13-2**), degenerative diseases (e.g., amyotrophic lateral sclerosis), metabolic disorders, and spinal cord injury.

The General Nature of Neurogenic Dysphagia

The neurological conditions outlined in the previous section can lead to a variety of sensorimotor problems in swallowing. At this point, we will look at common issues in each stage of the swallow.

Oral Preparatory Stage

In this stage, neurological injury can lead to weakness or impairment in the muscles of mastication, leading to chewing problems and prolonged oral preparation time. Chewing problems can put patients at risk for choking due to being unable to break down foods properly. People may also have difficulty controlling the bolus well enough during mastication, resulting in food or liquid spilling out of the mouth.

BOX 13-2 Toxin Exposure and Dysphagia: The Woman Who Drank Bleach

I received a request to complete a swallow evaluation on a 23-year-old woman who had attempted suicide. At first I was confused, wondering how a suicide attempt could impair swallowing. My mind raced through possibilities. Maybe she tried to hang herself and had injured her larynx or pharynx? Or perhaps she had attempted carbon monoxide poisoning and had an anoxic episode. As I perused her medical chart, I discovered the nature of her attempt and the cause of her swallowing problems: She had attempted suicide by drinking bleach **FIGURE 13-8**. The bleach had badly burned her oral, pharyngeal, laryngeal, and esophageal regions, resulting in severe edema.

She was able to generate some evidence of a swallow at bedside, so we took her to radiology and performed a VSS. The burns and edema were so significant that they greatly impaired her sensorimotor abilities in the oral and pharyngeal phases of the swallow, putting her at risk for aspiration. The patient was put on a nasogastric tube in order to receive nutrition and hydration. She would need to heal before she could safely swallow again.

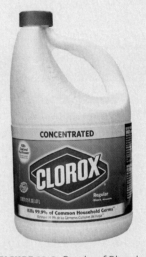

FIGURE 13-8 Bottle of Bleach.

Oral Stage

Motor problems can lead to paresis or paralysis in the orbicularis oris muscle, resulting in drooling. People may experience pocketing of food in the cheek due to impaired buccinator and risorius muscles. This pocketing (what I call "chipmunking" to patients) is dangerous, especially when there is sensory loss in the cheek. A person may not realize there is food in the cheek and may lie down to sleep, causing food to dislodge and be aspirated. In the oral stage, weak tongue muscles lead to impaired bolus control in the oral cavity. There can be great difficulty in forming the bolus, placing it on the tongue, forming the ramp, and then moving the bolus from the front of the mouth to the back of the mouth (i.e., anterior-to-posterior transport). Because of these problems, tongue pumping is often seen in the oral stage of swallow. This is a compensatory strategy (though often very inefficient) for moving the bolus to the pharynx. A sensory issue that may occur is a hyperactive gag response that triggers when utensils (e.g., fork, spoon) are used. Food itself may trigger the gag, making oral nutrition and hydration challenging.

Pharyngeal Stage

The pharyngeal stage of the swallow can be either delayed, weak, or completely absent, which can put a patient at risk for aspiration. These issues can result from oral, pharyngeal, laryngeal, and/or esophageal dysfunction of the musculature. Damage to the brainstem NTS and/or NA can result in the swallow response being absent. Weak pharyngeal constrictors lead to a lack of pharyngeal squeezing, causing food and liquids to pool in the valleculae and/or pyriform sinus. In addition to the issues with the swallow response, a lack of laryngeal elevation and closure can also result in aspiration. Laryngeal elevation may be impaired because of suprahyoid muscle weakness. Impairment to the intrinsic laryngeal adductors results in a lack of glottal closure. Weakness to the soft palate musculature results in incomplete velopharyngeal closure and nasal regurgitation of foods and liquids.

Esophageal Stage

The upper esophageal sphincter may be dysfunctional, resulting in the bolus not efficiently entering into the esophagus and pooling in the pyriform sinuses. Damage to any of the nerves that innervate esophageal peristalsis can result in dismotility. With this kind of damage, spasms may also occur in the esophagus that can be painful. **Achalasia** is a condition in which smooth esophageal muscle fails to relax, resulting in pain and regurgitation.

Specific Neurological Conditions Involving Dysphagia

Stroke and Traumatic Brain Injury

Stroke is the main cause of dysphagia. It can result in oral transit problems, delayed triggering of the

pharyngeal swallow, pooling of material in the pharynx, penetration of the airway, and aspiration. The severity of the swallowing deficits will vary based on the extent of the stroke, the number of strokes, and the location of the lesion. Brainstem strokes often are the most debilitating due to the location of the swallowing centers in it. With brainstem strokes, the entire swallow response may be absent. The positive side is that most patients make significant recovery over time (Corbin-Lewis, Liss, & Sciortino 2005). Predictors for long-term dysphagia include dysphonia, dysarthria, abnormal gag reflex, abnormal volitional cough, cough after swallow, and voice change after swallow. Patients with four or more of these factors have a poor prognosis for oral intake (Schroeder, Daniels, McClain, Corey, & Foundas, 2006).

Although stroke damage is typically focal in nature, traumatic brain injury (TBI) is diffuse, involving large portions of the cerebral cortex and subcortical white matter. TBI patients may experience oral mobility issues, delayed pharyngeal swallow, and aspiration (Lazarus & Logemann, 1987). Poor prognostic factors for TBI patients include increased age, low score on the Rancho Levels of Cognitive Functioning scale, tracheostomy tube placement, and aphonia (Mandaville, Ray, Robertson, Foster, & Jesser, 2014).

Multiple Sclerosis

Multiple sclerosis (MS) is a progressive, degenerative, demyelinating disease caused by an abnormal immune response. Dysphagia is a common symptom of MS, occurring in 33% to 43% of MS patients (Thomas & Wiles, 1999). Pharyngeal stage problems are the most common issue with MS patients, probably due to swallow delay and poor pharyngeal squeezing. These issues put MS patients at risk for aspiration (Abraham & Yun, 2002; Poorjavad et al., 2010).

Extrapyramidal Disorders

Parkinson Disease

Parkinson disease (PD) is another progressive, degenerative nervous system disease caused by degeneration of the midbrain's substantia nigra and a loss of the neurotransmitter dopamine. The three main symptoms of PD are bradykinesia, rigidity, and tremor. Dysphagia is a common complication in PD, affecting an estimated 40% to 90% of PD patients (Leopold & Kagel, 1997; Muller et al., 2001; Rosenbek & Jones, 2006).

In terms of swallowing, PD patients have mastication problems due to muscle rigidity in the oral preparatory stage. It is common to see tongue pumping in the oral stage due to this same rigidity issue. This results in poor anterior-to-posterior movement of the bolus. Drooling is evident due to poor labial seal. In the pharyngeal stage, PD patients often have delayed swallow responses and rigidity in the pharynx. This rigidity leads to a poor pharyngeal squeeze and residue material being left in the pharynx. Laryngeal elevation is reduced and the cough response is often suppressed in PD (Tjaden, 2009).

Huntington Disease

Huntington disease (HD) is a progressive, degenerative, inherited disease of the basal ganglia. Patients with HD suffer from dyskinesias, especially chorea. They have balance issues, resulting in falls, as well as speech and emotional issues. Dementia is an inevitable consequence of the disease (Corbin-Lewis, Liss, & Sciortino, 2005).

Swallowing is impaired by the chorea. Patients will orally hold onto the bolus, a phenomenon known as squirreling. Bolus formation and transport are typically poor. In the pharyngeal stage, swallowing is often delayed, with pooling and laryngeal penetration and possible aspiration. The continuous movements of the head exacerbate these issues (Kagel & Leopold, 1992; Leopold & Kagel, 1985).

Amyotrophic Lateral Sclerosis

Amyotrophic lateral sclerosis (ALS) is a progressive, degenerative disease of both the upper and lower motor neurons. About 1 in 10 cases is genetic, but the remaining cases have an unknown etiology.

The oral stage is typically the first swallowing stage to be affected in ALS. Patients experience a loss of lip and tongue movement, making bolus formation and transport challenging. Early pharyngeal issues include delayed swallow response and poor pharyngeal squeeze. As the disease progresses, patients experience poor airway protection and subsequent aspiration. Eventually ALS patients will not be able to swallow safely and will require long-term means of nutrition and hydration. It is the SLP's job to determine the timing of transition from oral feedings to nonoral options (Chapman, 2013).

Guillain-Barré Syndrome

Guillain-Barré syndrome (GBS) is a peripheral nerve disease of unknown origin. Patients experience a rapid onset of whole-body paralysis, including the muscles of respiration. With supportive care, patients will spontaneously recover over time. All stages of the swallow are affected as GBS progresses, with the patient eventually being unable to swallow. The SLP has to evaluate people with GBS on both ends of the disease—on the front end for when they no longer can eat by mouth and on the back end as they improve and can possible eat safely again.

Myasthenia Gravis

Most of the neurological diseases surveyed so far have been progressive, with the exception of most stroke and TBI cases. Myasthenia gravis (MG) is also a progressive, degenerative neurological disease of the neuromuscular junction. Postsynaptic acetylcholine receptors are impaired by the body's autoimmune system, leading to muscle fatigue and weakness. When muscles are rested, patients typically recover some level of strength. Swallowing is most at risk during periods of muscle use that lead to this fatigue and weakness. Symptoms of dysphagia include the logical result of weakness, including pharyngeal dismotility, pharyngeal pooling of material, aspiration, and poor esophageal motility in the cervical esophagus (Corbin-Lewis, Liss, & Sciortino, 2005).

Cervical Spinal Cord Injury

Spinal cord injury (SCI) is not typically associated with dysphagia, but SCI in the higher cervical regions can lead to impaired motor and sensory abilities in the neck. C1 innervates the geniohyoid, a laryngeal elevator. This function demonstrates that the cervical spinal cord is involved with normal swallowing.

Kirshblum, Johnston, Brown, O'Connor, and Jarosz (1999) found that 22.5% of the 187 patients with SCI studied had symptoms of dysphagia. Wolf and Meiners (2003) examined 51 patients with cervical spinal cord injury (CSCI) and found that 41% had severe dysphagia and 39% had mild dysphagia. Severe dysphagia was characterized by impairments in mastication, sensation, swallow reflex, and cough reflex. These problems led to massive aspiration of both saliva and food. Mild dysphagia was characterized by normal sensation, mastication, and swallow reflex, but mild aspiration of liquids was noted. The cough response was intact, and subjects were able to clear the aspirated materials. Both of these studies indicate that people with CSCI are at risk for dysphagia and should undergo routine evaluation for possible issues.

▶ Conclusion

Like language, our ability to swallow is something we probably take for granted. Our ability to eat is intimately connected to our social life. Just think about how many conversations you have over a meal. Now imagine losing the ability to swallow. What impact would that have on your social interactions?

Eating is also important to religious communities. Jewish people celebrate a number of religious feasts, including the feasts of Passover, Trumpets, and Tabernacles. Consider the Christian tradition and the importance of the Lord's Supper that reminds Christians of Christ's death, but also the unity Christians are to have with one another. Many other religions attach great importance to food and sharing a meal. How devastating might a swallow disorder be to a person of faith?

SUMMARY OF LEARNING OBJECTIVES

The following were the main learning objectives of this chapter. The information that should have been learned is below each learning objective.

1. The learner will briefly describe each stage of the normal swallow.
   - *Oral preparatory stage:* a voluntary swallowing stage that varies in length depending on the substance being eaten. Food is prepared for swallowing. Mastication occurs with solids.
   - *Oral stage:* a voluntary stage lasting approximately 1 second. It begins once mastication ceases. It involves moving the bolus posterior to the pharynx.
   - *Pharyngeal stage:* an essentially involuntary stage lasting approximately 1 second. The bolus is moved through the pharynx to the esophagus.
   - *Esophageal stage:* an involuntary stage that is variable in length (8–20 seconds) depending of the substance eaten. The bolus is moved through the esophagus to the stomach.

2. The learner will correctly identify the cranial nerves involved in each step of the normal swallow.
   - *Oral preparatory stage:* V, IX, VII
   - *Oral stage:* V, XII
   - *Pharyngeal stage:* V, VII, X, XI, XII
   - *Esophageal stage:* X

3. The learner will describe the main components of the central swallowing system.
   - *Nucleus tractus solitarius (NTS):* The NTS is located in the medulla and acts as a swallowing sensory center by receiving afferent information, such as touch and taste, from cranial nerves V, VII, IX, and X as well as sensory input from the respiratory and cardiovascular brainstem nuclei.
   - *Nucleus ambiguus (NA):* The NA is a motor swallowing center found in the medulla that innervates the swallowing muscles via cranial nerves in the peripheral swallowing system.
   - The NTS and NA together are sometimes referred to as the swallowing center of the medulla.
   - *Subcortical controls:* The hypothalamus regulates hunger and thirst, so it is connected to the eating and swallowing process. The thalamus relays the NTS's fibers to the primary sensory cortex for processing.
   - *Cortical controls:* the inferior primary motor cortex, claustrum, and others.

4. The learner will list neurological disorders that cause dysphagia and note the specific nature of the swallowing problem for each disorder.
   - *Stroke:* oral transit problems, delayed triggering of the pharyngeal swallow, pooling of material in the pharynx, penetration of the airway, and aspiration
   - *Traumatic brain injury:* oral mobility issues, delayed pharyngeal swallow, and aspiration
   - *Multiple sclerosis:* swallow delay, poor pharyngeal squeezing, aspiration risk
   - *Parkinson disease:* tongue pumping, poor anterior-to-posterior bolus movement, drooling, delayed swallow, poor pharyngeal squeeze, pooling of bolus in pharynx, reduced laryngeal elevation, and suppressed cough response
   - *Huntington disease:* squirreling, poor bolus formation and transport, swallow delay, pharyngeal pooling, laryngeal penetration, and aspiration
   - *Amyotrophic lateral sclerosis:* poor bolus formation and transport, delayed swallow, poor pharyngeal squeeze, eventual severe aspiration due to absent swallow response
   - *Guillain-Barré syndrome:* Devastates all stages of the swallow, but swallow improves as patient recovers from the condition

- *Myasthenia gravis:* pharyngeal dismotility, pharyngeal pooling of material, aspiration, and poor esophageal motility in the cervical esophagus

- *Cervical spinal cord injury:* impairments in mastication, sensation, swallow reflex, and cough reflex; possible aspiration

KEY TERMS

Achalasia
Aspiration
Bolus
Claustrum
Cricopharyngeus

Deglutition
Dysphagia
Esophageal stage
Nucleus ambiguus (NA)
Nucleus tractus solitarius (NTS)

Oral preparatory
  stage
Oral stage
Peristalsis
Pharyngeal stage

DRAW IT TO KNOW IT

1. Draw sagittal sections of the head and illustrate the oral, pharyngeal, and esophageal stages of the swallow.

QUESTIONS FOR DEEPER REFLECTION

1. List and describe the four stages of the normal swallow, including their timing and major events.
2. List and describe the function(s) of central swallow control structures.
3. How does neurological dysfunction affect the four stages of swallowing in general?

CASE STUDY

Les is a 54-year-old man who was referred to speech-language pathology due to gradual onset of swallowing and speech difficulty. In terms of swallowing, Les has begun to cough when drinking thin liquids as well as sometimes on his own saliva. In terms of speech, he reports that his tongue feels "thick and slow" and that his voice has become hoarse. Overall, Les demonstrates both upper motor neuron (UMN) and lower motor neuron (LMN) symptoms. His neurologist just diagnosed him with amyotrophic lateral sclerosis (ALS).

1. Given what you know about ALS, what stages of the swallow will be affected by this condition as it progresses?
2. What is the long-term prognosis for Les in terms of eating safely by mouth?

SUGGESTED PROJECTS

1. Obtain something to eat and drink. As you eat and drink, compare and contrast what your oral and pharyngeal cavities do as you swallow.
2. Choose one of the neurological conditions mentioned in this chapter and write a two- to three-page paper detailing the condition's effect on swallowing.
3. Survey a recent issue of the journal *Dysphagia*, choose an article of interest, read it carefully, and present the article in class.

REFERENCES

Abraham, S. S., & Yun, P. T. (2002). Laryngopharyngeal dismotility in multiple sclerosis. *Dysphagia, 17*(1), 69–74.

Chapman, B. (2013, April). *Dysphagia and communication management of the ALS patient*. Presentation at the 2013 annual meeting of the Indiana Speech-Language-Hearing Association. Retrieved from http://www.islha.org/Resources/Documents/Chapman-%20FINAL.pdf

Cola, M. G., Daniels, S. K., Corey, D. M., Lemen, L. C., Romero, M., & Foundas, A. L. (2010). Relevance of subcortical stroke in dysphagia. *Stroke, 41*(3), 482–486.

Corbin-Lewis, K. M., Liss, J. M., & Sciortino, K. F. (2005). *Clinical anatomy and physiology of the swallow mechanism.* Clifton Park, NY: Thompson-Delmar Learning.

Daniels, S. K., Ballo, L. A., Mahoney, M. C., & Foundas, A. L. (2000). Clinical predictors of dysphagia and aspiration risk: outcome measures in acute stroke patients. *Archives of Physical Medicine and Rehabilitation, 81*(8), 1030–1033.

Daniels, S. K., Brailey, K., & Foundas, A. L. (1999). Lingual discoordination and dysphagia following acute stroke: Analyses of lesion localization. *Dysphagia, 14*(2), 85–92.

Daniels, S. K., & Foundas, A. L. (1997). The role of the insular cortex in dysphagia. *Dysphagia, 12*(3), 146–156.

Daniels, S. K., & Foundas, A. L. (1999). Lesion localization in acute stroke patients with risk of aspiration. *Journal of Neuroimaging, 9*(2), 91–98.

Gerek, M., Atalay, A., Çekin, E., Ciyiltepe, M., & Ozkaptan, Y. (2005). The effectiveness of fiberoptic endoscopic swallow study and modified barium swallow study techniques in diagnosis of dysphagia. *Journal of Ear, Nose, and Throat, 15*(5–6), 103–111.

Hamdy, S., Mikulis, D. J., Crawley, A., Xue, S., Lau, H., Henry, S., & Diamant, N. E. (1999). Cortical activation during human volitional swallowing: An event-related fMRI study. *American Journal of Physiology—Gastrointestinal and Liver Physiology, 277*(1), G219–G225.

Kagel, M. C., & Leopold, N. A. (1992). Dysphagia in Huntington's disease: A 16-year retrospective. *Dysphagia, 7*(2), 106–114.

Kern, M. K., Jaradeh, S., Arndorfer, R. C., & Shaker, R. (2001). Cerebral cortical representation of reflexive and volitional swallowing in humans. *American Journal of Physiology—Gastrointestinal and Liver Physiology, 280*(3), G354–G360.

Kirshblum, S., Johnston, M. V., Brown, J., O'Connor, K. C., & Jarosz, P. (1999). Predictors of dysphagia after spinal cord injury. *Archives of Physical Medicine and Rehabilitation, 80*(9), 1101–1105.

Lazarus, C., & Logemann, J. A. (1987). Swallowing disorders in closed head trauma patients. *Archives of Physical Medicine and Rehabilitation, 68*(2), 79–84.

Leopold, N. A., & Kagel, M. C. (1985). Dysphagia in Huntington's disease. *Archives of Neurology, 42*(1), 57.

Leopold, N. A., & Kagel, M. C. (1997). Pharyngo-esophageal dysphagia in Parkinson's disease. *Dysphagia, 12*(1), 11–18.

Malandraki, G. A., Perlman, A. L., Karampinos, D. C., & Sutton, B. P. (2011). Reduced somatosensory activations in swallowing with age. *Human Brain Mapping, 32*(5), 730–743.

Mandaville, A., Ray, A., Robertson, H., Foster, C., & Jesser, C. (2014). A retrospective review of swallow dysfunction in patients with severe traumatic brain injury. *Dysphagia, 29*(3), 310–318.

Martin, R. E., Goodyear, B. G., Gati, J. S., & Menon, R. S. (2001). Cerebral cortical representation of automatic and volitional swallowing in humans. *Journal of Neurophysiology, 85*(2), 938–950.

Massey, B. T., & Shaker, R. (2003). Introduction to the field of deglutition and deglutition disorders. In A. L. Perlman & K. Schulze-Delrieu (Eds.), *Deglutition and its disorders: Anatomy, physiology, clinical diagnosis, and management* (pp. 1–14). San Diego, CA: Singular Publishing Group.

Mosier, K., & Bereznaya, I. (2001). Parallel cortical networks for volitional control of swallowing in humans. *Experimental Brain Research, 140*(3), 280–289.

Muller, J., Wenning, G. K., Verny, M., McKee, A., Chaudhuri, K., & Jellinger, K., . . . Litvan, I. (2001). Progression of dysarthria and dysphagia in postmortem-confirmed parkinsonian disorders. *Archives of Neurology, 58*(2), 259.

Polverino, M., Polverino, F., Fasolino, M., Andò, F., Alfieri, A., & De Blasio, F. (2012). Anatomy and neuro-pathophysiology of the cough reflex arc. *Multidisciplinary Respiratory Medicine, 7*(1), 1–5.

Poorjavad, M., Derakhshandeh, F., Etemadifar, M., Soleymani, B., Minagar, A., & Maghzi, A. (2010). Oropharyngeal dysphagia in multiple sclerosis. *Multiple Sclerosis, 16*(3), 362–365.

Rosenbek, J. C., & Jones, H. N. (2006). Dysphagia in patients with motor speech disorders. In G. Weismer (Ed.), *Motor speech disorders* (pp. 221–260). San Diego, CA: Plural Publishing.

Schroeder, M. F., Daniels, S. K., McClain, M., Corey, D. M., & Foundas, A. L. (2006). Clinical and cognitive predictors of swallowing recovery in stroke. *Journal of Rehabilitation Research and Development, 43*(3), 301–309.

Thomas, F., & Wiles, C., (1999). Dysphagia and nutritional status in multiple sclerosis. *Journal of Neurology, 246*, 677–682.

Tjaden, K. (2009). Speech and swallowing in Parkinson's disease. *Topics in Geriatric Rehabilitation, 24*(2), 115–126.

Wolf, C., & Meiners, T. H. (2003). Dysphagia in patients with acute cervical spinal cord injury. *Spinal Cord, 41*(6), 347–353.

Zald, D. H., & Pardo, J. V. (1999). The functional neuroanatomy of voluntary swallowing. *Annals of Neurology, 46*(3), 281–286.

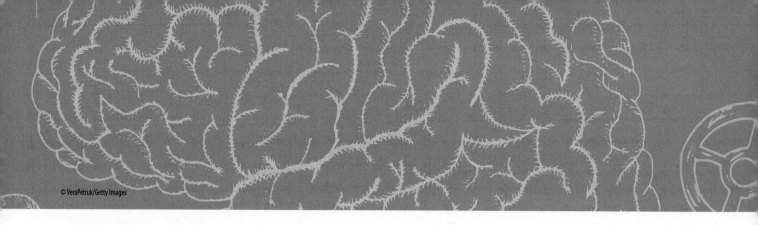
© VeraPetruk/Getty Images

CHAPTER 14

The Neurology of Cognition

CHAPTER PREVIEW

In this chapter we will consider the neurology of cognition. We all have the ability to think and remember, but how does this happen? What neurological structures are behind our thinking?

IN THIS CHAPTER

In this chapter, we will . . .

- Define *cognition*
- Describe the mental processes involved in cognition
- Survey three components of our cognitive abilities: attention, memory, and executive functions
- Review the neurology of attention, memory, and executive functions
- Consider disorders in the area of attention, memory, and executive functions

LEARNING OBJECTIVES

1. The learner will define the term *cognition* and list various cognitive functions.
2. The learner will define the following: *attention*, *memory*, and *executive function*.
3. The learner will describe the neural basis of attention, memory, and executive functions.
4. The learner will list and describe select disorders of attention, memory, and executive functions.

▶ Introduction

If there is one experience that truly tests and shapes our cognition, it is (or should be) college. What is this thing called cognition? **Cognition** is the mental process of knowing in which we acquire and act upon knowledge. This mental process is made up of at least five general functions: perceiving, remembering, comprehending, judging, and reasoning. **Perception** refers to recognizing if information is present, whether it be auditory, visual, or other information. **Remembering** is storing the information. After it is stored, the information has to be understood (**comprehension**). At this point, **judgment** occurs as one determines the accuracy or correctness of the information. Finally, **reasoning** takes place, as evidenced through either drawing conclusions or making arguments.

There are numerous specific cognition functions worth mentioning. These include attention, orientation, memory, new learning, thought organization, reasoning, problem solving, and executive functions. These cognitive functions can be conceptualized through a pyramid (**FIGURE 14-1**). Attention forms the base of the cognitive functions on top of which orientation, memory, learning new information (i.e., new learning), thought organization, reasoning, and problem solving are built. Finally, executive functions reside at the top, ordering all of the other cognitive components for goal-directed behavior. In this chapter, one example will be surveyed from each level of this pyramid. More specifically, attention, memory, and executive functions will be explored, as well as some select disorders of cognition and communication.

▶ Attention

Types of Attention

The neural system behind consciousness makes humans generally aware of themselves and their environment. Building upon consciousness is another cognitive ability—attention. **Attention** is a person's focus on a stimulus in the environment. It involves engaging a stimulus over time as well as disengaging from other stimuli (Ward, 2008). It is a very useful cognitive process because it helps us detect important stimuli in our environment and helps us react quickly to them. Attention can be either **bottom-up attention** (nonvolitional), driven by some characteristic of the stimulus itself, or **top-down attention** (volitional), driven by a person's will. For example, if there is a dog in the room (i.e., the stimulus), I can voluntarily choose to look at the dog (top-down). If the dog suddenly barks, then my attention might be involuntarily drawn to look at the dog (bottom-up).

Attention forms the foundation for our other cognitive and language abilities. For example, if one cannot attend to the professor's lecture, how will one remember anything about it? Attention can be directed toward various types of stimuli, including auditory and/or visual stimuli (e.g., the professor talking and writing on the board). Before talking about the neural basis of attention, different types of attention will be surveyed using a clinical model developed by Sohlberg and Mateer (1989) (**FIGURE 14-2**).

- *Focused attention:* Focused attention is the general ability to focus on a specific stimulus, whether it is auditory, visual, tactile, or the like.
- *Sustained attention:* Sustained attention allows humans to focus on a specific stimulus over a certain amount of time. For example, visual sustained attention is crucial for reading this text and gathering all its wisdom.
- *Selective attention:* Selective attention or vigilance is the ability to focus on a certain stimulus while ignoring competing stimuli. Using the example of reading this text, a student would be using selective attention if he or she maintains attention on reading while ignoring his or her roommate's phone conversation.

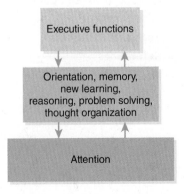

FIGURE 14-1 Organization of cognitive functions.

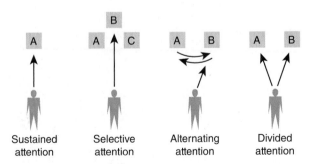

FIGURE 14-2 Types of attention. (Note: Focused attention is involved in each of these.)

■ *Alternating attention:* Alternating attention is exhibited when a person shifts focus from one task to another task. A student might read his or her book, then shift attention to writing an essay, and then shift back to reading the book.

■ *Divided attention:* Divided attention is the ability to focus on two stimuli at the same time. For example, a person might drive and talk on a cell phone at the same time, though this example may be problematic because driving becomes an automatic task that draws less on our attentional resources. It is also problematic because doing both is illegal in many states. A better example comes from the study by Spelke, Hirst, and Neisser (1976), who studied divided attention by having subjects read stories while also writing down words dictated to them. They found that divided attention abilities could be improved through practice. Wang and Tchernev (2012) found the opposite regarding media multitasking—that this behavior degrades cognitive performance. Students might want to consider this when they are tempted to text or use social media in class.

Neural Mechanisms of Attention

Right Posterior Parietal Lobe

The posterior parietal cortex is known to disengage our attention from a stimulus (Wright & Ward, 2008) (**FIGURE 14-3**). **Neglect syndrome** is a condition of disengagement in which a patient ignores stimuli (e.g., objects or people) in one visual field or the other.

The patient has not lost visual abilities in one visual field, which would be a condition called *hemianopsia*, but rather simply does not pay attention to either the right or left side of space. Studies have shown that neglect is caused, at least in part, by damage to the posterior right hemisphere (Heilman & Van Den Abell, 1980; Katz, Hartman-Maeir, Ring, & Soroker, 1999; Vallar & Perani, 1986). The right hemisphere processes visual-spatial information, and this particular part of the right hemisphere analyzes the *where of vision* (i.e., objects' positions in space), which is the dorsal stream of vision. If this ability were damaged, then a patient would not attend to objects in one side of space.

Superior Colliculi

The superior colliculi are located in the midbrain and play an important role in vision. Specifically, they contain a topographic map of the world we see and help direct the head and eyes to new stimuli found in the peripheral vision. In other words, the superior colliculi assist our eyes in shifting attention to a new stimulus (Wright & Ward, 2008). For example, as the author sits at his computer typing, the office door is in the right visual field. As one of the author's children walks down the hallway by the door, the author's visual attention is stimulated and he looks over and attends to his child (most of the time!).

Pulvinar Nucleus

The pulvinar nucleus is located in the thalamus and is a prime candidate in attention because of its

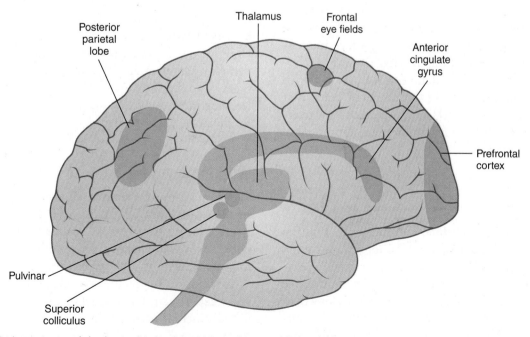

FIGURE 14-3 Attention and the brain. (Note: this is a lateral view of the right hemisphere.)

numerous reciprocal connections to the frontal, temporal, parietal, and occipital lobes as well as sub-cortical structures, like the superior colliculus. Specifically, it helps to engage and maintain attention to a new stimulus while also suppressing information from stimuli that are not needed, a process called *filtering* (Ward, 2008). Damage to the pulvinar nucleus can result in both temporal and spatial attention problems, though usually not as severe as damage to the cortical area.

Frontal Eye Fields

The frontal eye fields are located in the prefrontal cortex in Brodmann area (BA) 8. They are important in visual attention and eye movements. When damaged, the eyes deviate toward the side of injury and/or display rapid, irregular movement during focusing activities, which is called saccadic eye movements. As Ramat, Leigh, Zee, and Optican (2007) explain, "Saccades are rapid eye movements that redirect the fovea from one object to another" (p. 10). The fovea of the eye is that part of the retina packed with cones that is responsible for high-acuity central vision.

Attention-Deficit/Hyperactivity Disorder

Attention-deficit/hyperactivity disorder (ADHD) is a chronic, genetic condition characterized by inattention, hyperactivity, and impulsivity. It affects approximately 6% to 7% of children. Symptoms include distractibility, trouble staying on task, boredom, daydreaming, trouble following directions, fidgeting, nonstop talking, and impatience. Several genes related to dopamine are affected, and many patients with ADHD take medications like Ritalin, which increase the effect of dopamine and reduce inattention, hyperactivity, and impulsivity. The use of stimulant medications like Ritalin is controversial, with some patients complaining that the drug dulls their senses. Others believe ADHD medications are over-prescribed and that some children are simply more active than others are.

▶ Memory

Two stories of extraordinary memory are a fitting way to begin a discussion on the topic of memory. S. (1886–1958), a Russian man, remembered everything. His doctor, A. R. Luria, tested his remarkable memory over a 30-year period. The good doctor would give S. lists of words that were sometimes 70 words long, and S. could not only immediately remember

all the words but also recall them some 15 years later. S.'s memory was so good that he quit his job and became a mnemonist—a professional stage performer who did memory tricks for a living. As a university student reading about S. one is probably envious, but there was a dark side to remembering everything. He had trouble following stories and integrating new information into older information. In addition, there are many things that we would like to forget in our lives, but S. remembered it all.

Compare the story of S. with the story of H. M. (1926–2008). At around age 10 years, H. M. began experiencing serious epileptic seizures, perhaps due to a bicycle accident he suffered a few years earlier. Even with anticonvulsant drugs, H. M.'s seizures grew more serious over the years to the point where he could not work anymore. It was the early 1950s and the only option left for him was surgery. At 27 years old, H. M.'s medial temporal cortex was bilaterally removed. This removal included the temporal lobe's parahippocampal gyrus and hippocampal complex. After surgery, he appeared to be the same in personality and intelligence, but a serious memory problem resulted from his surgery. H. M. could not remember some events preceding his surgery (retrograde amnesia), but, more dramatically, could not remember anything that occurred after the surgery (anterograde amnesia). He was frozen in 1953 where Eisenhower was always president, the Cold War was in its early throes, and his mother was always alive. Even though H. M. had these terrible memory deficits, there was an aspect of memory that was still a strength—procedural memory.

The cases of S. and especially H. M. have taught the world much about memory, challenging some long-held false beliefs. What is long-term memory? How long is short-term memory? In patients with dementia, is all memory impaired or only certain types? Can one learn new things and not be aware of learning these things? In this section, new paradigms for memory will be reviewed.

Working Memory

When speaking of memory, almost everyone thinks in terms of long- and short-term memory. Today, neuroscientists conceive of memory in three categories: working memory, short-term memory, and long-term memory. The terms short term and working memory are sometimes used synonymously, but some experts, such as Baddeley (2012), believe there is a distinction between the two. He believes short-term memory is about temporary storage, whereas

working memory (WM) is more about manipulation. In other words, WM can be thought of as a system in the mind that allows for the manipulation of information. Think of it as a scratch pad where verbal and nonverbal problems are worked out. WM involves the use of executive functions, attention, and short-term memory storage. The neuroanatomical structures involved in WM consist of a network that includes the prefrontal cortex, cingulate cortex, and parietal lobe.

Different types of WM have been proposed (**FIGURE 14-4**). *Executive attention control* is a type of WM that controls our attention to select a stimulus and suppress other stimuli that might compete with it, which allows us the cognitive space to manipulate or work out the information from the selected stimulus. For example, if someone were to give you a math problem, you would use this form of WM to focus on the problem while suppressing other stimuli (e.g., the TV, the dog barking). Another type of WM is our *visuospatial sketchpad,* which we use to temporally store visual features of objects, like color, shape, location, and orientation. You might practically use this WM in describing an object (e.g., a flower) to a friend. In the realm of speech-language pathology and audiology, the *phonological loop* (sometimes called the phonological buffer) is an important type of WM focused on assembling phonemes and keeping them in WM long enough that we can turn them into speech sounds. It also is important for temporarily holding auditory information long enough that we can process and attach meaning to it. Executive attention control WM is the boss of these two types of WM (visuospatial sketchpad and phonological loop) in that it allocates space for them as needed.

Short-Term Memory

Short-term memory is storage for small amounts of information needed for a short time (seconds).

In terms of elements, it is usually described as holding seven elements total plus or minus two. For example, an acquaintance might give you her phone number and you store it long enough to type it in your phone or write it down on a piece of paper. The information in this temporary storehouse will quickly decay unless rehearsed using a memory strategy, like rehearsal. One theory to how it works is called the **synaptic theory**, which states that short-term memory works through neurotransmitter release (acetylcholine) but decays as neurotransmitter uptake occurs. As mentioned earlier, WM and short-term memory are sometimes lumped together; however, neuroscientists view them as distinct types of memory, associating short-term primarily with holding information, and WM with actively manipulating information.

Long-Term Memory

Many times short-term memories undergo memory consolidation (often during sleep), which means they are converted into long-term storage. **Long-term memory** involves memories that last for days, weeks, months, and even years. An example might be the trip to the Grand Canyon you took with your family when you were 10 years old. Long-term memory can be broken down into two major categories, declarative memory and nondeclarative memory (**FIGURE 14-5**).

Declarative Memory

Declarative memory (or explicit memory) is the conscious, willful recall of memories. The name "declarative" is descriptive of the type of memory; you consciously declare facts or events to others. It involves two subtypes, episodic memory and semantic memory. **Episodic memory** is memory for space–time episodes in life, like the trip to the Grand Canyon. It often integrates autobiographical memory by placing you as an actor in your memories. **Semantic memory** is recall of facts and general knowledge. For example, recalling that George Washington was the first president of the United States is a semantic memory feat. Episodic memory is personal, whereas semantic memory is impersonal. Both of these memory types depend on the medial temporal lobe, which contains the hippocampal structures (**FIGURE 14-6**).

Nondeclarative Memory

Nondeclarative memory (or implicit memory) is a type of memory that cannot be consciously brought

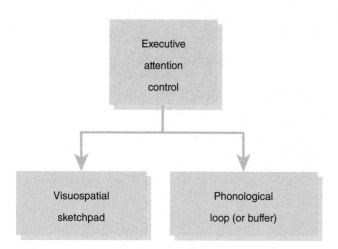

FIGURE 14-4 Types of working memory.

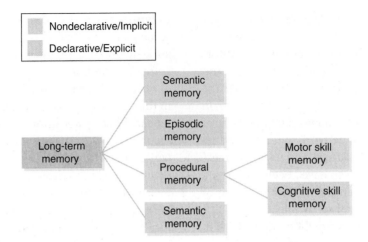

FIGURE 14-5 Types of long-term memory.

Data from Henke, K. (2010). A model for memory systems based on processing modes rather than consciousness. *Nature Reviews Neuroscience, 11*(7), 523–532.

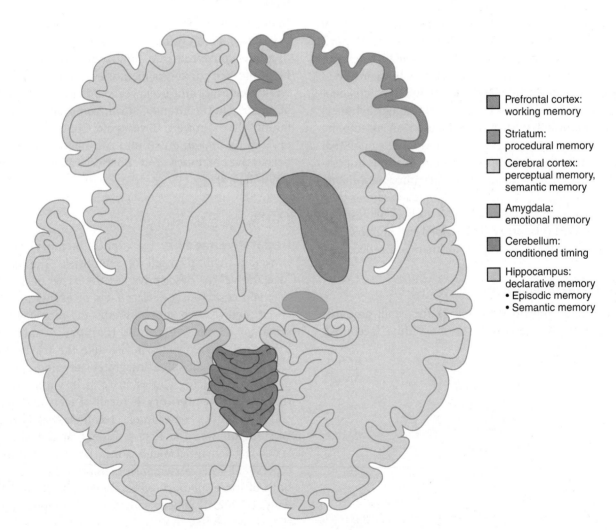

FIGURE 14-6 A transverse section of the brain illustrating important brain structures in memory.

Data from Eichenbaum, H. (2008). Memory. *Scholarpedia, 3*(3), 1747.

into awareness. It involves learning, but being unaware of that learning. One type of nondeclarative memory is **procedural memory**, which is memory for skills and habits, like riding a bike (a motor skill) or doing an algebra problem (a cognitive skill). Somewhere one learns how to do these activities, and once learned, one does not need to consciously recall memories to do them. Although H. M. could not make new declarative memories, his procedural memory was intact because his basal ganglia (specifically, the striatum) was neurologically intact. This type of memory is also a strength in patients with dementia and can be harnessed through techniques like spaced retrieval training to teach these kind of patients new skills (**BOX 14-1**).

Another type of nondeclarative memory is **priming memory**. This type of memory takes advantage of unconscious associations between objects. For example, showing a person the word "red" might enable the person to more quickly recognize the word "apple" because *red* and *apple* are linked together. A baseball analogy would be that *red* serves to bring *apple* up "on deck" while other less-related words stay in the dugout. Priming memory appears dependent neurologically on the neocortex (i.e., the six layers of the cerebral cortex) (Henke, 2010).

Neural Basis for Long-Term Memory

The medial temporal lobe is a key area in declarative memory. This area includes the parahippocampal gyrus, hippocampus, and rhinal cortices. The rhinal cortices occupy BAs 28 and 34–36 and include the entorhinal and perirhinal cortices. These structures in the medial temporal lobe are crucial for explicit memory consolidation (i.e., making long-term declarative memories); the case of H. M. illustrates the devastation that can occur if these structures are removed or damaged. The flow of information through the medial temporal lobe occurs like this:

Cortical areas

↓

Parahippocampal and rhinal cortices

↓

Hippocampus

Damage to the rhinal cortex causes severe damage to the ability to recognize objects (a semantic memory task), but damage to the hippocampus does not have this effect. Thus, it appears that the rhinal cortices are

BOX 14-1 Spaced Retrieval Training

Spaced retrieval training (SRT) is a compensatory memory technique that helps people with memory problems learn new information through implicit memory, specifically procedural memory. In this method, the therapist helps the client learn important information (e.g., when to take a pill) through progressively increasing the time between learning trials. For example, if the therapist's goal is for the patient to learn the location of his or her room (e.g., room 121) to decrease wandering around the facility, the prompt would be, "What is your room number?" and the expected response would be "121." The prompt would be offered with progressively longer delays, and if the client were to fail at a level, the therapist would go back to the previous successful time interval and move on from that point. An example of the process might look this this:

Trial 1 (0 seconds)
    Therapist: "What is your room number?"
    Client: "121." (correct)
Trial 2 (after 10 seconds)
    Therapist: "What is your room number?"
    Client: "121." (correct)
Trial 3 (after 30 seconds)
    Therapist: "What is your room number?"
    Client: "121." (correct)
Trial 4 (after 60 seconds)
    Therapist: "What is your room number?"
    Client: "100." (incorrect)
Trial 5 (after 30 seconds)
    Therapist: "What is your room number?"
    Client: "121." (correct)

SRT is an appropriate compensatory treatment method for people with declarative memory problems due to conditions like Alzheimer disease, who need to learn information through intact implicit memory routes. It has been found to be an effective memory strategy for these kinds of patients (see Brush & Camp, 1998; Han et al., 2017; Hopkins, Lyle, Hieb, & Ralston, 2016; Karpicke & Roediger, 2007; McKitrick & Camp, 1993; Oren, Willerton, & Small, 2014; Schacter, Rich, & Stampp, 1985). Try SRT the next time you need to memorize important facts for class, and see if it works for you.

crucial for semantic memory and the hippocampus is central for episodic memory.

So far, declarative memory has been discussed, but what about nondeclarative memory such as procedural memory? Does it operate on the same medial temporal lobe circuit, or does it utilize other brain structures? The answer is the latter. Nondeclarative memory depends on the basal ganglia, specifically the striatum of the basal ganglia, which includes the caudate nucleus and the putamen. The striatum is located in an important motor loop between the cortex and the thalamus; thus, motor repetition can lead to the establishment of new motor patterns without a person being conscious of this kind of learning. H. M.'s medial temporal cortices were removed and he suffered from profound amnesia, but his basal ganglia were not disturbed and he could still learn through his procedural memory.

▶ Executive Functions

The word *executive* features prominently in the familiar term *chief executive officer*. This term conjures up images of the boss who is in control of the various aspects of a business. In a neurological sense, executive functions are the boss of human cognition. **Executive functions** order and manage all other cognitive functions (e.g., attention, memory) for the purpose of setting and attaining goals.

The prefrontal cortex is an important neuroanatomical structure for executive functions. Restraint, initiative, and order are important functions of the prefrontal cortex and, thus, of executive function (**TABLE 14-1**). Blumenfeld (2010) defines **restraint** as the "inhibition of inappropriate behaviors" (p. 908), which includes the following areas:

- *Judgment:* making reasonable decisions (discernment, wisdom)
- *Foresight:* seeing or knowing beforehand (anticipate, envision)
- *Perseverance:* holding to a course of action without giving up (steadfastness)
- *Delaying gratification:* holding off on things you want
- *Inhibiting socially inappropriate responses:* for example, pinching someone
- *Self-governance:* governing or ruling oneself and one's life
- *Concentration:* focusing on a stimulus

Initiative involves "the motivation to pursue positive or productive activities" (Blumenfeld, 2010, p. 908) and involves the following:

- *Curiosity:* desiring to know and learn, especially about new, strange things
- *Spontaneity:* engaging in unpremeditated actions
- *Motivation:* having incentive to act
- *Drive:* pressing or pushing toward action and goals

TABLE 14-1 The Three Main Components of Executive Functions (Restraint, Initiative, and Order) and Their Subcomponents

Restraint	Initiative	Order
Judgment	Curiosity	Abstract reasoning
Foresight	Spontaneity	Working memory
Perseverance	Motivation	Perspective taking
Delaying gratification	Drive	Planning
Inhibiting socially inappropriate responses	Creativity	Insight
Self-governance	Shifting cognitive set	Organization
Concentration	Mental flexibility	Sequencing
	Personality	Temporal order

Data from Blumenfeld, H. (2010). *Neuroanatomy through clinical cases*. Sunderland, MA: Sinauer Associates.

- *Creativity:* having the imagination and ability to create things
- *Shifting cognitive set:* shifting thinking from one set of rules to another
- *Mental flexibility:* handling different situations in different ways, especially to respond effectively to new, complex, and problematic situations (e.g., adapting to change, taking risks, solving problems in new ways)
- *Personality:* having distinctive qualities, character, or traits

Lastly, Blumenfeld (2010) defines **order** as "the capacity to correctly perform sequencing tasks and a variety of other cognitive operations" (p. 908). Order involves the following:

- *Abstract reasoning:* thinking about and cognitively manipulating events, things, or concepts that are not in one's immediate presence or environment
- *WM:* immediately storing information needed for ongoing cognitive operations
- *Perspective taking:* stepping into another's shoes and seeing his or her perspective
- *Planning:* working out a program for action beforehand
- *Insight:* discerning the true nature of a situation
- *Organization:* pulling together items into an orderly whole
- *Sequencing:* logically ordering one thing after another (e.g., washing a car)
- *Temporal order:* Logically ordering space–time events (e.g., telling a story)

In thinking about how the executive functions control goal-directed behavior, many of the listed functions are crucial to this task. For example, under restraint, one would need foresight to see potential obstacles in attaining a goal as well as perseverance and concentration. Initiative might contribute drive and mental flexibility if obstacles are encountered. Lastly, order would add planning, organization, and sequencing in setting and attaining goals.

There are many disorders that can disrupt executive functions, including ADHD, depression, learning disabilities, dementia, cerebroventricular accidents, and traumatic brain injury. Signs of executive function problems are evident in the three categories presented earlier—restraint, initiative, and order. More specifically, those with executive function problems will have trouble planning projects and projecting the time needed to complete them,

organizing thoughts logically in verbal and/or written tasks, and finding the motivation necessary to complete projects. These people will also sometimes struggle with being socially appropriate, which can lead to social isolation.

▶ Cognitive-Communicative Disorders

Right Hemisphere Disorder

Historically, researchers in neuroscience have been more interested in left hemisphere function than right hemisphere function. In the 1870s, John Hughlings Jackson (1835–1911) was one of the early pioneers in exploring right hemisphere function, but he was followed by a great period of silence until the mid-20th century. Why this silence? It was thought that the right hemisphere was of little importance to communication and, thus, was not important overall.

In the 20th century, interest in this neglected half of the brain increased. Visual spatial deficits related to the right hemisphere were reported in the 1940s followed by an interest in communication problems in the 1960s and 1970s. Profiles of right hemisphere damage began to appear in the 1980s. Public awareness of right hemisphere damage also increased in the 1970s and 1980s through two famous cases. One of these involved the Supreme Court judge William O. Douglas (1898–1980), who suffered a right hemisphere stroke with left hemiparesis in 1974 but appeared to recover well, as he could still talk and write. He returned to the bench after his stroke, but observers of the Supreme Court noticed his communication rambled on and he often asked irrelevant questions; moreover, he denied having deficits, even his left hemiparesis. The other case involved James Brady (1940–2014), an aide to President Ronald Reagan, who was shot in the 1981 assassination attempt on the president. Damage was done to the right hemisphere, but Brady was not like Douglas in his symptomology. His conversations were relevant, coherent, and full of humor. Brady is remembered for the federal gun control legislation that bore his name—the Brady Handgun Violence Prevention Act—enacted in 1993 that mandated federal background checks and a 5-day waiting period for gun purchases.

Right hemisphere disorder (RHD) leads to deficits in two main areas—communication and cognition. Communication problems can be divided into linguistic and extralinguistic deficits. Linguistic deficits include rambling speech, poor coherence in producing and comprehending conversation and narratives, poor comprehension of abstract language and humor, and poor pragmatic skills. Extralinguistic deficits include **aprosody** and a lack of producing and interpreting emotion. In terms of cognition, we will consider the three cognitive areas we have discussed in this chapter—attention, memory, and executive functions—and look at how they are affected in RHD.

Attention

All forms of attention discussed in this chapter may be affected in RHD. This includes sustained, selective, alternating, and divided attention. This impaired attention may affect communication. For example, a person with RHD might not be able to sustain attention in a conversational situation and miss important information from the speaker. In addition, patients with RHD may also suffer neglect, which can impair reading and writing.

Memory

Gillespie, Bowen, and Foster (2006) performed a review of the literature on RHD and memory deficits. They found that RHD patients demonstrated deficits

in episodic memory, most likely due to attentional problems. Logic would dictate that improvements in attention would result in improvements in episodic memory in this population.

Executive Functions

People with RHD often suffer deficits in restraint, initiative, and order. Under restraint, they may demonstrate poor judgment and lack foresight in how their actions affect others. In terms of order, the case of William O. Douglas illustrated his denial of his deficits. This denial is called **anosognosia**, and this lack of insight (a subcomponent of order) is a major executive function issue in some people with RHD. (Note: Remember that James Brady did not suffer from this symptom.) This denial can be of cognitive-communicative deficits, but also physical problems, like hemiparesis.

Synthesis and inference are also executive function areas of struggle in RHD. These deficits are classified under order, specifically involving organization, sequencing, and temporal order. The Cookie Theft picture from the *Boston Diagnostic Aphasia Examination* is shown in **FIGURE 14-7**. Normally, if prompted to tell a story about this picture, a person without RHD would incorporate all the elements in the picture and produce something like the following:

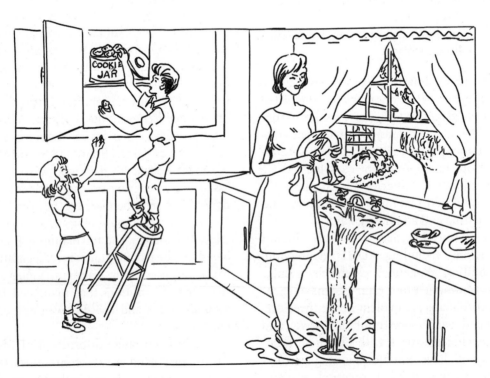

FIGURE 14-7 The Cookie Theft picture.

Goodglass, H., & Kaplan, E. (2001). *The assessment of aphasia and related disorders* (3rd ed.). Austin, TX: Pro-Ed.

One day a woman was doing dishes in the kitchen. She began daydreaming about being outside in the nice weather. Because of her daydreaming, she did not realize that the water was overflowing from the sink onto the floor. Also, she did not notice her son, Mikey, stealing cookies from the cookie jar. His sister, Cindy, wants Mikey to give her a cookie too. As Mikey begins to take a cookie, he loses his balance on the stool and is about to fall onto the floor. The mom is going to be really upset when she sees the chaos in the kitchen. Mikey will have to apologize to his mom and be disciplined, but then all will be forgiven. The end.

Now compare a narrative from a patient with RHD:

Well, this is a scene in a house. It looks like a fine spring day. The window is open. I guess it's not Minnesota, or the flies and mosquitos would be flying in. Outside I see a tree and another window. Looks like the neighbors have their windows closed. There's a woman near the window wearing what appears to be an inexpensive pair of shoes. She's holding something that looks like a plate. On the counter there, there's a hat and two caps that look like they would fit on a child's head.

There is no synthesis of the picture elements into an organized, cohesive narrative in the RHD example. Instead, the focus is on the details (e.g., "inexpensive shoes"), not the whole. There are even times the patient misperceives elements in the picture, like seeing a hat instead of a plate. This focus on the details at the expense of the whole picture can be a significant problem in telling stories to others or in having coherent and cohesive conversations.

Traumatic Brain Injury

Traumatic brain injury (TBI) results when extreme forces injure the brain after a motor vehicle accident, fall, assault, bomb blast, or collision in sports (see **BOXES 14-2** and **14-3**). The injury sustained can involve penetration of the skull (open head injury) or the brain coming in contact with the inside of the skull (closed head injury). Symptoms of TBI can include headache and nausea as well as cognitive, speech, and/or language problems.

Attention

One of the main cognitive symptoms of TBI is attention problems, which can involve focused, sustained, selective, alternating, and divided attention. Related, TBI patients have poor ability to tune out distractions. In addition, overall cognitive processing speed is slowed by TBI (Ben-David, Nguyen, & van Lieshout, 2011). These problems can lead to vocational and educational issues, because a lack of attention impairs both memory and executive functions, and slowed thinking makes these pursuits frustrating.

Memory

The majority of patients (75%) with TBI report problems with memory (Thomsen, 1984). Because of the diffuse nature of TBI, these memory problems can occur in both declarative and nondeclarative memory. A deficit in memory is called amnesia (Greek for "forgetfulness"). There are two main types of amnesia, anterograde and retrograde (**FIGURE 14-8**). Retrograde amnesia is a loss of some or all memory before the brain injury, while anterograde amnesia is a loss of some or all memory between the brain injury and the present. Anterograde amnesia is the loss of the ability to make new memories post-accident, like in the case of H. M.

Executive Functions

In addition to attention and memory, patients with TBI struggle with executive functions. These struggles can impair all three main areas of executive function (restraint, initiative, and order). In terms of restraint, patients will sometimes have difficulty inhibiting socially inappropriate behaviors. For example, they may make sexually explicit statements or inordinately use foul language. Initiative and order deficits can especially impair their ability to set, attain, and evaluate progress on goals. Goal-directed behavior is a part of everyday life. For example, when

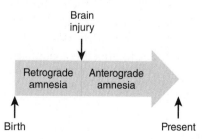

FIGURE 14-8 Two types of amnesia, retrograde and anterograde amnesia.

BOX 14-2   Traumatic Brain Injury in the Military due to Blast Injuries

In modern warfare, most head injuries to soldiers are the result of explosions rather than gunshot wounds. During the second Gulf War, many soldiers died or were injured by improvised explosive devices. When soldiers are exposed to bomb blasts, a series of tissue injuries will result due to the primary, secondary, tertiary, and quaternary levels of blast damage (**FIGURE 14-9**). The primary level of the blast involves the bomb's shock wave, which compresses and releases tissue in the body, including brain tissue. This can lead to concussions. The secondary level of damage results from flying shrapnel, causing open head injuries. The tertiary level of damage occurs when soldiers are knocked off their feet by the explosion. They may suffer a closed head injury due to hitting their head on the group or on an object. Lastly, quaternary levels of damage involve anything not covered under the categories of primary through tertiary levels of damage. This damage might include smoke inhalation or burns from the blast.

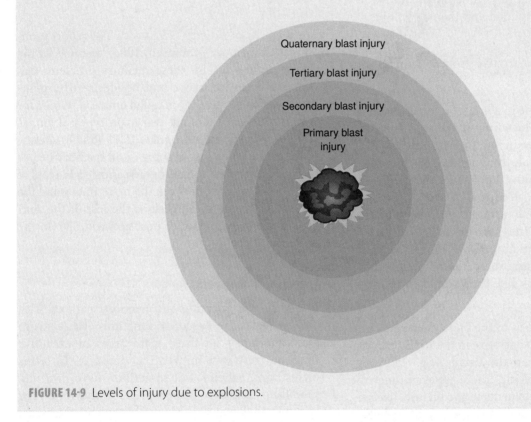

FIGURE 14-9 Levels of injury due to explosions.

a college student wakes up in the morning, one of the first things he or she will do is think about what needs to be accomplished during the day and how it will get done. At the end of the day, most will think back and assess how well these goals were achieved and what is left to be done. This skill is often seriously impaired in TBI due to difficulty formulating and initiating goals as well as behavior that might interfere with these goals.

Dementia

We experience significant changes to our bodies as we age. Not only do we lose hair, teeth, and bone mass,

but our brains change as well. Most people experience a decline in cognitive abilities as they age. More specifically, they experience increasing problems with WM, long-term memory, and verbal fluency. These problems are the result of structural changes in the brain. The brain shrinks with age, and the size of the ventricles increases. Some of this shrinkage is due to neuronal death, but most of it is due to myelin breaking down, the thinning of dendrites, and the loss of synapses.

Some people experience a faster than normal decline in their cognitive abilities. This is usually due to some kind of neurological pathology, such as mild cognitive impairment (MCI). People with MCI have

BOX 14-3 Football and Chronic Traumatic Encephalopathy

In 2002, Dr. Bennet Omalu, a neuropathologist, performed an autopsy on a 50-year-old former National Football League (NFL) player named Mike Webster, who had died of a heart attack. Because of Webster's young age, but poor physical appearance, Dr. Omalu decided to remove and examine Webster's brain. Using a microscope, Dr. Omalu found clumps of tau proteins throughout Webster's brain, a finding similar to what is found in the brains of Alzheimer patients (**FIGURE 14-10**). Webster had suffered from amnesia, depression, and executive function issues for years, and Dr. Omalu's findings helped explain Webster's deteriorating condition. He named the condition chronic traumatic encephalopathy (CTE), a condition caused by the thousands of subconcussive hits football players suffer, especially linemen like Mike Webster. Dr. Omalu examined four more former NFL players who had suffered from similar symptoms and found the condition in them also. Since 2002, the brains of 111 former NFL players have been examined, and CTE has been found in 110 of them (Mez et al., 2017). A book about CTE in NFL players has been written called *League of Denial*. The PBS program *Frontline* produced a documentary film based on this book, also called *League of Denial*. There has even been a big-budget movie starring Will Smith called *Concussion* that dramatizes Dr. Omalu's discovery of CTE and the subsequent pushback by the NFL.

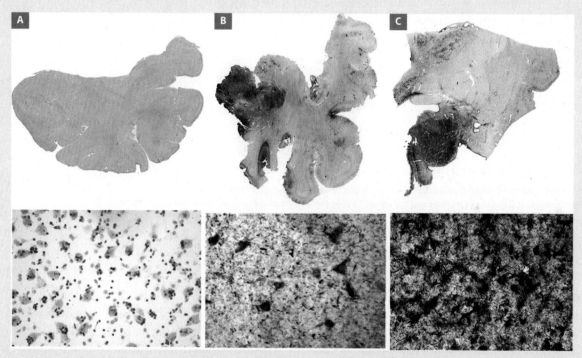

FIGURE 14-10 Chronic traumatic encephalopathy shown in immunostained sections of the medial temporal lobe; dark brown color indicates tau protein. **A.** Top: Whole brain section from a 65-year-old control subject showing no abnormal tau protein deposition. Bottom: Microscopic section showing no abnormal tau protein deposition. **B.** Top: Whole brain section from John Grimsley (former NFL player) showing abundant tau protein deposition in the brain. Bottom: Microscopic section showing numerous tau-containing neurofibrillary tangles in the brain. **C.** Top: Whole brain section from a 73-year-old world champion boxer with end-state CTE and dementia showing very severe tau protein deposition. Bottom: Microscopic section showing abundant tau-containing neurofibrillary tangles.

mild cognitive issues that concern them but do not interfere with their daily life. Unfortunately, about 65% of people with MCI develop Alzheimer disease (AD), which as it progresses, seriously disrupts daily life (Sanes & Jessell, 2013).

Dementia is a group of progressive neurological disorders that lead to cognitive decline. AD is the most well-known and common form of dementia (**BOX 14-4**). AD is a neurological condition in which patients experience a relentless decline in their cognitive abilities that

BOX 14-4 Types of Dementia

Dementia is a term that describes several conditions of progressive, irreversible cognitive decline. The most well-known form of dementia is Alzheimer disease (AD), named after the German psychiatrist Alois Alzheimer, who first published on the condition. AD accounts for approximately 70% of dementia cases. Vascular dementia is another type of dementia that is caused by small strokes. It accounts for 17% of dementia cases. The remaining 13% of cases are other types of dementia, such as frontotemporal dementia (FTD) (Plassman et al., 2007). FTD involves deterioration of the frontal and temporal lobes, whereas AD affects the hippocampus and more posterior parts of the brain and then progresses forward over time. FTD affects people younger than 65 years of age, while AD's onset occurs after age 65 years.

Primary progressive aphasia (PPA) is associated with FTD, as one of the first signs of FTD is language issues. In comparison, in AD the initial signs are impaired cognition and memory. There are at least three subtypes of PPA (**FIGURE 14-11**). The first is fluent semantic dementia (SD), which is characterized by fluent language and semantic paraphasias. The second type is progressive nonfluent aphasia (PNFA), which involves labored speech, agrammatism, and phonological paraphasias. The final form is logopenic variant of PPA (LV-PPA). It includes anomia, impaired repetition, and phonological paraphasias. Patients with this logopenic variant can be both fluent when not having word retrieval problems and nonfluent when experiencing anomia. Recently, a possible fourth form of PPA has been described called mixed PPA; it combines features from SD, PNFA, and LV-PPA.

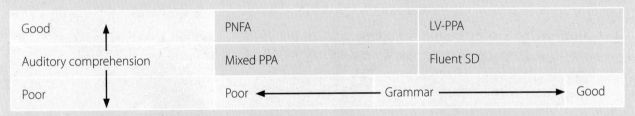

FIGURE 14-11 Types of primary progressive aphasia.

LV-PPA, logopenic variant of PPA; PPA, primary progressive aphasia; PNFA, progressive nonfluent aphasia; SD, semantic dementia.

Data from Mesulam, M. M. (2016). Primary progressive aphasia and the left hemisphere language network. *Dementia and Neurocognitive Disorders, 15*(4), 93–102.

results in difficulty completing activities of daily living. It is characterized by three changes to the brain. First, the brain atrophies at a greater rate than what is seen in normal aging (**FIGURE 14-12**). Second, brain tissue is characterized by amyloid plaques that surround and choke nervous system cells (**FIGURE 14-13**). These plaques are toxic to neural cells, causing inflammation and impairing their function. Third, neuron cell bodies develop neurofibrillary tangles in them. These tangles also interfere with normal neuronal function. These three signs of AD do not occur throughout the whole brain evenly, but rather occur in specific areas. The area most affected is the hippocampus and entorhinal area, critical structures for declarative memory. This explains why the first signs of AD are these types of memory issues.

Attention

Alertness and sustained attention are relatively intact in AD until the later stages of the disease (McGuinness,

Barrett, Craig, Lawson, & Passmore, 2010). Both selective and divided attention have been shown to be impaired in most forms of dementia, including AD (Baddeley, Baddeley, Bucks, & Wilcock, 2001). This impairment can show up practically in the inability to resist distraction from competing stimuli.

Memory

In terms of memory, AD affects WM (Baddeley, Baddeley, Bucks, & Wilcock, 2001) and declarative memory abilities (Bayles, 1991; Salmon & Bondi, 2009). Previously we had seen that WM is dependent on the prefrontal cortex, cingulate cortex, and parietal lobe. As these areas are affected by AD, WM becomes impaired. Also, the hippocampus is one of the first brain structures to be damaged in AD, leading to episodic memory problems followed later by semantic memory issues. Compare AD to another progressive neurological disease, Huntington disease (HD).

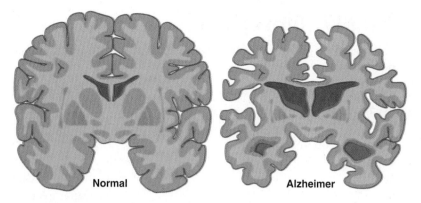

FIGURE 14-12 Atrophy of the brain in Alzheimer disease compared to a normal, healthy brain.

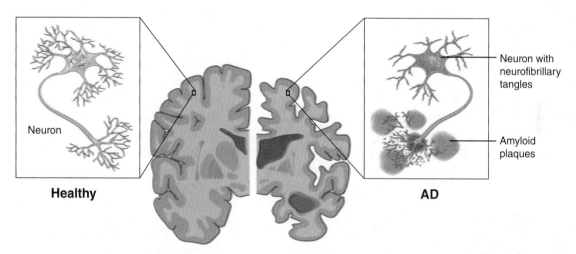

FIGURE 14-13 An example of a healthy neuron compared to a neuron in a brain with Alzheimer disease that has neurofibrillary tangles and amyloid plaques.

This condition is genetic, following an autosomal-dominant inheritance pattern in which children of those affected have a 50% chance of inheriting the disease. Like patients with AD, patients with HD develop dementia and memory problems, but their issues are with nondeclarative procedural memory. HD attacks the basal ganglia's striatum, which is preserved in AD. Procedural memory is a strength in dementia until the late stages of the disease.

Executive Functions

Executive dysfunction is a common feature of AD, especially later in the disease (Perry & Hodges, 1999). Restraint, initiative, and order all become progressively impaired. In terms of restraint, AD patients struggle with self-governance and judgment, making them safety risks if left unattended. Initiative to communicate can wain as the disease becomes worse, and when they do speak, their thoughts can lack order and be confusing to the listener.

▶ Conclusion

As a university student, your cognitive abilities should be working at a high level. The different forms of attention mentioned in this chapter are important for class lectures, reading, and other activities. Memory is critical for learning new information (declarative memory) and in learning new skills (nondeclarative memory). Executive functions are also essential for the many exams, quizzes, papers, and projects. In many ways, setting and achieving realistic goals is as important as acquiring knowledge and skills.

How about the patient population? Cognitive skills are necessary not only for college but also for life in general. All occupations require some degree of restraint, initiative, and order. Healthy human relationships require these too. Many patients, after a stroke or TBI, will struggle with these very processes, and it falls to many speech-language pathologists to help patients learn ways to compensate for cognitive impairment, especially in how it affects communication.

SUMMARY OF LEARNING OBJECTIVES

The following were the main learning objectives of this chapter. The information that should have been learned is listed below each learning objective.

1. The learner will define the term *cognition* and list various cognitive functions.
   - *Cognition:* the mental process of knowing, in which we acquire and act upon knowledge
   - *Perceiving:* recognizing if information is present, whether it be auditory, visual, or other information
   - *Remembering:* storing the information perceived
   - *Comprehending:* understanding the information that has been stored
   - *Judging:* assessing the accuracy or correctness of the information
   - *Reasoning:* either drawing conclusions or making arguments
2. The learner will define the following: *attention, memory,* and *executive function.*
   - *Attention:* a person's focus on a stimulus in the environment. The types of attention include focused, sustained, selective, alternating, and divided.
   - *Memory:* storing information. The types of memory include working memory (WM), short-term memory, and long-term memory. Long-term memory includes declarative or explicit memory (includes episodic and semantic) and nondeclarative or implicit memory (includes procedural memory).
   - *Executive function:* functions that order and manage all other cognitive functions (e.g., attention, memory) for the purpose of setting and attaining goals.
3. The learner will describe the neural basis of attention, memory, and executive functions.
   - *Attention:* right posterior parietal lobe (disengage attention), superior colliculus (assist in shifting attention), pulvinar nucleus (engage and maintain attention), and frontal eye fields (visual attention)
   - *Memory:* WM (prefrontal cortex, cingulate cortex, and parietal lobe), short-term memory (acetylcholine), long-term declarative memory (medial temporal lobe, parahippocampal gyrus, hippocampus, rhinal cortices, and diencephalon), and long-term nondeclarative memory (striatum of the basal ganglia)
   - *Executive functions:* prefrontal cortex
4. The learner will list and describe select disorders of attention, memory, and executive functions.
   - *Attention-deficit/hyperactivity disorder:* chronic, genetic condition characterized by inattention, hyperactivity, and impulsivity.
   - *Right hemisphere disorder:* Caused by damage to the right hemisphere, which results in both cognitive (attention, memory, and executive functions) and communicative (linguistic and extralinguistic) deficits.
   - *Traumatic brain injury:* a condition where patients can have deficits in attention, memory, and executive functions due to a traumatic blow to the head. Speech and language may also be affected, depending on the injury.
   - *Dementia:* the title for a category of irreversible, progressive neurocognitive disorders, the most famous of which is Alzheimer disease (AD). In AD, the hippocampus is one of the first brain structures to be damaged, leading to episodic memory problems followed later by semantic memory issues. Procedural memory is a strength. *By comparison, in Huntington disease* the basal ganglia degenerate, resulting in nondeclarative memory issues (i.e., procedural memory).

KEY TERMS

Anosognosia
Aprosody
Attention
Bottom-up attention
Cognition
Comprehension
Declarative memory
Dementia
Episodic memory

Executive functions
Initiative
Judgment
Long-term memory
Neglect syndrome
Nondeclarative memory
Order
Perception
Priming memory

Procedural memory
Reasoning
Remembering
Restraint
Semantic memory
Short-term memory
Synaptic theory
Top-down attention
Working memory (WM)

DRAW IT TO KNOW IT

1. Draw an illustration that would explain the different types of attention discussed in this chapter.
2. Draw a rough sketch of the right hemisphere and label the parts important in attention (see Figure 14-3).
3. Look at Figure 14-6 and sketch this transverse view of the brain. Highlight and label important memory areas.

QUESTIONS FOR DEEPER REFLECTION

1. List the different types of attention and give illustrations of how you use these in everyday life.
2. What are the cognitive functions, and how do you use them in everyday life?
3. List the neurological structures associated with attention, memory, and executive functions.
4. Define and provide examples of the following: restraint, initiative, and order.

CASE STUDY

Barry is a 61-year-old male who suffered a (R) cerebrovascular accident (CVA). He spent 3 days in acute care, but then was released home by his physician due to "the patient having no significant residual effects from the CVA". Once home, Barry's wife began to notice that he was different. Though he could talk fluently and understand what people said to him, he now appeared to ramble on in conversation. Once a gripping storyteller, he now verbally wandered in telling stories, perseverating on details and not telling the overall story arc. In conversation, he is pragmatically awkward as shown by dominating conversations, ignoring hints and requests from others for repairs, and lacking an ability to effectively use facial expression and emotion with others. In addition to all this, his wife reports he denies having any problems at all after his stroke.

1. Based on the limited information above, what cognitive-communicative diagnosis do you think is most likely in Barry's case? What factors led you to this conclusion?
2. What is the medical term for denial of deficits?
3. What would your counseling look like to Barry's wife?

SUGGESTED PROJECTS

1. Read Chapter 8 of Oliver Sacks's book *The Man Who Mistook His Wife for a Hat*. Write a one- to two-page summary of this story of neglect.
2. Think about the following cognitive processes: perceiving, remembering, comprehending, judging, and reasoning. Think about your life as a student and give concrete examples of how you use these processes on a daily basis.
3. Think about executive functions and describe how you engage in goal-directed behavior on a daily basis. Write up your thoughts and share in class.
4. Test your divided attention by attempting to read and talk to a friend at the same time. Write a paragraph describing how successful/unsuccessful you were in doing this.
5. Write a case of someone who has suffered a traumatic brain injury who now has executive function and memory problems.

REFERENCES

Baddeley, A. D. (2012). Working memory: Theories, models, and controversies. *Annual Review of Psychology, 63*, 1–29.

Baddeley, A. D., Baddeley, H. A., Bucks, R. S., & Wilcock, G. K. (2001). Attentional control in Alzheimer's disease. *Brain, 124*(8), 1492–1508.

Bayles, K. A. (1991). Alzheimer's disease symptoms: Prevalence and order of appearance. *Journal of Applied Gerontology, 10*(4), 419–430.

Ben-David, B. M., Nguyen, L. L., & van Lieshout, P. H. (2011). Stroop effects in persons with traumatic brain injury: Selective attention, speed of processing, or color-naming? A meta-analysis. *Journal of the International Neuropsychological Society, 17*(2), 354–363.

Blumenfeld, H. (2010). *Neuroanatomy through clinical cases*. Sunderland, MA: Sinauer Associates.

Brush, J. A., & Camp, C. J. (1998). Using spaced retrieval as an intervention during speech-language therapy. *Clinical Gerontologist, 19*(1), 51–64.

Gillespie, D. C., Bowen, A., & Foster, J. K. (2006). Memory impairment following right hemisphere stroke: A comparative meta-analytic and narrative review. *The Clinical Neuropsychologist, 20*(1), 59–75.

Han, J. W., Son, K. L., Byun, H. J., Ko, J. W., Kim, K., & Hong, J. W., . . . Kim, K. W. (2017). Efficacy of the Ubiquitous Spaced Retrieval-based Memory Advancement and Rehabilitation Training (USMART) program among patients with mild cognitive impairment: A randomized controlled crossover trial. *Alzheimer's Research & Therapy, 9*(1), 39.

Heilman, K. M., & Van Den Abell, T. (1980). Right hemisphere dominance for attention: The mechanism underlying hemispheric asymmetries of inattention (neglect). *Neurology, 30*(3), 327–327.

Henke, K. (2010). A model for memory systems based on processing modes rather than consciousness. *Nature Reviews Neuroscience, 11*(7), 523–532.

Hopkins, R. F., Lyle, K. B., Hieb, J. L., & Ralston, P. A. (2016). Spaced retrieval practice increases college students' short and long-term retention of mathematics knowledge. *Educational Psychology Review, 28*(4), 853–873.

Karpicke, J. D., & Roediger III, H. L. (2007). Expanding retrieval practice promotes short-term retention, but equally spaced retrieval enhances long-term retention. *Journal of Experimental Psychology: Learning, Memory, and Cognition, 33*(4), 704.

Katz, N., Hartman-Maeir, A., Ring, H., & Soroker, N. (1999). Functional disability and rehabilitation outcome in right hemisphere damaged patients with and without unilateral spatial neglect. *Archives of Physical Medicine and Rehabilitation, 80*(4), 379–384.

McGuinness, B., Barrett, S. L., Craig, D., Lawson, J., & Passmore, A. P. (2010). Attention deficits in Alzheimer's disease and vascular dementia. *Journal of Neurology, Neurosurgery & Psychiatry, 81*(2), 157–159.

McKitrick, L. A., & Camp, C. J. (1993). Relearning the names of things: The spaced-retrieval intervention implemented by a caregiver. *Clinical Gerontologist, 14*(2), 60–62.

Mez, J., Daneshvar, D. H., Kiernan, P. T., Abdolmohammadi, B., Alvarez, V. E., & Huber, B. R., . . . Cormier, K. A. (2017). Clinicopathological evaluation of chronic traumatic encephalopathy in players of American football. *JAMA, 318*(4), 360–370.

Oren, S., Willerton, C., & Small, J. (2014). Effects of spaced retrieval training on semantic memory in Alzheimer's disease: A systematic review. *Journal of Speech, Language, and Hearing Research, 57*(1), 247–270.

Perry, R. J., & Hodges, J. R. (1999). Attention and executive deficits in Alzheimer's disease: A critical review. *Brain, 122*(3), 383–404.

Plassman, B. L., Langa, K. M., Fisher, G. G., Heeringa, S. G., Weir, D. R., & Ofstedal, M. B., . . . Steffens, D. C. (2007). Prevalence of dementia in the United States: The aging, demographics, and memory study. *Neuroepidemiology, 29*(1–2), 125–132.

Ramat, S., Leigh, R. J., Zee, D. S., & Optican, L. M. (2006). What clinical disorders tell us about the neural control of saccadic eye movements. *Brain, 130*(1), 10–35.

Salmon, D. P., & Bondi, M. W. (2009). Neuropsychological assessment of dementia. *Annual Review of Psychology, 60*, 257–282.

Sanes, J. R., & Jessell, T. M. (2013). The aging brain. In E. R. Kandel, J. H. Schwartz, T. M. Jessell, S. A. Siegelbaum, & A. J. Hudspeth (Eds.), *Principles of neural science* (pp. 1328–1346). New York, NY: McGraw-Hill Medical.

Schacter, D. L., Rich, S. A., & Stampp, M. S. (1985). Remediation of memory disorders: Experimental evaluation of the spaced-retrieval technique. *Journal of Clinical and Experimental Neuropsychology, 7*(1), 79–96.

Sohlberg, M. M., & Mateer, C. A. (1989). *Introduction to cognitive rehabilitation: Theory and practice.* New York, NY: Guilford Press.

Spelke, E., Hirst, W., & Neisser, U. (1976). Skills of divided attention. *Cognition, 4*(3), 215–230.

Thomsen, I. V. (1984). Late outcome of very severe blunt head trauma: A 10-15 year second follow-up. *Journal of Neurology, Neurosurgery & Psychiatry, 47*(3), 260–268.

Vallar, G., & Perani, D. (1986). The anatomy of unilateral neglect after right-hemisphere stroke lesions. A clinical/CT-scan correlation study in man. *Neuropsychologia, 24*(5), 609–622.

Wang, Z., & Tchernev, J. M. (2012). The "myth" of media multitasking: Reciprocal dynamics of media multitasking, personal needs, and gratifications. *Journal of Communication, 62*(3), 493–513.

Ward, L. M. (2008). Attention. *Scholarpedia, 3*(10), 1538.

Wright, R. D., & Ward, L. M. (2008). *Orienting of attention.* New York, NY: Oxford University Press.

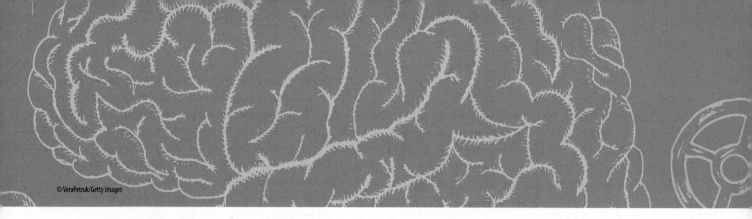
© VeraPetruk/Getty Images

CHAPTER 15

The Neurology of Emotion

CHAPTER PREVIEW

Emotion may seem like a strange topic to include when discussing neuroanatomy for communication sciences and disorders. It is a relevant topic for two reasons. First, our patients are emotional beings and will express emotion to us at some point in time. Second, some of our patients, like those with autism, will have difficulty with their emotions or reading the emotions of others. Thus, the topic of emotion is a highly relevant topic for speech-language pathologists and audiologists, especially as it intersects with counseling patients and their caregivers.

IN THIS CHAPTER

In this chapter, we will . . .
- Define what emotions are
- Consider the concept of emotional intelligence
- Survey three theories of emotion
- Explore the neurology of emotion
- Survey examples of emotional disorders

LEARNING OBJECTIVES

1. The learner will define what emotion and emotional intelligence are.
2. The learner will describe three theories of emotion.
3. The learner will list and describe neural structures involved with emotional processing.
4. The learner will describe three conditions in which there is a disruption in emotion: Klüver-Bucy syndrome, autism, and lability.
5. The learner will describe the connection between patient emotions, like fear, and the need for counseling in speech-language pathology and audiology.

▶ Introduction

In its various iterations, the *Star Trek* series has explored the balance between rational thought and emotions. Vulcans, a humanoid species, have learned to suppress their emotions over many centuries in order to live by logic. They at times despise humans, who to them are ruled by their emotions. One of the fun parts of the series is to see Vulcans begin to get in touch with their suppressed emotions and become more like humans. Dr. Spock, who is part human and part Vulcan, is one of the best examples of this struggle. To appreciate emotions, think about what life would be like without them. What would it be like not to experience happiness, sadness, or anger? What would it be like to be Vulcan?

What is **emotion**? To answer this question, we can view emotion objectively or we can view it subjectively. Objectively, emotions can be defined as a certain set of physiological responses to certain stimuli. For example, if I encounter a rattlesnake coiled and ready to strike, my heart starts beating fast, my muscles get tense, and I flee from danger. All these responses can be either observed directly or measured in some way. Subjectively, emotion can also refer to a conscious internal experience of feelings. When I see the snake, I have an internal, conscious feeling of fear. When I see my wife, I have an internal, conscious feeling of love. As we shall see, theorists have taken one definition or the other in exploring the topic of emotion. For our purposes, we will define emotion as both the subjective, conscious affective experience (e.g., fear, joy) and the parallel objective, physiological reactions (e.g., change in blood pressure) to stimuli in the environment.

The purpose of this chapter is to explore the neural basis of emotion. It might seem curious to discuss the neurology of emotion, but many speech-language pathologists (SLPs) and audiologists work with people with autism, who have differences in emotional processing. Having a basic understanding of emotion and its neuroanatomy will be helpful in understanding, being empathetic toward, and helping this population.

▶ Emotional Intelligence

More and more, emotions are being seen as a very important part of being human. For years, scientists have talked a lot about intelligence quotients (i.e., a person's IQ score), but a new breed of affective neuroscientists, like Daniel Goleman, are reminding the rest of us that humans possess multiple intelligences, one of which is **emotional intelligence (EI)**. The subject of EI has become popularized only in recent decades. It is our ability to understand our own emotions as well as those of others that guides us in our personal relationships. It is a concept that has been around for a long, long time. Aristotle in *The Nicomachean Ethics* stated:

> Those who are not angry at the things they should be angry at are thought to be fools, and so are those who are not angry in the right way at the right time, or with the right persons; for such a man is thought not to feel things nor to be pained by them, and, since he does not get angry, he is thought unlikely to defend himself.
>
> (Book 4, Chapter 5)

Salovey and Mayer (as cited in Colman, 2014c) formally defined EI along four competencies:

> (a) the ability to perceive, appraise, and express emotions accurately, (b) the ability to access and evoke emotions when they facilitate cognition, (c) the ability to comprehend emotional messages and to make use of emotional information, and (d) the ability to regulate one's own emotions to promote growth and well-being.
>
> (Colman, 2014c)

Think of how important each of these competencies is to being an SLP or audiologist. Our patients will express emotion to us at some point about their speech, language, cognitive, or hearing loss, and we need to be able to read the intents of our patients' messages. Some of these intents will be informational (e.g., "Could you explain what the larynx is?"), but other messages will be emotional (e.g., "I am so frustrated with these new hearing aids. All the kids are teasing me about them."). Our ability to perceive, appraise, and comprehend our patients' emotions (e.g., "this is sadness") and emotional messages is critical not only for establishing rapport, support, and trust in the clinical relationship but also for making appropriate referrals to other professionals (e.g., psychologist).

As clinicians, we must also consider our own emotions. We are emotional creatures and, as clinicians, we need to be able to perceive, appraise, and comprehend our own emotions as well as regulate them appropriately so they do not overburden our patients. In essence, we want to be able to *hold* our patients emotionally so their emotions do not overwhelm us but also regulate our own emotions so as not to create unhealthy emotional bonds that might overwhelm them. At times, some clinicians have developed an unhealthy attachment to their patients, finding satisfaction for the clinician's own emotional needs. This is not good for our patients or us.

Our emotional life, as well as that of the people with whom we work, is important. Through EI, we navigate the patient–clinician relationship. Many patients and caregivers report that they want clinicians who are not only competent but also empathetic and supportive. To be this type of clinician, we must take advantage of our EI. We must also realize that EI can be impaired in our patients through various neuropathologies. It is the neurological side of emotion to which we now turn.

▶ Theories of Emotion

Theorists of emotion have asked the question: What is the relationship between emotional experience and emotional expression? In other words, which comes first—the internal subjective emotional experience or the external objective physiological expression? In the 19th century, William James (1842–1910) and Carl Lange (1834–1900) proposed a theory called the **James-Lange theory**. It proposed that physiological responses (e.g., trembling) to external stimuli lead to emotional experience (Colman, 2014d). This theory can be represented as follows:

Environment → Trembling → Afraid

James and Lange defined emotion as the external, physiological status of the body (e.g., trembling) and a person's interpretation of the body's status. For example, if a wild bear approached you, you would begin to tremble. As you trembled, you would say to yourself, "I am trembling. I must be afraid!" This theory proposes that your feelings are never directly connected to the external stimulus (e.g., the bear), but rather are directly tied to your physiological state. What if you were angry, with your heart pounding and your face red? If these emotional expressions were removed, what would be left? Would you still "feel" angry if the physiological feelings were removed? James and Lange would say, "No!"

In the early 20th century, Walter Cannon (1871–1945) challenged the James-Lange theory. After some modification by his student Philip Bard (1898–1977), the **Cannon-Bard theory** of emotion became popular. It theorized that an external stimulus simultaneously triggers a physiological response and an emotional experience, both occurring independently of each other (Colman, 2014a). The Cannon-Bard theory can be represented in this way:

Environment → Trembling and Afraid

Using our example of the bear again, as the bear approaches you, you would simultaneously start to tremble and feel afraid. In other words, your feelings (e.g., fear) are tied directly to the external stimulus. Could a person have an emotional experience with no physiological response? Cannon and Bard would respond, "Yes!" For example, there might be a person with locked-in syndrome who experiences emotion but does not express emotion physiologically (i.e., no trembling). Another example is sleep: The body is in a state of rest, but we can experience vivid emotions connected to our dreams.

One last theory of emotion is the **two-factor theory** (or cognitive-appraisal theory) proposed by Stanley Schachter and Jerome Singer in the 1960s. This theory states that emotion is based on two factors—a physiological state and the interpretation of that state (Colman, 2014b). It can be represented this way:

Trembling → Environment → Afraid

For example, you begin to tremble, so you look to the environment to discover a stimulus that explains why you are trembling. You then see a bear and decide that the trembling is due to the bear.

These three theories differ neurologically. The James-Lange theory posits that the viscera and sensory system are the center of the emotional system. In contrast, the Cannon-Bard theory hypothesizes that the thalamus is the center of the emotional system, sending two parallel yet independent signals. One of these signals goes to the cortex where a subjective emotional experience occurs; the other goes to the sympathetic nervous system via the hypothalamus to induce a physiological response. The two-factor theory relies heavily on the autonomic nervous system and the cognitive aspects of the cortex. It does not address known areas of emotional processing, such as the amygdala.

Which of these three theories is correct? It appears that there are elements of truth in all three theories. For example, it is possible to force yourself to smile a lot and find that happy feelings begin to arise over time; the physiological experience has given rise to the emotional experience (James-Lange). It is equally possible to have an internal emotional experience but have or not have a physiological response (Cannon-Bard). Finally, we may at times look to the environment for an explanation of a physiological response we are having and frame that response emotionally (e.g., fear) based on the environmental stimulus (two-factor).

Setting these theories aside and stepping back, what is the relationship between emotion and our neurological system? Is emotion reducible to the viscera? Or the thalamus? Or the autonomic nervous system? What are the components of the nervous system that process and help us express our emotions?

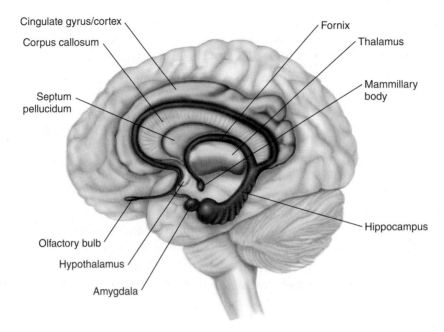

FIGURE 15-1 Major limbic structures.

▶ The Neural Basis of Emotion

The Limbic System

An American neuroscientist named James Papez (1883–1958) built on the work of Cannon and Bard and proposed that a series of structures known as the limbic system was the brain's emotional system. In addition to emotion, the limbic system is involved in olfaction, memory, and homeostasis. Blumenfeld (2010) suggests these four limbic functions can be remembered by the acronym **HOME**: **H**omeostasis, **O**lfaction, **M**emory, and **E**motion. We have all had the experience of smelling something that evoked both memory and emotion; it is the limbic system that integrates the neurological structures behind these experiences.

The limbic system is located between the thalamus and the medial walls of the cerebral hemispheres (**FIGURE 15-1**). The name *limbic*, which is Latin for "border," was given by Paul Broca for the cortical area that is a part of this system.

Papez proposed that a number of structures are involved in this system, not just the thalamic structures. His proposal became known as the **Papez circuit**. This circuit includes the sensory cortex, cingulate cortex, hippocampus, hypothalamus, and anterior thalamic nuclei (**FIGURE 15-2**). According to Papez, the body's sensory experiences are sent to the thalamus and then are routed to the hypothalamus. The hypothalamus then sends ascending fibers through the anterior thalamus and cingulate cortex to the sensory cortex, resulting in conscious emotional experience,

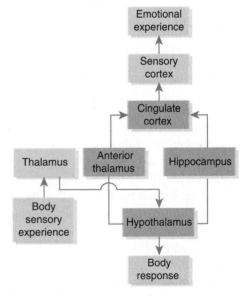

FIGURE 15-2 The Papez circuit. Note: The purple boxes indicate the basic components of the Papez circuit.

Data from Dalgleish, T. (2004). The emotional brain. *Nature Reviews Neuroscience, 5*, 583–589.

especially the coloring of that experience (positive versus negative emotions). To complete the circuit, fibers then descend through the hippocampus, back to the hypothalamus, and to the body, leading to physiological responses (e.g., increased heart rate) (LeDoux & Damasio, 2013). The connections between cortical structures and the hypothalamus are bidirectional, meaning that the two influence each other. This means that both the James-Lange and Cannon-Bard theories are probably correct. Emotional experience can cause

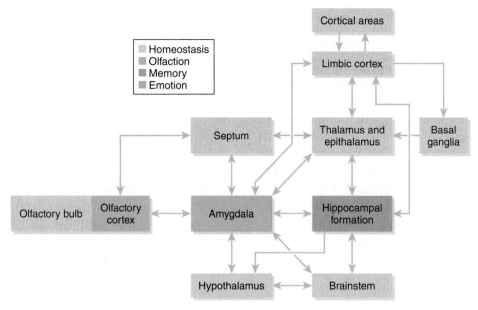

FIGURE 15-3 Overview of the limbic circuitry.

emotional expression, and emotional expression can cause emotional experience.

The Papez circuit continues to have explanatory power in neuroscience. Today, this system is known to involve more structures than Papez theorized, including the olfactory bulb, hypothalamus, amygdala, septal nuclei, anterior nucleus of the thalamus, piriform olfactory cortex, hippocampal formation, and limbic cortex (**FIGURE 15-3**) (Castro, Merchut, Neafsey, & Wurster, 2002). Though the hippocampus is classified as a memory structure by many, there is a clear connection between emotion and memory, because many of our strongest memories have a strong emotional component to them.

The Amygdala

The Papez circuit theory predicts that if any damage occurs within the circuit, there will be effects on emotional behavior. This has not always been found to be true, but one area that clearly results in changes in emotional behavior when damaged is the amygdala. The term **amygdala** is Greek for "almond," and there are two of these almond-shaped nuclei deep in our brains. The amygdala is clearly involved in fear and aggression.

The amygdala is situated in the medial temporal lobe and is made up of two groups of nuclei: the corticomedial group and the basolateral group. The corticomedial group is related to olfaction, whereas the basolateral group has extensive cortical connections that are both afferent and efferent. Afferent connections include the olfactory tract, the limbic cortex, and nuclei (solitary and parabrachial) involved with taste

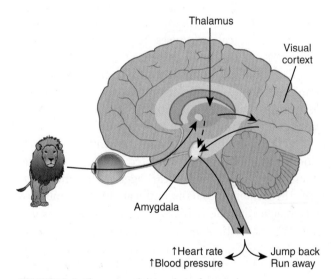

FIGURE 15-4 The amygdala's role in fear and self-preservation.

and general visceral functions. Efferent connections are made with the hypothalamus, limbic cortex, and various autonomic nervous system centers (Castro et al., 2002).

The amygdala is a central structure in our ability to preserve ourselves and respond to environmental danger. **FIGURE 15-4** illustrates this function by showing how the amygdala might protect us if we were to spot a ferocious lion. It would increase our heart rate and blood pressure via the hypothalamus and invoke a flight response away from danger.

Other behaviors the amygdala directs include feeding and drinking, fighting, mating, maternal care, and our response to physical or emotional stress.

The amygdala is also important in emotional learning and emotional memory. These processes are *implicit* in nature, meaning that this learning and memory occur unconsciously. Emotional learning and memory can become explicit in times of danger, though. In these situations, those structures involved in explicit memory (e.g., hippocampus) are brought online to record the experience so it can be consciously recalled later (LeDoux & Damasio, 2013). For example, when this author was a child, he touched the engine of a running tractor, resulting in burns to his hands. It is safe to say that a strong emotional memory was formed that day and he never touched a running engine again!

Studies have shown that damage to the amygdala flattens emotions and produces difficulty recognizing facial emotions in others. When the amygdala is bilaterally damaged, subjects will have an explicit memory of a conditioning experience (e.g., electrical shock), but no physiological responses (e.g., avoidance) when the source of the shock is displayed. For example, if I were the subject, I could tell you about my experience touching the tractor's engine, but you could not record any physiological responses (e.g., increased blood pressure) if a running engine were brought into the room. In contrast, patients with bilateral hippocampi damage have physiological responses (and implicit learning) when the source of the shock is displayed, but no explicit recall of the experience.

If the opposite occurs and the amygdala's function is altered or overstimulated in some way, the result may be abnormal fear, aggression, and anxiety. Thus, the amygdala is implicated in a number of psychiatric disorders, including depression, anxiety, and posttraumatic stress disorder (PTSD) (LeDoux & Damasio, 2013). It is also involved in positive experiences, like pleasure and rewards. Pleasurable experiences induced through alcohol and drugs can result in addictions. The architecture of structures like the amygdala can change when substances are abused, resulting in anxiety and stress as levels of these substances decrease in the body. This stress and anxiety can then only be eased by the continued, and often increased, abuse of these substances.

The Cingulate Cortex

The cingulate cortex is an arch-shaped band of cortical tissue located in the medial region of the cerebral cortex (Figure 15-3). Superior to the cingulate cortex is the cingulate sulcus, and above the cingulate sulcus are the lobes of the brain. Inferior to the cingulate is the corpus callosum.

Papez (1937) was one of the first to theorize that the cingulate cortex is important in emotional processing and social behavior, but the exact nature of this processing has proven elusive. Lesion studies in animals have demonstrated that damage to the cingulate cortex results in decreases in social behavior, reduced time spent with others, and a decrease in vocalizations. Subjects also demonstrate an increase in time with inanimate objects (Hadland, Rushworth, Gaffan, & Passingham, 2003). Activation in the cingulate has been noted when subjects are exposed to negative emotion, such as pictures of angry faces (Blair, Morris, Frith, Perrett, & Dolan, 1999; Etkin, Egner, & Kalisch, 2011; Lane, Chua, & Dolan, 1999). The resolution of emotional conflict and thus the regulation of emotions have been associated with activation of the anterior cingulate cortex (Etkin, Egner, & Kalisch, 2011; Etkin, Egner, Peraza, Kandel, & Hirsch, 2006). The anterior cingulate cortex also seems to play a role in attention, especially in filtering out irrelevant information, even perhaps irrelevant emotional signals (Kozlovskiv, Vartanov, Nikonova, Pyasik, & Velichkovsky, 2012; Mohanty et al., 2007).

It is difficult to separate emotion from cognition. The cingulate cortex plays a role in cognition through its connections with the prefrontal cortex. For example, activations have also been noted in tasks that require **theory of mind (ToM)** abilities (Frith & Frith, 1999; Gallagher et al., 2000). ToM is the ability to understand that I have a mind, that you have a mind, and that our minds are different from one another. This ability is obviously important in having empathy for others.

Damage to the cingulate cortex has been associated with disorders such as depression and schizophrenia. Drevets, Savitz, and Trimble (2008) have reported abnormal reduction in cingulate tissue near the genu of the corpus callosum associated with mood disorders like major depression and bipolar disorder. Adams and David (2007) found that the cingulate was either underactive or overactive in people with schizophrenia in comparison to normal subjects, but psychiatric medications returned the cingulate to normal activation patterns.

The Insular Cortex

The insular cortex is located at the medial temporal lobes and has many connections to structures involved in emotional processing, including the amygdala, hypothalamus, and other areas. It plays a role in the expression of some negative emotions, like disgust (Jezzini, Caruana, Stoianov, Gallese, & Rizzolatti, 2012). It also plays an important role in emotional awareness, a key ability in EI (Craig, 2009). Lamm and Singer (2010) concluded that the insula is involved in empathy, compassion, fairness, and cooperation. These are all important intrapersonal abilities that would flow from emotional awareness of self and others. This obviously relates to ToM.

The Prefrontal Cortex

The **prefrontal cortex** plays an important role not only in cognition but also in emotion. This is not surprising given the heavy interconnectedness between it and other limbic areas, especially the anterior cingulate cortex. People who have experienced prefrontal cortex damage often have impaired abilities in social emotions. Because of this, they may experience the loss of stable social relationships with spouses and friends (LeDoux & Damasio, 2013). One patient I had several years ago had prefrontal cortex damage after a minor car accident. He reported that after the accident, he did not love his wife anymore. His wife reported that he did not have any interest in her or their son since the accident. The husband alienated all of their friends, and the marriage eventually ended in divorce.

The ventromedial region of the prefrontal cortex (Brodmann areas [BAs] 10, 11, 12), the anterior cingulate cortex (BAs 25, 32), and the amygdala appear to be critically important in emotion. Lesions in the prefrontal cortex can result in a disconnection with the anterior cingulate and amygdala and a flattening of emotional responses. Patients will no longer have physiological emotional reactions to stimuli that people normally have (LeDoux & Damasio, 2013). Some people become the opposite though—explosively emotional. Several studies have found that people with prefrontal cortex damage have difficulty reading facial emotions and identifying vocal expressions of emotion (Blair & Cipolotti, 2000; Hornak, Rolls, & Wade, 1996; Hornak et al., 2003).

▸ Disorders of Emotion

Klüver-Bucy Syndrome

Though very rare in humans, **Klüver-Bucy syndrome** has been induced through experiments performing bilateral amygdalectomies on wild rhesus monkeys (Dicks, Myers, & Kling, 1969). After the surgery, the monkeys were released into the wild and 2 weeks later were found dead. They had either starved, drowned, or been killed by other animals. After their surgery, the monkeys could not see or avoid potentially dangerous situations. Those running the experiment concluded that the monkeys had lost their ability to fear and that fear is tied to having intact amygdalae. Klüver-Bucy

syndrome is caused by bilateral damage to the amygdala and results in diminished fears, overeating, oral fixation, heightened sex drive, and visual agnosia. In humans, the condition has been documented as occurring after temporal lobectomies, encephalitis, or bilateral stroke (Victor & Ropper, 2001).

One famous case of living without amygdalae is the case of S. M., who unlike the rhesus monkeys is still alive today. Her case was first described in 1994 by Adolphs, Tranel, Damasio, and Damasio. S. M. has a rare genetic condition called Urbach-Wiethe disease, of which there have been only about 400 reported cases worldwide since the early 20th century. It results in skin wrinkles, lesions, and scars; hoarse voice due to thickened vocal cords; and papules (i.e., skin bumps) around the eyelids. In addition, the condition hardens tissues in the medial temporal lobes. In S. M.'s case, this hardening began happening when she was a young girl, most prominently in the amygdalae. She was referred to a neurologist when she was 20 years of age and met Dr. Daniel Tranel. They began a professional relationship that remains in place to this day. Computed tomography and magnetic resonance imaging revealed that both amygdalae had almost completely calcified. Behaviorally, experiments showed that S. M. did not have any kind of fear response. Experimenters exposed her to items such as snakes and spiders as well as horror films and observed she did not exhibit fear. Instead, interest and curiosity were observed. S. M. has no fear of strangers, cannot read fear or other negative emotions on other people's faces, and tends to be very positive about people and situations. As such, S. M. is at great risk of being taken advantage of by others, and the researchers who have been studying her are very careful in not revealing her identity or where she lives. She has already been the victim of violent crime but has never demonstrated any of the normal behavioral fear or distress responses to those situations.

Most of us would do anything to rid ourselves of fear, but the case of S. M. shows that the right amount of fear helps us negotiate a sometimes dangerous world. Too much fear can paralyze us in life (e.g., PTSD), but too little can leave us open to being abused by others. As stated by Feinstein, Adolphs, and Tranel (2016), "When it comes to survival, no other emotion is as imperative as fear" (p. 7).

Autism

Autism is a neurological developmental disorder that occurs in 1 in 59 children in the United States (Centers for Disease Control and Prevention, 2018). The disorder is characterized by problems in social interaction, communication problems, and stereotyped behaviors, all of which are diagnosed before a child is 3 years of age. Autism is five times more likely in boys than in girls. Twin studies have demonstrated that if one twin has autism, there is a 60% to 96% chance that the other twin will have it as well, suggesting a strong genetic causal component.

It has been argued that children with autism have brains that differ from the brains of their typical counterparts in significant ways. The cerebral cortex, hippocampus, basal ganglia, corpus callosum, brainstem, cerebellum, and amygdala are all thought to have neuroanatomical differences in autism. One theory is neuron overgrowth in these areas leading to overconnectivity between brain areas. In addition, both the amygdala and the fusiform gyrus may show underactivation in these children (Corbett et al., 2009). This may explain at least in part why children with autism process emotion differently than do typical children. A recent, large-scale study by Haar, Berman, Behrmann, and Dinstein (2016) has challenged these neurological difference theories put forward by previous small-scale studies. These researchers report that people with autism have the same basic brain anatomy as people without autism. They acknowledge that while many subgroups of people with autism do have brain differences, the vast majority of people with autism have brains that are fundamentally the same as anyone else's.

Both aggression and difficulty interpreting the emotional behavior of others have been frequently reported in cases of autism (Amaral, Schumann, & Nordahl, 2008; Schumann et al., 2004). People with autism have a kind of *emotional agnosia* when it comes to reading the emotions of other people, whether they are expressed as facial expression, vocal intonation, or body language. Because of possible dysfunction in both the amygdala and fusiform gyrus, it is not surprising that these children experience these issues. If neurological difference theories do prove true, the dysfunction in the amygdala leads to emotional processing problems, and the dysfunction in the fusiform gyrus leads to a kind of prosopagnosia, or face blindness, to facial emotions (not a real prosopagnosia because they can still recognize familiar faces). This inability to read people's emotions is thought to be related to their deficits in ToM (Hobson, 1995). Children with autism have obvious difficulty in reading the mental states of others and typically fail ToM tests. The result of these deficits is a lack of empathy toward others (Clark, Winkielman, & McIntosh, 2008).

Rizzolatti and Craighero (2004) made an interesting discovery regarding the mirror-neuron system that may have application to autism. Motor command neurons are found in the premotor cortex and they fire when a person performs a certain action, like raising his or her hand. What Rizzolatti and Craighero discovered was that about 20% of these neurons also fire when we watch someone else carry out a motor command. These are called **mirror neurons** because they mirror what other people do, and they are important in our ability to watch others and learn new skills.

Mirror neurons are also found in the somatosensory cortex and work in the same way with touch. The mirror neurons fire when I am being touched, but they also fire when I see someone else being touched. This is a form of empathy. Ramachandran (2009) summarizes the functions of these neurons as follows:

> The mirror neuron system underlies the interface allowing you to rethink about issues like consciousness, representation of self, what separates you from other human beings, what allows you to empathize with other human beings, and also even things like the emergence of culture and civilization, which is unique to human beings.

Lability

Emotional lability (or emotionalism) is an involuntary display of emotion that can sometimes be the result of a neuropathology. As human beings mature, their ability to control their emotions matures as well. The degree to which this is true depends on culture, gender, and ethnicity (Victor & Ropper, 2001).

As we have seen, there are connections between the cortex, especially the prefrontal cortex, and the cingulate cortex, amygdala, and hypothalamus. The prefrontal cortex acts as a regulator of our emotions; when there is damage to it, a person's emotional life may change. Some patients experience flatness to their emotional life, whereas others experience "emotional incontinence" after a stroke or traumatic brain injury. A sudden outburst of laughing or crying might occur, though patients will report later that they did not feel particularly happy or sad when the outburst occurred. Patients report that these episodes are "both distressing and socially disabling" (House, Dennis, Molyneux, Warlow, & Hawton, 1989, p. 994). This sudden and seemingly strange display of emotion can shock many clinicians. When an episode occurs, it is best to stop all activities and allow the patient a few moments to compose himself or herself, after which many patients can usually resume therapy tasks. Trying to delve into why the person was crying is often not helpful or productive, because there is no underlying reason for it.

► Working With Patients' Emotions: Counseling

A Tale of Two Minds

Daniel Goleman (1995) said that every person has two minds, one that is thinking in nature and another that is feeling. Tanner (1980), understanding the feeling mind, stated that SLPs should regard their clients as being in a state of grief over their communication loss. Several researchers have written about stages of grief connected to the death of a loved one (Kübler-Ross, 1969; Maciejewski, Zhang, Block, & Prigerson, 2007; Powers & Singer, 1993; Schneider, 1984), but others have confirmed that grief can occur when a patient has experienced a disability, like a communication disorder (Davis, 1987; Riesz, 2004; Robinson, Clare, & Evans, 2005; Rybarczyk, Edwards, & Behel, 2004; Sanders & Adams, 2005). Death grief is often thought of as being temporary, whereas grief associated with disease and disability is often chronic and episodic (Friehe, Bloedow, & Hesse, 2003; Kurtzer-White & Luterman, 2003). According to Spillers (2007), "Grief is a normal human response to loss, and loss permeates disability. Grief allows a person to separate from the loss and make some sense out of it" (p. 191).

Various researchers have explored different dimensions of grief associated with the loss associated with disability. Gilhome-Herbst and Humphrey (1980) found that 27% of their subjects were in a state of denial about their diagnoses. Martin, George, O'Neal, and Daly (1987) discovered that two of the most common reactions to a diagnosis of hearing loss are sorrow and depression. Clark (1990a) reported that patients often intellectualize their diagnoses in order to keep their condition at a distance. Kurtzer-White and Luterman (2003) stated that parents of children with hearing loss often feel overwhelmed and inadequate. Luterman (2001) reported two additional patient responses to communication loss, namely vulnerability and confusion. Friehe, Bloedow, & Hesse (2003) also reported confusion as well as shock and fear.

The Therapist's Response to Patient Loss

In light of these patient reactions, our therapy plans should include "the facilitation of the grieving process and the ultimate acceptance of the loss by the patient" (Tanner, 1980, p. 928). However, patients often report that professionals do not understand their emotional difficulties in adjusting to a communication disorder (Martin, Krall, & O'Neal, 1989). For example, a patient might report feeling depressed because of his or her diagnosis of dysarthria; the clinician may respond that dysarthria is a term that describes slurred speech and that the patient will need to learn some speech techniques to reduce the slurring. In this example, the patient is using his or her feeling mind while the clinician is responding to the patient's thinking mind. In other words, the clinician has not correctly read and matched the patient's communication intent (i.e., poor EI), resulting in a well-intentioned but useless patient pep talk (Clark, 1990b). The clinician is playing the part of the expert instead of connecting to his or her patient on an emotional level (Beazely & Moore, 1995). The danger of not connecting on this emotional level is the development of patient stress, both in the clinician–patient relationship and within the patient's family (Zraick & Boone, 1991).

Counseling as a Critical Skill in Medicine

Physicians have long recognized the importance of patient counseling in establishing patient trust (Epstein et al., 2007; Fiscella, Meldrum, & Franks, 2004). Part of this counseling includes physicians understanding patients' feelings. Unfortunately, patient concerns are not always expressed in a straightforward manner. In fact, they often use "affectively loaded questions" and statements, which "are often superficially straightforward, but reflect underlying feelings of fear, anger, or apprehension that should be addressed" (Epstein et al., 2007, p. 1731). Patients leave it up to the physician to explore these topics further, and if physicians do not, patients then assume that these emotions are either not important or the physician does not care (Salmon, Peters, & Stanley, 1999; Seaburn et al., 2005). When physicians do take interest in patients' emotions, patients report higher satisfaction in that they trust and feel more supported by their physicians. Unfortunately, researchers have shown the reality to be that "patient concerns are minimized" and "expressions of empathy and support are uncommon" (Epstein et al., 2007, p. 1732).

As in medicine, counseling is seen as crucial to a patient's and family's adjustment to a communication disorder (Toner & Shadden, 2002). The American Speech Language Hearing Association (2004), in its statements on preferred practice patterns and scope of practice for SLPs, stated that counseling is part of the SLP's responsibilities in the rehabilitative process.

Training Particular Counseling Skills

A crucial part of entering the patient's inner world through counseling is the skill of being empathetic

(Riley, 2002). In fact, patients and caregivers have reported that they want not only skillful clinicians, "but also an empathetic, supportive counselor" (Luterman & Kurtzer-White, 1999, p. 16). The *Merriam-Webster's Collegiate Dictionary* (2007) defines **empathy** as "the action of understanding, being aware of, being sensitive to, and vicariously experiencing the feelings, thoughts, and experience of another of either the past or present without having the feelings, thoughts, and experience fully communicated in an objectively explicit manner."

Margulies (1984) divided empathy into two modes. First, there is *resonant empathy*, which is a form of empathy in which the clinician listens attentively to the patient's expressions of emotions. Second, there is *imaginative empathy*, in which the clinician uses his or her imagination to step into the patient's shoes and construct what the patient's inner world might be like. To be effective SLPs and audiologists, clinicians must have not only resonant empathetic skills, but also knowledge about the possible emotions, struggles, and other characteristics of a patient to effectively engage the patient in imaginative empathy.

Important clinical skills in both resonant and imaginative empathy include the abilities to pay attention, listen well, and determine and match patients' communicative intents (Eagen, 2001; Ivey, 2001). According to Holland (2005), good listening "involves sensitivity to both what a message's manifest (surface) content and its latent (deeper emotional) content are, and whether or not these two messages are in agreement" (p. 13). Caldwell (2004) describes these clinical communication skills as "the currency of therapy" and states that "high-quality, non-judgmental attention can be a balm directly applied to a client's wound, which soothes immediately and heals over time" (p. 35). Luterman (2006) describes the role of the counselor as follows:

> The counseling relationship is not a conventional one; it places a different set of demands on the professional. It is a relationship that requires deep, selfless listening. The professional must be willing to put aside his or her agenda and listen to the client. Therefore, the professional can have no point of view other than trying to hear and understand where the client is coming from, and in many cases, reflect that back to the client. Within a counseling relationship, there is the understanding that wisdom resides within the client; therefore, all professional judgments are suspended. Because nonjudgmental listening offers a high degree of emotional safety for the client, he or she can begin the process of resolving problems. When interacting with clients, professionals must learn to listen for the "faint knocking" that is the client's affect because clients are often unaware of how they feel. By listening deeply we can elicit the feelings and provide the support. (p. 9)

▶ Conclusion

Emotions are not a typical topic of study in the field of communication disorders, but much is communicated through emotion. Sometimes emotions can even betray a person by contradicting the very thing the person is saying (e.g., saying "I'm just fine" while gritting teeth and red faced). As clinicians, we will encounter many patients and caregivers going through the stages of grief. Others will be struggling with emotional deficits due to neurological disorders. Clinicians must stand ready to understand not only their own emotions but also the emotions of their patients. By doing this, we will be the supportive and empathetic counselors our patients desire.

SUMMARY OF LEARNING OBJECTIVES

The following were the main learning objectives of this chapter. The information that should have been learned is below each learning objective.

1. The learner will define what emotion and emotional intelligence are.
   - *Emotion:* Objectively, emotions can be defined as a certain set of physiological responses to certain stimuli. Subjectively, emotion can also refer to a conscious internal experience of feelings.
   - *Emotional intelligence (EI):* Colman (2014c) defines EI along four competencies:

□ The ability to perceive, appraise, and express emotions accurately

□ The ability to access and evoke emotions when they facilitate cognition

□ The ability to comprehend emotional messages and to make use of emotional information

□ The ability to regulate one's own emotions to promote growth and well-being

2. The learner will describe three theories of emotion.

   • *James-Lange theory:* Proposes that physiological responses (e.g., trembling) to external stimuli lead to emotional experience (Environment → Trembling → Afraid).

   • *Cannon-Bard theory:* Theorizes that an external stimulus simultaneously triggers a physiological response and an emotional experience, both occurring independently of each other (Environment → Trembling and Afraid).

   • *Two-factor theory:* States that emotion is based on two factors: a physiological state and the interpretation of that state (Trembling → Environment → Afraid).

3. The learner will list and describe neural structures involved with emotional processing.

   • *Limbic system:* Proposed by Papez (1937) to be the brain's emotional system.

   • *Amygdala:* Directs feeding and drinking, fighting, mating, maternal care, our response to physical or emotional stress, emotional learning, and emotional memory.

   • *Cingulate cortex:* important in emotional processing and social behavior.

   • *Insular cortex:* Plays a role in the expression of some negative emotions, like disgust, and also emotional awareness.

   • *Prefrontal cortex:* important for reading facial emotions and identifying vocal expressions of emotions. Damage can leave a person flat or explosively emotional.

4. The learner will describe three conditions in which there is a disruption in emotion: Klüver-Bucy syndrome, autism, and lability.

   • *Klüver-Bucy syndrome:* a condition caused by bilateral damage to the amygdala, resulting in diminished fears, overeating, oral fixation, heightened sex drive, and visual agnosia

   • *Autism:* a condition that involves emotional issues, namely aggression and difficulty interpreting the emotional behavior of others

   • *Lability:* an involuntary display of emotion that can sometimes be the result of a neuropathology

5. The learner will describe the connection between patient emotions, like fear, and the need for counseling in speech-language pathology and audiology.

   • Communication disorders are a form of loss, and with that loss comes a patient grieving process.

   • Grief due to a communication disorder involves many emotions, such as fear, shame, guilt, and worry.

   • Clinicians should be ready to enter grieving patients' worlds by using their feeling mind (EI) and using empathy as a tool to connect with patients and patient emotions.

   • This process is called counseling, and it is a critical skill found in the scope of practice for both speech-language pathologists and audiologists scope.

   • The purpose of counseling is for the patient to adjust in a healthy manner to his or her new communication disorder.

KEY TERMS

Amygdala	Emotional lability	Mirror neurons
Autism	Empathy	Papez circuit
Cannon-Bard theory	HOME	Prefrontal cortex
Emotion	James-Lange theory	Theory of mind (ToM)
Emotional intelligence (EI)	Klüver-Bucy syndrome	Two-factor theory

DRAW IT TO KNOW IT

1. Draw the Papez circuit from memory as presented in Figure 15-2. Indicate the basic components of this circuit.

QUESTIONS FOR DEEPER REFLECTION

1. Compare and contrast the three theories of emotion presented in this chapter.
2. List the neuroanatomical areas known to be involved in emotion and state their contribution to it.
3. Describe the emotional challenges people with autism face.
4. Explain how you might handle a patient who demonstrates emotional lability.

CASE STUDY

Ana is a 54-year-old female who suffered a (L) cerebrovascular accident (CVA) approximately 3 weeks ago. She spent a few days in acute care, but now is receiving physical therapy (PT), occupational therapy (OT), and speech therapy (ST) in the hospital's acute rehabilitation (AR) unit. One of Ana's behaviors you have observed in therapy is that Ana will suddenly burst out crying during therapy and that these outbursts do not seem connected to anything specific in therapy. Ana is scheduled to be discharged from the AR in 2 days to her home. Home health PT, OT, and ST have been ordered for Ana.

1. What label would you give to Ana's crying outbursts?
2. What counsel would you give to Ana's home health ST?

SUGGESTED PROJECTS

1. Pick a partner from class and use your smartphone to make a movie in which you and your partner describe and act out the three theories of emotion presented in this chapter.
2. Access the "How Emotionally Intelligent Are You?" test online (Cherry, 2016). Take the test to determine your emotional intelligence.
3. Write a three- to four-page paper on the emotional life and challenges of those with autism.
4. Write a two- to three-page paper on mirror neurons using three or four scholarly resources.
5. Read Temple Grandin's book *Thinking in Pictures* and write a two- to three-page reflection paper on it. Half your paper should be a summary of the book and the other half should include your reflections/reactions to the book.
6. Read the original article about S. M. in Adolphs, Tranel, Damasio, and Damasio (1994), and give a 10-minute oral presentation of the case to your class.

REFERENCES

Adams, R., & David, A. S. (2007). Patterns of anterior cingulate activation in schizophrenia: A selective review. *Neuropsychiatric Disease and Treatment, 3*(1), 87–101.

Adolphs, R., Tranel, D., Damasio, H., & Damasio, A. (1994). Impaired recognition of emotion in facial expressions following bilateral damage to the human amygdala. *Nature, 372*(6507), 669.

Amaral, D. G., Schumann, C. M., & Nordahl, C. W. (2008). Neuroanatomy of autism. *Trends in Neurosciences, 31*(3), 137–145.

American Speech Language Hearing Association. (2004). *Scope of practice in speech language pathology*. Rockville, MD: Author.

Beazely, S., & Moore, M. (1995). *Deaf children, their families, and professionals: Dismantling barriers*. London, UK: David Fulton Publishers.

Blair, R. J. R., & Cipolotti, L. (2000). Impaired social response reversal: A case of acquired sociopathy. *Brain, 123*(6), 1122–1141.

Blair, R. J. R., Morris, J. S., Frith, C. D., Perrett, D. I., & Dolan, R. J. (1999). Dissociable neural responses to facial expressions of sadness and anger. *Brain, 122*, 883–893.

Blumenfeld, H. (2010). *Neuroanatomy through clinical cases*. Sunderland, MA: Sinauer Associates.

Caldwell, C. (2004, July-August). Caring for the caregiver: The art of oscillating attention. *Psychotherapy Networker*, 34–35.

Castro, A. J., Merchut, M. P., Neafsey, E. J., & Wurster, R. D. (2002). *Neuroscience: An outline approach*. St. Louis, MO: Mosby.

Centers for Disease Control and Prevention (CDC). (2018). *Autism spectrum disorder (ASD): Data and statistics*. CDC, Division of Birth Defects, National Center on Birth Defects and Developmental Disabilities. Retrieved from http://www.cdc.gov/ncbddd/autism/data.html

Cherry, K. (2016). *How emotionally intelligent are you?* Very Well Mind. Retrieved from https://www.verywellmind.com/how-emotionally-intelligent-are-you-2796099

Clark, J. G. (1990a, June/July). Emotional response transformations: Redirections and projections. *ASHA, 28*, 67–68.

Clark, J. G. (1990b). The "don't worry, be happy" professional response. *Hearing Journal, 43*(1), 21–23.

Clark, T. F., Winkielman, P., & McIntosh, D. N. (2008). Autism and the extraction of emotion from briefly presented facial expressions: Stumbling at the first step of empathy. *Emotion, 8*(6), 803–809.

Colman, A. M. (2014a). Cannon-Bard theory. In A. M. Colman (Ed.), *Oxford dictionary of psychology*. Oxford, UK: Oxford University Press.

Colman, A. M. (2014b). Cognitive-appraisal theory. In A. M. Colman (Ed.), *Oxford dictionary of psychology*. Oxford, UK: Oxford University Press.

Colman, A. (2014c). Emotional intelligence. In A. M. Colman (Ed.), *Oxford dictionary of psychology*. Oxford, UK: Oxford University Press.

Colman, A. (2014d). James-Lange theory. In A. M. Colman (Ed.), *Oxford dictionary of psychology*. Oxford, UK: Oxford University Press.

Corbett, B. A., Carmean, V., Ravizza, S., Wendelken, C., Henry, M. L., Carter, C., & Rivera, S. M. (2009). A functional and structural study of emotion and face processing in children with autism. *Psychiatry Research: Neuroimaging, 173*(3), 196–205.

Craig, A. D. (2009). How do you feel—now? The anterior insula and human awareness. *Nature Reviews Neuroscience, 10*, 59–70.

Dalgleish, T. (2004). The emotional brain. *Nature Reviews Neuroscience, 5*, 583–589.

Davis, B. H. (1987). Disability and grief. *Social Casework: The Journal of Contemporary Social Work, 68*, 352–357.

Dicks, D., Myers, R. E., & Kling, A. (1969). Uncus and amygdala lesions: Effects on social behavior in the free-ranging rhesus monkey. *Science, 165*(3888), 69–71.

Drevets, W. C., Savitz, J., & Trimble, M. (2008). The subgenual anterior cingulate cortex in mood disorders. *CNS Spectrums, 13*(8), 663.

Eagen, G. (2001). *The skilled helper*. Monterey, CA: Brooks/Cole Publishing.

Empathy. (2007). *Merriam-Webster's collegiate dictionary* (11th ed.). Springfield, MA: Merriam-Webster.

Epstein, R., Hadee, T., Carroll, J., Meldrum, S., Lardner, J., & Shields, C. (2007). "Could this be something serious?" Reassurance, uncertainty, and empathy in response to patients' expressions of worry. *Journal of General Internal Medicine, 22*, 1731–1739.

Etkin, A., Egner, T., & Kalisch, R. (2011). Emotional processing in anterior cingulate and medial prefrontal cortex. *Trends in Cognitive Sciences, 15*(2), 85–93.

Etkin, A., Egner, T., Peraza, D. M., Kandel, E. R., & Hirsch, J. (2006). Resolving emotional conflict: A role for the rostral anterior cingulate cortex in modulating activity in the amygdala. *Neuron, 51*(6), 871–882.

Feinstein, J. S., Adolphs, R., & Tranel, D. (2016). A tale of survival from the world of patient S. M. In D. G. Amaral & R. Adolphs (Eds.), *Living without an amygdala* (pp. 1–38). New York, NY: The Guilford Press.

Fiscella, K., Meldrum, S., & Franks, P. (2004). Patient trust: Is it related to patient-centered behavior of primary care physicians? *Medical Care, 42*, 1049–1055.

Friehe, M. J., Bloedow, A., & Hesse, S. (2003). Counseling families of children with communication disorders. *Communication Disorders Quarterly, 24*, 211–220.

Frith, C. D., & Frith, U. (1999). Interacting minds: A biological basis. *Science, 286*, 1692–1695.

Gallagher, H. L., Happe, F., Brunswick, N., Fletcher, P. C., Frith, U., & Frith, C. D. (2000). Reading the mind in cartoons and stories: An fMRI study of theory of mind in verbal and non-verbal tasks. *Neuropsychologia, 38*, 11–21.

Gilhome-Herbst, K. & Humphrey, C. (1980). Hearing impairments and mental state in the elderly living at home. *British Medical Journal, 281*, 903–905.

Goleman, D. (1995). *Emotional intelligence*. New York, NY: Bantam Books.

Hadland, K. A., Rushworth, M. F. S., Gaffan, D., & Passingham, R. E. (2003). The effect of cingulate lesions on social behaviour and emotion. *Neuropsychologia, 41*(8), 919–931.

Haar, S., Berman, S. Behrmann, M., & Dinstein, I. (2016). Anatomical abnormalities in autism? *Cerebral Cortex, 26*(4), 1440–1452.

Hobson, R. P. (1995). *Autism and the development of mind*. New York, NY: Psychology Press.

Holland, A. L. (2005, Winter). Counseling families and adults with speech and language disorders: The view from a wellness perspective. *CSHA Magazine, 35*, 12–16.

Hornak, J., Bramham, J., Rolls, E. T., Morris, R. G., O'Doherty, J., Bullock, P. R., & Polkey, C. E. (2003). Changes in emotion after circumscribed surgical lesions of the orbitofrontal and cingulate cortices. *Brain, 126*(7), 1691–1712.

Hornak, J., Rolls, E. T., & Wade, D. (1996). Face and voice expression identification in patients with emotional and behavioural changes following ventral frontal lobe damage. *Neuropsychologia, 34*(4), 247–261.

House, A., Dennis, M., Molyneux, A., Warlow, C., & Hawton, K. (1989). Emotionalism after stroke. *British Medical Journal, 298*(6679), 991.

Ivey, A. (2001). *Intentional interviewing in counseling* (4th ed.). Belmont, CA: Brooks/Cole Publishing.

Jezzini, A., Caruana, F., Stoianov, I., Gallese, V., & Rizzolatti, G. (2012). Functional organization of the insula and inner perisylvian regions. *Proceedings of the National Academy of Sciences, 109*(25), 10077–10082.

Kozlovskiy, S. A., Vartanov, A. V., Nikonova, E. Y., Pyasik, M. M., & Velichkovsky, B. M. (2012). The cingulate cortex and human memory processes. *Psychology in Russia, 5*, 231–243.

Kübler-Ross, E. (1969). *On death and dying*. New York, NY: MacMillan.

Kurtzer-White, E., & Luterman, D. (2003). Families and children with hearing loss: Grief and coping. *Mental Retardation and Developmental Disabilities Research Reviews, 9*, 232–235.

Lamm, C., & Singer, T. (2010). The role of anterior insular cortex in social emotions. *Brain Structure and Function, 214*(5–6), 579–591.

Lane, R. D., Chua, M. L., & Dolan, R. J. (1999). Common effects of emotional valence, arousal, and attention on neural activation during visual processing of pictures. *Neuropsychologia, 37*, 989–998.

LeDoux, J. E., & Damasio, A. R. (2013). Emotions and feelings. In E. R. Kandel, J. H. Schwartz, T. M. Jessell, S. A. Siegelbaum, & A. J. Hudspeth (Eds.), *Principles of neural science* (pp. 1079–1094). New York, NY: McGraw-Hill Medical.

Luterman, D. (2001). *Counseling persons with communication disorders and their families* (4th ed.). Austin, TX: Pro-Ed.

Luterman, D. (2006). The counseling relationship. *The ASHA Leader, 11*(8–9), 33–38.

Luterman, D., & Kurtzer-White, E. (1999). Identifying hearing loss: Parents' need. *American Journal of Audiology, 8*(1), 13–18.

Maciejewski, P. K., Zhang, B., Block, S. D., & Prigerson, H. G. (2007). An empirical examination of the stage theory of grief. *Journal of the American Medical Association, 297*, 716–723.

Margulies, A. (1984). Toward empathy: The uses of wonder. *The American Journal of Psychiatry, 141*, 1025–1033.

Martin, F. N., George, K. A., O'Neal, J., & Daly, J. A. (1987, June/July). Audiologists' and parents' attitudes regarding counseling of families of hearing-impaired children. *ASHA, 29*, 27–33.

Martin, F. N., Krall, L., & O'Neal, J. (1989, February/March). The diagnosis of acquired hearing loss: Patient reactions. *ASHA, 31*, 47–50.

Mohanty, A., Engels, A. S., Herrington, J. D., Heller, W., Ringo Ho, M. H., & Banich, M. T., . . . Miller, G. A. (2007). Differential engagement of anterior cingulate cortex subdivisions for cognitive and emotional function. *Psychophysiology, 44*(3), 343–351.

Papez, J. W. (1937). A proposed mechanism of emotion. *Archives of Neurological Psychiatry, 38*, 725–743.

Powers, L., & Singer, G. (1993). *Families, disability, and empowerment: Active coping skills and strategies for family interventions.* Baltimore, MD: Brookes Publishing.

Ramachandran, V. S. (2009). *Vilayanur Ramachandran: The neurons that shaped civilization* [Video]. Retrieved from https://www.ted.com/talks/vs_ramachandran_the_neurons_that_shaped_civilization

Riesz, E. D. (2004). Loss and transitions: A 30-year perspective on life with a child who has Down syndrome. *Journal of Loss and Trauma, 9*, 371–382.

Riley, J. (2002). Counseling: An approach for speech-language pathologists. *Contemporary Issues in Communication Science and Disorders, 29*(1), 6–16.

Rizzolatti, G., & Craighero, L. (2004). The mirror-neuron system. *Annual Review of Neuroscience, 27*, 169–192.

Robinson, L., Clare, L., & Evans, K. (2005). Making sense of dementia and adjusting to loss: Psychological reactions to a diagnosis of dementia in couples. *Aging & Mental Health, 9*, 337–347.

Rybarczyk, B., Edwards, R., & Behel, J. (2004). Diversity in adjustment to a leg amputation: Case illustrations of common themes. *Disability and Rehabilitation, 26*, 944–953.

Salmon, P., Peters, S., & Stanley, I. (1999). Patients' perceptions of medical explanations for somatisation disorders: Qualitative analysis. *British Medical Journal, 318*, 372–376.

Salovey, P., & Mayer, J. D. (1990). Emotional intelligence. *Imagination, Cognition and Personality, 9*(3), 185–211.

Sanders, S., & Adams, K. B. (2005). Grief reactions and depression in caregivers of individuals with Alzheimer's disease: Results from a pilot study in an urban setting. *Health and Social Work, 30*, 287–295.

Schneider, J. (1984). *Stress, loss, and grief.* Baltimore, MD: University Park Press.

Schumann, C. M., Hamstra, J., Goodlin-Jones, B. L., Lotspeich, L. J., Kwon, H., & Buonocore, M. H., . . . Amaral, D. G. (2004). The amygdala is enlarged in children but not adolescents with autism: The hippocampus is enlarged at all ages. *Journal of Neuroscience, 24*(28), 6392–6401.

Seaburn, D. B., Morse, D., McDaniel, S. H., Beckman, H., Silberman, J., & Epstein, R. M. (2005). Physician responses to ambiguous patient symptoms. *Journal of General Internal Medicine, 20*, 525–530.

Spillers, C. S. (2007). An existential framework for understanding the counseling needs of clients. *American Journal of Speech-Language Pathology, 16*(3), 191–197.

Tanner, D. C. (1980). Loss and grief: Implications for the speech-language pathologist and audiologist. *ASHA, 22*, 916–928.

Toner, M. A., & Shadden, B. B. (2002). Counseling challenges: Working with older clients and caregivers. *Contemporary Issues in Communication Science and Disorders, 29*(2), 68–78.

Victor, M., & Ropper, A. H. (2001). *Principles of neurology* (7th ed.). New York, NY: McGraw-Hill Medical.

Zraick, R. I., & Boone, D. R. (1991). Spouse attitudes toward the person with aphasia. *Journal of Speech and Hearing Research, 34*(1), 123–128.

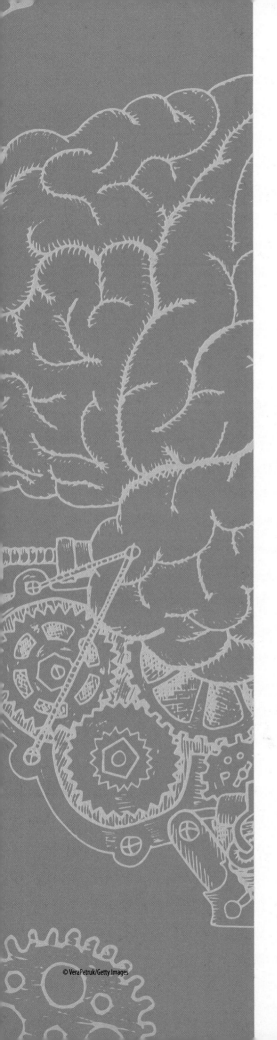

PART IV

Practicing Neuroanatomy

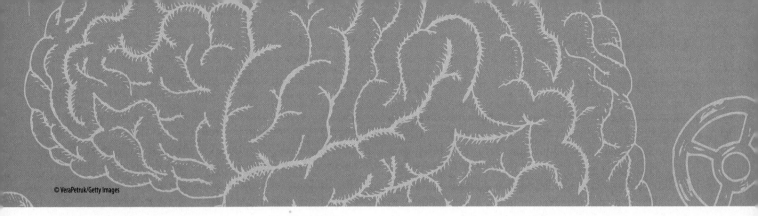

© VeraPetruk/Getty Images

CHAPTER 16

The Neurological Exam

CHAPTER PREVIEW

To complete our journey into the world of neuroscience, we will explore how to evaluate the nervous system. We will first survey how a neurologist performs a neurological exam and then look for areas of overlap with methods used by communication disorders professionals.

IN THIS CHAPTER

In this chapter, we will . . .

- Explain what a neurological exam is and list what tools are needed for it
- List and explain the different parts of the neurological exam
- Compare and contrast the neurological exams used by neurologists with those used by communication disorders professionals
- Explore the salient signs of neurological injury

LEARNING OBJECTIVES

1. The learner will define what a neurological exam is.
2. The learner will list the steps of the neurological exam and the tools involved.
3. The learner will list and define signs of neurological injury.

▶ Introduction

Hippocrates (460–370 BCE) was an ancient Greek physician best known for developing the oath that doctors still make today, the Hippocratic Oath (**BOX 16-1**). In a time when gods and goddesses were seen as the causes of illness, Hippocrates believed that diseases had natural causes (e.g., diet, the environment, living habits). He developed this belief out of his powers of observation. In other words, he believed that observation of the patient was critical to good medical care. Lloyd (1984) summarizes the Hippocratic tradition of observation, using quotes from the Ancient Greek text *Prognosis,* as follows:

> First he should examine the patient's face, for example the colour and texture of the skin, and especially the eyes, where he should consider whether "they avoid the glare of light, or weep involuntarily," whether "the whites are livid," whether the eyes "wander, or project, or are deeply sunken," and so on. (p. 152)

Following in the Hippocratic tradition, there is no real substitute for a careful, systematic examination of people with neurological conditions. In fact, Blumenfeld (2010) remarked that before the neuroimaging era, "great clinicians could pinpoint a lesion in the nervous system with often astounding accuracy" (p. 50). Many students rush to get through a patient examination in order to get to the fun stuff—therapy. What they soon learn is that good therapy is built on a good evaluation. It is in the process of evaluating people that both their strengths and their weaknesses are identified. Through this process, weaknesses can be addressed, often using the remaining strengths. In this chapter, the components of a careful neurological exam by a neurologist will be surveyed, and points of overlap with an exam by a communication disorders professional will be considered.

▶ The Neurological Exam

A **neurological exam** is a systematic examination of the nervous system. The nervous system is a series of organs that make communication possible throughout the body. The neurological exam is a tool used to explore and identify any pathology affecting the proper functioning of these organs. This exam is *systematic,* meaning that it involves a method or ordered plan. Neurological exams are typically performed by **neurologists**, who are doctors with specialized training in nervous system anatomy and physiology as well as its pathologies. We will explore how a neurologist goes about his or her examination of the nervous system and identify areas of overlap with the examination that a speech-language pathologist (SLP) or audiologist would perform.

BOX 16-1 The Hippocratic Oath

I swear by Apollo the physician, and Asclepius, and Hygieia and Panacea and all the gods and goddesses as my witnesses, that, according to my ability and judgment, I will keep this Oath and this contract:

To hold him who taught me this art equally dear to me as my parents, to be a partner in life with him, and to fulfill his needs when required; to look upon his offspring as equals to my own siblings, and to teach them this art, if they shall wish to learn it, without fee or contract; and that by the set rules, lectures, and every other mode of instruction, I will impart a knowledge of the art to my own sons, and those of my teachers, and to students bound by this contract and having sworn this Oath to the law of medicine, but to no others.

I will use those dietary regimens which will benefit my patients according to my greatest ability and judgment, and I will do no harm or injustice to them.

I will not give a lethal drug to anyone if I am asked, nor will I advise such a plan; and similarly I will not give a woman a pessary [medical device] to cause an abortion.

In purity and according to divine law will I carry out my life and my art.

I will not use the knife, even upon those suffering from stones, but I will leave this to those who are trained in this craft.

Into whatever homes I go, I will enter them for the benefit of the sick, avoiding any voluntary act of impropriety or corruption, including the seduction of women or men, whether they are free men or slaves.

Whatever I see or hear in the lives of my patients, whether in connection with my professional practice or not, which ought not to be spoken of outside, I will keep secret, as considering all such things to be private.

So long as I maintain this Oath faithfully and without corruption, may it be granted to me to partake of life fully and the practice of my art, gaining the respect of all men for all time. However, should I transgress this Oath and violate it, may the opposite be my fate.

The Tools of the Neurological Exam

A neurologist typically uses seven tools in a neurological exam (**FIGURE 16-1**):

1. The *reflex hammer* is used to elicit deep tendon reflexes. One well-known deep tendon reflex is the patellar or knee reflex, which involves a slight kick elicited by striking the knee just below the patella. Examples of other common reflexes associated with communication structures can be found in **BOX 16-2**.

2. A *pin* is used to test sensory abilities, light touch, and some reflexes. For example, sensory functions of the foot are tested by lightly touching the parts of the foot and asking the patient if they can feel the pin. This occurs often with diabetics who suffer from peripheral neuropathy.

3. An *ophthalmoscope* is used to observe the structure of the eye and test the pupillary light reflex, which is the reduction in the size of the pupil with the introduction of light.

4. *Visual acuity cards* are used to test a patient's visual abilities.

5. *Cotton swabs* are used to test the corneal reflex (i.e., when the eye blinks in response to something coming near it).

6. *Tuning forks,* one tuned to 256 hertz (Hz) and the other to 512 Hz, are used to test a patient's sense of vibration as well as hearing. In terms of hearing, the Rinne test is completed by striking the 512-Hz tuning fork and placing it on the mastoid bone behind the ear. The patient then reports the point when he or she cannot hear the sound anymore. The tuning fork is then

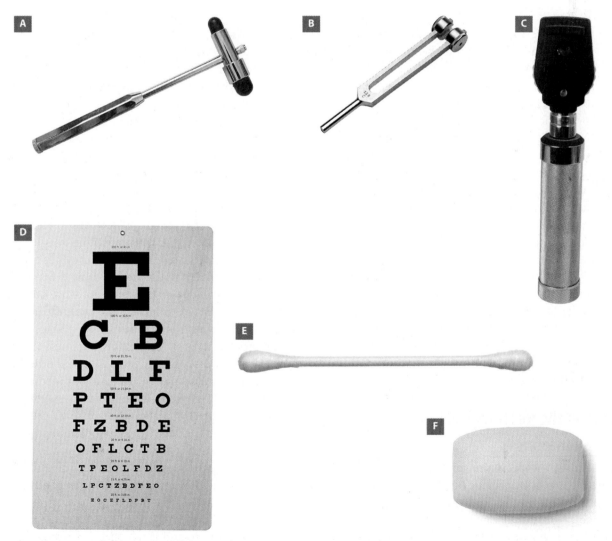

FIGURE 16-1 Seven tools are used in the neurological exam. One of the tools, the pin, is not pictured. The other tools are shown as follows: **A.** Reflex hammer. **B.** Tuning fork. **C.** Ophthalmoscope. **D.** Visual acuity card. **E.** Cotton swab. **F.** Soap.

BOX 16-2 Examples of Reflexes Associated With Communication and Swallowing Structures

Acoustic reflex: The middle ear muscles contract in response to increased sound intensities. This reflex functions to protect middle-ear bones. It appears at birth and persists into adulthood.

Tongue reflex: The tongue thrusts when touched. This reflex appears at birth and disappears between 12 and 18 months.

Jaw jerk reflex: The mandible elevates after a light tap below the lower lip. This reflex is normally absent or only slight. It appears at birth and persists into adulthood.

Rooting reflex: An infant turns his or her mouth toward anything that might come near the mouth. This reflex appears at birth and disappears between 3 and 6 months.

Suckling reflex: An infant displays bursts of rhythmic sucking in response to a finger or nipple near the mouth. This reflex appears at birth and disappears between 6 and 12 months.

Swallowing reflex: Pharyngeal muscles contract to move a bolus through the pharynx to the esophagus. This reflex appears at birth and persists into adulthood.

Bite reflex: When pressure is applied to the gums, the jaw closes and the infant bites down. This reflex appears at birth and disappears between 9 and 12 months.

Gag reflex: When the posterior pharyngeal wall is touched, a vomit-like response occurs, without actual vomiting. This reflex appears at birth and persists into adulthood.

Cough reflex: The vocal cords enable a rapid release of air from lungs. This reflex functions to protect the airway by kicking foreign substances away. It appears at birth and persists into adulthood.

---

held to the ear on the same side, and the patient is asked if it can be heard and if it is louder or softer than behind the ear. The sound should be louder when the tuning fork is next to the ear than behind it. If it is not, then the patient may have a conductive or middle ear hearing loss. A Weber test is done by striking the 256-Hz tuning fork and placing it on the center of the head. If the sound is louder in the affected ear, then the loss is conductive (middle ear); if softer, then the loss is sensorineural (inner ear). Normal hearing results in the sound being heard in the middle.

7. A *bar of soap* is often used to test a patient's sense of smell, although some neurologists prefer to use a small vial of coffee grounds. The neurologist asks the patient to close his or her eyes and then places the bar of soap or vial of grounds below the nostrils and asks the patient to identify the scent.

The Steps of the Neurological Exam

Step 1: The Interview

As mentioned at the beginning of this chapter, the neurological exam is systematic in that it follows a certain set of steps. The neurologist begins this systematic review by first interviewing the patient and/or the patient's family to understand the circumstances of the illness and the patient's symptoms. A **symptom** refers to a patient's subjective report of what he or she is experiencing during the illness. This can be compared to a **sign**, which is an observation made by an observer, sometimes through use of equipment such as a thermometer or blood pressure reader. Thus, a patient may report "feeling hot" (a symptom), whereas a nurse might report that the patient's temperature is 101°F (38.3°C) on the thermometer (a sign).

Neurologists differ in how they interview patients, but a common way to begin is to ask why the patient is in the hospital or why the patient has come to see the doctor. This line of questioning is meant to elicit the patient's *chief complaint*. Next, questions involving the *history of the present illness* are typically asked, such as, "When did your symptoms begin?," "How long have they lasted?," and "Do they get better or worse?" A patient's *past medical history* is then explored, which includes questions about what other illnesses he or she has experienced and the treatment involved in those conditions. Questions may expand to the patient's family and their history of illness (i.e., *family history*) because many illnesses are inherited. In addition, the patient may be asked about medications he or she is taking and allergies he or she may have. Sometimes questions about the patient's *social history* will be asked (i.e., activities or hobbies) as well as *environmental history*, focusing on the particular environments the patient spends time (e.g., chemical plant, dry cleaners). The neurologist will then conduct a *review of systems* where the patient is asked if he or she has any problems with his or her lungs, digestion system, and so on, and if so, what symptoms are being experienced. (Note: The *review of systems* can be done through an intake form before a patient sees the doctor.)

Step 2: The Physical Exam

The physical exam begins by the neurologist introducing himself or herself to the patient and observing whether the patient is awake, alert, and responsive. Personal hygiene and dress are examined to determine if the patient is capable of self-care. The neurologist then proceeds with an examination of the head, ears, eyes, nose, and throat, which is known as a HEENT exam. Major systems (e.g., heart, lungs) are examined using a stethoscope. The patient's body posture and motor activity are observed. If the patient leans to one side, there may be weakness issues. **Dyskinesias** (i.e., movement problems) may indicate nervous system damage. Height and weight are measured to determine if the patient is obese or cachectic (i.e., ill health with emaciation), and vital signs (e.g., blood pressure) are taken. A dysmorphic examination is performed, noting any abnormalities of face or body shape (e.g., low-set ears or wide-set eyes).

Step 3: The Neurological Exam Proper

In many ways, this part of the exam began with the interview and physical exam as the neurologist observed the patient's mental status and motor activity. During the neurological exam proper, the neurologist performs a more formal assessment of mental status and motor activity as well as reflexes, senses, and equilibrium.

Mental status is the degree of cognitive competence a person has. The neurologist will often begin informally assessing this area by considering the patient's expressive and receptive language abilities. To do so, the neurologist asks the patient to name items, repeat words, follow commands, read, and write. He or she also tests the patient's orientation to person, place, time, and purpose (e.g., "Why are you in the hospital?"). To test long-term memory, three unrelated words are usually given, which the patient is asked to recall after 5 minutes. Short-term memory is assessed by asking the patient to recall strings of numbers. Attention and math are evaluated by asking the patient to count backward by 7 from 100. Abstract reasoning is tested by asking the patient to interpret proverbs (e.g., Please explain this proverb: "The grass is always greener on the other side of the fence."). Formal testing of these abilities can also be done through published tests, such as the Mini-Mental State Examination, the Short Portable Mental Status Questionnaire, and the Galveston Orientation and Amnesia Test.

After assessing the patient's mental status, the neurologist conducts a **cranial nerve** evaluation. Humans have 12 pairs of cranial nerves that control motor, sensory, and other functions of the head and neck. Some of the conditions associated with cranial nerve damage will be explored later in this chapter.

Motor testing involves observing posture and how well the patient moves his or her limbs. Neurological damage will sometimes result in **paresis** (i.e., weakness) or **plegia** (i.e., paralysis), so the neurologist needs to determine whether these problems exist; if they do, physical and/or occupational therapy can then be ordered. **Reflexes**, which are the lightning-quick, unconscious responses our body makes to stimuli, are assessed at this time, as is sensation in terms of touch, pain, temperature, and vibration. A patient's **equilibrium** (i.e., coordination and balance) is tested by observing **gait** (i.e., walking) and **diadochokinetic rates** (i.e., rapid, alternating motor movements such as quickly saying "pa-ta-ka" as fast as possible).

Step 4: Laboratory Tests

Hematological tests (i.e., blood tests) are routinely ordered to assess a patient's red and white blood cell counts, among other factors. In addition, neuroimaging studies, which allow neurologists to see visual representations of the nervous system, are routinely ordered when nervous system damage is suspected. Because SLPs and audiologists are often consumers of neuroimaging study reports, which are available in the patient's medical record, a basic understanding of these techniques is important.

▶ A Comparison of Neurological Exams by Neurologists and SLPs/Audiologists

Like neurologists, SLPs and audiologists conduct interviews with their patients, asking questions about the chief complaint, history of the present illness, past medical history, review of communication systems, family history, social and environmental history, and allergies and medications. There are many commonalities with the physical exam as well. The neurologist, SLP, and audiologist all assess the patient's level of consciousness and personal hygiene and dress. They perform a similar HEENT exam, with the exception of the eye exam. Professionals in communication disorders evaluate major communication systems instead of other major body systems. They should also observe posture, motor activity, and dysmorphic signs. In terms of the neurological exam, both types of professionals conduct a mental state evaluation. SLPs and audiologists also test the cranial nerves, but typically only those relevant to speech, hearing, and swallowing. They test reflexes related to communication and observe, and perhaps even formally assess, the patient's equilibrium. Although professionals in communication disorders do not order laboratory tests, they are consumers of the data from these examinations, especially neuroimaging data.

▶ Signs of Neurological Disease

The neurological examination, especially the neurological exam proper, will reveal certain signs of neurological disease. In this section, we will further explore some of the signs mentioned in the preceding sections that may stand out during a neurological exam. These signs are arranged in the following categories, reflecting the order given in the neurological exam proper: cranial nerve, motor, reflex, sensory, and other miscellaneous signs, including signs found in the areas of speech and language.

Cranial Nerve Signs

Cranial nerve I is called the olfactory nerve. The term **olfaction** refers to our sense of smell, which involves specialized sensory cells in the nose that receive odor molecules. These molecules trigger a nerve impulse that is sent through cranial nerve I to the olfactory bulb, a part of the central nervous system that lies just inferior to the brain's frontal lobes. The nerve impulse finally reaches the olfactory cortex of the temporal lobe where the olfactory impulse is processed and interpreted (e.g., noxious versus pleasant). Damage to cranial nerve I through mechanisms like traumatic brain injury (TBI) can result in **anosmia** (i.e., an inability to smell), hyperosmia (i.e., abnormally sensitive smell), or hyposmia (i.e., decreased sense of smell). Zasler, Costanzo, and Heywood (1990) found that the severity of TBI correlated with the amount of olfactory dysfunction. Specifically, 27% of patients with mild TBI and 67% of patients with moderate to severe TBI had some form of olfactory impairment.

Cranial nerves II–IV and VI are all involved in vision, with cranial nerve II being the main conduit for visual information and cranial nerves III, IV, and VI controlling various aspects of eye movement. Cranial nerve II is the optic nerve (**FIGURE 16-2**), and damage to it can lead to decreased vision and blindness. More specifically, injury to the optic nerve anterior to the optic chiasm (i.e., where the optic tracts cross) results in the loss of a visual field; lesions posterior to the optic chiasm result in contralateral homonymous **hemianopsia** (i.e., one-sided visual loss). This condition involves partial blindness to half of each visual field opposite to the side where the lesion occurred. Lesions at the optic chiasm lead to a loss of peripheral

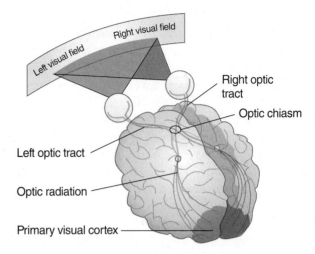

FIGURE 16-2 The visual system.

vision in both visual fields. Damage to cranial nerves III, IV, and/or VI, which are usually tested together, can result in loss of the **pupillary light reflex** (i.e., when the pupils change in size as light is introduced or removed), deviation of gaze, **diplopia** or double vision, and **nystagmus**, which involves involuntary eye movements, sometimes called dancing eyes.

Damage to cranial nerve VII, IX, X, or XII will impair functions related to speech and swallowing. Damage to cranial nerve VII leads to facial plegia or paresis and loss of taste. Often plegia and paresis are on one side of the face only, resulting in conditions called *hemiplegia* and *hemiparesis,* where the prefix *hemi-* refers to one sided. Injury to cranial nerves IX and X can result in an absent gag response, absent swallow, loss of soft palate movement, and loss of voice. Cranial nerve XII impairment often results in loss of tongue movement and the wasting away or atrophy of the tongue, with possible **fasciculation**, a term referring to muscle twitches. These twitches resemble snakes squirming in a bag. Injury to cranial nerve XI results in a droopy shoulder due to impaired function of the sternocleidomastoid muscle.

Cranial nerve VIII is an important nerve for transmitting hearing and balance information from the inner ear to the brain. Harm to this nerve results in hearing loss, **vertigo** (i.e., dizziness), loss of equilibrium, and **tinnitus**, which is ringing in the ears.

A cranial nerve evaluation form can be found in **BOX 16-3**. Function is recorded in the blanks as either *N* for normal or *A* for abnormal. Numbers with *A* in the blank should be circled next to the appropriate cranial nerve at the bottom of the form, which indicates which cranial nerve may be impaired. (Note: Only the cranial nerves involved in speech and hearing are tested, with the exception of cranial nerve II for vision.) An example of a normal cranial nerve exam can be found in **BOX 16-4**.

BOX 16-3 Cranial Nerve Evaluation

Evaluate the following cranial nerve functions. Place an *N* on the line to indicate normal function or an *A* to indicate abnormal function.

Head and Neck:
1. Facial symmetry: Upper: _____ Lower: _____
2. Chin erect _____
3. Shoulder symmetry at rest _____
4. Shoulder symmetry shrugging _____
5. Head rotation _____
6. Visual fields intact _____

Lips:
7. Rest symmetry _____
8. Smile symmetry _____
9. Pursing symmetry _____
10. Diadochokinesis /p/ _____

Mandible:
11. Deviation when depressed _____
12. Diadochokinesis /j/ _____
13. Lateral resistive strength _____
14. Opening/closing ability _____

Teeth:
15. Present (upper/lower) _____ Dentures (upper/lower) _____
16. Occlusions or deviations present _____

Tongue:
17. Tremors: Resting _____ Other movements _____ Atrophy _____
18. Protrusion _____
19. Elevation _____
20. Lateral movement _____
21. Protrusion resistive strength (use tongue depressor) _____
22. Lateral resistive strength (use tongue depressor) _____
23. Blade diadochokinesis /t/ _____
24. Back diadochokinesis /k/ _____
25. Rapid alternating movements /p t k/ _____
26. Taste on posterior third of tongue _____

Velum:
27. Rest symmetry _____
28. Elevation on phonation (say "ah") _____
29. Gag reflex (touch back of throat with tongue depressor) _____
30. Palatal reflex (touch palate with tongue depressor) _____

Pharynx:
31. Posterior wall constrictions (say forceful "eee") _____
32. Dysphagia: Liquids _____ Solids _____

Larynx:
33. Phonation ("ah") _____
34. Length of prolonged "ah" in seconds _____
35. Voice quality (breathy, hoarse, harsh, strangled) _____
36. Cough _____
37. Vary: Pitch _____ Volume _____

(continues)

BOX 16-3 Cranial Nerve Evaluation   *(continued)*

Cranial Nerve Assessment (circle numbers that were rated as abnormal):
II (Optic): 6
V (Trigeminal): 11 12 13 14
VII (Facial): 1 2 7 8 9 10
IX (Glossopharyngeal): 24 26 27 28 29 30
X (Vagus): 31 32 33 34 35 36 37
XI (Spinal accessory): 3 4 5
XII (Hypoglossal): 17 18 19 20 21 22 23

BOX 16-4 Example of a Normal Cranial Nerve Exam

CN I: Olfaction normal. Patient able to identify a bar of soap while eyes closed.
CN II: Vision normal. Visual acuity appears to be 20/20 as tested by Snellen eye chart. Pupils equally round and responsive to light stimulation.
CN III, IV, VI: Eye movements are normal. No nystagmus or ptosis.
CN V: Sensory function of face is normal in all three CN V branch areas. Motor function is normal for mastication.
CN VII: Motor function of face muscles is normal. Face is symmetrical.
CN VIII: Hearing equity is normal bilaterally as tested by portable audiometer. Vestibular function appears intact.
CN IX: The velum and uvula elevate symmetrically. Gag reflex is intact. Timely swallow response can be palpated.
CN X: Voice function normal for age and sex in terms of phonation quality, pitch, and intensity.
CN XI: Shoulders are symmetrical upon rest and upon shrugging.
CN XII: Tongue function normal for protrusion, retraction, and lateralization. Resistive strength appears normal for speech and swallowing.

Motor Signs

One of the most common motor signs after neurological injury is muscle weakness, also known as *paresis*. Extreme weakness is called *plegia*. After a stroke, many people will suffer paresis or plegia on one side of the body or the other. When this happens, it is called hemiparesis or hemiplegia. Because of contralateral innervation, the paresis or plegia will be on the opposite side of the body from the damage. For example, someone with left hemisphere damage may have right hemiparesis or hemiplegia. Weakness is a characteristic in both upper motor neuron (UMN) and lower motor neuron (LMN) damage; however, LMN lesions result in decreased muscle tone and reflexes as well as muscle atrophy and fasciculations. UMN lesions lead to increased muscle tone and exaggerated reflexes, but no atrophy or fasciculations.

Movement disorders in general are grouped under the term *dyskinesias*. The various movement disorders that fit within this category are typically involuntary and can be slow or fast in their movement (**FIGURE 16-3**). Beginning with the slowest and moving to the fastest, **bradykinesia** is a term that literally means slowed

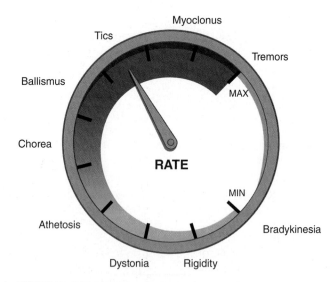

FIGURE 16-3 Dyskinesias compared.

movements. Related to bradykinesia are the terms *hypokinesia* (decreased movement) and *akinesia* (absent movement). Hemiparesis and hemiplegia were defined in the previous section; hemiparesis can be thought of as a form of hypokinesia and hemiplegia a form of akinesia. **Rigidity** denotes stiff muscles that resist passive movement to a limb. **Dystonia** is a dyskinesia in which sustained muscle contractions result in distorted body postures. Some patients experience **athetosis**, slow twisting movements of hands and feet, or **chorea** (which comes from the Greek word for "dance"), which is quick movements of the hands or feet that have a dance-like quality. These two conditions can occur together, resulting in *choreoathetosis*. **Ballism** is a rare movement disorder involving the quick flinging of the limbs. It generally occurs on one side of the body and is thus called **hemiballismus**. Some patients experience tics, which are repetitive involuntary motor and/or vocal behaviors associated with conditions like Tourette syndrome. Other patients may experience **myoclonus**, or sudden involuntary muscle jerks. Common myoclonic experiences include hiccups or a sudden jerk when falling asleep, but more consistent and extreme experiences can occur after neurological injury.

The most well-known dyskinesia is probably **tremor**. Tremors are involuntary, rhythmic shaking in which the shaking oscillates at a certain frequency. There are several different types of tremors. Intention tremors occur only when a patient initiates purposeful action; in contrast, resting tremors occur only when a limb is at rest and disappear when the limb is put to purposeful action. Parkinson patients often demonstrate a resting tremor known as a "pill-rolling" tremor in which the thumb oscillates against the index and/or middle fingers as if the patient had clay between them and was trying to roll it into a ball.

In addition to dyskinesias, gait disorders (i.e., walking problems) can occur with neurological injury (Ryan, 2009). For example, patients with Parkinson disease demonstrate a shuffling gait (i.e., Parkinsonian gait), moving through a series of slow, shuffling steps while having a stooped posture and little arm swinging (**FIGURE 16-4**). Another example of a gait disorder is scissors gait, seen most often in patients with paraparesis (i.e., weakness in both legs). This gait involves stiff-looking legs, toes that scrape the ground, and legs that often cross in front of each other (**FIGURE 16-5**).

Reflex Signs

Reflexes are lightning-quick body responses to environmental stimuli. They may be absent, diminished, or exaggerated due to neurological injury. Their assessment can help in locating where damage is located in the nervous system.

In addition to the reflexes mentioned in Box 16-2 are reflexes like the corneal, light, plantar, and patellar reflexes. The corneal and light reflexes both involve the eyes. When we close our eyes as a foreign object

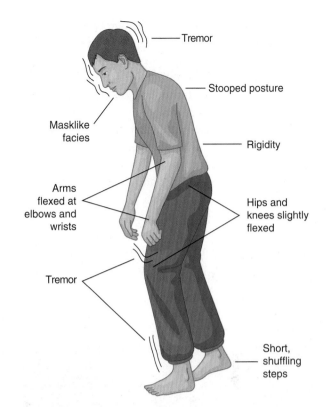

FIGURE 16-4 Parkinsonian gait.

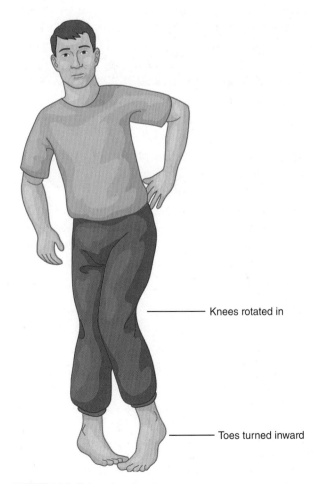

FIGURE 16-5 Scissors gait.

moves toward them, we are experiencing the corneal reflex that is meant to protect our eyes. The light reflex is also called the pupillary light reflex, which involves the expansion or contraction of the pupil to light (**FIGURE 16-6**). A lack of pupillary contraction to light can indicate neurological injury.

The plantar reflex is elicited by stroking the bottom of the foot with a blunt object, such as the handle end of a reflex hammer (**FIGURE 16-7**). A normal response is for the toes to curl and the foot to pull away. Adult patients with neurological injury either will not respond or their big toe will dorsiflex and the other toes will fan out in what is known as a positive Babinski sign. This sign can indicate a UMN lesion. A negative Babinski sign in an adult is consistent with a normal plantar reflex.

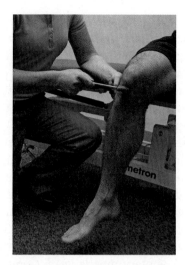

FIGURE 16-8 A physician testing a patient's patellar reflex.

The patellar reflex is one of the most recognized reflexes. A doctor tests it by tapping the patient's knee with a small hammer, causing the knee to jerk in a normal nervous system (**FIGURE 16-8**). This test evaluates the reflex arc.

Sensory Signs

Our experiences of touch, pain, temperature, vibration, and proprioception are all mediated through the **somatosensory system**. The first part of this compound word—*somato*—comes from the Greek word *soma*, which means "body," so the seemingly complex term *somatosensory* simply means the body-sensory system. Neurological injury can affect our sensory system in profound ways. Some patients may experience abnormal amounts of chronic or acute pain. Other patients may experience **paresthesias** (from the Greek: *para* = beside; *aesthesia* = sensation), which include tingling, prickling, or burning sensations. These are also common experiences when one of our limbs falls asleep and we experience first numbness and then a "pins and needles" sensation. Still other patients may suffer from **anesthesia** (from the Greek: *an* = without; *aesthesia* = sensation), in which body parts feel numb. Obviously, this experience can be induced through drugs for the purpose of surgery or dental work, for which we are all thankful.

The conditions discussed so far in this section deal with the loss of feeling, but some patients experience too much sensation in the form of pain. Pain is the unpleasant sensory experience with an emotional component associated with damage to the body. All of us have experienced *acute pain*, such as stepping on a piece of glass, and this type of pain plays an important

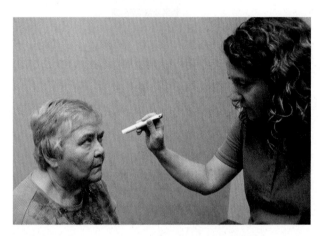

FIGURE 16-6 A clinician testing a woman's pupillary reflex.

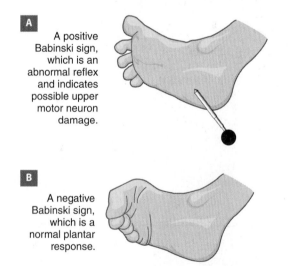

A
A positive Babinski sign, which is an abnormal reflex and indicates possible upper motor neuron damage.

B
A negative Babinski sign, which is a normal plantar response.

FIGURE 16-7 Testing of the plantar reflex. **A.** A positive Babinski sign, which is an abnormal reflex in an adult and indicates possible upper motor neuron damage. **B.** A negative Babinski sign, which is a normal plantar response in an adult.

role in telling us when something is wrong with our body. *Chronic pain*, which is often associated with neurological injury, serves no purpose. This pain can involve nerve injury affecting a specific anatomical structure, like the back or a limb. Chronic pain conditions, like fibromyalgia (a chronic condition involving pain throughout the body, especially in response to pressure), involve more diffuse, whole-body pain. Pain medications and protocols have made such improvements today that patients should never have to suffer from chronic pain conditions when under the care of healthcare professionals who have expertise in treating pain (Chelimsky, 2009).

Headaches are painful experiences located in the cranial area and are one of the most common symptoms of neurological disease patients report. Most headaches are not indicative of a serious pathology, but some can be a red flag for a life-threatening condition. Headaches do not involve the brain itself, because the brain has no pain receptors of its own, but rather are sensory experiences associated with scalp, skull, meninges (i.e., layers of tissue around the brain), or blood vessels. Vascular and tension headaches make up the two general types of headache. Vascular headaches, like migraines, are not well understood, but are thought to be caused by a mixture of environmental and genetic factors. Tension headaches involve prolonged contraction of neck and scalp muscles. These are typically the type of headache reported by people after a motor vehicle accident (Blumenfeld, 2010; Slevin & Ryan, 2009).

Changes in special sensory functions, like vision and hearing, can also result from neurological damage. These have already been discussed under cranial nerves.

Other Signs

There are many other signs of neurological dysfunction that may be apparent upon examination. Patients may have muscle tone issues and experience **hypertonia** (too much tone, resulting in spastic muscles) or **hypotonia** (too little tone, resulting in flaccid muscles). Hypotonia is also known as "rag doll" where the patient is floppy and unsteady like a child's doll. Muscle strength may be reduced or lost, and range of motion of limbs may be reduced. All these conditions can lead to problems in walking or gait and with posture.

Some patients may experience syncope due to neurological problems. **Syncope** is an episode of fainting in which a person loses consciousness. This complete loss of consciousness happens suddenly but

is brief in nature and is accompanied by hypotonia. It is often caused by an interruption of blood flow to the cerebrum but can also be caused by a lack of oxygen or glucose, neurotoxins (e.g., lead poisoning), or seizures. Syncope should be differentiated from dizziness, in which a person may feel close to losing consciousness but ultimately does not experience it (Massey, 2009).

Seizures are electrical storms in the brain; there are two basic types, partial and generalized seizures (**FIGURE 16-9**). The main distinction between these two types of seizures is the extent of the abnormal electrical activity. Partial seizures are focal in nature, meaning they are confined to specific areas of the brain, whereas generalized seizures involve the whole brain (**FIGURES 16-10** and **16-11**). There are several subtypes of both partial and generalized seizures; the most common are compared in **TABLE 16-1**. Seizures can be caused by a variety of factors, including high fevers, toxins, head trauma, alcohol or drug withdrawal, and strokes. Approximately 10% to

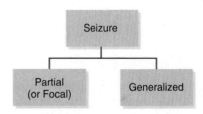

FIGURE 16-9 International classification of epileptic seizures.

Data from Holmes, G. L. (1997). *Classification of seizures and the epilepsies*. In: S. C. Schachter & D. L. Schomer (Eds.). *The comprehensive evaluation and treatment of epilepsy* (pp. 1–36). San Diego, CA: Academic Press, with permission from Elsevier.

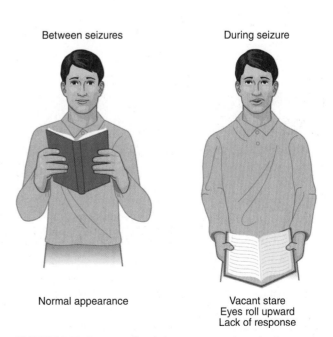

FIGURE 16-10 A generalized absence or petit mal seizure.

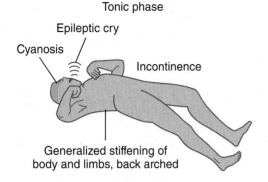

Tonic phase

Epileptic cry

Cyanosis

Incontinence

Generalized stiffening of
body and limbs, back arched

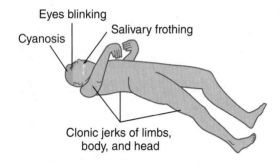

Clonic phase

Eyes blinking

Salivary frothing

Cyanosis

Clonic jerks of limbs,
body, and head

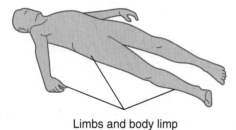

Postictal confusional fatigue

Limbs and body limp

FIGURE 16-11 A generalized tonic–clonic seizure, more popularly known as a grand mal seizure.

15% of the population will experience at least one seizure in their lifetime, and 1% of the population suffers from a seizure disorder like epilepsy. Different phases of a seizure are experienced, including the aura, ictal, postictal, and interictal phases; *aura* refers to a preliminary sense a seizure is coming, and *ictal* (from the Latin *ictus*, meaning "a blow") refers to the physiological event (**FIGURE 16-12**) (Blumenfeld, 2010; Massey, 2009).

Our sense of balance and orientation in space is controlled through the vestibular system (**FIGURE 16-13**). Anatomically, this system is housed in the inner ear in the form of three mazes or labyrinths called the semicircular canals. Dizziness is the disagreeable experience of spatial disorientation. There are four general types of dizziness:

- *Vertigo:* the sensation of a room spinning
- *Disequilibrium:* the feeling of unsteadiness while standing or walking, which often results in falls
- *Presyncope:* the feeling that one is going to faint and lose consciousness
- *Psychogenic dizziness:* the feeling of being separated from one's body, associated with stress and anxiety and often related to crowds and confined spaces

There are many possible causes of dizziness, ranging from head trauma to inner ear infections to psychological issues (Lanska, 2009b).

Neurological injury may also affect sleep. Some patients may experience insomnia (i.e., the inability to fall asleep), whereas others may experience hypersomnolence (i.e., excessive sleepiness) (Kovacevic-Ristanovic & Kuzniar, 2009).

Mental changes are common in neurological disorders. Patients may experience acute

TABLE 16-1 Comparison of the Most Common Seizure Types

Seizure	Types	Consciousness	Extent of Brain Involved	Duration
Partial	Simple	Preserved	Focal	10–30 seconds
	Complex	Lost	Focal	30–120 seconds
	Evolving	Eventually lost	Focal	Variable
Generalized	Absence (petit mal)	Preserved	Diffuse	10 seconds or less
	Tonic–clonic (grand mal)	Lost	Diffuse	30–120 seconds

Data from Blumenfeld, H. (2010). *Neuroanatomy through clinical cases.* Sunderland, MA: Sinauer Associates.

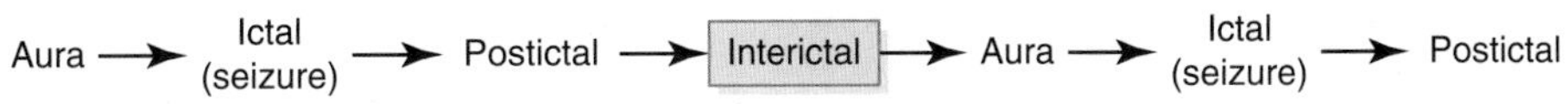

Aura → Ictal (seizure) → Postictal → Interictal → Aura → Ictal (seizure) → Postictal

FIGURE 16-12 Phases of a seizure.

confusional states, such as lethargy or delirium. Lethargic patients tend to be sleepy, confused, and uninterested in what is going on around them. Delirious patients are the opposite in that they are often apprehensive or angry. There are also chronic confusional states, like dementia. In dementia, a person experiences slow cognitive decline, which may or may not be reversible. Alzheimer disease, an irreversible condition, is the most recognized form of dementia. Related to these states are other emotional problems that may arise, such as anxiety or depression (Lanska, 2009a).

Neurological damage may also lead to changes in speech and language abilities. Language is the code we use to communicate through speaking and writing. Patients with neurological injury may have difficulty understanding language (**receptive aphasia**) or expressing language (**expressive aphasia**).

Speech is the motor production or execution of language. Some patients' motor speech systems become impaired and they experience apraxia of speech (difficulty accessing the motor plans and programs for speech) or dysarthria (difficulty executing the movements for speech).

▶ Conclusion

Sometimes ancient wisdom is some of the best wisdom. In light of this, we should remember Hippocrates's sage advice about the power of observation and the wisdom of completing a careful, systematic examination of the communication system. Many students put their faith in formal tests and the score they generate, which are valuable clinical instruments. But, there is no substitute for careful clinical observation.

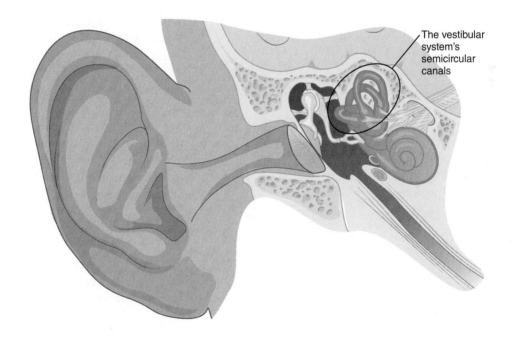

The vestibular system's semicircular canals

FIGURE 16-13 The vestibular system's semicircular canals.

SUMMARY OF LEARNING OBJECTIVES

The following were the main learning objectives of this chapter. The information that should have been learned is below each learning objective.

1. The learner will define what a neurological exam is.
   - A neurological exam is a systematic examination of the nervous system.
2. The learner will list the steps of the neurological exam and the tools involved.
   - Steps in the neurological exam:
     - □ Step 1: the interview
     - □ Step 2: the physical exam
     - □ Step 3: the neurological exam proper
     - □ Step 4: laboratory tests
   - Tools in the neurological exam:
     - □ Reflex hammer
     - □ Pin
     - □ Ophthalmoscope
     - □ Visual acuity cards
     - □ Cotton swabs
     - □ Tuning fork
     - □ Bar of soap
3. The learner will list and define signs of neurological injury.
   - *Anosmia:* inability to smell
   - *Hyperosmia:* abnormally sensitive smell
   - *Hyposmia:* decreased sense of smell
   - *Hemianopsia:* one-sided visual loss
   - *Diplopia:* double vision
   - *Nystagmus:* involuntary eye movements, usually shaking
   - *Plegia:* paralysis
   - *Paresis:* weakness
   - *Fasciculation:* muscle twitches
   - *Vertigo:* dizziness
   - *Tinnitus:* ringing in the ears

- *Bradykinesia:* slowed movements
- *Hypokinesia:* decreased movement
- *Akinesia:* absent movement
- *Rigidity:* stiff muscles that resist passive movement
- *Dystonia:* distorted body postures
- *Athetosis:* slow, twisting movements of the hands and feet
- *Chorea:* quick movements of the hands and feet with a dance-like quality
- *Ballism:* quick flinging of the limb(s)
- *Myoclonus:* sudden involuntary jerking movements
- *Tremor:* involuntary rhythmic shaking
- *Gait disorders:* problems with walking
- *Paresthesia:* abnormal sensations
- *Anesthesia:* loss of feeling; numbness
- *Pain:* unpleasant sensory experience with an emotional component associated with damage to the body
- *Headaches:* painful experiences located in the cranial area
- *Hypertonia:* too much muscle tone
- *Hypotonia:* too little muscle tone
- *Syncope:* fainting
- *Seizures:* electrical storms in the brain
- *Dizziness:* disagreeable experience of spatial disorientation; vertigo
- *Aphasia:* acquired multimodality language loss
- *Apraxia of speech:* difficulty pulling up the motor plans for speech
- *Dysarthria:* difficulty executing the movements for speech

KEY TERMS

Anesthesia
Anosmia
Athetosis
Ballism
Bradykinesia
Chorea
Cranial nerve
Diadochokinetic rates
Diplopia
Dyskinesias
Dystonia
Equilibrium
Expressive aphasia
Fasciculation

Gait
Hemianopsia
Hemiballismus
Hypertonia
Hypotonia
Mental status
Myoclonus
Neurological exam
Neurologists
Nystagmus
Olfaction
Parasthesias
Paresis
Plegia

Pupillary light reflex
Receptive aphasia
Reflexes
Rigidity
Seizures
Sign
Somatosensory system
Symptom
Syncope
Tinnitus
Tremor
Vertigo

DRAW IT TO KNOW IT

1. Draw a simple sketch of the visual system (see Figure 16-2), and identify the optic tracts.
2. Draw a simple sketch of a person with Parkinson disease (see Figure 16-4), and write a detailed description under the sketch of the Parkinsonian gait.

QUESTIONS FOR DEEPER REFLECTION

1. Compare and contrast the neurological exam of a neurologist with that of a professional in communication disorders.
2. In your opinion, why is there no substitute for careful clinical observation by a trained professional?
3. How might you apply the information presented in this chapter to a patient interaction?

CASE STUDY

Juan is a 47-year-old male with the diagnosis of traumatic brain injury (TBI). He has been referred to you, one of the hospital SLPs, for a speech and swallowing evaluation. As part of your evaluation, you completed the cranial nerve examination (Box 16-3) and found that he had bilateral difficulty with the following items on the form: 7, 8, 9, 10, 18, 19, 20, 21, 22, 23, 24, 25.

1. What cranial nerves would you report are impaired?
2. How would impairment to these cranial nerves affect his speech and swallowing?

SUGGESTED PROJECTS

1. Pick a partner in class and perform the cranial nerve evaluation (see Box 16-3). Make a list of questions regarding things you do not understand, and ask your professor.
2. Review the parts of the neurological interview. Create a fictitious patient and create a script with your questions and your patient's answers. Be creative and have fun.
3. Visit the *Neuroanatomy Through Clinical Cases* website and watch videos of Dr. Blumenfeld performing a neurological examination (Blumenfeld, n.d.).

REFERENCES

Blumenfeld, H. (2010). *Neuroanatomy through clinical cases* (2nd ed.). Sunderland, MA: Sinauer Associates.

Blumenfeld, H. (n.d.). *Neuroanatomy through clinical cases* (2nd ed.) website. Sunderland, MA: Sinauer Associates. Retrieved from http://www.neuroexam.com

Chelimsky, T. C. (2009). Pain. In J. Corey-Bloom & R. David (Eds.), *Clinical adult neurology* (pp. 149–165). New York, NY: Demos Medical.

Kovacevic-Ristanovic, R., & Kuzniar, T. J. (2009). Sleep disorders. In J. Corey-Bloom & R. David (Eds.), *Clinical adult neurology* (pp. 167–184). New York, NY: Demos Medical.

Lanska, D. J. (2009a). Acute confusional states. In J. Corey-Bloom & R. David (Eds.), *Clinical adult neurology* (pp. 185–200). New York, NY: Demos Medical.

Lanska, D. J. (2009b). Vertigo and other forms of dizziness. In J. Corey-Bloom & R. David (Eds.), *Clinical adult neurology* (pp. 93–111). New York, NY: Demos Medical.

Lloyd, G. E. R. (1984). *Hippocratic writings*. New York, NY: Penguin Classics.

Massey, A. D. (2009). Syncope and seizures. In J. Corey-Bloom & R. David (Eds.), *Clinical adult neurology* (pp. 81–91). New York, NY: Demos Medical.

Ryan, S. J. (2009). Disorders of gait. In J. Corey-Bloom & R. David (Eds.), *Clinical adult neurology* (pp. 113–121). New York, NY: Demos Medical.

Slevin, J. T., & Ryan, M. (2009). Headaches. In J. Corey-Bloom & R. David (Eds.), *Clinical adult neurology* (pp. 123–147). New York, NY: Demos Medical.

Zasler, N. D., Costanzo, R. M., & Heywood, P. A. (1990). Neuroimaging correlates of olfactory dysfunction after traumatic brain injury. *Archives of Physical Medicine and Rehabilitation, 71*, 814.

Glossary

A

Abduct To move structures apart.

Absolute refractory period The time after a neuron fires when it is unresponsive because sodium channels are inactivated.

Acetylcholine (ACh) A rapid-fire neurotransmitter of the peripheral nervous system's neuromuscular junction that causes muscle tissue to contract. It has a restricted role in the central nervous system, being found only in the brainstem, the base of the forebrain, and the basal ganglia. It is thought to regulate central nervous system neuronal activity, especially in alertness, attention, memory, and learning.

Achalasia A condition of the esophagus in which smooth esophageal muscle fails to relax, resulting in pain and regurgitation.

Action potential A rapid change in membrane polarity, which moves or propagates like a wave down the axon.

Activity barriers Difficulties in executing activities, especially skills of daily living like walking or eating.

Adduct To bring structures together.

Afferent communication Bottom-up or ascending (body to the brain) sensory communication.

Agraphia An acquired disorder of writing.

Agyria/lissencephaly A condition in which the brain lacks its characteristic sulci and gyri and looks rather smooth in appearance. The condition is associated with severe motor, intellectual, and psychological disability.

Akinesia A loss of voluntary movement.

Akinetic mutism A condition in which patients are passive and do not move or talk.

Alexia An acquired disorder of reading.

All-or-none principle A principle stating that when a threshold is reached, a neuron will depolarize and fire at a fixed strength. If the threshold is not met, the neuron will not fire.

Allographic agraphia A reading problem caused by left parieto-occipital lesions resulting in errors in lowercase versus uppercase letters (e.g., mR. sMitH). It can also include confusion of print and cursive scripts.

Alpha motor neurons Neurons that innervate extrafusal muscle fibers, which leads to muscle contraction.

Alzheimer disease A progressive neurological disease that results in a general intellectual decline.

Amygdala Paired almond-shaped nuclei situated in the medial temporal lobe that are involved in fear and aggression.

Amyotrophic lateral sclerosis (ALS) The most well-known type of motor neuron disease. It is characterized by progressive weakness that often begins in the hands, feet, or mouth, but then involves the rest of the body. Also known as Lou Gehrig disease.

Anarthria Having no speech at all. Compare to dysarthria.

Anatomical position The starting position to describe anatomical features and positions.

Anatomy The structure of the body.

Anencephaly A severe neural tube defect in which neurological development ceases at the brainstem, leaving the infant without cerebral hemispheres and thus without higher cortical functions.

Anesthesia A lack of sensation (numbness).

Aneurysm An abnormal ballooning of a weakened artery wall that can rupture.

Angiography An invasive neuroimaging technique that uses iodine and x-rays to produce pictures of the blood vessels.

Anomia Impairment in the ability to name objects. It is a symptom of aphasia.

Anosmia An inability to smell.

Anosognosia A disorder of executive function in which a person lacks insight into his or her deficits.

Anterior Toward the belly.

Anterior (ventral) corticospinal tract A nerve tract that originates in the motor and premotor areas of the frontal lobe and then courses ipsilateral down the spinal cord, inputting at the ventral horn. It controls the trunk muscles.

Anterior reading system A neural system involving Broca's area as well as the ventral and dorsal premotor areas that plays an important role in word analysis in terms of spoken language and articulation; it also plays a role in silent reading.

Anton syndrome A rare condition in which patients have visual loss and visual anosognosia (i.e., denial of visual deficits) due to damage to the visual cortex. Also known as cortical blindness.

Aphasia An acquired multimodality language disorder.

Apraxia of speech (AOS) A motor speech disorder involving difficulty planning or programming the articulators for speech in the absence of muscle weakness.

Apraxic agraphia A problem in writing due to damage to the superior parietal lobe, premotor cortex, and supplementary motor area that results in people not being able to call up the motor plans for writing.

Aprosody A lack of melodic contour (or prosody) in speech; monotone.

Arachnoid mater The middle layer of the meninges that is made up of a thin, delicate connective tissue.

Arachnoid space An actual space below the arachnoid mater and above the pia mater.

Aspiration Penetration of food or liquid below the vocal cords, providing a clear path to the lungs.

Astereognosis Difficulty recognizing three-dimensional forms via touch, often due to damage to the primary sensory cortex.

Astrocyte A star-shaped nervous system cell that nourishes neurons and helps to maintain the neuronal environment.

Astrocytoma An abnormal mass of astrocyte cells.

Ataxic dysarthria A form of dysarthria caused by cerebellar damage and characterized by harsh voice, monopitch, loud voice, imprecise consonants, and irregular breakdown in articulation. People with this form of dysarthria often sound drunk in their speech.

Athetosis Slow, twisting movements of the hands and feet.

Attention A person's focus on a stimulus in the environment.

Attentional alexia A condition in which the person can read single words, but when there are multiple words on a page the person becomes distracted and unable to read. Usually caused by damage to the prefrontal cortex, which helps mediate attention.

Audition The process of hearing whereby acoustic or sound energy waves are changed into neural impulses.

Auditory association cortex An area in the superior temporal lobe involved in auditory processing and attaching meaning to spoken words. Also known as Wernicke's area.

Auditory brainstem response (ABR) A test that evaluates the integrity of cranial nerve VIII and the central auditory pathway without depending on a voluntary response from the patient.

Auditory processing disorder (APD) A condition that can be thought of as dyslexia of the ears in that there is difficulty processing and interpreting auditory symbols, similar to how people with dyslexia have difficulty interpreting written symbols.

Autism A neurological developmental disorder that occurs in 1 in 68 children in the United States and is characterized by problems in social interaction, communication problems, and stereotyped behaviors, all of which are diagnosed before a child is 3 years of age.

Autonomic nervous system That part of the motor nervous system involved in body functions that happen automatically and without conscious control. Contrast with the *somatic nervous system*.

Axoaxonic synapse A synapse that involves the axon of one neuron connecting and sending a chemical signal to the axon of another neuron. These are usually regulatory in nature.

Axodendritic synapse A synapse that involves the axon of one neuron connecting and sending a chemical signal to the dendrite of another neuron. These are usually excitatory in nature.

Axons Neurites that send signals away from the neuron's cell body.

Axosomatic synapse A synapse that involves the axon of one neuron connecting and sending a chemical signal to the soma of another neuron. These are usually inhibitory in nature.

B

Babinski sign A sign elicited when scratching the bottom of the foot. In a healthy adult, a normal (negative) Babinski sign occurs when the toes curl and withdraw from the scratching. An abnormal (positive) Babinski occurs when the big toe extends and the other toes flare out, indicating upper motor neuron damage.

Ballism A quick flinging of a limb or limbs.

Basal ganglia A group of subcortical gray matter structures including the caudate nucleus, globus pallidus, and putamen. It is a key component of the motor system. Damage results in dyskinesias.

Benedikt syndrome A condition caused by damage to the midbrain, resulting in contralateral hemiparesis and ataxic tremor.

Binaural hearing Hearing with two ears that allows us to determine the location of a sound.

Blood–brain barrier (BBB) A barrier located in the walls of the central nervous system's blood vessels that protects the brain from foreign invaders, hormones, antibodies, and other substances that might adversely affect it.

Bolus A food or liquid ball that is swallowed by a person.

Bottom-up attention A type of attention that is nonvolitional and driven by some characteristic of the stimulus itself.

Bradykinesia A dyskinesia involving slowed movements.

Brain death A state in which a person has no purposeful responses to stimuli, no brainstem reflexes, and no sleep–wake cycle, and there are flat electroencephalographic patterns.

Brainstem Three-part structure that is continuous with the spinal cord and lies inferior to the cerebral hemispheres. It consists of the medulla, pons, and midbrain, which together control many basic life functions and reflexes.

Broca's aphasia A type of aphasia in which people have limited verbal output that is agrammatic in nature.

Broca's area An area named after Paul Broca located in the inferior frontal gyrus of the frontal lobe (areas 44 and 45) that is involved in language processing and speech production.

Brodmann map A map of the human brain in which the cerebral cortex is divided into 52 areas based on differences in gross anatomy and cellular structure with the thought that each of these areas is responsible for certain functions.

C

Cannon-Bard theory A theory of emotion that states that an external stimulus simultaneously triggers a physiological response and an emotional experience, both occurring independently of each other.

Carotid arteries The main arteries that run up the anterolateral part of the neck and feed the brain blood.

Caudal Latin for "tail"; it means inferior.

Caudate nucleus One of the three structures that make up the basal ganglia. It has a functional relationship with the putamen, together forming the striatum.

Cell doctrine The belief that the brain's ventricles (i.e., cells) have psychic gases (or humors) in them responsible for mental functions.

Cell theory A theory that states that all organic beings (humans, animals, and plants) are composed of individual cells.

Cells The fundamental units of an organism.

Central Toward the center.

Central agraphia A reading problem involving impairment in the underlying linguistic reading system.

Central alexia A linguistic problem that affects the underlying reading system.

Central auditory system The auditory system that involves hearing structures found centrally in the head, including areas in the brainstem, the thalamus, and the cerebral cortex.

Central fissure A deep groove in the brain that separates the frontal lobe from the parietal lobe.

Central nervous system (CNS) The part of the nervous system made up of the brain and spinal cord.

Centrosome A cell structure that directs the growth of the cell through cell division.

Cerebellar circuit A neural circuit involving the cerebellum, premotor cortex, and precentral gyrus that integrates proprioceptive and kinesthetic information into motor activity so that motor movements are smooth and precise.

Cerebellar hemispheral syndrome A condition of the cerebellum that can be caused by stroke, tumor, and multiple sclerosis that primarily affects the ipsilateral limbs, causing tremor, dysmetria, and dysdiadochokinesia.

Cerebellar peduncles Nerve tracts that make communication between the cerebellum and other nervous system structures possible.

Cerebellum A structure that lies just posterior to the pons and is involved in the coordination and precision of fine motor movement.

Cerebral hemispheres The areas of the brain, divided into left and right cerebral hemispheres, that control higher cortical functions such as cognition and language as well as planning motor function and interpreting sensory experiences.

Cerebral palsy (CP) A nonprogressive neurological brain disorder that develops before birth (prenatal), during birth (perinatal), or shortly after birth (postnatal) and that affects movement, posture, balance, and sometimes speech and swallowing. *Cerebral* refers to the brain and *palsy* refers to paralysis or uncontrolled movements. CP can be caused by a lack of oxygen, premature birth, infections, brain hemorrhages, jaundice, and head injury.

Cerebral peduncles Portion of the midbrain that includes everything except the tectum.

Cerebral spinal rhinorrhea A condition caused by trauma to the nose resulting in cerebral spinal fluid leaking through the nose.

Cerebral vascular accident (CVA) An event that involves some kind of interruption to the brain's blood supply, whether a blockage or a hemorrhage. Popularly known as a stroke.

Cerebrospinal fluid (CSF) A clear, colorless fluid found in the brain's ventricles and the arachnoid space of the meninges. It cushions brain tissue, reduces the brain's weight through buoyancy, removes waste, and transports nutrients and hormones to the brain.

Chorea Means "like a dance"; quick movements of the hands or feet that have a dance-like quality.

Choroid plexus A structure located in each ventricle that produces cerebrospinal fluid.

Cingulate cortex An area located in the medial surface of the brain between the corpus callosum and the cingulate sulcus. It is a part of the limbic system, our emotional processing center.

Circle of Willis A circular array of blood vessels at the base of the brain that helps to equalize blood flow and pressure. The carotid and vertebral arteries feed this system.

Circumventricular organs (CVOs) Highly vascular brain structures that lack a normal blood–brain barrier and, thus, are routes around the blood–brain barrier.

Claustrum A sheet-like membrane of neurons under the cortex that appears to provide some level of cortical control of swallowing.

Clonus Involuntary muscle contractions, which can have a rhythmic quality; one common example is hiccups.

Closed head injury A type of traumatic brain injury that involves forces that cause damage to the brain, but without penetrating the skull; compare to open head injury.

Cochlear nucleus (CN) A collection of specialized auditory cells located at the cerebellopontine area where cranial nerve VIII inputs.

Cognition The mental process of knowing in which we acquire and act upon knowledge.

Coma A state in which a person does not respond purposefully to stimuli or have a sleep–wake cycle but does demonstrate brainstem reflexes and electroencephalographic (EEG) patterns, though the EEG is severely depressed.

Commissurotomy A surgical procedure in which the corpus callosum is severed. This procedure is usually performed to help people with severe epilepsy.

Comprehension The understanding of information acquired through perception and remembered.

Computed tomography (CT) A neuroimaging technique that passes x-rays through the human body that reflect off different densities of tissue, bone, and fluid in different ways, producing an image.

Conduction aphasia A type of aphasia in which people have difficulty repeating words said to them but have preserved speech fluency as well as auditory comprehension.

Connectionism The belief that there are centers in the brain responsible for certain functions, but that these areas are connected together and work cooperatively.

Consciousness The ability to be aware of self and surroundings.

Constitution view A belief regarding human constitution that humans are material only but are different from animals because people have a first-person perspective (i.e., extended consciousness).

Content The meaning of words. Also known as semantics.

Contralateral Opposite side.

Contralateral innervation The fact that, due to decussation of motor tracts, the right side of the brain controls the left side of the body and the left side of the brain controls the right side of the body.

Contrecoup damage A brain injury caused by the rebounding of the brain to the opposite site of the skull, causing a second area of damage.

Core consciousness From a neuroscience perspective, a type of consciousness involving our sense of ourselves in the here and now (i.e., at this very moment), objects in the world, and our relationship to those objects.

Corona radiata Means "radiating crown"; a fan-shaped sheet of axons between the thalamus and cortical surface.

Coronal A body section that splits a structure into front and back portions.

Corpus callosum A band of axonal fibers that connects the two cerebral hemispheres, allowing them to communicate with each other.

Coup damage The initial brain injury caused by the brain banging up against the inside of the skull; compare to contrecoup damage.

Cranial nerve A nerve that arises directly from the brain or brainstem that helps in information exchange between the brain and head and neck structures. Humans have 12 pairs of cranial nerves.

Creature consciousness From a philosophical perspective, the consciousness of whole organisms involving both wakefulness and core consciousness.

Cricopharyngeus A muscle at the top of the esophagus that relaxes, allowing the bolus to enter the esophagus.

Crus cerebri The anterior portion of the midbrain's cerebral peduncles.

Cytoskeleton A cell structure made up of microtubules that transport molecules around the cell.

D

Declarative memory The conscious, willful recall of memories. Memory for facts (semantic memory) and space–time events (episodic memory). Also known as explicit memory.

Decussation The point where a contralateral tract crosses from left to right (or right to left).

Deep agraphia A writing disorder characterized by semantic paraphasias (i.e., substituting one word for another) and spelling errors, especially homophones (e.g., *night* versus *knight*). Also known as semantic agraphia.

Deep alexia A condition in which people recognize words as other words (e.g., *scale* is perceived as *skate*). Also known as semantic alexia.

Deep cerebral veins Veins in the brain that collect blood from subcortical gray matter structures, like the thalamus and hippocampus.

Deglutition The act of swallowing.

Dementia A group of progressive neurological disorders (e.g., Alzheimer disease) that lead to cognitive decline.

Dendrite A neurite that receives signals and sends them to the neuron's cell body.

Depolarization The balancing of charge and concentration gradients in an axon resulting in an action potential.

Dermatome A specific skin region associated with a specific spinal nerve.

Diadochokinesia The ability to make rapid, alternating motor movements (e.g., saying "pa-ta-ka" quickly).

Diadochokinetic rates Rapid, alternating motor movements, such as saying "pa-ta-ka" as fast as possible.

Diencephalon A neurodevelopmental term for a set of brain structures found superior to the midbrain. Includes the thalamus, subthalamus, hypothalamus, and epithalamus.

Diffuse damage Traumatic brain injury that tends to be widespread in nature.

Diplopia Double vision, or seeing two images simultaneously.

Disfluency Any interruption in the smoothness with which sound, words, and sentences flow during oral language.

Distal The part of the limb farthest from its attachment.

Dopamine A neurotransmitter that plays a role in motor control as well as our reward system.

Dorsal Toward the back.

Dorsal column medial lemniscal pathway A sensory pathway that involves fine touch (as is found in the hands and mouth), vibratory sense, and proprioception.

Dorsal columns Nerve tracts that reside in the dorsal area of the spinal cord but have their origin at the dorsal root ganglion. The dorsal columns relay fine and discriminative touch, pressure, and proprioceptive sensory information to the brainstem, then the thalamus, and finally the sensory cortex for final processing.

Dorsal induction A neurodevelopmental period (3–7 weeks' gestation) in which the neural tube is formed.

Dualist A person who believes that humans are two substances, a material body (with a brain) and an immaterial soul (with a mind).

Dura mater The outermost layer of the meninges that adheres to the inner surface of the skull.

Dynamic polarization of neurons A theory that information flows only one way through a neuron, beginning with dendrites, then through the cell body, and finally through the axon.

Dysarthria Speech that is slurred and/or uncoordinated due to central or peripheral nervous system problems that affect one or more of the following: respiration, phonation, resonance, or articulation. Involves weakness in the speech muscles.

Dyskinesia A movement disorder involving involuntary movements (e.g., tremor).

Dyslexia A term for developmental problems in acquiring reading skills.

Dysphagia A condition in which a person has difficulty swallowing. It can involve any of the swallowing stages (oral preparatory, oral, pharyngeal, and/or esophageal).

Dystonia A dyskinesia in which sustained muscle contractions result in distorted body postures.

E

Ectoderm An embryonic layer that later turns into the skin and nervous system.

Efferent communication Top-down or descending (i.e., brain to the body) motor communication.

Electroencephalography (EEG) A temporal resolution neuroimaging technique that measures the neuronal electrical activity through electrodes placed on the scalp.

Embolus A type of ischemic clot that originates somewhere else in the body and then lodges in a cerebral blood vessel; compare to a thrombus.

Emergent dualism A belief regarding human constitution that the human mind emerges or arises from a combination of many brain activities.

Emotion Defined objectively, a certain set of physiological responses to certain stimuli. Defined subjectively, a conscious internal experience of feelings.

Emotional intelligence (EI) Our ability to understand our own emotions as well as those of others that guides us in our personal relationships.

Emotional lability An involuntary display of emotion that can sometimes be the result of a neuropathology.

Empathy The action of understanding, being aware of, being sensitive to, and vicariously experiencing the feelings, thoughts, and experiences of another of either the past or present without having the feelings, thoughts, and experience fully communicated in an objectively explicit manner

Encephalocele A rare malformation of the skull in which a malformed portion of the brain, usually the occipital lobe, protrudes from the skull in a sac.

Endoplasmic reticulum A cell structure that acts as a production plant for proteins needed by the cell.

Enteric nervous system A part of the autonomic nervous system that manages the gastrointestinal system.

Entorhinal cortex A major input/output relay between the cerebral cortex and the hippocampus.

Epidural hematoma A hemorrhage that occurs between the skull and the outer layer of the meninges (dura mater).

Epidural space A potential space between the skull and the dura mater.

Epinephrine A neurotransmitter involved in regulating heart rate, blood pressure, and breathing and in the fight-or-flight response.

Episodic memory A type of declarative memory for space–time episodes in life, like a family trip.

Epithalamus A part of the diencephalon that regulates genital development, the sleep–wake cycle, and optic reflexes.

Equilibrium A person's sense of coordination and balance.

Esophageal stage A stage of the normal swallow that is involuntary and variable in length (8–20 seconds), depending on the substance eaten. After the bolus enters the esophagus, peristaltic waves move the bolus to the stomach in conjunction with gravity.

Executive functions The human capacity to order and manage all other cognitive functions (e.g., attention, memory) for the purpose of setting and attaining goals.

Expressive aphasia An acquired language loss in speaking and/or writing.

Extended consciousness From a neuroscience perspective, a type of consciousness involving our sense of self in the flow of time. We think of ourselves in the past and anticipate ourselves living in a future (i.e., autobiographical self).

Extension The act of straightening a joint.

Extra-axial hemorrhage A type of hemorrhagic stroke that involves bleeding in or around the meninges; compare to an intra-axial hemorrhage.

Extrapyramidal system An indirect motor system that controls involuntary movements involved in posture, muscle tone, and reflexes as well as the coordination or modulation of movements.

F

Fasciculation Involuntary muscle fiber twitches.

Fissures Deep grooves in the brain.

Flaccid dysarthria A type of dysarthria caused by lower motor neuron damage in the pyramidal system, resulting in speech that is breathy in voice, monopitch, and hypernasal and that uses short phrases and imprecise consonants.

Flexion The act of bending a joint.

Fluency The smoothness with which sound, words, and sentences flow during oral language.

Fluency shaping A type of stuttering therapy that focuses on fluency itself and strategies that promote more fluent speech; compare to stuttering modification.

Focal damage Brain damage due to cerebral vascular accidents that tends to be focused to a particular area of the brain.

Form The structure of language. Also known as grammar.

Friedreich ataxia An inherited, progressive neurological disorder caused by an autosomal recessive inheritance pattern resulting in cerebellar dysfunction. Symptoms include progressive muscle weakness in the limbs, loss of coordination, dysmetria, dysarthria, curvature of the spine, and vision and hearing issues.

Frontal lobe An area of the cerebral cortex that lies at the front of the brain, just above the eyes, with the posterior border being the central fissure. Overall, its main functions include reasoning, planning, and voluntary motor movement.

Functional imaging A class of neuroimaging techniques that reveal the physiology of the brain.

Functional magnetic resonance imaging (fMRI) A neuroimaging technique that combines the advantages of magnetic resonance imaging with the advantages of positron emission tomography, showing both the anatomy and physiology of the brain by measuring blood oxygenation.

Function barriers Problems in body function or alterations in body structure, such as paralysis and blindness.

G

Gait A person's walking ability/characteristics.

Gait ataxia A condition in which the person walks with a wide base or the feet wide apart, giving the person more stability.

Gamma-aminobutyric acid (GABA) The main inhibitory neurotransmitter of the central nervous system. In addition to controlling information flow in the nervous system, GABA plays a role in the sleep–wake cycle.

Gamma motor neurons Neurons that innervate intrafusal muscle spindles, which is important for proprioception and reflexes.

General somatic afferent (GSA) fibers A type of spinal nerve fiber that carries sensory information from the skin.

General somatic efferent (GSE) fibers A type of spinal nerve fiber that carries motor information to skeletal muscles.

General visceral afferent (GVA) fibers A type of spinal nerve fiber that carries sensory information from the lungs and digestive tract.

General visceral efferent (GVE) fibers A type of spinal nerve fiber that carries motor information to smooth muscle, the heart, and glands.

Geniculocalcarine tract A visual neural tract that runs from the lateral geniculate nucleus of the thalamus and projects to the occipital lobe where visual information is processed.

Genu A bend where the internal capsule passes between the thalamus and the basal ganglia.

Glasgow Coma Scale (GCS) A 15-point scale that attempts to measure a patient's level of consciousness in three areas: eyes, motor, and verbal.

Glial cell A nervous system cell that anchors, nourishes, insulates, and protects neurons. Some may also play a role in neural transmission.

Global aphasia A form of nonfluent aphasia in which a person has little to no verbal output, poor auditory comprehension, and poor repeating skills.

Globus pallidus One of the three structures that make up the basal ganglia. It has an anatomical relationship with the putamen, together forming the lenticular nucleus.

Glutamate The major excitatory chemical of synaptic activity in the central nervous system. It plays a role in synaptic plasticity, learning, and memory, which is the same role acetylcholine plays in the peripheral nervous system.

Golgi apparatus The cell's mail office that packages and sends sugars and proteins out of the cell.

Gradient A sloping or imbalance of some sort.

Graphemic agraphia A reading problem due to lesions to the left prefrontal cortex and left parietal lobe resulting in patients omitting, substituting, adding, or transposing letters.

Graphemic buffer agraphia A type of agraphia in which a person cannot hold written forms in the linguistic working memory long enough to write the word. Shorter words are easier to write than are longer words because shorter words require less graphemic buffer space.

Guillain–Barré syndrome (GBS) A rapid, progressive demyelinating disease of the peripheral nervous system from which most patients will recover.

Gyri Hills or raised-up portions of the cerebral cortex. Singular term is *gyrus*.

H

Hematoma A collection of blood in a tissue (e.g., subdural hematoma).

Hemianopsia One-sided visual loss.

Hemiballismus The flinging of a limb, occurring on only one side of the body.

Hemiplegia Weakness of one side of the body.

Hemispheric specialization The fact that, in terms of function, each hemisphere is not a mirror image of the other; rather, the two hemispheres function uniquely (e.g., language is a left hemisphere function in most people).

Hemorrhagic CVA A type of stroke that involves a blood vessel bursting and spilling blood into brain tissue or into the meningeal layers.

Hippocampus An S-shaped structure important for declarative memory, which is our memory for facts (semantic memory) and space–time events (episodic memory).

Holism The belief that the whole brain is involved in a mental function, not just a discrete part of the brain.

Holistic dualism A belief regarding human constitution that human persons are integrated wholes. In other words, bodily existence is what it is to be human, and there is no separation between material and immaterial because they are intertwined.

Holmes rebound phenomenon A reflex can be elicited by the patient holding out one of his or her arms while the examiner tries to push down on it. The rebound phenomenon occurs when the examiner lets go of the patient's arm, which then bounces up significantly.

Holoprosencephaly A failure in brain cleavage resulting in impaired cerebral hemisphere development.

HOME An acronym for the functions of the limbic system: Homeostasis, Olfaction, Memory, and Emotion.

Homeostasis The body's maintenance of the status quo (stability and constancy).

Hydrocephalus A condition in which cerebrospinal fluid accumulates in the brain ventricles, causing brain tissue to be compressed against the skull.

Hyperkinetic dysarthria A type of dysarthria due to extrapyramidal damage in the basal ganglia. Speech is characterized by a harsh voice, monopitch, loud voice level, imprecise consonants, and distorted vowels.

Hypersomnia Excessive daytime sleepiness that can sometimes be a result of thalamic damage.

Hypertonia Too much tone in muscles, resulting in spastic muscles.

Hypokinetic dysarthria A type of dysarthria due to extrapyramidal damage in the midbrain's substantia nigra, which affects dopamine production. Speech includes breathy voice, monopitch, reduced syllable stress, variable speech rate, and imprecise consonants.

Hypomyelination A recessive genetic disorder in which children have a reduced ability to produce myelin, resulting in slowed development and paresis, muscle atrophy, neuropathy, cataracts, dysarthria, and mild to moderate intellectual disability.

Hypothalamus A part of the diencephalon that regulates various body functions (e.g., body temperature).

Hypotonia Too little tone in muscles, resulting in flaccid muscles.

I

Idealism A belief regarding human constitution that the immaterial is all there is and that things in the material world (if there is a material world) are created from the immaterial. Priority is given to the mind.

Incidence The number of new cases per year in a given population.

Infarct A region of dead brain tissue after a neurological event like a stroke.

Inferior From a low position.

Inferior colliculus The auditory center of the midbrain that regulates the acoustic startle reflex, which is when we suddenly move in response to an unanticipated sound.

Initiative The motivation to pursue positive or productive activities.

Inner ear That part of the ear involved in mechanical energy being changed or transduced into hydraulic energy at the oval window and then electrochemical energy at the organ of Corti.

Insular cortex A structure that is folded up and located deep within the lateral sulcus. It contains a posterior-dorsal portion involved in sensorimotor functions and an anterior part specializing in orofacial programs and emotions.

Intellectual disability A condition formerly known as mental retardation in which a person demonstrates sub-average intelligence during development that leads to difficulties functioning in his or her environment (e.g., home, school).

Internal capsule A narrow space between the caudate nucleus and the lenticular nucleus.

Interneurons Neurons that connect neurons together.

Intra-axial hemorrhage A type of hemorrhagic stroke that involves bleeding from a ruptured blood vessel inside the brain; compare to an extra-axial hemorrhage.

Ionotrophic receptor A type of postsynaptic receptor that directly opens or closes ion channels.

Ipsilateral Same sided.

Ischemic CVA A type of stroke that involves a loss of blood flow to the brain due to a blockage of some sort.

J

James–Lange theory A theory of emotion that proposes that physiological responses (e.g., trembling) to external stimuli lead to emotional experience.

Judgment A determination of the correctness of information perceived, remembered, and comprehended.

K

Kinesthesia The brain's awareness of the position and movement of the articulators through sense organs embedded in muscles called proprioceptors.

Klüver–Bucy syndrome A condition caused by bilateral damage to the amygdala and that results in diminished fears, overeating, oral fixation, heightened sex drive, and visual agnosia.

L

Language A generative and dynamic code containing universal characteristics whereby ideas about the world are expressed through a conventional system of arbitrary symbols for communication.

Lateral Away from the body's midline.

Lateral corticospinal/corticobulbar tract A nerve tract that originates in the motor cortex of the frontal lobe, decussates at the lower medulla–spinal cord juncture, and then inputs along the spinal cord at the ventral horns. Functionally, it is responsible for contralateral movement of the body.

Lateral fissure A deep groove in the brain that separates the frontal lobe from the parietal and temporal lobes.

Lateral geniculate body (LGB) An important thalamic visual center that relays visual information from the optic tracts to the primary visual cortex of the occipital lobe.

Lateral lemniscus A tract of six auditory pathways/axons that travels from the cochlear nuclear complex and superior olivary complex to the inferior colliculus in the midbrain.

Lateral superior olivary complex (LSOC) The peripheral part of the olivary complex that specializes in higher frequency hearing.

Lateral vestibulospinal tract An ipsilateral neural tract that descends from the vestibular nuclear complex and terminates in the thoracic and lumbar levels of the spinal cord. The tract stimulates extensor leg muscles in order to maintain a balanced posture, especially when bending over (vestibulospinal reflex).

Law of specific nerve energies A statement that the origin of the sensation (e.g., visual or tactile) does not determine our sensory experience, but rather the pathway it is carried on determines it.

Lenticular nucleus A collection of similar cells involving the globus pallidus and the putamen.

Limbic lobe An arc-shaped brain region on the medial surface of the cerebral hemispheres that involves the cingulate gyrus and other brain structures.

Lissencephaly A condition caused by a lack of reelin, resulting in the brain having a smooth appearance with no characteristic hills and valleys.

Locked-in syndrome (LIS) A condition caused by damage to the ventral pons resulting in quadriplegia and cranial nerve paralysis. Fully aware, conscious people are locked inside bodies that do not work and cannot respond to stimuli. Some patients can communicate through eye blinking.

Long-term memory A type of memory that involves memories that last for days, weeks, months, and even years.

Longitudinal fissure A deep groove that separates the left and right cerebral hemispheres.

Lower motor neurons (LMNs) That part of the pyramidal tract that runs from the brainstem through the cranial (or spinal) nerves, thus being housed entirely within the peripheral nervous system.

Lysosomes The garbage collectors of the cell, which use enzymes to break down and recycle used molecules.

M

Macropsia A condition due to dorsal stream of vision damage where things look abnormally large.

Magnetic resonance imaging (MRI) A neuroimaging technique that uses a magnetic current to flip protons within the body's water molecules. The signal that is produced through this process is picked up by the MRI's receiver coils and the data are formed into three-dimensional images.

Medial Toward the body's midline.

Medial geniculate body (MGB) An important thalamic auditory center that relays auditory information from subcortical midbrain structures (i.e., inferior colliculus) to the primary auditory cortex of the temporal lobe.

Medial superior olivary complex (MSOC) The center part of the olivary complex that specializes in low-frequency hearing, specifically integrating low-frequency hearing from the right and left ears to create binaural hearing.

Medial vestibulospinal tract Neural tracts that input in the lower motor neuron portions of the cervical spinal cord, resulting in our ability to rotate our head in one direction and our body in the other direction.

Medulla The most inferior part of the brainstem. About 80% of motor fibers cross, or decussate, at this level, and various life function centers are located in it, including cardiac, vasoconstrictor, respiratory, and swallowing centers.

Membrane In human and animal cells, a double-walled structure (bilipid membrane) made up of lipids and proteins that when bonded together are called lipoproteins.

Meniere disease An ear disorder caused by a buildup of inner ear fluid leading to sensorineural hearing loss.

Meninges A three-layer membrane that surrounds and protects the cerebral hemispheres and the spinal cord.

Meningitis An inflammation of the meninges.

Mental-state consciousness From a philosophical perspective, consciousness as it relates to particular mental states and processes; essentially the same as extended consciousness.

Mental status The degree of cognitive competence a person has (e.g., orientation).

Mesencephalon A neurodevelopmental term for those embryonic structures that will develop into the midbrain.

Metabotrophic receptors A type of postsynaptic receptor that uses a secondary messenger (a molecule called a G-protein) to open or close ion channels.

Metastatic brain tumor A tumor that originates somewhere else in the body and migrates to the brain.

Metencephalon A neurodevelopmental term for those embryonic structures that will develop into the pons and cerebellum.

Microcephaly Abnormally small brain mass due to faulty proliferation of nervous system cells during the neural proliferation stage of development (3–4 months' gestation).

Microglia A central nervous system cell thought to defend nervous system structures by warding off foreign invaders.

Micropsia A condition due to dorsal stream of vision damage where objects look abnormally small.

Microtubules Components of a cell's cytoskeleton that facilitate intracellular transport of molecules within the cell.

Midbrain A brainstem structure that lies inferior to the diencephalon and superior to the pons and that contains the cerebral peduncles, tectum, and substantia nigra.

Middle ear That part of the ear involved in acoustic energy being changed or transduced into mechanical energy by the tympanic membrane. This mechanical energy is then transmitted through the ossicular chain (malleus, incus, and stapes) to the cochlea.

Midsagittal A body plane or section that cuts an organ in equal right and left portions.

Mind–brain debate The debate about whether humans have a mind and a brain or just a brain that is either the same thing as the mind or that gives rise to a mind.

Minimally conscious state (MCS) A state in which a person responds purposefully, but inconsistently, to stimuli and does demonstrate brainstem reflexes, a sleep–wake cycle, and electroencephalographic patterns. The condition is thought to be a state between persistent vegetative state and normal consciousness.

Mirror neuron A specialized neuron in the premotor cortex that fires when we watch someone else carry out a motor command, which is important in our ability to watch others and learn new skills.

Mitochondria The cell's energy factory where oxygen and sugars are metabolized by enzymes and their energy powers the cell.

Mixed dysarthria A mixture of two or more of the pure dysarthrias due to damage to multiple motor systems.

Molecules Substances that consist of two or more atoms held together by a chemical bond.

Monist A person who believes that humans are one substance, a material body (with a brain/mind).

Morphology The study of a language's word structure; a component of language form.

Motor neurons Multipolar neurons that connect to body structures (e.g., muscles) involved with movement.

Motor speech disorder (MSD) Disorders of the speech system, including the different types of dysarthria and apraxia of speech.

Motor units The motor neuron and the fibers (extrafusal versus intrafusal) it innervates.

Multiple sclerosis (MS) A condition in which the myelin sheath around the axon is damaged by an autoimmune response, impairing the ability of neurons to communicate with other neurons and muscles.

Myasthenia gravis (MG) A progressive autoimmune disease of the neuromuscular junction that affects women in their 30s and men in their 50s. The body's antibodies block postsynaptic acetylcholine receptors at the neuromuscular junction, resulting in muscle weakness and fatigue.

Myelencephalon A neurodevelopmental term for those embryonic structures that will develop into the medulla.

Myelin/myelination A fatty, white coating that covers axons and aids neural transmission.

Myelitis A general term for inflammation of the spinal cord.

Myoclonus Sudden involuntary muscle jerks.

N

Neglect alexia A condition that occurs usually because of damage to the right hemisphere. Sufferers will fail to identify the initial portions of a word or sentence as they try to read.

Neglect syndrome A condition of disengagement in which a patient ignores stimuli (e.g., objects or people) in one visual field or the other, but retains an intact visual system.

Neoplasms An abnormal massing of cells.

Nervous system A series of organs that make communication between the brain and body possible in order for humans to interact with the world around them.

Neural plate An embryonic structure formed around the third week of development when the dorsal ectoderm thickens.

Neural tube A tube from which the brain and spinal cord will develop. It forms around the fourth week of development when the neural plate bends and wraps around itself.

Neural tube defects (NTDs) Conditions in which the neural tube's neuropores fail to close properly, resulting in a defect of the neural tube.

Neurites Projections (i.e., axons and dendrites) from a neuron's cell body.

Neuroanatomy The study of the nervous system's structure.

Neurogenesis A process at the heart of the neural proliferation stage involving the birth of new neurons.

Neurological disorder A disease of the nervous system that impairs a person's health, resulting in some level of disability.

Neurological exam Systematic examination of the nervous system.

Neurologist A doctor with specialized training in nervous system anatomy, physiology, and pathology.

Neurology The study of the anatomy, physiology, and pathology of the nervous system.

Neuroma An abnormal mass of nerve tissue.

Neuron A nervous system cell with specialized projections that transfers information throughout the body via an electrochemical process.

Neuron doctrine The belief that each neuron is a separate cell and the fundamental building block of the nervous system.

Neuropathology The study of diseases of the nervous system.

Neurophysiology The study of how neurons function.

Neuroplasticity The adaptive capacity of the human brain, meaning that the brain is always changing, rewiring itself in response to internal and external influencers.

Neuropores Openings at the ends of the neural tube.

Neurotransmitter A chemical messenger that transmits messages through the synaptic cleft from the presynaptic membrane to the postsynaptic membrane.

Neurulation The process of forming the neural tube.

Noise-induced hearing loss Hearing loss in the inner ear induced by loud noise, usually due to damage in the hair cells located in the organ of Corti.

Nondeclarative memory A type of memory that cannot be consciously brought into awareness. It involves learning, but being unaware of that learning. Also known as implicit memory.

Nonreductive materialism A belief regarding human constitution that experiences (e.g., beauty) cannot be reduced to mere neurological processes, but rather, other processes (psychological, philosophical, and theological) are needed to explain these complex, nonreducible experiences.

Nonsemantic reading A form of alexia in which the person can read real and nonwords, and regular and irregular words without difficulty; however, they do not comprehend what they are reading. Also known as reading without meaning.

Norepinephrine A neurotransmitter that modulates attention, the sleep–wake cycle, and mood.

Nucleolus A component of the nucleus that directs the creation of proteins using the RNA needed to build and repair the cell.

Nucleus That part of the cell that contains DNA, which is the genetic code that regulates the maintenance of the cell and production of new cells.

Nucleus ambiguus (NA) A set of specialized cells located in the medulla that acts as a motor swallowing center that innervates the swallowing muscles via cranial nerves in the peripheral swallowing system.

Nucleus tractus solitarius (NTS) A set of specialized cells located in the medulla that acts as a swallowing sensory center by receiving afferent information, such as touch and taste, from cranial nerves V, VII, IX, and X as well as sensory input from the respiratory and cardiovascular brainstem nuclei and then transferring this information to the nucleus ambiguus.

Nystagmus Involuntary eye movements; sometimes called dancing eyes.

O

Occipital lobe An area of the cerebral cortex that lies posterior to the parietal and temporal lobes and makes up the very back part of the brain. Its main function is visual processing.

Occipitotemporal reading system A posterior neural reading system involving the left inferior occipital area, left inferior-posterior temporal area, and fusiform gyrus that is concerned with visual word form recognition (i.e., sight-reading), rapid access to whole words, and integration of printed letters with their corresponding sounds (i.e., grapheme-to-phoneme conversion).

Ocular apraxia A disorder due to damage to the dorsal stream of vision involving difficulty voluntarily directing one's gaze to a certain object.

Olfaction The sense of smell.

Oligodendroglia A central nervous system cell that produces and coats axons with myelin.

Open head injury A type of traumatic brain injury in which some object (e.g., bullet, shell fragment, rock) penetrates the skull and causes damage to the brain; compare to a closed head injury.

Optic ataxia A disorder due to damage to the dorsal stream of vision involving difficulty visually guiding the hand to touch an object.

Optic chiasm A structure between the optic nerves and the optic tracts where optic nerve fibers from the nasal retinas cross.

Oral preparatory stage A stage in the normal swallow that is voluntary and variable in length depending on the substance being eaten. In this stage, food is placed in the mouth and is prepared for swallowing through chewing.

Oral stage A stage in the normal swallow that is voluntary, lasting approximately 1 second. It begins once mastication ceases and ends once the bolus reaches the oropharynx.

Order The capacity to correctly perform sequencing tasks.

Organ A group of tissues that together carry out certain functions (e.g., heart, brain).

Outer ear The portion of the ear that includes the pinna (or auricle) and the external auditory meatus. It is involved in the hearing process that involves the pinna locating, collecting, and funneling acoustic energy (i.e., sound) to the middle ear via the external auditory meatus.

P

Palinopsia A recurring ghost image due to damage to the dorsal stream of vision.

Palsy A condition that involves paralysis, weakness, or even uncontrolled movements (e.g., shaking).

Papez circuit A set of structures (i.e., the sensory cortex, cingulate cortex, hippocampus, hypothalamus, and anterior thalamic nuclei) that make up the human emotional system.

Parasagittal A body plane or section that cuts an organ into uneven left and right portions (i.e., not right in the middle of the organ).

Paresthesias Sensations that include such experiences as tingling, prickling, or burning.

Parasympathetic nervous system A part of the autonomic nervous system that calms and relaxes the body through slowing the heart and lowering blood pressure. It is sometimes referred to as the "rest and digest" system.

Paresis Weakness in a muscle or limb.

Parietal lobe An area of the cerebral cortex that lies posterior to the central fissure and superior to the lateral fissure. Its main functions include sensory perception and interpretation.

Parietotemporal reading system A posterior neural reading system involving the angular gyrus (Brodmann area 39), the supramarginal gyrus (Brodmann area 40), and the posterior part of the superior temporal lobe that focuses on word analysis and the comprehension of written and spoken language.

Parkinson disease A degenerative disorder of the central nervous system characterized by tremors.

Participation barriers Problems with involvement in any area of life, such as participating in education and employment.

Pathology The study of disease processes that affect both anatomy and physiology.

Perception Recognizing whether information is present, whether it be auditory, visual, or other information.

Peripheral Toward the outer surface.

Peripheral agraphia Writing problems due to visuospatial processing and attention problems.

Peripheral alexia Reading problems due to visuospatial processing and attention problems.

Peripheral auditory system An auditory system that involves hearing structures found on the periphery of the head, including the outer, middle, and inner ear as well as cranial nerve VIII.

Peripheral nervous system (PNS) The part of the nervous system made up of the cranial and spinal nerves.

Peripheral neuropathy An inflammation of the peripheral nervous system that results in degeneration of the spinal nerves, usually in the hands and feet.

Peristalsis Involuntary, sequential, wavelike contractions of smooth muscle.

Persistent vegetative state (PVS) A state in which a person does not respond purposefully to stimuli, but does demonstrate brainstem reflexes, a sleep–wake cycle, and electroencephalographic patterns.

Pharyngeal stage A stage in the normal swallow that is essentially involuntary and lasts approximately 1 second. The bolus is moved from the oral cavity, through the pharynx, to the esophagus by pharyngeal squeezing action.

Phineas Gage A 19th-century railroad worker who suffered severe brain injury, yet survived. His case taught neuroscientists much about the functioning of the prefrontal cortex because Gage experienced significant personality changes after his accident.

Phonological agraphia A relatively mild form of agraphia in which patients can write regular and irregular words but have difficulty with nonwords or nonconcrete words (e.g., the word *pride*).

Phonological alexia A relatively mild form of dyslexia that usually does not affect the reading of real words, but rather the real difficulty comes in reading/sounding out new or nonwords (i.e., pseudowords).

Phonological dyslexia A type of central dyslexia that is a relatively mild form of dyslexia involving reading/sounding out new or nonwords (i.e., pseudowords).

Phonology The study of a language's sound structure; a component of language form.

Phrenic nerve A nerve that originates mainly from the fourth cervical spinal nerve but receives some help from the third and fifth cervical spinal nerves. It innervates the diaphragm, which, along with other muscles, is crucial for supplying the air power for speech.

Phrenology A study based on the belief that bumps on the skull correspond to certain brain areas (and only those areas) that perform certain mental functions.

Physiology The study of the body's function.

Pia mater The innermost layer of the meninges that adheres closely to the gyri and sulci of the cerebral cortex.

Pineal gland An endocrine gland located in the epithalamus.

Pituitary gland An endocrine gland associated with the hypothalamus that regulates growth, stress, reproduction, and lactation.

Planum temporale A triangular auditory area that lies posterior to the auditory cortex and makes up the heart of Wernicke's area (Brodmann area 22). It is involved in the processing of auditory information.

Plegia Paralysis of a muscle or limb.

Plexus A branching network of sensory and motor nerve fibers that arise from the ventral rami of the spinal cord.

Polymicrogyria A condition associated with errors in cortical organization in which children have too many folds (gyri) in the cerebral hemispheres.

Pons A brainstem structure that lies superior to the medulla and inferior to the midbrain. It acts as a bridge, relaying neural fibers between the cerebrum, cerebellum, and lower structures like the medulla and spinal cord. It contains cranial nerve nuclei and other nuclei that help regulate respiration, swallowing, hearing, eye movements, and facial expression and sensation.

Positron emission tomography (PET) A spatial resolution neuroimaging technology that shows brain activity based on the brain's glucose metabolism.

Posterior Toward the back.

Pragmatics The practical use of language in everyday life (e.g., conversation).

Prefrontal cortex An area in the anterior frontal lobe that plays an important role in cognition, personality, and emotion.

Prefrontal lobotomy A surgical procedure done to help psychiatric patients that disconnects the prefrontal cortex from the rest of the brain, resulting in passivity and a lack of rational decision-making abilities and action based more on impulse.

Prevalence The total number of current cases in a given population at a point in time.

Primary brain tumor A brain tumor that originates in the brain.

Primary cerebellar agenesis A rare condition in which a person is born without a cerebellum.

Priming memory A form of nondeclarative memory that takes advantage of unconscious associations between objects for learning.

Procedural memory A type of nondeclarative memory for skills and habits, like driving a car or riding a bike.

Pronate When the face/ventral surface is down.

Proprioception The body's eyes for itself or the brain's ability to know where the different parts of the body (arms, legs) are in space at a given time.

Prosencephalon A neurodevelopmental term for the forebrain, which will develop into the diencephalon (i.e., thalamic structures) and telencephalon (i.e., cerebral hemispheres).

Prosopagnosia A disorder due to damage to the ventral stream of vision involving an inability to recognize familiar faces.

Proximal The point nearest a limb's attachment.

Ptosis Drooping of the eyelids.

Pupillary light reflex A reflex in which the pupils change in size as light is introduced or removed.

Pure alexia A condition in which the person has difficulty reading, but writing ability is left intact. Also known as alexia without agraphia, verbal alexia, or letter-by-letter reading.

Pure word deafness A rare type of auditory agnosia resulting from damage to Brodmann areas 41 and 42. Sufferers have a pure deficit whereby they cannot understand speech; however, they do not have difficulties with speaking, reading, or writing. Patients report that they can hear the person talking but cannot understand what is being said.

Putamen One of the three structures that make up the basal ganglia. It has a functional relationship with the caudate nucleus, forming the striatum, and an anatomical relationship with the globus pallidus, forming the lenticular nucleus.

Pyramidal neurons The primary neurons found in the pyramidal tract, which are pyramid shaped.

Pyramidal system A direct, voluntary motor system that controls gross motor movement.

R

Radical dualism A belief regarding human constitution that is similar to substance dualism, but the emphasis is on the soul; the soul *is* the human person and the body is just a mechanism the soul inhabits for a time. This is the "ghost in the machine" view.

Rancho Levels of Cognitive Functioning (RLCF) An eight-level scale that describes the process of recovery from brain injury.

Reasoning The process of acting on information perceived, remembered, comprehended, and judged by drawing conclusions or by making arguments.

Receptive aphasia An acquired language loss in listening and understanding and/or reading.

Red nucleus A paired structure located in the tegmentum of the midbrain next to the substantia nigra. It receives connections from the cerebral cortex, and its axons give rise to the rubrospinal tract that descends from the brainstem and inputs into the spinal cord's ventral horn cells. This tract modulates flexor tone in the upper extremities and probably participates in activities such as babies' ability to crawl and arm swinging in walking.

Reductive materialism A belief regarding human constitution that all of life is reduced to the material and to naturalistic explanations. In this view, the mind is reduced to the brain.

Reflex A lightning-quick, unconscious response our body makes to environmental stimuli.

Reflex arc A neural pathway that controls reflexes. When a stimulus occurs, a sensory signal is sent to the spinal cord, which in turn responds and sends a motor signal back to the muscle to move.

Relative refractory period The time when a neuron will respond to another stimulus, but that stimulus must be stronger than normal due to sodium channels still being in recovery mode.

Remembering The storing of perceived information.

Restraint The inhibition of inappropriate behaviors.

Reticular activating system A system that begins in the midbrain's reticular formation and radiates out to the cerebral cortex through the thalamus; activates and coordinates the cerebral cortex for conscious experience.

Reticular formation A series of nuclei in the center of the brainstem important in cortical wakefulness.

Reticulospinal tract A nerve tract that is involved in muscle tone in the trunk muscles as well as the proximal limbs and overall helps to control a person's posture and facilitate gait.

Rhombencephalon A neurodevelopmental term for those embryonic structures that will develop into pons, medulla, and cerebellum (i.e., the myelencephalon and metencephalon). Also known as the hindbrain.

Ribosomes Cell structures found in the endoplasmic reticulum that are the primary place for protein synthesis.

Rigidity Stiff muscles that resist passive movement of a limb.

Rubrospinal tract A nerve tract that begins in the midbrain, where it decussates and courses down the brainstem and spinal cord until inputting into the ventral horn of the spinal cord. In terms of function, it modulates flexor tone in the upper extremities.

S

Sagittal A body section that divides the body or a specific anatomical structure into left and right portions.

Satellite cells A peripheral nervous system cell that surrounds and nourishes neurons.

Schizencephaly A rare condition characterized by abnormal openings or clefts in the cerebral hemispheres.

Schwann cells Peripheral nervous system cells that produce and coat axons with myelin.

Seizures Electrical storms in the brain.

Semantic agraphia A disorder of writing in which a person has difficulty spelling homophones.

Semantic memory A type of declarative memory involving the recall of facts and general knowledge.

Sensorineural hearing loss A hearing loss caused by problems with either the inner ear, the vestibulocochlear nerve (cranial nerve VIII), or the central processing areas of the cerebral cortex.

Sensory neurons Unipolar or bipolar neurons that connect to sensory structures in the body.

Serotonin A neurotransmitter with both excitatory and inhibitory effects on the nervous system. It plays a role in arousal in the sleep–wake cycle.

Short-term memory A type of memory that involves storage for small amounts of information needed for a short time, such as seconds.

Sign An observation made by an observer sometimes involving equipment, such as a thermometer or blood pressure reader.

Simultanagnosia A disorder due to damage to the dorsal stream of vision in which a patient cannot put the parts of a visual scene together into a comprehensive whole.

Soma A neuron's cell body.

Somatic nervous system A part of the nervous system that voluntarily and consciously coordinates the body's skeletal muscles for movement. Contrast with the *autonomic nervous system*.

Somatosensory system The body sensory system that mediates our experiences of touch, pain, temperature, vibration, and proprioception.

Spastic dysarthria A type of dysarthria due to upper motor neuron damage in the pyramidal system, resulting in stiff, rigid muscles. Speech is characterized by a harsh/strained voice, monopitch intonation, hypernasality, slow speech rate, and imprecise consonants.

Spatial agraphia A reading problem due to right hemisphere damage in which people have difficulty writing on a straight line and/or may write on one side of the paper or the other and/or will make extra marks on a letter.

Spatial resolution A class of neuroimaging techniques that show the location of brain activity.

Special somatic afferent (SSA) fibers Nerve fibers that conduct visual and auditory information from the eyes and inner ear to the appropriate cerebral cortex area

Special visceral afferent (SVA) fibers Nerve fibers that relay special sense information like smell and taste.

Special visceral efferent (SVE) fibers Nerve fibers that control glands in the head and neck.

Spina bifida (SB) A condition in which a neural tube defect affects the posterior neuropore, resulting in the development of a cyst on the lower back that may or may not affect the spinal cord.

Spinal cord A structure consisting of neural tracts housed in the vertebral column that connects the brain to the body, acting as the information superhighway of the body.

Spinal cord injury (SCI) Traumatic injury to the spinal cord that can result in either paresis or paralysis.

Spinocerebellar tracts Two nerve tracts (dorsal and ventral) that lie on the lateral edge of the spinal cord. They have their origin in the dorsal root ganglions and ascend to input into the cerebellum. They convey proprioceptive information about the body to the cerebellum.

Spinothalamic tract A nerve tract that lies in the lateral ventral portion of the spinal cord. It originates in the dorsal horns and then ascends through the spinal cord and brainstem to the thalamus. The thalamus then relays this tract to the sensory cortex. Functionally, this tract sends the following sensory information: pain, temperature, and crude touch.

Strabismus Crossed vision due to poor eye teaming.

Striatum A functional unit of the caudate nucleus and putamen involved in motor activity.

Structural imaging A class of neuroimaging techniques that reveal the anatomy of the brain.

Stuttering A type of fluency disorder in which the smoothness of speech is interrupted beyond the normal disfluencies all people experience. The interruptions often occur within words, though there may be whole-word or between-word disfluencies as well.

Stuttering modification A type of stuttering treatment that focuses on the moment of stuttering and training patients to stutter more easily and with less tension; compare to fluency shaping.

Subarachnoid hematoma A type of hemorrhage that occurs in the arachnoid space, the space below the arachnoid mater.

Subarachnoid space A space below the arachnoid mater that is occupied by blood vessels, spider-web-like support structures, and cerebrospinal fluid.

Subdural hematoma A type of hemorrhage that occurs between the dura mater and the middle layer of the meninges (arachnoid mater).

Subdural space A potential space between the dura mater and the arachnoid mater.

Substance dualism A belief regarding human constitution that humans are both material and immaterial and that the immaterial can exist apart from the material for a time. In this view, the brain is material and the mind is immaterial.

Substance P A type of neurotransmitter that sensitizes mammals to pain. It causes inflammation at an injury site, which leads to healing.

Substantia nigra A dopamine-producing area located in the midbrain.

Subthalamus A part of the diencephalon that regulates and coordinates motor function.

Sulci Grooves or valleys in the brain that are not as deep as fissures. Singular term is sulcus.

Superficial cerebral veins Veins in the brain that collect blood from the cerebral cortex and subcortical white matter.

Superior From a high position.

Superior colliculi The visual center of the midbrain that receives input from the retinas and the primary visual cortex.

Superior olivary complex (SOC) An area in the pons that is important in integrating auditory information.

Supine When the face/ventral surface is up.

Surface agraphia A writing disorder caused by damage to extrasylvian temporoparietal regions of the left hemisphere. It involves impairments in spelling irregular words (e.g., island), but spelling of regular words is preserved.

Surface alexia Difficulty reading words with irregular print-to-sound correspondences (e.g., island).

Sympathetic nervous system A part of the autonomic nervous system that excites the body for action by increasing heart rate, blood pressure, and adrenaline. It triggers what is known as our "fight-or-flight" response.

Symptom A patient's subjective report of what he or she is experiencing during an illness (e.g., "my stomach hurts").

Synapse A connection between a neuron and another neuron, muscle, or gland.

Synaptic pruning A process in which extra synaptic connections are eliminated during the cortical organization and synapse formation stage of neural development age (5 months to teen years).

Synaptic theory A theory of short-term memory that states that short-term memory works through neurotransmitter release (acetylcholine) but decays as neurotransmitter uptake occurs.

Synaptogenesis The formation of synapses between neurons during the cortical organization and synapse formation stage of neural development age (5 months to years postnatal).

Syncope An episode of fainting in which a person loses consciousness.

Syntax The study of a language's phrase and sentence structure; a component of language form.

System A group of organs that together carry out certain functions (e.g., circulatory, digestive, reproductive).

T

Tectospinal tract A nerve tract that coordinates the movement of the head and neck with the eyes.

Tectum The roof of the midbrain that is responsible for auditory and visual reflexes.

Tegmentum The posterior portion of the midbrain's cerebral peduncles, which contains several cranial nerve nuclei.

Telencephalon A neurodevelopmental term for the cerebral hemispheres.

Temporal lobe An area of the cerebral cortex that lies inferior to the parietal lobe and posterior to the frontal lobe. Its main functions include the processing of auditory information (including speech) and some memory functions.

Temporal resolution A class of neuroimaging techniques that deal with the time between when a stimulus is introduced and the brain's response to it.

Thalamic aphasia A type of aphasia with fluent verbal output and semantic paraphasias, auditory comprehension that is less severe than one would expect for the severity of verbal output, and minimally impaired or even intact repetition.

Thalamic pain syndrome A condition caused by damage to the thalamus resulting in burning or tingling sensations and possibly hypersensitivity to things that would not normally be painful, such as light touch or temperature change.

Thalamus A part of the diencephalon that acts as a relay station for sensory fibers.

Theory of mind (ToM) The human ability to understand that I have a mind, you have a mind, and that our minds are different from one another. In short, the capacity to be other-minded.

Thrombus A type of ischemic clot in which the blockage originates within a cerebral blood vessel itself; compare to an embolus.

Tics Repetitive involuntary motor and/or vocal behaviors associated with conditions like Tourette syndrome.

Tinnitus The sensation of ringing in the ears.

Tissue A group of similar cells that come together to carry out certain functions (e.g., muscle tissue, nervous tissue).

Tonotopic organization The basilar membrane's and auditory cortex's arrangement or organization by tones (i.e., different areas being sensitive to different sound frequencies).

Top-down attention A type of attention that is volitional and driven by a person's will.

Transcortical sensory aphasia (TSA) A fluent form of aphasia similar to Wernicke's aphasia but with paraphasias and echolalia, or repeating what other people say. Unlike people with Wernicke's, patients with TSA can repeat words said to them. Auditory comprehension is poor, as is reading and writing.

Transducer A device that changes energy from one form to another (e.g., the ear).

Transient ischemic attack (TIA) A type of ischemic stroke involving a temporary loss of blood flow to the brain but with stroke symptoms resolving in a matter of minutes or within 24 hours.

Transport The moving of a substance from point A to point B. May be passive (i.e., no energy expended) or active (i.e., energy expended) in nature.

Transverse A body section that splits a structure into top and bottom portions.

Traumatic brain injury (TBI) Some type of traumatic blow to the brain that impairs the functioning of the brain.

Tremor Involuntary, rhythmic shaking in which the shaking oscillates at a certain frequency.

Trephination The process of creating a hole in the skull through cutting, scraping, and/or drilling in order to relieve neurological problems.

Trephine Trephination instruments, usually sharp stones, used to create holes in skulls.

Two-factor theory This theory states that emotion is based on two factors—a physiological state and the interpretation of that state. Also known as the cognitive-appraisal theory.

U

Unilateral upper motor neuron (UMN) dysarthria A milder form of dysarthria caused by unilateral UMN damage that affects only one side of the face and mouth. It usually has minimal impact on speech because the person still has one functional side of the face and mouth.

Upper motor neurons (UMNs) That part of the pyramidal tract that runs from the cortex to the brainstem, thus being entirely housed within the central nervous system.

V

Venous system A waste disposal system in the brain that moves deoxygenated blood away from the brain as well as used cerebrospinal fluid from the ventricular system.

Ventral Toward the stomach.

Ventral induction A neurodevelopmental period in which the face and brain develop out of the superior end of the neural tube.

Ventricles Spaces in the brain that contain cerebrospinal fluid.

Vermal syndrome A condition caused by damage to the cerebellum's vermis, resulting in trunk muscle unsteadiness, tremor, postural issues, and gait ataxia.

Vertebral arteries Arteries that run up the cervical vertebral column and supply the brainstem, cerebellum, and temporal lobe with blood.

Vertebral column A bony cylinder of 32 to 34 segments that surrounds and protects the spinal cord.

Vertigo The sensation of dizziness.

Vestibular nucleus (VN) A structure consisting of four nuclei (superior, inferior, medial, and lateral [Deiter] nuclei) on each side of the brainstem whose axons make connections with various nervous system structures.

Vestibulocollic reflex A reflex that allows people to rotate their head in one direction and their body in the other direction.

Vestibulo-ocular reflex A reflex mediated by various brainstem auditory nuclei that allows a person to keep his or her eyes fixed on a target while moving the head.

Vestibulospinal reflex A reflex that occurs when the leg extends in response to bending over, helping to maintain a balanced posture.

Vestibulospinal tract An ipsilateral neural tract that originates in the medulla and courses down the spinal cord until inputting into the ventral horn of the spinal cord. Functionally, this tract controls extensor tone, which is the amount of tension present in muscles when a joint is extended. It also mediates the vestibulospinal reflex.

Visceral sensory system The part of the sensory nervous system that mediates general sensory information like stretch, pain, temperature, and irritation in the internal organs as well as sensations like nausea and hunger, for the brain.

Visual alexia An impairment in the way written words are perceived and analyzed during reading. It manifests as letter or syllable substitutions, additions, or omissions.

Visual anosognosia A denial of visual deficits.

W

Wallenberg syndrome A disorder of the medulla involving contralateral loss of pain and temperature in the body, ipsilateral loss of pain and temperature in the face, vertigo, ataxia, paralysis of the ipsilateral palate and vocal cord, and dysphagia.

Wallerian degeneration A degenerative process that occurs after an axon is crushed or cut.

Weber syndrome A condition caused by damage to the midbrain resulting in contralateral hemiplegia and ipsilateral oculomotor paralysis with ptosis.

Wernicke's aphasia A form of fluent aphasia due to damage to Wernicke's area that results in severe auditory comprehension deficits, verbal jargon, and poor repetition abilities.

Wernicke's area Named after Karl Wernicke, Brodmann area 22, which is involved in attaching meaning to auditory information, especially speech and language.

Wernicke-Geschwind model A model of language function that uses a connectionist framework, connecting the following structures in language tasks: Broca's area, the arcuate fasciculus, Wernicke's area, the angular gyrus, and the supramarginal gyrus.

Working memory (WM) A system in the mind that allows temporary memory space for the manipulation of information, like a scratch pad.

Index

Note: Page numbers followed by *b*, *f*, or *t* indicate materials in boxes, figures, or tables respectively.